PDR®
2007
FIRST
EDITION

PDR®
Lab Advisor

THOMSON

PDR

DIRECTOR, EDITORIAL SERVICES: Bette LaGow
MANAGER, PROFESSIONAL SERVICES: Michael DeLuca, PharmD, MBA
DRUG INFORMATION SPECIALISTS: Majid Kerolous, PharmD; Nermin Shenouda, PharmD; Greg Tallis, RPh
PRODUCTION EDITOR: Elise Philippi
PROJECT MANAGER: Christina Klinger
DIRECTOR OF OPERATIONS: Robert Klein
MANAGER, PRODUCTION PURCHASING: Thomas Westburgh
PRODUCTION DESIGN SUPERVISOR: Adeline Rich
SENIOR ELECTRONIC PUBLISHING DESIGNER: Livio Udina
ELECTRONIC PUBLISHING DESIGNERS: Deana DiVizio, Carrie Faeth, Monika Popowitz

EXECUTIVE VICE PRESIDENT, PDR: Kevin Sanborn
VICE PRESIDENT, PDR SERVICES: Brian Holland
VICE PRESIDENT, MARKETING: William T. Hicks
DIRECTOR, PRODUCT MANAGEMENT: Swan Oey

CHIEF MEDICAL OFFICER, THOMSON HEALTHCARE: Rich Klasco, MD, FACEP

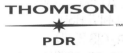

How to Use this Book

PDR Lab Advisor allows you to quickly review pertinent information on any of more than 600 laboratory tests—helping you to choose the right test for the suspected condition, then interpret and manage the results.

This guide is divided into two sections. First is a list of lab tests by indication, with the page numbers for the corresponding test. Following this you'll find comprehensive information on more than 600 tests, organized alphabetically. Included in each description is:

- Test definition
- Synonyms
- Reference range
- Indications (with detailed results interpretation)
- Abnormal results
- Collection/storage information
- LOINC codes

The following key refers to the "Strength of Recommendation" and "Strength of Evidence" sections under "Indications":

STRENGTH OF RECOMMENDATION
Class I - Recommended
The given test or treatment has been proven to be useful, and should be performed or administered.

Class IIa - Recommended, In Most Cases
The given test or treatment is generally considered to be useful, and is indicated in most cases.

Class IIb - Recommended, In Some Cases
The given test or treatment may be useful, and is indicated in some, but not most, cases.

Class III - Not Recommended
The given test or treatment is not useful, and should be avoided.

Class Indeterminant - Evidence Inconclusive

STRENGTH OF EVIDENCE
Category A
Category A evidence is based on data derived from: Meta-analyses of randomized controlled trials with homogeneity with regard to the directions and degrees of results between individual studies. Multiple, well-done randomized clinical trials involving large numbers of patients.

Category B
Category B evidence is based on data derived from: Meta-analyses of randomized controlled trials with conflicting conclusions with regard to the directions and degrees of results between individual studies. Randomized controlled trials that involved small numbers of patients or had significant methodological flaws (e.g., bias, drop-out rate, flawed analysis, etc.). Nonrandomized studies (e.g., cohort studies, case-control studies, observational studies).

Category C
Category C evidence is based on data derived from: Expert opinion or consensus, case reports or case series.

No Evidence

LAB TESTS BY INDICATION

ALPHABETICAL LIST OF LAB TESTS

17 Hydroxyprogesterone measurement, amniotic fluid

TEST DEFINITION

Measurement of amniotic fluid 17-hydroxyprogesterone for prenatal diagnosis of congenital adrenal hyperplasia

REFERENCE RANGE

- Amniotic fluid: 0.21-4.96 ng/mL
  Please refer to your institution's reference ranges as lab normals may vary.

INDICATIONS

Prenatal screen for fetuses with a family history of congenital adrenal hyperplasia
   Strength of Recommendation: Class IIb
   Strength of Evidence: Category B
   Results Interpretation:
   Abnormal laboratory findings
   Elevated amniotic fluid levels of 17-hydroxyprogesterone are strongly correlated with congenital adrenal hyperplasia.
   Timing of Monitoring
   Amniotic fluid may be tested for 17-hydroxyprogesterone from 13 to 18 weeks of gestation.

CLINICAL NOTES

Prenatal diagnosis by assaying amniotic fluid 17-hydroxyprogesterone levels has largely been supplanted by molecular genetic analysis on fetal DNA extracted from chorionic villus cells or amniocentesis.

COLLECTION/STORAGE INFORMATION

- Specimen Collection and Handling:
  - If mothers are on corticosteroids, stop treatment 5 to 7 days prior to the amniocentesis.
  - Avoid contamination with blood or meconium.
  - Freeze samples immediately at -20°C until analysis.

17 Hydroxyprogesterone measurement, serum

TEST DEFINITION

Measurement of serum 17-hydroxyprogesterone levels in serum for evaluation of 21-hydroxylase deficiency-congenital adrenal hyperplasia

REFERENCE RANGE

- Premature infants: 26-568 ng/dL (0.8-17 nmol/L)
- Newborn infants (3 days): 7-77 ng/dL (0.2-2.3 nmol/L)
  Please refer to your institution's reference ranges as lab normals may vary.

INDICATIONS

Screening in newborns for 21-hydroxylase deficiency-congenital adrenal hyperplasia
   Strength of Recommendation: Class IIa
   Strength of Evidence: Category B
   Results Interpretation:
   Positive laboratory findings
   Moderately elevated 17-hydroxyprogesterone (17-OHP) levels are normally defined as 40 ng/dL or greater in term infants and 65 ng/dL or greater in premature infants. Levels of 100 ng/dL or higher in term infants and 200 ng/dL or higher in premature infants are considered extremely elevated. Levels greater than 90 ng/mL are associated with severe forms of congenital adrenal hyperplasia (CAH). Follow-up testing is necessary for

levels between 40 ng/mL and 89 ng/mL as these values may indicate less severe forms of 21-hydroxylase deficiency-congenital adrenal hyperplasia (21-OH-D-CAH). Timely clinical reexamination in conjunction with retesting is recommended if 21-OH-D-CAH is suspected.

Interpretation of results is complicated by many factors including the lack of consistent screening guidelines for CAH, the inconsistency in the timing of sample collection after birth, the differences in normal ranges depending on the assay used, and the differing levels of expertise of the laboratory personnel performing the test, and the clinicians performing the clinical exam and interpreting the laboratory results.

Timing of Monitoring

In European countries and the United States blood spots are most often taken after the first 2 days of life; retesting in the United States is done in 1 to 2 weeks.

CLINICAL NOTES

Prematurity, low birth weight, pain, illness, or stress can cause false positive results.

COLLECTION/STORAGE INFORMATION

- Obtain specimen in newborns by capillary heel stick.
- Early morning specimens are preferred.

LOINC CODES

- Code: 14569-8 (*Short Name* - 17-OHP SerPl-sCnc)
- Code: 1668-3 (*Short Name* - 17OHP SerPl-mCnc)
- Code: 27996-8 (*Short Name* - 17OHP BS SerPl-mCnc)
- Code: 32538-1 (*Short Name* - 17OHP 2H p chal SerPl-sCnc)

17-Hydroxypregnenolone measurement

TEST DEFINITION

Measurement of 17-hydroxypregnenolone in plasma for the evaluation and management of congenital adrenal hyperplasia

REFERENCE RANGE

- Prepubertal child (2 years to 8 years): $\leq$100 ng/dL ($\leq$3.0 nmol/L)
- Adult Male: 41-183 ng/dL (1.2-5.5 nmol/L)
- Adult Female:
- Follicular: 45-1185 ng/dL (1.3-35.7 nmol/L)
- Luteal: 42-450 ng/dL (1.3-13.5 nmol/L)
- Postmenopausal: 18-48 ng/dL (0.5-1.4 nmol/L)
  Please refer to your institution's reference ranges as lab normals may vary.

INDICATIONS

Suspected or known congenital adrenal hyperplasia
    Strength of Recommendation: Class IIb
    Strength of Evidence: Category C
Results Interpretation:
Increased level (laboratory finding)

Elevated plasma levels of 17-hydroxypregnenolone are seen with patients who have poorly controlled or untreated congenital adrenal hyperplasia (CAH) due to 21-hydroxylase deficiency and $3_{|fb}$ -hydroxysteroid dehydrogenase-isomerase deficiency. Increased plasma levels may be due to a phenomenon of product inhibition or because the $3_{|fb}$ hydroxysteroid dehydrogenase enzyme system is saturated.

CAH can be recognized in adolescents and young adults in conjunction with complaints of hirsutism, menstrual irregularity, and infertility.

COLLECTION/STORAGE INFORMATION

- Store serum sample frozen at $-20°C$

LOINC CODES

- Code: 25316-1 (*Short Name* - 17-OH-Pregnenolone Ser-sCnc)
- Code: 6765-2 (*Short Name* - 17-OH-Pregnenolone Ser-mCnc)
- Code: 16297-4 (*Short Name* - 17OH-Preg Ur-mCnc)
- Code: 21037-7 (*Short Name* - 17OH-Preg 24H Ur-mRate)

21-Hydroxylase antibody assay

TEST DEFINITION

Detection of 21-hydroxylase antibody in serum for diagnosis and monitoring of patients with autoimmune adrenal insufficiency

REFERENCE RANGE

Adults and Children (upper limits of normal): index value of 0.6 to 2.6
Please refer to your institution's reference ranges as lab normals may vary.

INDICATIONS

Suspected adrenal hypofunction
Results Interpretation:
Positive immunology findings
A positive 21-hydroxylase antibody titer is diagnostic for autoimmune adrenal disease, and may be a useful screening marker for distinguishing autoimmune from non-autoimmune primary adrenal insufficiency.
The simultaneous detection of 21-hydroxylase antibody and adrenal cortex antibody may potentially serve as the 'gold standard' approach for diagnosing autoimmune variants of primary adrenal insufficiency.
Polyglandular autoimmune syndrome type II consists of adrenal failure with autoimmune thyroid disease and/or type I diabetes mellitus. Onset usually is seen in adulthood and accounts for up to 50% of cases of idiopathic adrenal failure. It is associated with antibodies against the adrenal 21-hydroxylase enzyme, in conjunction with HLA-B8 (DW3) and HLA-DR3 haplotypes.

Suspected autoimmune polyglandular syndrome type II
Strength of Recommendation: Class I
Strength of Evidence: Category B
Results Interpretation:
Positive immunology findings
A positive 21-hydroxylase antibody titer, in combination with thyroiditis and diabetes mellitus type I, is diagnostic for autoimmune polyglandular syndrome type II.

CLINICAL NOTES

21-hydroxylase antibody assays using [125] I labeling appear to be more sensitive than assays using [35] S.

COLLECTION/STORAGE INFORMATION

- Store serum at −20°C.

LOINC CODES

- Code: 17781-6 (*Short Name* - 21Hydroxylase Ab Ser-aCnc)

24 hour urine calcium output measurement

TEST DEFINITION

Measurement of calcium in urine for evaluation of urinary calcium excretion

SYNONYMS

- 24 hour urine calcium output

REFERENCE RANGE

- Adults: <300 mg/24 hours (<7.5 mmol/24 hours) with low dietary calcium intake of 200 mg/24 hours
- Children: Up to 6 mg/kg/24 hours (0.15 mmol/kg/24 hours)
  Please refer to your institution's reference ranges as lab normals may vary.

INDICATIONS

Nephrolithiasis related to suspected hypercalciuria
>   **Strength of Recommendation:** Class IIa
>   **Strength of Evidence:** Category B
>   **Results Interpretation:**
>   **Hypercalciuria**
>   Hypercalciuria is defined as a calcium level greater than 300mg/24 hours. Idiopathic hypercalciuria is the most common abnormal metabolic finding in patients with calcium nephrolithiasis. It occurs in up to 40% of such patients, and of these patients, 40% to 70% have a relative who also has nephrolithiasis.

Suspected primary hyperparathyroidism
>   **Strength of Recommendation:** Class IIa
>   **Strength of Evidence:** Category C
>   **Results Interpretation:**
>   **Hypercalciuria**
>   Hypercalciuria, defined as urine calcium level greater than 300 mg/24 hours, is found in up to 30% of patients with primary hyperparathyroidism. Elderly women are most frequently affected with primary hyperparathyroidism, but urine calcium levels can vary and frequently are not elevated in elderly patients.
>   Normal to high urinary calcium levels can suggest sporadic adenoma or multiple endocrine neoplasia Type 1. Normal to low urinary calcium levels can suggest familial hypocalciuric hypercalcemia or neonatal severe primary hyperparathyroidism.
>   In asymptomatic patients with known hyperparathyroidism who are at least 50 years of age, surgery is not indicated if their serum calcium concentration is 1 to 1.6 mg/dL (0.25 to 0.4 mmol/L) above the upper limit of normal, if a urinary calcium level is less than 400 mg (100 mmol) per day, if a creatinine clearance is at least 70% of normal, or if a z score is higher than -2 for bone mass.

ABNORMAL RESULTS

- Results increased in:
  - Malignancies
  - Immobilization
  - Granulomatosis

CLINICAL NOTES

>   This test requires strict patient compliance.
>   Calcium and protein intake or phosphate excretion can alter urinary calcium excretion.

COLLECTION/STORAGE INFORMATION

- Specimen Collection and Handling:
  - Discard first morning void; collect all other voids that day plus the first morning void of the following day
  - Collect 24-hour urine specimen in a bottle containing preservative (usually hydrochloric acid); acidify specimen to pH less than 2
  - Avoid specimen contamination with stool in children

LOINC CODES

- Code: 14637-3 (*Short Name* - Calcium 24H Ur-sRate)
- Code: 18488-7 (*Short Name* - Calcium 24H Ur-mCnc)
- Code: 25362-5 (*Short Name* - Calcium 24H Ur-sCnc)
- Code: 6874-2 (*Short Name* - Calcium 24H Ur-mRate)
- Code: 1993-5 (*Short Name* - Calcium Cl 24H Ur-vRate)

24 hour urine citrate output measurement

TEST DEFINITION
Measurement of citrate excretion in urine for the evaluation and management of nephrolithiasis

SYNONYMS
- 24 hour urine citrate output

REFERENCE RANGE
- Males: >450 mg per day
- Females: >550 mg per day
  Please refer to your institution's reference ranges as lab normals may vary.

INDICATIONS
Recurrent nephrolithiasis
  Strength of Recommendation: Class IIa
  Strength of Evidence: Category C
  Results Interpretation:
  Decreased urine citrate level
   Hypocitraturia is defined as urinary citrate excretion levels less than 320 mg per day. It is found in 20% to 63% of patients with recurrent calcium nephrolithiasis.
   Hypocitraturia is more frequent in elderly patients.
   Decreased urinary citrate levels have been associated with indinavir-induced renal stones.
   Other etiologies related to hypocitraturia include: urinary tract infections, intracellular acidosis, bowel disease, ileostomy, and chronic laxative use.
  Frequency of Monitoring
   Patients who are being treated for recurrent urolithiasis related to hypocitraturia should have 24-hour urine collections for citrate at 1 to 2 month intervals until desired treatment effect is achieved, then yearly for continued monitoring.

COLLECTION/STORAGE INFORMATION
- The 24-hour urine sample should be refrigerated during the collection period and can be frozen at −20°C until the time of assay.

LOINC CODES
- Code: 14650-6 (*Short Name* - Citrate 24H Ur-sRate)
- Code: 25876-4 (*Short Name* - Citrate 24H Ur-sCnc)
- Code: 6687-8 (*Short Name* - Citrate 24H Ur-mRate)

24 hour urine copper output measurement

TEST DEFINITION
Measurement of copper in urine, primarily for the detection and monitoring of Wilson's disease

SYNONYMS
- 24 hour urine copper output

REFERENCE RANGE
- Adults and Children: <40 mcg/24 hours (<0.6 micromoles/24 hours)
- Adults and Children: 2-80 mcg/L (0.03-1.26 micromoles/L)
  Please refer to your institution's reference ranges as lab normals may vary.

INDICATIONS

Suspected Wilson's disease
>**Strength of Recommendation:** Class IIa
>**Strength of Evidence:** Category C

Results Interpretation:

Elev urine levels of drugs, medicaments & biolog substances

A urine copper level greater than 100 mcg in 24 hours is a presumptive diagnosis of Wilson's disease. A urine copper level greater than 40 mcg in 24 hours needs further evaluation..

In children, a penicillamine challenge with a 24-hour urine test may assist in the diagnosis of Wilson's disease. The D-penicillamine test has been standardized only in the pediatric population. A urine copper level greater than 1,600 mcg in 24 hours (25 micromoles/24 hours) after D-penicillamine challenge provides evidence of Wilson's disease.

Frequency of Monitoring

In very young siblings of patients with Wilson's disease, urine copper levels are recommended every few years until 20 years of age. If the level remains normal, Wilson's disease is considered ruled out. If urine copper level is elevated to above 50 mcg/day, further evaluation is needed.

ABNORMAL RESULTS

- Results increased in:
  - Chronic active hepatitis
  - Biliary cirrhosis
  - Primary sclerosing cholangitis
  - Autoimmune hepatitis
  - Proteinuria
  - Rheumatoid arthritis
- Results decreased in :
  - Protein malnutrition

CLINICAL NOTES

Spot urines are not recommended to check copper levels due to variability of copper content.

COLLECTION/STORAGE INFORMATION

- Specimen Collection and Handling:
  - Collect 24-hour urine in plastic or acid-washed glass container
  - Acidify to pH 2.0 with hydrochloric acid

LOINC CODES

- Code: 5633-3 (*Short Name* - Copper 24H Ur-mRate)
- Code: 21219-1 (*Short Name* - Copper 24H Ur-mCnc)
- Code: 29942-0 (*Short Name* - Copper/creat 24H Ur-mRto)
- Code: 25879-8 (*Short Name* - Copper 24H Ur-sCnc)

24 hour urine magnesium output measurement

TEST DEFINITION

Measurement of magnesium in urine, after administration of magnesium loading dose, for evaluation and management of electrolyte imbalances

SYNONYMS

- 24 hour urine magnesium output

REFERENCE RANGE

- With intravenous magnesium sulfate preload:
- Adults: 18-30 mmol/24 hours
  Please refer to your institution's reference ranges as lab normals may vary.

INDICATIONS

Suspected hypomagnesemia in chronic pancreatitis
> **Strength of Recommendation:** Class IIb
> **Strength of Evidence:** Category B
> **Results Interpretation:**
> **Urine electrolyte levels - finding**
> Increased magnesium retention, determined by decreased levels in a 24-hour urine magnesium load test, may indicate hypomagnesemia in patients with chronic pancreatitis, even when serum magnesium levels are normal.

Suspected hypomagnesemia
> **Strength of Recommendation:** Class IIb
> **Strength of Evidence:** Category B
> **Results Interpretation:**
> **Urine electrolyte levels - finding**
> Decreased magnesium urine excretion (compared with baseline level), after administration of a magnesium loading dose, may indicate systemic hypomagnesemia.
> After administration of a magnesium loading dose, increased magnesium urine excretion, compared to a baseline level, may suggest underlying conditions that could contribute to systemic hypomagnesemia.

TEST COMPLICATIONS

- Cardiac arrest
- Hypermagnesemia
- Diarrhea
- Respiratory depression

CLINICAL NOTES

This test requires strict patient compliance and is not recommended for routine analysis.

COLLECTION/STORAGE INFORMATION

- Collect baseline urine sample prior to magnesium administration.
- Collect 24-hour urine specimen in metal free container without preservatives.
- Acidify urine to pH 1.

LOINC CODES

- Code: 2599-9 (*Short Name* - Magnesium 24H Ur-sRate)
- Code: 25954-9 (*Short Name* - Magnesium 24H Ur-sCnc)
- Code: 24447-5 (*Short Name* - Magnesium 24H Ur-mRate)
- Code: 32024-2 (*Short Name* - Magnesium 24H Ur-mCnc)

24 hour urine sodium output measurement

TEST DEFINITION

Measurement of sodium in urine for evaluation of intravascular volume status

SYNONYMS

- 24 hour urine sodium output

REFERENCE RANGE

- Adults (varies with intake): 100-260 mEq/24-hours (100-260 mmol/24-hours)
- Full term neonates 7 to 14 days old: Sodium clearance is about 20% of adult values
- Females 6 to 10 years: 20-69 mEq/day (20-69 mmol/day)
- Males 6 to 10 years: 41-115 mEq/day (41-115 mmol/day)
- Females 10 to 14 years: 48-168 mEq/day (48-168 mmol/day)
- Males 10 to 14 years: 63-177 mEq/day (63-177 mmol/day)
  Please refer to your institution's reference ranges as lab normals may vary.

INDICATIONS
Suspected acute renal failure
    Strength of Recommendation: Class IIa
    Strength of Evidence: Category C
Results Interpretation:
Sodium level - finding
    In acute tubular necrosis, urinary sodium concentrations are usually greater than 40 mmol/L
    Urinary sodium concentrations are usually less than 20 mmol/L in prerenal azotemia

Suspected hyponatremia
    Strength of Recommendation: Class IIa
    Strength of Evidence: Category C
Results Interpretation:
Decreased sodium level
    Without the influence of diuretics, urine sodium concentration will be low (usually less than 10-20 mEq/L) in cases of hypovolemic hyponatremia secondary to extrarenal loss and in hypervolemic states associated with edema and third spacing.
    A urinary sodium concentration less than 30 mEq/L suggests a saline-responsive hyponatremic patient.
Sodium level - finding
- Causes of high urine sodium levels (greater than 40 mEq/L) include the following:
  - Diuretic overuse
  - Primary adrenal insufficiency
  - Sodium-losing renal diseases
  - Proximal renal tubular acidosis
  - SIADH
- Urine sodium may be increased despite hypovolemia in patients with severe metabolic alkalosis in whom bicarbonaturia obligates excretion of an accompanying cation (eg, sodium).

ABNORMAL RESULTS
- Results decreased in:
  - Overhydration

COLLECTION/STORAGE INFORMATION
- Specimen Collection and Handling:
  - Discard the first morning specimen, then collect all urine including the final specimen voided at the end of the 24 hour period
  - Refrigerate 24-hour urine specimen immediately after collection
  - Deliver specimen to lab within 1 hour of collection

LOINC CODES
- Code: 26761-7 (*Short Name* - Sodium Cl 2H Ur-vRate)
- Code: 21525-1 (*Short Name* - Sodium 24H Ur-sCnc)
- Code: 21526-9 (*Short Name* - Sodium 24H Ur-mCnc)
- Code: 21527-7 (*Short Name* - Sodium 24H Ur-mRate)
- Code: 13809-9 (*Short Name* - Sodium/creat 24H Ur-mRto)
- Code: 2956-1 (*Short Name* - Sodium 24H Ur-sRate)

5-Hydroxyindoleacetic acid measurement

TEST DEFINITION
    Measurement of 5-hydroxyindoleacetic acid (5-HIAA) in urine or plasma for the evaluation of carcinoid tumors

REFERENCE RANGE
- Urine
- Qualitative: <25 mg/day (<131 micromol/day)
- Quantitative: <6 mg/24 hours (<31 micromol/24 hours)
- Plasma: 27-70 nmol/L
Please refer to your institution's reference ranges as lab normals may vary.

INDICATIONS
Patients with carcinoid syndrome with suspected or known carcinoid disease
> **Strength of Recommendation:** Class IIa
> **Strength of Evidence:** Category B
> **Results Interpretation:**
> **Increased level (laboratory finding)**
>> A 24-hour urine collection for 5-hydroxyindoleacetic acid (5-HIAA) is often used to support the diagnosis of carcinoid syndrome and has a moderate sensitivity and specificity. Some data suggest that an 8-hour overnight urine or plasma 5-HIAA may be used in lieu of a 24-hour urine collection.
>> There appears to be a nonsignificant trend toward higher levels of urinary 5-HIAA in patients with distant disease vs patients with local or regional disease.
>> Urinary 5-HIAA levels are higher in patients with carcinoid heart disease and may be predictive of progressive cardiac involvement.

COLLECTION/STORAGE INFORMATION
- Have patient abstain from prescription medications and over-the counter drugs for 72 hours prior to the test.
- Collect a 24-hour urine or random urine sample.
- Acidify 24-hour urine collection with hydrochloric acid, boric acid, or glacial acetic acid.
- Store acidified urine at 4°C for 2 weeks and at −20°C for longer periods.
- Avoid serotonin-containing foods before and during collection.
- Collect plasma in heparinized tube following overnight fast.

LOINC CODES
- Code: 1692-3 (*Short Name* - 5HIAA CSF-mCnc)
- Code: 1693-1 (*Short Name* - 5HIAA Ser-mCnc)

AD7c neural thread protein measurement, cerebrospinal fluid

TEST DEFINITION
Measurement of AD7c-neural thread protein (AD7c-NTP) in cerebrospinal fluid as a diagnostic and prognostic marker in the evaluation of Alzheimer's disease (AD)

SYNONYMS
- AD7c NTP measurement, cerebrospinal fluid

REFERENCE RANGE
Normal range has not been established.
Please refer to your institution's reference ranges as lab normals may vary.

INDICATIONS
Suspected Alzheimer disease
> **Results Interpretation:**
> **Increased AD7c neural thread protein level**
>> AD7c-neural thread protein (AD7c-NTP) levels are elevated in cerebrospinal fluid (CSF) of patients with Alzheimer disease (AD).
>> Elevated AD7c-NTP level in CSF correlates with the severity of dementia.
>> Low levels of AD7c-NTP in CSF may reflect early disease or severe end-stage disease.

CLINICAL NOTES
The AD7c-neural thread protein (AD7c-NTP) can be excreted in the urine, potentially providing a future noninvasive biomarker to detect early Alzheimer's disease (AD).

COLLECTION/STORAGE INFORMATION
- Specimen Collection and Handling:
  - Obtain cerebrospinal fluid by lumbar puncture.

• Store the sample at -80°C in the original containers or in screwcapped glass vials.

LOINC CODES
• Code: 28560-1 (*Short Name* - Neuronal Thread Prot CSF-mCnc)

AD7c neural thread protein measurement, urine

TEST DEFINITION
Measurement of AD7c neural thread protein (NTP) in urine for the diagnosis and management of Alzheimer's disease

SYNONYMS
• AD7c neural thread protein, urine
• AD7c-NTP, urine

INDICATIONS
Suspected Alzheimer disease
    Strength of Recommendation: Class IIb
    Strength of Evidence: Category B
    Results Interpretation:
    Increased AD7c neural thread protein level
    Chronically elevated levels of urinary AD7c-NTP are suggestive of Alzheimer disease (AD) and justify further testing to confirm diagnosis.
    Elevated urinary AD7c-NTP levels are chronic in persons with AD and may increase further during the clinical course.
    Elevations of urinary AD7c-NTP correlate with the severity of dementia in AD.
    Frequency of Monitoring
    Aat least 2 urinary AD7c-NTP level measurements several months apart should be performed to confirm chronically elevated levels in patients with Alzheimer disease.

COLLECTION/STORAGE INFORMATION
• Specimen Collection and Handling:
    • Collect a sterile urine specimen in a sterile plastic container.
    • Specimen is stable for up to 24 hours at 4°C before processing.
    • Unprocessed and processed urine samples are stable for 3 months at temperatures of -20°C and -80°C, respectively.

ANA measurement

TEST DEFINITION
Measurement of antinuclear antibodies (ANA) in serum for evaluation of autoimmune and connective tissue diseases

SYNONYMS
• ANA - Anti-nuclear antibody level
• Anti-nuclear antibody level
• Anti-nuclear antibody measurement

REFERENCE RANGE
• Adults: Negative at 1:40 dilution
    Please refer to your institution's reference ranges as lab normals may vary.

INDICATIONS
Monitoring disease activity in multiple sclerosis
Results Interpretation:
Antinuclear antibody positive

Antinuclear antibodies (ANA) are detected in 10% to 80% of multiple sclerosis (MS) patients, depending on the method used to detect ANA. ANA may be produced during MS exacerbations as a byproduct of systemic immune dysfunction, and their occurrence correlates well with MS disease activity; however, the prognostic or therapeutic significance of positive ANA remains to be determined.

MS patients with elevated anticardiolipin antibodies display atypical features and slower disease progression. These patients may be more prone to thrombotic events.

Suspected and known rheumatoid arthritis
Results Interpretation:
Increased level (laboratory finding)

Antinuclear antibodies (ANA) may be useful in screening for systemic lupus erythematosus and other autoimmune and connective tissue disorders. ANA assays are positive in up to 30% of rheumatoid arthritis (RA) patients with a positive rheumatoid factor test. However, these ANAs are not directed against specific nuclear antigens that are usually tested in the ANA profile (anti-SSA, anti-SSB, anti-Smith, anti-RNP, and anti-double stranded DNA antibodies).

Suspected autoimmune thyroid disease
Strength of Recommendation: Class IIb
Strength of Evidence: Category B
Results Interpretation:
Positive immunology findings

The presence of antinuclear antibodies may indicate autoimmune thyroid disease.

Suspected scleroderma (systemic sclerosis)
Strength of Recommendation: Class IIa
Strength of Evidence: Category B
Results Interpretation:
Positive immunology findings

The presence of serum antinuclear antibodies (ANA) may be predictive of systemic sclerosis. Different serotype variants appear to be associated with different clinical manifestations.

Approximately 40% of patients with scleroderma and associated conditions will test positive for ANA. In patients with progressive systemic sclerosis, approximately 96% have ANA when the Hep-2 substrate is used, and the ANA serotype variant SCL-70 has been found in 20% of these patients.

Suspected Sj|f-gren's syndrome
Strength of Recommendation: Class IIb
Strength of Evidence: Category C
Results Interpretation:
Positive immunology findings

Antinuclear antibodies (ANA) measurement is one of the several criteria used to diagnose Sj|f-gren's syndrome. A positive test is a dilution greater than or equal to 1 in 40.

Suspected systemic lupus erythematosus
Strength of Recommendation: Class I
Strength of Evidence: Category B
Results Interpretation:
Antinuclear antibody positive

An abnormal titer of antinuclear antibody (ANA) by immunofluorescence or an equivalent assay is 1 of 11 American College of Rheumatology (ACR) criteria for the diagnosis of systemic lupus erythematosus (SLE). A patient with 4 of the 11 criteria can be diagnosed with SLE with a specificity of approximately 95% and a sensitivity of 85%. Patients with positive ANA alone, without organ system involvement or typical laboratory findings, are unlikely to have SLE. Patients with a negative ANA have a very low probability of having SLE.

Antinuclear antibody (ANA) testing is not specific for systemic lupus erythematosus (SLE), as ANA is detected in numerous autoimmune, rheumatic and infectious disorders. ANA is also detectable in normal individuals, especially children and the elderly. Nevertheless, ANA is the best single test for ruling out the diagnosis of SLE.

Antinuclear antibodies (ANA) are frequently present for years prior to development of clinical illness. An abnormal ANA titer is present in 76% of patients at SLE onset and in 94% of patients at any time after SLE onset.

COMMON PANELS
- Arthritis panel
- Collagen/Lupus panel

CLINICAL NOTES
Accuracy of the antinuclear antibody test depends on each laboratory using a cutoff based on their conditions of assay.

Substantial variability exists between laboratories due to immunologic reagents and laboratory conditions.

The ANA test is frequently over-ordered. The test has excellent sensitivity and acceptable specificity, but its positive predictive value is often low because of overuse in low-risk populations, with a false-positive of 20% or more.

Several patterns of fluorescence in the ANA can be seen microscopically; however, these patterns are not diagnostic of different related diseases.

COLLECTION/STORAGE INFORMATION
- Specimen Collection and Handling:
    - Collect serum in red top tube.
    - Store sample at -20°C.

Acetaminophen blood measurement

TEST DEFINITION
Measurement of acetaminophen level in plasma or serum for the evaluation and management of potential toxicity

SYNONYMS
- Paracetamol: blood level
- Paracetamol blood measurement

REFERENCE RANGE
Adults and Children: 10-30 mcg/mL (66-199 micromole/L)
Please refer to your institution's reference ranges as lab normals may vary.

INDICATIONS
Suspected acute acetaminophen (paracetamol) poisoning
      Strength of Recommendation: Class I
      Strength of Evidence: Category B
      Results Interpretation:
      Blood drug level high

When reliable information is available, children with a single acetaminophen ingestion of less than 150 to 200 mg/kg, and adults with less than 7.5 g, do not require assessment for toxicity.

Acetaminophen levels obtained 4 to 16 hours after a single ingestion are most predictive of potential hepatotoxicity. Levels obtained earlier may not reflect complete absorption and should not be used to predict toxic effects. Nevertheless, a negligible acetaminophen level at 2 to 4 hours after ingestion adequately rules out toxicity.

Acetaminophen levels above the 'possible risk' line (ie, the line that extends from 140 mg/L at 4 hours to 50 mg/L at 10 hours) on a modified Rumack-Matthew nomogram predict potential hepatotoxicity.

Do not delay NAC therapy for lack of an acetaminophen level. Administer loading dose, then discontinue NAC if the level comes back below the treatment line. Do not discontinue NAC therapy if the initial acetaminophen level is above the treatment line and subsequent levels fall below the treatment line.

No standard guidelines exist for assessing patients with repeated supratherapeutic ingestion of acetaminophen. However, the Rocky Mountain Poison and Drug Center has not identified any patient presenting with a history of chronic acetaminophen overdosing who required NAC therapy, if the acetaminophen level was less than 10 mg/L and the AST level was less than 50 International Units/L.

Frequency of Monitoring

If the initial acetaminophen level is above the 'treatment line' and NAC therapy is started, the value of subsequent acetaminophen levels is unclear. The standard protocol has been to continue the entire NAC regimen (eg, oral NAC every 4 hours for 72 hours) regardless of subsequent acetaminophen levels. Based on a retrospective case series of 75 patients, an alterative protocol includes stopping NAC therapy if serial serum acetaminophen levels become nondetectable and there is no evidence of hepatotoxicity (ie, elevated AST or ALT level) at 36 hours following ingestion.

Timing of Monitoring

The serum/plasma acetaminophen level in a blood sample drawn at least 4 hours after a single ingestion of acetaminophen is the most reliable predictor of potential hepatotoxicity and need for N-acetylcysteine (NAC) therapy.

In a study of serum acetaminophen levels drawn less than 4 hours after ingestion, NAC therapy was needed only in patients with acetaminophen levels greater than 200 mcg/mL (200 mg/L); however, further studies are needed before acetaminophen levels drawn less than 4 hours after ingestion are used to guide therapy.

CLINICAL NOTES

Blood levels peak within 30 minutes to 2 hours of ingestion of a therapeutic dose. Acetaminophen absorption is slower in neonates, possible secondary to prolonged gastric emptying.

COLLECTION/STORAGE INFORMATION

- Collect 7 mL of whole blood in plain (red top) tube

Acetylcholine receptor antibody assay

TEST DEFINITION

Detection of acetylcholine receptor antibody in serum for the evaluation and management of myasthenia gravis

REFERENCE RANGE

- Adults and children: <0.03 nmol/L
  Please refer to your institution's reference ranges as lab normals may vary.

INDICATIONS

Suspected and known myasthenia gravis
   Strength of Recommendation: Class IIa
   Strength of Evidence: Category B
   Results Interpretation:
   Positive immunology findings

A positive anti-acetylcholine receptor (AChR) antibody titer is suggestive of generalized myasthenia gravis (MG) and increased titers are associated with clinical deterioration. In the approximately 9% of MG patients who are titer-negative, the disease is mild, of early onset, or confined to the extraocular muscles. False positives are rare. Male MG patients may have antibody titer levels 25% lower than females.

COLLECTION/STORAGE INFORMATION

- Collect serum in red-top or serum separator tube.
- Store frozen at -20°C or refrigerate with preservatives.

LOINC CODES

- Code: 8058-0 (*Short Name* - AChR Ab Ser-aCnc)
- Code: 20427-1 (*Short Name* - AChR Ab Ser-sCnc)

Acetylcholinesterase measurement, amniotic fluid

TEST DEFINITION
Measurement of acetylcholinesterase in amniotic fluid for the prenatal detection of neural tube defects

SYNONYMS
- AChE-AF measurement

REFERENCE RANGE
- Normal range by method:
- Polyacrylamide gel electrophoresis: Negative
- AE-2 immunoassay: Negative
- Inhibition assay: 5.17 ± 2.63 milliunits/mL (5.17 ± 2.63 units/L)
  Please refer to your institution's reference ranges as lab normals may vary.

INDICATIONS
Suspected fetal neural tube defect
>   **Strength of Recommendation:** Class IIb
>   **Strength of Evidence:** Category B
>   **Results Interpretation:**
>   **Increased acetylcholinesterase level**

Historically, amniocentesis has been performed in women with a positive maternal serum alpha-fetoprotein (AFP). If the AFP in amniotic fluid is elevated, an acetylcholinesterase assay is run. If both the amniotic fluid AFP and acetylcholinesterase are elevated, this is considered diagnostic for a neural tube defect.

Given that acetylcholinesterase levels in amniotic fluid may be elevated in fetal malformations other than those caused by neural tube defects, a high acetylcholinesterase/pseudocholinesterase ratio may be helpful in distinguishing those cases with neural tube defects.

More recently, advanced ultrasound technology has demonstrated such high sensitivity and specificity for detecting neural tube defects that performing an amniocentesis to obtain an acetylcholinesterase level is often not necessary. Amniocentesis may still be done when the maternal serum AFP level is very high, the ultrasound is indeterminate, the woman is at particularly high risk (eg, those with a prior history of having a fetus with a neural tube defect), or genetic analysis is indicated.

>   **Timing of Monitoring**

False-positive results in the amniotic fluid acetylcholinesterase assay may occur more frequently at 11 to 14 weeks' gestation than at 15 to 20 weeks' gestation.

CLINICAL NOTES
Contaminating the specimen with blood (which usually occurs during amniocentesis) or freezing the sample (which can induce hemolysis) may cause false-positive results due to the release of red blood cell acetylcholinesterase. This problem may be avoided by using a monoclonal antibody assay that can distinguish between brain and erythrocyte acetylcholinesterase.

COLLECTION/STORAGE INFORMATION
- Specimen Collection and Handling:
  - Do not freeze specimen.

LOINC CODES
- Code: 30106-9 (*Short Name* - AChE Amn Ql)

Acetylcholinesterase, red blood cell measurement

TEST DEFINITION

Measurement of erythrocyte acetylcholinesterase (AChE) enzyme to evaluate suspected organophosphate toxicity.

SYNONYMS

- Acetylcholinesterase, RBC measurement
- Cholinesterase, erythrocytic measurement
- Red cell cholinesterase measurement

REFERENCE RANGE

Adults and Children: 12.5 ± 1.3 units/mL packed RBC
Please refer to your institution's reference ranges as lab normals may vary.

INDICATIONS

Suspected organophosphate poisoning.
Strength of Recommendation: Class IIb
Strength of Evidence: Category C
Results Interpretation:
Decreased erythrocyte acetylcholinesterase activity

Symptomatic patients with organophosphate poisoning usually have depression of blood cholinesterase activities in excess of 50% of the pre-exposure value. Depressions in excess of 90% may occur in severe poisonings.

Alternatively, moderate to severe organophosphate poisoning has been diagnosed in patients with 'normal' red blood acetylcholinesterase (AChE) activity. In these patients AChE levels were decreased as much as 50% but were still within the normal range.

COLLECTION/STORAGE INFORMATION

-
- Collect venous blood in either an EDTA-containing (lavender-top) or heparin-containing (green-top) tube.
- Add 200 microL blood in 20 mL ice-cold diluting reagent and centrifuge to isolate plasma fraction.
- Freeze at -20 °C until ready to assay.
- Keep the thawed samples on ice until analysis.

LOINC CODES

- Code: 23839-4 (*Short Name* - Cholinesterase RBC Calc-aCnc)
- Code: 2099-0 (*Short Name* - Cholinesterase RBC-cCnc)

Acetylcholinesterase/pseudocholinesterase ratio

TEST DEFINITION

A calculated ratio of acetylcholinesterase to pseudocholinesterase in amniotic fluid, used to distinguish fetal open neural tube defects from ventral wall defects

REFERENCE RANGE

- Negative
Please refer to your institution's reference ranges as lab normals may vary.

INDICATIONS
Suspected fetal neural tube defect
> **Strength of Recommendation:** Class IIa
> **Strength of Evidence:** Category B
Results Interpretation:
Positive laboratory findings
> In the absence of blood contamination, an elevated acetylcholinesterase/pseudocholinesterase ratio in amniotic fluid can distinguish between open neural tube defects and ventral wall defects in the fetus.
Timing of Monitoring
> The acetylcholinesterase/pseudocholinesterase ratio test should be performed on amniotic fluid between gestational weeks 15 and 20.

ABNORMAL RESULTS
• Sample visibly contaminated with fetal blood

COLLECTION/STORAGE INFORMATION
• Do not freeze specimen and avoid hemolysis.

Acid fast stain method, Nocardia species

TEST DEFINITION
Detection of *Nocardia* species in biological samples for the evaluation and management of infectious diseases

SYNONYMS
• Acid fast stain

REFERENCE RANGE
• Negative
Please refer to your institution's reference ranges as lab normals may vary.

INDICATIONS
Suspected nocardiosis as a result of *Nocardia* infection
> **Strength of Recommendation:** Class IIb
> **Strength of Evidence:** Category B
Results Interpretation:
Positive laboratory findings
> In the presence of a positive Gram stain, a positive modified acid-fast stain on branching, beaded filaments is suggestive of *Nocardia*.
> *Nocardia* filaments may or not be acid-fast. Therefore, diagnosis of nocardial infection should not be based solely on modified acid-fast testing.
> The modified acid-fast test is useful in differential diagnoses between *Nocardia* and *Actinomyces* infections.
Negative laboratory findings
> A negative modified acid-fast result may not rule out *Nocardia* infection.

COLLECTION/STORAGE INFORMATION
• Specimen Collection and Handling
  • Specimens may include:
    • Sputum
    • Transtracheal aspirates
    • Bronchial washings
    • Surgical specimens
    • Exudate
  • Send macroscopically-noted granules to the laboratory for examination.

LOINC CODES
- Code: 32189-3 (*Short Name* - AFB Stn Fld)
- Code: 6655-5 (*Short Name* - AFB Kinyoun Stn Tiss)
- Code: 641-1 (*Short Name* - AFB Mod Kinyoun Stn Gast)
- Code: 6656-3 (*Short Name* - AFB Mod Kinyoun Stn Tiss)
- Code: 640-3 (*Short Name* - AFB Kinyoun Stn Gast)
- Code: 11479-3 (*Short Name* - AFB Stn Tiss)
- Code: 24002-8 (*Short Name* - AFB Stn Bro)
- Code: 11476-9 (*Short Name* - AFB Stn Gast)
- Code: 11545-1 (*Short Name* - AFB Stn XXX)

Acid fast stain method, Parasite

TEST DEFINITION
Identification of coccidian parasites in stool for the evaluation of chronic diarrhea

SYNONYMS
- Acid fast stain

REFERENCE RANGE
Negative
Please refer to your institution's reference ranges as lab normals may vary.

INDICATIONS
Suspected parasitic infection with coccidian parasites *(eg, Cryptosporidium, Cyclospora*, **or** *Isospora belli*) **causing chronic diarrhea**
>**Strength of Recommendation:** Class IIa
>**Strength of Evidence:** Category C
>**Results Interpretation:**
>**Feces: parasite present**
>> A positive acid-fast stain identifies *Cryptosporidium, Cyclospora*, or *Isospora belli* as the cause of chronic diarrhea.
>
>**Frequency of Monitoring**
>> Submit 1 stool specimen each day for 3 days before ruling out parasitic infection.

CLINICAL NOTES
Acid-fast stain is the only reliable stain for detecting the coccidian parasites *Cryptosporidium, Cyclospora*, and *Isospora belli* in stool.

Modified acid-fast stain effectively detects *Cryptosporidium* in stool, but enzyme-linked immunosorbent-based immunoassay formats or immunofluorescent assays providing visualization of fecal oocysts are more sensitive.

COLLECTION/STORAGE INFORMATION
- Specimen Collection and Handling:
  - Collect fresh random stool in a container with a lid.
  - Collect 1 specimen per day for 3 days.
  - Ensure specimen is free of urine, water, and soil.
  - Transport to lab immediately.
  - Avoid collecting specimens within one week of the use of oily laxatives, antidiarrheal medication, antacids, or barium.

LOINC CODES
- Code: 32189-3 (*Short Name* - AFB Stn Fld)
- Code: 6655-5 (*Short Name* - AFB Kinyoun Stn Tiss)
- Code: 641-1 (*Short Name* - AFB Mod Kinyoun Stn Gast)
- Code: 6656-3 (*Short Name* - AFB Mod Kinyoun Stn Tiss)
- Code: 640-3 (*Short Name* - AFB Kinyoun Stn Gast)
- Code: 11479-3 (*Short Name* - AFB Stn Tiss)

- Code: 24002-8 (*Short Name* - AFB Stn Bro)
- Code: 11476-9 (*Short Name* - AFB Stn Gast)
- Code: 11545-1 (*Short Name* - AFB Stn XXX)

Acid mucopolysaccharides measurement, quantitative

TEST DEFINITION
Quantification of acid mucopolysaccharides in random urine specimens

REFERENCE RANGE
- Urinary glycosaminoglycan (GAG) concentration: 7.1-54.3 mg/mmol creatinine (dimethylmethylene blue/creatinine ratio [DMB/CRE])
- Mucopolysaccharidoses (MPS) type not found (negative) with two-dimensional electrophoresis method
Please refer to your institution's reference ranges as lab normals may vary.

INDICATIONS
Suspected mucopolysaccharidosis
     Strength of Recommendation: Class IIa
     Strength of Evidence: Category B
Results Interpretation:
Mucopolysaccharidosis
     Urine dimethylmethylene blue-based (DMB), expressed as the DMB creatinine ratio (GAG mg/mmol creatinine), quantifies urinary glycosaminoglycans (GAG); it is used as a reference for MPS diagnosis, but cannot differentiate between MPS types. The DMB/creatinine ratio should be considered only for estimating the amount of GAG's in a sample, and is not a definitive basis for the diagnosis of MPS.
     Two-dimensional electrophoresis (2D-EP) testing differentiates MPS types and clearly separates GAG types; it is a reliable first screening method.
     Once MPS type is identified in the initial screening tests, enzymatic assay must be performed to measure specific enzyme activity and confirm the diagnosis of MPS.
     The DMB ratio is age dependent and varies between MPS types; DMB ratios have been shown to be the highest in the first year of life.

CLINICAL NOTES
     Because of variable levels of glycosaminoglycans (GAG) in mucopolysaccharidoses (MPS), MPS screening tests (including the spot and turbidity tests) are not specific or sensitive in the preliminary diagnosis of MPS. There is a high rate of false negative results in the spot test (up to 32%) and a high rate of false positive results with the turbidity test; as a result, neither testing method is recommended for the screening of MPS.
     The diagnosis of MPS is possible during the prenatal period, although testing is typically done during early childhood.

COLLECTION/STORAGE INFORMATION
- Specimen Collection and Handling:
  - Obtain random urine
  - Avoid adding preservatives to urine specimen
  - Store samples frozen at -20°C until further analysis

Actinomyces culture

TEST DEFINITION
Detection of *Actinomyces* species by culture for the evaluation of actinomycosis infection

REFERENCE RANGE
No growth
Please refer to your institution's reference ranges as lab normals may vary.

INDICATIONS
Suspected actinomycotic infection
> **Strength of Recommendation:** Class IIa
> **Strength of Evidence:** Category C
> **Results Interpretation:**
> **Positive laboratory findings**
>> Detection of *Actinomyces* species

CLINICAL NOTES
The *Actinomyces* species are normal inhabitants of the oropharynx, gastrointestinal tract, and female genital tract. Therefore, sputum or cervico-vaginal secretions are seldom cultured to identify invasive disease.

COLLECTION/STORAGE INFORMATION
Specimen Collection and Handling:
Optimize recovery of the actinomycosis microorganisms with proper collection and handling of specimens and by collecting culture specimens prior to antibiotic use.
Collect specimen from draining sinuses, pleural fluid, or lung tissue.
Place specimen in an anaerobic transport vial or on swabs in anaerobic transport tubes.
Do not place specimen in formalin.
Do not refrigerate specimen.
Transport to the lab as soon as possible.
Inform the lab that actinomycosis is suspected.

LOINC CODES
· Code: 9816-0 (*Short Name* - Actinomyces XXX Cult)

Adenosine deaminase measurement, cerebrospinal fluid

TEST DEFINITION
Measurement of adenosine deaminase in cerebrospinal fluid for the evaluation and management of tuberculous meningitis

REFERENCE RANGE
· 0-2.1 units/L
Please refer to your institution's reference ranges as lab normals may vary.

INDICATIONS
Suspected or known tuberculous meningitis
> **Strength of Recommendation:** Class IIb
> **Strength of Evidence:** Category B
> **Results Interpretation:**
> **Increased adenosine deaminase level**
>> Measurement of adenosine deaminase (ADA) in cerebrospinal fluid (CSF) is one method for early diagnosis and follow-up of tuberculosis meningitis (TBM), especially in areas of increased prevalence.
>> The definitive criterion for the diagnosis of TBM is detection of *M. Tuberculosis* in CSF. When ADA in CSF is greater than 15 units/L, TBM should be suspected, although experts do not agree on a cut-off value for ADA in CSF.
>> ADA value increases in the first 10 days of therapy for disease, follows a gradual decline on days 10 to 20, and normalizes after several months of treatment. ADA value increases in patients who develop complications during the course of therapy for TBM.

Opinions vary on the value of ADA in CSF to diagnose TBM. False positives may occur in pyogenic meningitis or lymphomatous infiltration of the meninges. Some experts recommend ADA in CSF levels to be used in the differential diagnosis of TBM versus neurobrucellosis or other forms of aseptic meningitis.

Neurologic diseases associated with HIV infection may cause an increased ADA level in CSF, as may an inflammatory response secondary to infections or lymphoma. False-positives may be found in patients with cytomegalovirus and meningitis caused by other organisms.

COLLECTION/STORAGE INFORMATION
- Obtain sample by lumbar puncture.
- Process immediately or store specimen at -20°C.
- Samples may be stored frozen at -70°C for up to 2 years.

Adenosine deaminase measurement, peritoneal fluid

TEST DEFINITION
Measurement of adenosine deaminase in peritoneal fluid for the evaluation of tuberculous peritonitis

REFERENCE RANGE
- Range varies based on the cut-off value used in studies
Please refer to your institution's reference ranges as lab normals may vary.

INDICATIONS
Suspected tuberculous peritonitis
   Strength of Recommendation: Class IIb
   Strength of Evidence: Category B
   Results Interpretation:
   Increased adenosine deaminase level
   In areas with a high prevalence of tuberculosis, adenosine deaminase (ADA) is used as a rapid diagnostic test for tuberculous peritonitis and can also distinguish tuberculosis from other causes of ascites.

   ADA levels in ascitic fluid, in conjunction with mycobacterial culture and response to anti-tuberculosis therapy, can direct initiation of medication treatment for tuberculosis.

   ADA is a marker of immune response. Due to immunosuppression associated with advanced liver disease, or a dilutional occurrence associated with malnutrition, ADA in peritoneal fluid is limited when used as a diagnostic aid.

   HIV status does not appear to affect ADA levels in tuberculous peritonitis.

COLLECTION/STORAGE INFORMATION
- Obtain specimen by paracentesis.

Adenosine deaminase measurement, pleural fluid

TEST DEFINITION
Measurement of adenosine deaminase in pleural fluid

INDICATIONS
Suspected tuberculosis in patients with pleural effusion
   Strength of Recommendation: Class IIa
   Strength of Evidence: Category B

Results Interpretation:
Increased adenosine deaminase level

According to some experts, a pleural fluid deaminase (ADA) level greater than 70 units/L strongly suggests the diagnosis of pleural tuberculosis (TB), while a level less than 40 units/L virtually rules out the diagnosis. The patient's immune status and the prevalence of disease also need to be considered, however.

ADA levels may be lower in immunosuppressed patients.

If the ADA level is less than 45 units/L in immunocompetent patients with an idiopathic pleural effusion and a positive purified protein derivative (PPD) test, some experts recommend that treatment for TB should not be initiated.

If the ADA level is greater than 47 units/L in patients with a pleural exudate, some experts recommend treating for TB once empyema has been ruled out as a potential etiology. In a high prevalence setting, biopsy may not be necessary if the ADA level is greater than 47 units/L and the patient is younger than 35 years.

COLLECTION/STORAGE INFORMATION

- Collect pleural fluid specimen by thoracentesis.
- Place fluid in heparinized tube.
- May store in refrigerator for up to 2 days
- May store samples at -80°C for 6 months

Adenovirus antibody assay

TEST DEFINITION

Detection and measurement of serum antibodies to adenovirus

SYNONYMS

- Serologic test for Adenovirus

REFERENCE RANGE

- Adults and Children: Negative
  Please refer to your institution's reference ranges as lab normals may vary.

INDICATIONS

Acute respiratory disease with suspected adenovirus etiology
> **Strength of Recommendation:** Class IIa
> **Strength of Evidence:** Category B

Results Interpretation:
Serology positive

A 4-fold or greater change between the titer levels of acute phase and convalescent phase is considered diagnostic for adenovirus respiratory infections.

Positive serology findings may indicate prior adenovirus infection. For patients who have military service experience, positive serology may also reflect vaccination against adenovirus.

Adenovirus types 4 and 7 may cause an acute respiratory disease (ARD) syndrome.

Prevalence of positive serology results for adenovirus types 4 and 7 increases with patient age.

Serology assays for adenovirus may be genus-specific or type-specific (there are at least 49 known serotypes of adenovirus).

Negative laboratory findings

Negative serology findings may indicate lack of immunity against adenovirus.

Timing of Monitoring

Serologic testing should be performed at the onset of acute illness and during the convalescent phase (eg, 2 to 4 weeks later).

COLLECTION/STORAGE INFORMATION

- Specimen Collection and Handling:
  - Collect blood for serum testing.
  - Label the specimen as 'acute phase' or 'convalescent phase.'
  - Freeze specimens that are not tested immediately.

LOINC CODES

- Code: 31282-7 (*Short Name* - CAdV1 Ab Ser Ql)
- Code: 7805-5 (*Short Name* - HAdV Ab Ser-aCnc)
- Code: 24249-5 (*Short Name* - HAdV Ab sp1 Titr Ser)
- Code: 13915-4 (*Short Name* - HAdV IgM Titr Ser)
- Code: 13914-7 (*Short Name* - HAdV IgG Ser-aCnc)
- Code: 24175-2 (*Short Name* - HAdV Ab sp1 Titr Ser CF)
- Code: 5042-7 (*Short Name* - HAdV IgM Ser-aCnc)
- Code: 31217-3 (*Short Name* - HAdV Ab Fld-aCnc)
- Code: 5041-9 (*Short Name* - HAdV Ab Titr Ser CF)
- Code: 23685-1 (*Short Name* - CAdV1 Ab Ser Ql Nt)
- Code: 29314-2 (*Short Name* - HAdV Ab Titr Fld CF)
- Code: 13913-9 (*Short Name* - HAdV Ab Titr Ser IF)
- Code: 23950-9 (*Short Name* - HAdV Ab Titr CSF CF)
- Code: 22080-6 (*Short Name* - HAdV Ab Titr Ser)

Adrenal antibody test

TEST DEFINITION

Detection of antiadrenal autoantibodies in serum for the evaluation and monitoring of patients with autoimmune adrenocortical insufficiency

SYNONYMS

- Adrenal autoantibodies
- Adrenal autoantibody level
- Antibody to adrenal antigen measurement

REFERENCE RANGE

- Adults: Negative at 1:10 dilution
  Please refer to your institution's reference ranges as lab normals may vary.

INDICATIONS

Autoimmune adrenocortical insufficiency
    Strength of Recommendation: Class IIa
    Strength of Evidence: Category B
Results Interpretation:
Adrenal antibodies present
The presence of circulating adrenal cell autoantibody (ACA) at low titers is not diagnostic of autoimmune Addison's disease (AAD), and does not always signify progression to clinical AAD. The development of persistently high ACA titers of greater than 1:16 in patients with no known adrenocortical failure signifies an increased risk for the development of adrenal failure (6% to 19% per year) and suggests the need to monitor adrenal cortex function. The simultaneous detection of ACA and 21-hydroxylase autoantibodies (21OHAb) can be used routinely to differentiate autoimmune from non-autoimmune primary adrenal insufficiency and both ACA and 21-OHAb titers are significantly associated with the progression of autoimmune adrenal disease.

COLLECTION/STORAGE INFORMATION

- Store serum at $-20°C$

LOINC CODES

- Code: 5043-5 (*Short Name* - Adrenal Ab Titr Ser IF)
- Code: 14232-3 (*Short Name* - Adrenal Ab Ser Ql)

Adrenocorticotropic hormone measurement

TEST DEFINITION

Measurement of ACTH (adrenocorticotropic hormone) level in serum or plasma to evaluate disorders of the hypothalamic-pituitary-adrenal (HPA) axis.

SYNONYMS

* ACTH measurement
* Adrenocorticotrophic hormone level
* Corticotropin measurement

REFERENCE RANGE

* Adults: 6-76 pg/mL
  Please refer to your institution's reference ranges as lab normals may vary.

INDICATIONS

Suspected adrenocorticotropin (ACTH)-independent Cushing's syndrome secondary to adrenal tumor
   Results Interpretation:
   Hypercortisolism due to adrenal neoplasm
      If the plasma cortisol level is greater than 15 mcg/dL (greater than 415 nmol/L) and the adrenocorticotropin (ACTH) level is less than 5 pg/mL, the patient has ACTH-independent (ie, primary adrenal) Cushing's syndrome.
      If the ACTH level is greater than 15 pg/mL (greater than 3.3 pmol/L) the cortisol secretion is ACTH dependent.
      Intermediate results, while usually reflective of ACTH dependent disease, require further evaluation.
   Timing of Monitoring
      The best time to assay adrenocorticotropin (ACTH) and cortisol concentrations in the workup of hypercortisolism is between midnight and 2 AM when levels are at their physiologic nadir.

Suspected adrenocorticotropin hormone (ACTH) dependent Cushing's syndrome, including Cushing's disease and ectopic ACTH secretion (EAS)
      Strength of Recommendation: Class IIa
      Strength of Evidence: Category B
   Results Interpretation:
   ACTH hypersecretion
      The evaluation of adrenocorticotropin (ACTH) levels following corticotropin releasing hormone (CRH) stimulation can aid in the differential diagnosis of hypercortisolism.
      Following corticotropin releasing hormone (CRH) stimulation testing, an increase in adrenocorticotropin (ACTH) levels of greater than 50% from baseline has an 86.5% probability of correctly differentiating between Cushing's disease and ectopic ACTH syndrome.
   Timing of Monitoring
      The optimal time to assay adrenocorticotropin (ACTH) and cortisol levels in the workup of hypercortisolism is between midnight and 2 AM when levels are at their physiologic nadir.

Suspected Cushing's disease due to Nelson syndrome
   Results Interpretation:
   ACTH hypersecretion
      In conjunction with patient history and physical examination, the finding of high adrenocorticotropin (ACTH) levels accompanied by minimal or absent endogenous cortisol will confirm the diagnosis of Nelson syndrome.
   Timing of Monitoring
      The best time to assay adrenocorticotropin (ACTH) and cortisol concentrations in the workup of hypercortisolism is between midnight and 2 AM when levels are at their physiologic nadir.

CLINICAL NOTES

* In patients with suspected adrenal insufficiency, adrenocorticotropin (ACTH) levels should be obtained between 8 AM and 10 AM when levels are at their physiologic peak.
* In patients with suspected Cushing's syndrome, levels should be drawn between 9 PM and midnight when they are at their physiologic nadir.

    • Because adrenocorticotropin hormone (ACTH) is subject to rapid proteolytic degradation in blood, it must be stored at -20°C if not analyzed immediately.
    • Avoid contact with glass because ACTH adsorbs to glass.

Aerobic microbial culture

TEST DEFINITION
Detection and identification of aerobic microorganisms using culture for suspected infection based on the appropriate specimen (eg, body fluids, wounds, soft tissue abscess).

REFERENCE RANGE
• Adults and Children: Negative or No Growth
Please refer to your institution's reference ranges as lab normals may vary.

INDICATIONS
Suspected bacterial infection.
Strength of Recommendation: Class IIa
Strength of Evidence: Category B
Results Interpretation:
Positive microbiology findings
The presence of aerobic organisms (*Streptococcus, Staphylococcus, Eikenella corrodens, Haemophilus, Corynebacterium, Gemella, Enterobacter cloacae, Neisseria*, and *Enterococcus*) in carefully obtained cultures can be indicative of bacterial infection.

In wound cultures, overgrowth with many species may limit the clinical usefulness of the culture. In vitro and in vivo antibiotic sensitivities are often poorly correlated. Multiple species, as well as strains of a single organism, in the same wound may complicate identification and subsequent sensitivity testing. For example, encapsulated and nonencapsulated vibrios with differing antibiotic sensitivity have been cultured from a single wound.

Bacterial cultures from various anatomical sites (eg, wound infections, soft tissue abscess) may be positive for both aerobic and anaerobic isolates.

Streptococcus spp., Staphylococcus spp., and *Corynebacteria* are commonly identified isolates, along with *Enterobacteriaceae* and *Haemophilus Influenzae*. Likely bacterial isolates vary according to anatomical site from which the specimen was taken

CLINICAL NOTES
If possible, a culture specimen should be collected prior to antibiotic therapy.

COLLECTION/STORAGE INFORMATION
• Specimen Collection and Handling:
    • Collect as much body fluid as possible in sterile tube or syringe prior to antibiotic therapy.
    • Avoid contamination of specimen with normal flora from the skin, rectum, vaginal tract or other body systems.
    • Transport specimen to lab immediately.
    • Samples are usually incubated at 35°C; and initially examined after 18 to 24 hours.

LOINC CODES
• Code: 17908-5 (*Short Name* - Tiss Aerobe Cult org #6)
• Code: 14478-2 (*Short Name* - Pen Aerobe Cult)
• Code: 17891-3 (*Short Name* - Nose Aerobe Cult org #5)
• Code: 627-0 (*Short Name* - Tiss Aerobe Cult)
• Code: 17887-1 (*Short Name* - Gen Aerobe Cult org #6)
• Code: 17933-3 (*Short Name* - Bld Aerobe Cult org #6)
• Code: 17875-6 (*Short Name* - Bone Aerobe Cult org #4)
• Code: 632-0 (*Short Name* - Wnd Aerobe Cult)
• Code: 595-9 (*Short Name* - Abs Aerobe Cult)
• Code: 617-1 (*Short Name* - Plc Aerobe Cult)

- Code: 629-6 (*Short Name* - Ulc Aerobe Cult)
- Code: 14475-8 (*Short Name* - Cvx Aerobe Cult)
- Code: 17877-2 (*Short Name* - Bone Aerobe Cult org #6)
- Code: 17950-7 (*Short Name* - Fld Aerobe Cult)
- Code: 17919-2 (*Short Name* - Shlw Wnd Aerobe Cult org #5)
- Code: 17917-6 (*Short Name* - Shlw Wnd Aerobe Cult org #3)
- Code: 17885-5 (*Short Name* - Gen Aerobe Cult org #4)
- Code: 17886-3 (*Short Name* - Gen Aerobe Cult org #5)
- Code: 17878-0 (*Short Name* - Bro Aerobe Cult org #2)
- Code: 17918-4 (*Short Name* - Shlw Wnd Aerobe Cult org #4)
- Code: 17931-7 (*Short Name* - Bld Aerobe Cult org #4)
- Code: 17889-7 (*Short Name* - Nose Aerobe Cult org #3)
- Code: 17953-1 (*Short Name* - Fld Aerobe Cult org #4)
- Code: 610-6 (*Short Name* - Fld Aerobe Cult)
- Code: 17880-6 (*Short Name* - Bro Aerobe Cult org #4)
- Code: 17884-8 (*Short Name* - Gen Aerobe Cult org #3)
- Code: 17955-6 (*Short Name* - Fld Aerobe Cult org #6)
- Code: 602-3 (*Short Name* - Bone Aerobe Cult)
- Code: 17890-5 (*Short Name* - Nose Aerobe Cult org #4)
- Code: 17951-5 (*Short Name* - Fld Aerobe BFld Cult org #2)
- Code: 17932-5 (*Short Name* - Bld Aerobe Cult org #5)
- Code: 17907-7 (*Short Name* - Tiss Aerobe Cult org #5)
- Code: 14477-4 (*Short Name* - Urth Aerobe Cult)
- Code: 17883-0 (*Short Name* - Gen Aerobe Cult org #2)
- Code: 605-6 (*Short Name* - Cnl Aerobe Cult)
- Code: 17954-9 (*Short Name* - Fld Aerobe Cult org #5)
- Code: 11261-5 (*Short Name* - GenV Aerobe Cult)
- Code: 17915-0 (*Short Name* - Shlw Wnd Aerobe Cult)
- Code: 620-5 (*Short Name* - Skn Aerobe Cult)
- Code: 17952-3 (*Short Name* - Fld Aerobe Cult org #3)
- Code: 17928-3 (*Short Name* - Bld Aerobe Cult)
- Code: 17916-8 (*Short Name* - Shlw Wnd Aerobe Cult org #2)
- Code: 17881-4 (*Short Name* - Bro Aerobe Cult org #5)
- Code: 17876-4 (*Short Name* - Bone Aerobe Cult org #5)
- Code: 607-2 (*Short Name* - Drn Aerobe Cult)
- Code: 17882-2 (*Short Name* - Bro Aerobe Cult org #6)
- Code: 17874-9 (*Short Name* - Bone Aerobe Cult org #3)
- Code: 17930-9 (*Short Name* - Bld Aerobe Cult org #3)
- Code: 17279-1 (*Short Name* - Plr Aerobe Cult)
- Code: 597-5 (*Short Name* - Asp Aerobe Cult)
- Code: 17873-1 (*Short Name* - Bone Aerobe Cult org #2)
- Code: 17909-3 (*Short Name* - Deep Wnd Aerobe Cult)
- Code: 10352-3 (*Short Name* - Gen Aerobe Cult)
- Code: 17892-1 (*Short Name* - Nose Aerobe Cult org #6)
- Code: 604-9 (*Short Name* - Bro Aerobe Cult)
- Code: 599-1 (*Short Name* - BBL Aerobe Cult)
- Code: 609-8 (*Short Name* - Eye Aerobe Cult)
- Code: 20694-6 (*Short Name* - Bacteria Embryo Aerobe Cult)
- Code: 634-6 (*Short Name* - XXX Aerobe Cult)
- Code: 17914-3 (*Short Name* - Deep Wnd Aerobe Cult org #6)
- Code: 17888-9 (*Short Name* - Nose Aerobe Cult org #2)
- Code: 17879-8 (*Short Name* - Bro Aerobe Cult org #3)
- Code: 10353-1 (*Short Name* - Nose Aerobe Cult)
- Code: 608-0 (*Short Name* - Ear Aerobe Cult)
- Code: 17929-1 (*Short Name* - Bld Aerobe Cult org #2)
- Code: 17920-0 (*Short Name* - Shlw Wnd Aerobe Cult org #6)

Alanine aminotransferase measurement

TEST DEFINITION
The measurement of alanine aminotransferase (ALT/SGOT) levels in serum for the evaluation and management of hepatic disease or injury

SYNONYMS
- ALT measurement
- Glutamic pyruvate transaminase measurement
- GPT measurement
- SGPT measurement

REFERENCE RANGE
- Adults: 0-35 units/L (0-0.58 microkat/L)
  Please refer to your institution's reference ranges as lab normals may vary.

INDICATIONS
Ehrlichiosis
    Results Interpretation:
    ALT/SGPT increased
    Mild to moderate elevations in serum alanine aminotransferase levels are a typical finding during the first week of illness, noted in 75% to 80% of patients.

Suspected cholecystitis
    Results Interpretation:
    ALT/SGPT increased
    ALT levels are often mildly elevated in acute cholecystitis, but marked elevation suggests alternative diagnoses such as hepatitis. The values typically return to normal within one week after symptoms resolve, unless suppuration ensues.
    Even without common bile duct obstruction or cholangitis, the ALT values are elevated in 40% to 75% of cases, usually to less than 5 times normal.

Suspected drug-induced liver disease
    Strength of Recommendation: Class I
    Strength of Evidence: Category C
    Results Interpretation:
    Raised hematology findings
    Hepatocellular or cytolytic injury is characterized by marked elevations in ALT levels. ALT values that are normal at baseline and rise 2- to 3-fold above normal should lead to enhanced vigilance with more frequent monitoring. ALT levels greater than 3 times the upper limit of the normal range may indicate of liver injury; however, elevated levels should be correlated with clinical symptoms. ALT values that rise 4 to 5 times above normal should prompt immediate discontinuation of the drug to avoid causing more severe injury.
    ALT values are more specific for liver damage than AST values and help to exclude the possible effect of alcohol injury on the liver.

Suspected liver disease
    Strength of Recommendation: Class IIa
    Strength of Evidence: Category B
    Results Interpretation:
    ALT/SGPT increased
    The traditional normal range cut-off value (40 International Units/L) is being reevaluated because it may lead to an underestimation of the prevalence of liver disease. One study suggests cut-off values of 19 units/L for women and 30 units/L for men. Another study identified the most beneficial cut-off value for predicting liver disease in men is 30 International Units/L; the cut-off value in women could not be established..

Suspected metabolic syndrome
    Strength of Recommendation: Class IIa
    Strength of Evidence: Category B

Results Interpretation:
ALT/SGPT increased

Increased alanine aminotransferase (ALT) levels is defined as levels greater than 43 International Units/L.

Metabolic syndrome is significantly associated with increased serum alanine aminotransferase (ALT) levels in person with and without other causes of chronic liver disease.

Suspected or known viral hepatitis
Results Interpretation:
ALT/SGPT increased

Alanine aminotransferase (ALT) increases variably in the prodromal phase of acute hepatitis, preceding the rise in bilirubin level. Peak ALT levels vary from 400 to 4000 IU or more in acute hepatitis; these levels are usually reached when the patient is clinically icteric and diminish during the recovery phase. Acute ALT levels do not correlate well with the degree of liver cell damage. Serologic testing for hepatitis may be indicated in outpatients with unexplained elevations in serum ALT

In acute hepatitis C, serum ALT levels are more than 7 times the upper limit of normal. Persistently elevated ALT in chronic hepatitis C is an indication to consider antiviral treatment.

Persistent or intermittent ALT elevations in chronic active hepatitis B suggest the need for further evaluation with a liver biopsy and consideration for treatment. ALT levels should be monitored periodically in hepatitis B carrier states, as liver disease may become active even years later.

Suspected viral hepatitis C infection

Strength of Recommendation: Class I
Strength of Evidence: Category B
Results Interpretation:
ALT/SGPT increased

Elevated alanine aminotransferase (ALT) levels are associated with chronic hepatitis C virus (HCV) infection in most patients. However, abnormal ALT levels can fluctuate significantly, and approximately one-third of patients with HCV have persistently normal ALT levels.

Frequency of Monitoring

Because a single alanine aminotransferase (ALT) level may not accurately reflect disease severity, serial ALT measurements are recommended as a general method for monitoring patients with hepatitis C virus (HCV).

COMMON PANELS

- Comprehensive metabolic panel
- Hepatic function panel

ABNORMAL RESULTS

- Results increased in:
  - Hispanics
  - Obesity
  - Hemolyzed sample
  - Cigarette smoking
  - Serum cholesterol concentration
  - Strenuous exercise in men

COLLECTION/STORAGE INFORMATION

- Collect 7 mL blood in red top tube
- Analyze specimen within 12 to 24 hours after collection

LOINC CODES

- Code: 16324-6 (*Short Name* - ALT RBC-cCnc)
- Code: 1741-8 (*Short Name* - ALT Amn-cCnc)
- Code: 25302-1 (*Short Name* - ALT Fld-cCnc)

Alanine measurement

TEST DEFINITION

Measurement of alanine in plasma for detection of acquired and hereditary amino acid disorders.

SYNONYMS
- Alanine level

REFERENCE RANGE
- Premature neonate, 1 day: 3.34 ± 0.45mg/dL (375 ± 50 micromol/L)
- Neonate, 1 day: 2.1-3.65 mg/dL (236-410 micromol/L)
- Infants 1 to 3 months: 2.45 ± 0.63 mg/dL (275 ± 71 micromol/L)
- Infants 2 to 6 months: 1.58-3.68 mg/dL (177-413 micromol/L)
- Infants 9 to 24 months: 0.88-2.79 mg/dL (99-313 micromol/L)
- Children 3 to 10 years: 1.22-2.72 mg/dL (137-305 micromol/L)
- Children 6 to 18 years: 1.72-4.86 mg/dL (193-545 micromol/L)
- Adults: 1.87-5.89 mg/dL (210-661 micromol/L)
  Please refer to your institution's reference ranges as lab normals may vary.

INDICATIONS
Suspected inborn error of metabolism
>**Strength of Recommendation:** Class IIa
>**Strength of Evidence:** Category C
>**Results Interpretation:**
>**Abnormal laboratory findings**
>Inherited amino acid disorders are directly related to the absence of an enzyme involved in the metabolism of one or more amino acids; therefore, an elevated plasma level of a particular amino acid is highly suggestive of an inherited metabolic defect. In the majority of cases amino acid and organic acid analysis together permit diagnostic confirmation in infants. Immediate treatment should be initiated when an inborn error of metabolism is suspected even if a definitive diagnosis has not yet been determined.
>Carbamoyl phosphate synthetase deficiency is associated with increased alanine, glutamine, glycine and lysine, and low or undetectable arginine and citrulline.

COLLECTION/STORAGE INFORMATION
- Specimen Collection and Handling:
  - Immediately place sample in ice water.
  - Isolate plasma sample and freeze it within 1 hour; sample stable for 1 week at -20°C.
  - Sample should be deproteinized and stored at -70°C for protracted periods of usage.

LOINC CODES
- Code: 27013-2 (*Short Name* - Alanine Amn-sCnc)
- Code: 22657-1 (*Short Name* - Alanine CSF-sCnc)
- Code: 22724-9 (*Short Name* - Alanine XXX-sCnc)
- Code: 12280-4 (*Short Name* - Alanine Amn-mCnc)
- Code: 1735-0 (*Short Name* - Alanine CSF-mCnc)
- Code: 32221-4 (*Short Name* - Alanine Vitf-sCnc)

Albumin measurement, serum

TEST DEFINITION
Measurement of albumin in serum for the evaluation of nutritional status or disease severity

SYNONYMS
- SA - Serum albumin
- Serum albumin
- Serum albumin level

REFERENCE RANGE
- Adults: 3.5-5.5 g/dL (35-55 g/L)
  Please refer to your institution's reference ranges as lab normals may vary.

INDICATIONS

Patients hospitalized with community-acquired pneumonia
Results Interpretation:
Decreased albumin

Chronic malnutrition is a major cause of decreased serum albumin in elderly patients with community-acquired pneumonia.

A decreased albumin level on admission is associated with poor prognosis, increased mortality, and colonization of the respiratory tract with the development of secondary infection. In survivors, a decreased albumin level is associated with a longer hospital stay, delayed recovery, and delayed resolution on chest films.

Hypocalcemia
Results Interpretation:
Decreased albumin

It has been observed that hypoalbuminemia is the most common cause of laboratory hypocalcemia. As a general rule, for every one-gram decrease in albumin below 4 g/dL, total serum calcium level falls 0.8 mg/dL. The ionized fraction of calcium remains normal, however, so symptoms of hypocalcemia do not develop.

In critically ill patients, the presence of ionized hypocalcemia and/or hypoalbuminemia on admission is associated with increased hospital mortality..

Pancreatitis
Results Interpretation:
Decreased albumin

Decreased serum albumin is more often an important factor in chronic pancreatitis. Progressive hypoalbuminemia, indicative of deteriorating nutritional status, may occur in patients with pancreatitis despite use of parenteral and enteral nutrition. An albumin level less than 3 g/dL has been associated with a poor prognosis.

Hypoalbuminemia is common in severe pancreatitis and has an associated mortality of 21%.

Suspected and known Kawasaki disease
Results Interpretation:
Decreased level (laboratory finding)

A serum albumin level of 3 mg/dL or less, in conjunction with other laboratory data, supports the diagnosis of Kawasaki disease.

Suspected hypercalcemia
Results Interpretation:
Abnormal laboratory findings

An alteration in the serum albumin level of 1 g/dL will cause a change in total calcium measurement of 0.8 mg/dL in the same direction. Ionized calcium concentration does not change.

Because a major portion of serum calcium is bound to albumin, changes from normal in the serum albumin level will result in corresponding predictable changes in the serum calcium level.

Suspected hypoalbuminemia
Strength of Recommendation: Class IIa
Strength of Evidence: Category C
Results Interpretation:
Decreased albumin

A decreased serum albumin level of less than 3.5 g/dL (35 g/L) indicates significant hypoalbuminemia.

A decrease in serum albumin may be seen in patients with chronic inflammatory diseases, hantavirus pulmonary syndrome, HIV infection (common), leishmaniasis (common), malaria (common), rheumatic fever (80% of patients), and inflammatory liver disease.

Hypoalbuminemia is a predictor of mortality and morbidity in end-stage renal failure patients undergoing dialysis therapy and is associated with subsequent development of vascular disease (eg, acute myocardial infarction, peripheral vascular disease).

Low serum albumin concentrations are a marker of an underlying disease process.

Suspected nutritional disorder
Strength of Recommendation: Class IIb
Strength of Evidence: Category C

Results Interpretation:
Decreased albumin

Serum albumin levels of 2.9 to 3.4 g/dL indicate mild malnutrition, levels of 2.3 to 2.8 g/dL indicate severe malnutrition, and levels below 2.2 g/dL indicate very severe malnutrition.

Decreased serum albumin levels seen in the presence of systemic inflammation and vascular disease and may be secondary to the underlying inflammatory state rather than to malnutrition.

Decreased serum albumin in adults is not the preferred biochemical marker of isolated protein-energy malnutrition.

Serum albumin normal

In the early stages of malnutrition, serum albumin levels can remain normal because of long half life of albumin (20 days).

A reduction (10%) in serum albumin level is not seen until the patient sustains a protein-deficient diet for two weeks.

During energy and protein deprivation, serum albumin levels may remain unchanged due to reduced synthesis and increased catabolism.

COMMON PANELS

- Bone and joint panel
- Comprehensive metabolic panel
- Enteral/Parenteral nutritional management panel
- Hepatic function panel
- Parathyroid panel
- Renal panel
- Transplant panel

ABNORMAL RESULTS

- Results increased in:
  - Dehydration
  - Hemoconcentration
- Results decreased in:
  - Increased loss via body surfaces (eg, burns, trauma)
  - Hypervolemia
  - Pregnancy

COLLECTION/STORAGE INFORMATION

- Collect specimen in a red top tube.

LOINC CODES

- Code: 21058-3 (*Short Name* - Alb 2H p PD Ser-mCnc)
- Code: 1751-7 (*Short Name* - Alb SerPl-mCnc)
- Code: 2862-1 (*Short Name* - Alb SerPl Elph-mCnc)

Aldosterone measurement, urine

TEST DEFINITION

Measurement of urinary aldosterone excretion rate in relation to sodium balance for the evaluation of aldosterone production

REFERENCE RANGE

- Adults (Random, low-sodium diet): 2.3-21 mcg/24 hours (6.38-58.25 nmol/24 hours)
  Please refer to your institution's reference ranges as lab normals may vary.

INDICATIONS

Suspected primary aldosteronism in hypertensive patients
      Strength of Recommendation: Class IIa
      Strength of Evidence: Category B

Results Interpretation:
Decreased level (laboratory finding)
   With the exception of glucocorticoid-remedial aldosteronism, urinary aldosterone excretion of less than 14 mcg/24 hours after sodium loading rules out primary aldosteronism.
Increased aldosterone level
   As part of the definitive diagnosis of aldosteronism, hypertensive patients with high aldosterone excretion following a 2 to 3 day high NaCl diet (2 to 3 g at each meal) should have a plasma renin level drawn.

COLLECTION/STORAGE INFORMATION
- Prior to sample collection, advise patient to avoid antihypertensive medications that can affect renin and aldosterone measurements
- Refrigerate sample during collection; freeze stored sample
- Add 50% acetic acid to final sample to achieve a pH between 2 and 4

LOINC CODES
- Code: 13482-5 (*Short Name* - Aldost/creat Ur-mRto)
- Code: 15010-2 (*Short Name* - Aldost Ur-sCnc)
- Code: 1764-0 (*Short Name* - Aldost Ur-mCnc)
- Code: 25845-9 (*Short Name* - Aldost 24H Ur-sCnc)
- Code: 31992-1 (*Short Name* - Aldost 24H Ur-mCnc)
- Code: 14587-0 (*Short Name* - Aldost 24H Ur-sRate)
- Code: 1765-7 (*Short Name* - Aldost 24H Ur-mRate)

Allergen specific IgE antibody measurement, Serum

TEST DEFINITION
   Measurement of allergen specific IgE antibody in serum to evaluate etiology of suspected atopy

REFERENCE RANGE
   The normal range, generally reported in kilo international units per liter (kIU/L or kU_A/L), is determined by the specific test technology and antigen being studied.
- Test Specific Normal Ranges:
- CAP® System: <0.35 kU_A/L
- AlaSTAT®: <0.35 kU_A/L
- CARLA®: <0.5 kU_A/L
- ENEA®: <0.36 kU_A/L
   Please refer to your institution's reference ranges as lab normals may vary.

INDICATIONS
Suspected allergy
   Strength of Recommendation: Class IIb
   Strength of Evidence: Category C
   Results Interpretation:
   Immunoglobulin level - finding
      A finding of allergen specific IgE antibodies may identify the cause of an allergic reaction.
      Allergen specific IgE testing is a safe and specific alternative when the more sensitive skin testing is contraindicated or indeterminate.
      Though not as sensitive as traditional allergen skin testing, current generation allergen specific IgE assays have improved utility. Quantified results allow the determination of highly specific cut points that have high predictive value in determining patients at risk for allergic response to clinical challenge. Particularly in the area of food specific allergens, IgE levels correlate well with clinical atopic sensitivity.
      Allergen specific IgE assays are preferred for patients with dermographism dermatitis, those who cannot discontinue antihistamines, or those who are afraid of skin testing. The assays are also preferred for infants with few suspected allergens, or patients with severe reactions.

CLINICAL NOTES

Because of significant variability between manufacturer's test technologies, results obtained by different methodologies and using proprietary antigen and anti-IgE antibody preparations, cannot be directly compared. Therefore it is necessary that results report the technology used, along with the quantitative interpretation.

COLLECTION/STORAGE INFORMATION

- Serum is stable for 1 week at 2°C to 8°C and up to 6 months at -20°C.

LOINC CODES

- Code: 16019-2 (*Short Name* - Silk IgE RAST QI)
- Code: 15594-5 (*Short Name* - White burrobrush IgE RAST QI)
- Code: 15674-5 (*Short Name* - Daisy IgE RAST QI)
- Code: 15844-4 (*Short Name* - Mexican tea IgE RAST QI)
- Code: 15896-4 (*Short Name* - Orris root IgE RAST QI)
- Code: 21104-5 (*Short Name* - Soybean dust IgE RAST QI)
- Code: 25525-7 (*Short Name* - S lacrymans IgE RAST QI)
- Code: 15778-4 (*Short Name* - Honeysuckle IgE RAST QI)
- Code: 21272-0 (*Short Name* - Fireweed IgE RAST QI)
- Code: 15825-3 (*Short Name* - Lycopodium IgE RAST QI)
- Code: 21508-7 (*Short Name* - Calif Sagbrsh IgE RAST QI)
- Code: 25744-4 (*Short Name* - Quinoa IgE RAST QI)
- Code: 15787-5 (*Short Name* - Horseradish IgE RAST QI)
- Code: 15817-0 (*Short Name* - Easter lily IgE RAST QI)
- Code: 15713-1 (*Short Name* - Fiscus IgE RAST QI)
- Code: 26026-5 (*Short Name* - HHPA IgE RAST QI)
- Code: 16094-5 (*Short Name* - Wingscale IgE RAST QI)
- Code: 16021-8 (*Short Name* - Silver IgE RAST QI)

Alpha-1-Fetoprotein measurement, amniotic fluid

TEST DEFINITION

Measurement of alpha-fetoprotein in amniotic fluid for detection of open neural tube defects

SYNONYMS

- Alpha-1-Foetoprotein measurement, amniotic fluid

REFERENCE RANGE

- Pregnancy:
- 15 weeks' gestation: 16.3 mcg/mL (16.3 mg/L)
- 16 weeks' gestation: 14.5 mcg/mL (14.5 mg/L)
- 17 weeks' gestation: 13.4 mcg/mL (13.4 mg/L)
- 18 weeks' gestation: 12 mcg/mL (12 mg/L)
- 19 weeks' gestation: 10.7 mcg/mL (10.7 mg/L)
- 20 weeks' gestation: 8.1 mcg/mL (8.1 mg/L)
- Twin pregnancy: Values are 2 times higher
- Blacks: Values are 15% higher
- Type 2 diabetes mellitus: Values are 20% lower
  Please refer to your institution's reference ranges as lab normals may vary.

INDICATIONS

Prenatal diagnosis of suspected neural tube defect
        Strength of Recommendation: Class IIb
        Strength of Evidence: Category C

Results Interpretation:
Amniotic fluid AFP - finding
Amniotic fluid alpha fetoprotein (AFP) values of 2 multiples of the median (MoM) or higher are seen in approximately 96% of pregnancies affected by open tube neural defects and 1% of unaffected pregnancies.

Elevated alpha-fetoprotein levels in amniotic fluid can also occur in ventral wall defects, congenital disorders, fetal bleeding, fetal demise, and nephrotic syndrome.

Level 2 ultrasound, a high-resolution scan performed by an experienced operator, has become the preferred method for identifying congenital anomalies, except in cases where chromosomal analysis is indicated.

Timing of Monitoring
The optimal time frame for testing alpha-fetoprotein in amniotic fluid is during the first part of the second trimester of pregnancy, between 14 and 16 weeks' gestation.

CLINICAL NOTES
The alpha fetoprotein assay is not done in isolation to identify neural tube defects. The result is interpreted in conjunction with confirmatory ultrasound.

COLLECTION/STORAGE INFORMATION
- Specimen Collection and Handling:
  - Collect a minimum of 3 to 4 mL of aminiotic fluid in a sterile syringe.
  - If the test is delayed, refrigerate sterile specimen up to a few hours. If longer delays occur, specimen should be frozen.
  - Avoid exposure to heat and light.

LOINC CODES
- Code: 15019-3 (*Short Name* - AFP Amn-sCnc)
- Code: 19171-8 (*Short Name* - AFP Amn-aCnc)
- Code: 1832-5 (*Short Name* - AFP Amn-mCnc)
- Code: 29253-2 (*Short Name* - AFP MoM adj Amn Calc)

Alpha-1-antitrypsin measurement

TEST DEFINITION
Measurement of alpha-$_1$-antitrypsin in serum for diagnosis and management of alpha-$_1$-antitrypsin deficiency

REFERENCE RANGE
- Adults 18 to 60 years of age (M-phenotype): 78-200 mg/dL (0.78-2.00 g/L)
- Adults older than 60 years of age: 115-200 mg/dL (1.15-2.00 g/L)
- Neonate: 145-270 mg/dL (1.45-2.70 g/L)
  Please refer to your institution's reference ranges as lab normals may vary.

INDICATIONS
Suspected alpha-1-antitrypsin deficiency
  Strength of Recommendation: Class I
  Strength of Evidence: Category B
  Results Interpretation:
  Lowered biochemistry findings
  Decreased alpha-$_1$-antitrypsin serum concentrations appear to be predictive of homozygous PiZZ phenotype for alpha-$_1$-antitrypsin deficiency. Homozygous PiZZ phenotype produces the most severe manifestations of the disease compared with other phenotypes.

The American Thoracic Society recommends that testing for alpha-$_1$-antitrypsin deficiency be conducted as one of the initial diagnostic steps for patients who present with chronic obstructive pulmonary dysfunction of unknown etiology or who present with unexplained hepatic disease.

ABNORMAL RESULTS
- Results increased in:
  - Acute inflammation
  - Pregnancy (especially 3rd trimester)

• Presence of rheumatoid factor

CLINICAL NOTES

Normal mean ranges for alpha$_1$ -antitrypsin may vary according to the purified protein preparation or trypsin preparation upon which the calibration standard is based.

COLLECTION/STORAGE INFORMATION

• Specimen Collection and Handling:
  • Serum, plasma:
    • Immediately separate serum prior to storage
    • Store in lavender-top (EDTA) tube
    • May store more than 7 days at $-4°C$, and for 3 months at $-70°C$
  • Cord blood:
    • Analyze while fresh or store at $-4°C$ for no more than 72 hours
    • May store at $-20°C$ for 6 months or at $-70°C$ indefinitely

LOINC CODES

• Code: 29146-8 (*Short Name* - A-1-AT Fld-mCnc)

Alpha-1-antitrypsin phenotyping

TEST DEFINITION

Alpha-1-antitrypsin (AAT) phenotyping of blood for the evaluation of genetic AAT deficiency and related diseases

SYNONYMS

• Alpha-1-Protease inhibitor

REFERENCE RANGE

• Phenotype MM
  Please refer to your institution's reference ranges as lab normals may vary.

INDICATIONS

Suspected alpha-1-antitrypsin deficiency
  Results Interpretation:
  Abnormal laboratory findings
    Individuals with serum alpha-1-antitrypsin (AAT) levels below 80 mg/dL should be phenotyped to screen for possible AAT deficiency.
    AAT has more than 90 phenotypes. The homozygous ZZ phenotype is associated with the most severe form of AAT deficiency, in which levels are only 10% to 15% of normal.
    SZ heterozygotes produce 40% of normal AAT levels and are at risk for symptomatic disease. SS homozygotes produce 60% of normal levels, and may be moderately symptomatic in some cases. MZ and MS heterozygotes have lower but adequate AAT levels. Though usually asymptomatic, they are carriers of the condition.
    AAT deficiency is associated with liver disease and early-onset COPD.

COLLECTION/STORAGE INFORMATION

• Dried blood samples can be stored up to one month at $-20°C$, up to one week at 4°C and only three days at room temperature.
• Collect plasma samples in a lavender top (EDTA) tube, or serum in a red top or marbled tube. Separate serum immediately. Specimen is stable 7 days at 4°C, and 3 months at -70°C.

LOINC CODES

• Code: 6770-2 (*Short Name* - A1AT Phenotyp SerPl IFE)

Alpha-1-fetoprotein measurement, serum

Test Definition
Measurement of alpha-fetoprotein (AFP) in serum for prenatal risk assessment or a tumor marker

Synonyms
- Serum alpha-fetoprotein

Reference Range
- Adults: <15 ng/mL (15 mcg/L)
- Fetal blood (first trimester): Peak 200-400 mg/dL (2-4 g/L)
- Pregnancy (2nd trimester):
- 14 weeks' gestation: Median 25.6 ng/mL (25.6 mcg/L)
- 15 weeks' gestation: Median 29.9 ng/mL (29.9 mcg/L)
- 16 weeks' gestation: Median 34.8 ng/mL (34.8 mcg/L)
- 17 weeks' gestation: Median 40.6 ng/mL (40.6 mcg/L)
- 18 weeks' gestation: Median 47.3 ng/mL (47.3 mcg/L)
- 19 weeks' gestation: Median 55.1 ng/mL (55.1 mcg/L)
- 20 weeks' gestation: Median 64.3 ng/mL (64.3 mcg/L)
- 21 weeks' gestation: Median 74.9 ng/mL (74.9 mcg/L)
- The multiple of the median (MoM) value is adjusted for maternal weight, race, diabetes mellitus, and twin pregnancy.
  Normal values are approximately 15% higher for blacks or African Americans than for whites
  Normal values are approximately 200% higher in women with twin pregnancy.
  Please refer to your institution's reference ranges as lab normals may vary.

Indications
Suspected hepatocellular carcinoma in patients with hepatic cirrhosis or type B viral hepatitis
> **Strength of Recommendation:** Class III
> **Strength of Evidence:** Category B
> **Results Interpretation:**
> **Serum alpha-fetoprotein level elevated**
>> Various cut-off values of 20 to 400 ng/mL have been used in screening for hepatocellular carcinoma (HCC). The diagnosis of HCC is confirmed noninvasively by the combination of an alpha fetoprotein higher than 400 ng/mL and an imaging technique that reveals a nodule greater than 2 cm with arterial hypervascularization.
>
>> **False Results**
>>> Cirrhosis or chronic hepatitis with reactivation may present with increased alpha fetoprotein (AFP) levels not related to hepatocellular carcinoma (HCC). Generally, the detection of HCC is not improved by an elevated AFP level if no liver nodule is demonstrable by ultrasonography.
>> **Frequency of Monitoring**
>>> The European Association for the Study of the Liver recommends surveillance every 6 months with serum alpha-fetoprotein and ultrasonography for patients with hepatic cirrhosis who are candidates for potentially curative treatment of hepatocellular carcinoma. Others suggest a 1-year screening interval.

Prenatal screening for open neural tube defects
> **Strength of Recommendation:** Class I
> **Strength of Evidence:** Category A
> **Results Interpretation:**
> **Serum alpha-fetoprotein level elevated**
>> A second-trimester maternal serum alpha fetoprotein assay is particularly useful for detecting fetal open neural tube defects. The detection rates for open neural tube defects depend on the cutoff value for the adjusted multiple of the median (MoM) serum alpha-fetoprotein concentration; the most commonly used cutoff is a MoM of 2.5 or higher. If the cutoff is 2.5 or higher, the detection rate for anencephaly is 90% and for open spina bifida is 80%; the false positive rate is 1.5%. If the cutoff MoM is 2 or higher, the detection rate for anencephaly is 95% and for open spina bifida is 85%; the false positive rate is 2.5%..
>> When the alpha-fetoprotein assay is used for prenatal screening, the laboratory results report should include absolute and median values, multiple of the median (MoM) calculations, MoM adjustments, and risk assessment.

Alpha-fetoprotein low

A low adjusted maternal serum multiple of the mean (MoM) alpha-fetoprotein level is also associated with adverse outcomes, including chromosomal defect (RR = 11.6) and fetal death (RR = 3.3).

Timing of Monitoring

Maternal blood specimens are obtained at 16 to 22 weeks gestational age.

Screening test for pregnancy complications and adverse neonatal outcomes

Strength of Recommendation: Class IIa

Strength of Evidence: Category A

Results Interpretation:

Serum alpha-fetoprotein level elevated

A high adjusted maternal serum alpha-fetoprotein (MS-AFP) multiple of the mean (MoM) value in the second trimester is associated with high-risk pregnancies and adverse neonatal outcomes; however, an elevated MS-AFP level is a nonspecific marker.

When the alpha-fetoprotein assay is for prenatal screening, the laboratory results report should include absolute and median values, multiple of the median (MoM) calculations, MoM adjustments, and risk assessment.

Although high adjusted maternal serum multiple of the median (MoM) alpha-fetoprotein (AFP) values are potentially associated with many adverse pregnancy outcomes, the relative risk (RR) for specific disorders is usually very low (eg, RR for neural tube defect is 224; RR for other major congenital defect is 4.7). Ventral abdominal wall defects are an exception; both omphalocele or gastroschisis are usually associated with elevated MS-AFP levels.

Timing of Monitoring

Maternal serum alpha-fetoprotein (AFP) assessment is typically performed at 15 to 20 weeks gestation.

Suspected testicular cancer.

Results Interpretation:

Serum alpha-fetoprotein level elevated

- Serum alpha-fetoprotein (AFP) levels are elevated in 70% of patients with embryonal carcinoma and 64% with teratoma, but are normal in patients with seminoma. When combined with human chorionic gonadotropin measurements, serum AFP measurements may enhance clinical staging and facilitate the differential diagnosis of subtypes of germ cell tumors.
- A moderately increased serum alpha-fetoprotein level in a patient with a histologic diagnosis of seminoma indicates nonseminomatous components, which require specific, nonseminomatous tumor therapy.
- In the American Joint Committee on Cancer (AJCC) serum tumor markers (S) classification system, serum alpha-fetoprotein (AFP) rankings include
  - S0: AFP level within normal limits
  - S1: AFP <1,000 ng/mL
  - S2: AFP 1,000 to 10,000 ng/mL
  - S3: AFP >10,000 ng/mL
- In germ cell tumors, the likelihood of an elevated serum alpha-fetoprotein level correlates with the clinical stage:
  - Stage I: 10% to 20%
  - Stage II: 20% to 40%
  - Stage III: 40% to 60%
- Serum alpha-fetoprotein (AFP) levels are included in the standard international prognostic classification system criteria for metastatic germ cell tumors:
  - Seminoma:
    - Good prognosis: AFP normal
    - Intermediate prognosis: AFP normal
    - Nonseminoma:
- Good prognosis: AFP <1,000 ng/mL
- Intermediate prognosis: AFP 1,000 to 10,000 ng/mL
- Poor prognosis: AFP >10,000 ng/mL

Frequency of Monitoring

After definitive therapy, serum alpha-fetoprotein (and other serum marker) measurements are indicated at every follow-up visit (eg, monthly in first year; bimonthly in second year).

Timing of Monitoring

Before diagnostic orchiectomy, evaluation includes measurements of the 3 major serum markers for testicular cancer (ie, alpha-fetoprotein [AFP], beta-human chorionic gonadotropin [beta-hCG], and lactate dehydrogenase [LDH]).

Abnormal Results

- Results increased in (during pregnancy):
  - Underestimation of gestational age, based on recall of the last menstrual period, is a common cause of false results. Whenever the adjusted maternal serum multiple of the mean (MoM) alpha-fetoprotein is 2 or higher, fetal ultrasonography (biparietal diameter) is indicated to confirm gestational age.
  - Comorbid hepatic disorder (eg, acute injury, fibrosis, chronic hepatitis)
  - Maternal blood sampled after insertion of amniocentesis needle
- Results decreased in (during pregnancy): Type 2 diabetes mellitus

Collection/Storage Information

- Specimen Collection and Handling:
  - Collect venous blood sample in a marble-top tube and avoid hemolysis
  - Keep at 2°C to 8°C if assay within 24 hours; otherwise freeze at -20°C or below
  - If the assay is for prenatal screening, include the following information with the specimen:
    - Gestational day when serum sample drawn
    - Maternal weight
    - Maternal race
    - Relevant demographic or medical information (eg, maternal diabetes mellitus, twin pregnancy)

LOINC Codes

- Code: 1834-1 (*Short Name* - AFP Ser-mCnc)
- Code: 19177-5 (*Short Name* - AFP Ser-sCnc)
- Code: 23811-3 (*Short Name* - AFP MoM adj Ser Calc)
- Code: 19176-7 (*Short Name* - AFP Ser-aCnc)
- Code: 31993-9 (*Short Name* - AFP Ser Ql)

Alpha-2 antiplasmin assay

Test Definition

Measurement of alpha-2 antiplasmin in plasma for the evaluation of suspected alpha-2 antiplasmin deficiency

Reference Range

- 80% - 130% (0.80 - 1.30)
  Please refer to your institution's reference ranges as lab normals may vary.

Indications

Suspected alpha-2 antiplasmin deficiency
    Strength of Recommendation: Class IIa
    Strength of Evidence: Category B
    Results Interpretation:
    Decreased level (laboratory finding)
        Alpha-2 antiplasmin levels less than 50% of normal are associated with an increased risk of life-threatening hemorrhagic diathesis.

Clinical Notes

Antigenic tests may have higher values than functional tests.

Collection/Storage Information

- Collect sample in a blue (buffered citrate) top tube.
- Sample is stable for 2 hours at 4°C.
- Avoid samples containing heparin.

LOINC Codes

- Code: 5965-9 (*Short Name* - Plasm Inhib PPP Chro-aCnc)
- Code: 28658-3 (*Short Name* - Plasm Inhib Act/Nor PPP Imm)
- Code: 27810-1 (*Short Name* - Plasm Inhib Act/Nor PPP Chro)

alpha-Amino-n-butyrate measurement

TEST DEFINITION
Measurement of alpha-amino-N-butyrate in plasma for detection of acquired and hereditary amino acid disorders.

REFERENCE RANGE
- Neonate, 1 day: 0.06-0.3 mg/dL (6-29 micromol/L)
- Infants 1 to 3 months: 0.16 ± 0.09 mg/dL (16 ± 9 micromol/L)
- Infants 2 to 6 months: <0.39 mg/dL (< 38 micromol/L)
- Children 2 to 17 years: Less than 0.01-0.4 mg/dL (1-39 micromol/L)
- Adults: 0.08-0.36 mg/dL (8-35 micromol/L)
  Please refer to your institution's reference ranges as lab normals may vary.

INDICATIONS
Suspected inborn error of metabolism
> **Strength of Recommendation:** Class IIa
> **Strength of Evidence:** Category C
> **Results Interpretation:**
> **Increased amino acid**
> Inherited amino acid disorders are directly related to the absence of an enzyme involved in the metabolism of one or more amino acids; therefore, an elevated plasma level of a particular amino acid is highly suggestive of an inherited metabolic defect. In the majority of cases amino acid and organic acid analysis together permit diagnostic confirmation in infants. Immediate treatment should be initiated when an inborn error of metabolism is suspected, even if a definitive diagnosis has not yet been determined.

COLLECTION/STORAGE INFORMATION
- Specimen Collection and Handling:
  - Immediately place sample in ice water.
  - Isolate plasma sample and freeze it within 1 hour; sample stable for 1 week at -20°C.
  - Sample should be deproteinized and stored at -70°C for protracted periods of usage.

LOINC CODES
- Code: 20634-2 (*Short Name* - A-Aminobutyr SerPl-sCnc)
- Code: 16345-1 (*Short Name* - A-Aminobutyr Ur Ql)
- Code: 32224-8 (*Short Name* - A-Aminobutyr Vitf-sCnc)
- Code: 25849-1 (*Short Name* - A-Aminobutyr/creat 24H Ur-sRto)
- Code: 26919-1 (*Short Name* - A-Aminobutyr/creat Ur-sRto)
- Code: 1787-1 (*Short Name* - A-Aminobutyr SerPl Ql)
- Code: 28590-8 (*Short Name* - A-Aminobutyr/creat Ur-Rto)
- Code: 13667-1 (*Short Name* - A-Aminobutyr/creat Ur-mRto)
- Code: 1790-5 (*Short Name* - A-Aminobutyr Ur-mCnc)
- Code: 1788-9 (*Short Name* - A-Aminobutyr SerPl-mCnc)
- Code: 1786-3 (*Short Name* - A-Aminobutyr CSF-mCnc)
- Code: 13383-5 (*Short Name* - A-Aminobutyr Amn-mCnc)
- Code: 25305-4 (*Short Name* - A-Aminobutyr 24H Ur-sRate)
- Code: 6870-0 (*Short Name* - A-Aminobutyr 24H Ur-mCnc)
- Code: 26794-8 (*Short Name* - A-Aminobutyr 24H Ur Ql)
- Code: 26586-8 (*Short Name* - A-Aminobutyr CSF-sCnc)
- Code: 25848-3 (*Short Name* - A-Aminobutyr 24H Ur-sCnc)
- Code: 27341-7 (*Short Name* - A-Aminobutyr Ur-sCnc)
- Code: 26819-3 (*Short Name* - A-Aminobutyr Amn-sCnc)
- Code: 32223-0 (*Short Name* - A-Aminobutyr Fld-sCnc)

Aluminum measurement, blood

TEST DEFINITION
Measurement of blood aluminum level for diagnosing aluminum accumulation, or therapeutic or occupational exposure

SYNONYMS
- Aluminium measurement, blood
- Blood aluminium
- Blood aluminium level
- Blood aluminum
- Blood aluminum level

REFERENCE RANGE
- Adults and Children:
- Serum: <5.41 mcg/L (<0.2 micromol/L)
- Plasma: 6-7 mcg/L (0.22-0.26 micromol/L)
- Plasma: <30 mcg/L (<1.11 micromol/L)
- Patients on hemodialysis:
- Serum: <116 mcg/L (<4.29 micromol/L); Range: 20-550 mcg/L (0.74-20.4 micromol/L)
  Please refer to your institution's reference ranges as lab normals may vary.

INDICATIONS
Suspected aluminum toxicity
   Strength of Recommendation: Class IIa
   Strength of Evidence: Category C
   Results Interpretation:
   Increased level (laboratory finding)
   An aluminum level greater than 100 mcg/L (3.7 micromol/L) has been associated with signs of toxicity, and patients should be monitored frequently for evidence of toxic exposure. Levels greater than 200 mcg/L (7.4 micromol/L) are usually associated with symptoms.
   Chronic dialysis patients with aluminum levels greater than 200 mcg/L have increased morbidity and mortality. Levels between 114 and 633 mcg/L have been associated with microcytic anemia and bone pain.
   Concurrent elevated serum aluminum levels (greater than 100 mcg/L) and low level in situ parathyroid hormone levels indicate possible osteomalacic osteodystrophy or low turn-over bone disease. A bone biopsy is indicated for serum aluminum levels between 200 and 500 mcg/L.

COLLECTION/STORAGE INFORMATION
- Specimen Collection and Handling:
  - Collect specimens in a metal-free container.
  - Store sample in plastic; avoid glass containers.
  - Transport sample immediately to lab.
  - Freeze serum or plasma specimens at -4°C to -10°C to store.

LOINC CODES
- Code: 5575-6 (*Short Name* - Aluminum RBC-mCnc)

Aluminum measurement, dialysis fluid

TEST DEFINITION
Measurement of the aluminum content of dialysate

REFERENCE RANGE
- Dialysate: <2 mcg of aluminum/L
  Please refer to your institution's reference ranges as lab normals may vary.

INDICATIONS
Routine testing for aluminum levels in dialysis fluid
    Strength of Recommendation: Class IIb
    Strength of Evidence: Category C
Results Interpretation:
Increased level (laboratory finding)
    Several large studies in Europe have shown an association between elevated aluminum concentrations in the water used for dialysis solution and an increased incidence of encephalopathy and osteomalacia.
    The standard in the USA and Europe, which has nearly eliminated dialysate-induced aluminum intoxication, is to treat the water used in dialysis to keep aluminum concentrations under 2 mcg/L. Unfortunately, in some parts of the world, the water used for dialysis is inadequately treated and continues to be a source of aluminum intoxication.
Frequency of Monitoring
    Monthly measurements of aluminum in water used for dialysis fluid is recommended.

LOINC CODES
- Code: 15113-4 (*Short Name* - Aluminum Diaf-sCnc)
- Code: 5572-3 (*Short Name* - Aluminum Diaf-mCnc)

Amino acids measurement, quantitative, urine

TEST DEFINITION
Measurement of amino acids in urine for detection of acquired and hereditary amino acid disorders

SYNONYMS
- Urine amino acid levels
- Urine amino acids

REFERENCE RANGE
Please refer to your institution's reference ranges as lab normals may vary.

INDICATIONS
Suspected inborn error of metabolism (IEM)
    Strength of Recommendation: Class IIa
    Strength of Evidence: Category C
Results Interpretation:
Increased amino acid
    Inherited amino acid metabolic disorders are directly related to the absence or abnormality of an enzyme required for the metabolism of one or more amino acids. Elevated urine levels of a particular amino acid are highly suggestive of an inherited defect in metabolism.
    The following inborn errors of amino acid metabolism should be suspected when a urine screen is abnormal:
- Primary overflow aminoacidurias (autosomal recessive disorders):
  - Phenylketonuria (excess of phenylalanine and its metabolites)
  - Tyrosinuria (excess tyrosine and its metabolites)
  - Alkaptonuria (excess homogentisic acid)
  - Homocystinuria (excess homocystine, methionine and its sulfoxide, or methylmalonic acid)
  - Histidinemia (excess pyruvic acid and other histidine metabolites, and imidazole)
  - Branched-chain ketoaciduria (maple syrup urine disease) (during acute attack excess leucine, isoleucine, alloisoleucine, valine, and corresponding ketoacids)
  - Nonketotic hyperglycinemia (excess glycine)
  - Propionic acidemia (excess glycine, propionate, hydroxypropionate, methylcitrate)
  - Methylmalonic acidemia (excess glycine, methylmalonic acid)
  - Cystathioninuria (excess cystathionine and cystathionine metabolites
  - Carnosinemia (excess carnosine)
  - Hyperprolinemia I & II (excess proline, free hydroxyproline, and glycine)
- Urea cycle disorders:
  - Citrullinemia (excess citrulline, glutamine)

- Argininosuccinic aciduria (excess argininosuccinic acid and its anhydride, citrulline)
- Argininemia (normal or excess arginine, cystine, and ornithine)
- Hyperornithinemia (excess ornithine, homocitrulline)
- Ornithine transcarbamylase deficiency (excess orotic acid, uridine, uracil)
- Carbamoylphosphate synthetase deficiency (excess glycine, glutamine)
- Primary renal aminoacidurias (autosomal recessive disorders):
  - Cystinuria, classic (abnormal level of lysine, ornithine, arginine, cystine)
  - Hypercystinuria (abnormal level of cystine)
  - Dibasic aminoaciduria and lysinuric protein intolerance (abnormal level of ornithine, lysine, arginine)
  - Hartnup disease (abnormal level of all neutral amino acids)
  - Iminoglycinuria (abnormal level of glycine, proline, free hydroxyproline)
  - Dicarboxylic aminoaciduria (abnormal level of glutamic acid and aspartic acid)
  - Methionine malabsorption (abnormal level of methionine, tyrosine, phenylalanine, and branched-chain amino acids; alpha-hydroxybutyric acid)

CLINICAL NOTES
Random urine samples should be collected at specific times as amino acid concentrations follow a circadian rhythm. Highest values occur midafternoon, lowest values in early morning.

COLLECTION/STORAGE INFORMATION
- Specimen Collection and Handling:
  - Collect a 24-hour urine specimen.
  - Add 20 mL of toluene at the beginning of collection; otherwise, keep the sample in a refrigerator during collection.
  - Store specimen at -20°C; for long periods store at -70°C.
  - For random urine, do not add any preservatives, and freeze sample within 3 hours of collection.

LOINC CODES
- Code: 18191-7 (*Short Name* - AA 24H Ur)
- Code: 15139-9 (*Short Name* - Ans+Car+Cyseine+His+Orn Ur Ql)
- Code: 12177-2 (*Short Name* - AA/creat Ur-Rto)
- Code: 15143-1 (*Short Name* - Asp+Cit+Gly+Hcys2+Hyp Ur Ql)

Amitriptyline measurement

TEST DEFINITION
Measurement of amitriptyline levels in serum or plasma to facilitate therapeutic or toxicity monitoring

REFERENCE RANGE
- Adults: 120-250 ng/mL (433-903 nmol/L)
  Please refer to your institution's reference ranges as lab normals may vary.

INDICATIONS
Drug level monitoring during amitriptyline therapy
  Strength of Recommendation: Class I
  Strength of Evidence: Category B
  Results Interpretation:
  Blood drug levels - finding
  Within a range of 0 to 250 ng/mL, a higher amitriptyline level appears to be associated with a lower depression score. The evaluation of amitriptyline's efficacy should be based on both blood concentration and clinical presentation.
  There is a wide variation among individuals in their ability to metabolize amitriptyline.
  A decrease in serum protein may alter the range of effective amitriptyline concentration.
  Blood drug level low
  A low amitriptyline concentration may be attributable to noncompliance or decreased bioavailability.
  Blood drug level high
  Higher drug concentrations of amitriptyline are associated with serious side effects, including convulsions and cardiac arrhythmias.

Suspected amitriptyline toxicity
    Strength of Recommendation: Class IIb
    Strength of Evidence: Category B
Results Interpretation:
Blood drug level high
- Toxic level (adults): >500 ng/mL (>1,805 nmol/L)
- The development of delirium is associated with tricyclic antidepressant plasma levels above 300 ng/mL.
- The development of seizures is associated with tricyclic antidepressant plasma levels above 1,000 ng/mL.
- Lethal tricyclic antidepressant levels reported from forensic studies have ranged from 1,100 to 21,800 ng/mL (4,000 to 80,000 nmol/L).
- Blood concentrations of amitriptyline may correlate with coma grade in patients who have overdosed.

COLLECTION/STORAGE INFORMATION
- Specimen Collection and Handling:
  - Draw serum or plasma in an EDTA tube.
  - Collect trough sample 12 hours after last dose.
  - Refrigerate immediately.
  - Store at -20°C for up to 4 months.

LOINC CODES
- Code: 19333-4 (*Short Name* - Amitrip CtOff Ur Scn-mCnc)
- Code: 3332-4 (*Short Name* - Amitrip SerPl Ql)
- Code: 16225-5 (*Short Name* - Amitrip Ur Ql Cnfrn)
- Code: 14597-9 (*Short Name* - Amitrip SerPl-sCnc)
- Code: 19331-8 (*Short Name* - Amitrip Ur Ql Scn)
- Code: 20515-3 (*Short Name* - Amitrip Ur Cnfrn-mCnc)
- Code: 16114-1 (*Short Name* - Amitrip Ur-mCnc)
- Code: 3333-2 (*Short Name* - Amitrip SerPl-mCnc)
- Code: 16360-0 (*Short Name* - Amitrip Peak SerPl-mCnc)
- Code: 29406-6 (*Short Name* - Amitrip Gast-mCnc)
- Code: 16361-8 (*Short Name* - Amitrip Trough SerPl-mCnc)
- Code: 3334-0 (*Short Name* - Amitrip Ur Ql)
- Code: 19334-2 (*Short Name* - Amitrip CtO Ur Cfm-mCnc)

Ammonia measurement, arterial

TEST DEFINITION
Measurement of ammonia in arterial blood to evaluate the severity of liver disease.

REFERENCE RANGE
- Adults and Children: 0-32 micromol/L
  Please refer to your institution's reference ranges as lab normals may vary.

INDICATIONS
Evaluation of severity of hepatic encephalopathy
    Strength of Recommendation: Class IIa
    Strength of Evidence: Category B
Results Interpretation:
Increased level (laboratory finding)
    There is substantial overlap between total arterial ammonia levels and various grades of hepatic encephalopathy.
    Patients with grade 1 or 2 hepatic encephalopathy usually have levels less than 150 micromol/L.

COLLECTION/STORAGE INFORMATION
- Collection and Handling:
  - Collect 3 mL of arterial blood in a lavender top tube
  - Place specimen immediately on ice

Ammonia measurement, venous

TEST DEFINITION
Measurement of ammonia in venous blood to assess the metabolism by, and accumulation of, ammonia in various organ systems

REFERENCE RANGE
- Adults: 10-80 mcg/dL (6-47 micromol/L)
- Neonates, 0 to 10 days (enzymatic): 170-341 mcg/dL (100-200 micromol/L)
- Infants and toddlers, 10 days to 2 years (enzymatic): 68-136 mcg/dL (40-80 micromol/L)
- Children, older than 2 years (enzymatic): 19-60 mcg/dL (11-35 micromol/L)
  Please refer to your institution's reference ranges as lab normals may vary.

INDICATIONS
Suspected hepatic encephalopathy in liver cirrhosis
  Strength of Recommendation: Class IIa
  Strength of Evidence: Category B
  Results Interpretation:
  Increased ammonia level
    Elevated levels of venous ammonia correlate with the severity of hepatic encephalopathy. There is no significant difference between the correlation of venous ammonia with hepatic encephalopathy and the correlation of arterial ammonia with hepatic encephalopathy.

Suspected inborn error of metabolism associated with hyperammonemia in children
  Strength of Recommendation: Class IIa
  Strength of Evidence: Category C
  Results Interpretation:
  Increased ammonia level
- Ammonia levels and associated signs:
  - 50 to 100 micromol/L: Usually asymptomatic
  - 100 to 200 micromol/L: Anorexia, vomiting, ataxia, irritability, hyperactivity
  - Above 200 micromol/L: Stage II coma, combative state followed by stupor
  - Above 300 micromol/L: Stage III coma, responsive only to painful stimuli
  - Above 500 micromol/L: Elevated intracranial pressure, stage IV coma, decerebrate posturing
  - Above 1000 micromol/L: About 50% survive
- Ammonia levels seen in inborn errors of metabolism:
  - Urea cycle defects: 500 to 2000 micromol/L
  - Organic acidemias: 100 to 1000 micromol/L
  - Transport defects of urea cycle intermediates: 100 to 300 micromol/L
  - Fatty acid oxidation defects: Normal to 300 micromol/L
  - Pyruvate metabolism disorders: Normal to 600 micromol/L
  Almost all patients with ammonia levels over 500 micromol/L have an inborn error of metabolism.

Suspected Reye's syndrome
  Strength of Recommendation: Class I
  Strength of Evidence: Category B
  Results Interpretation:
  Increased ammonia level
    Ammonia levels are elevated at least 150% in 90% of patients with Reye's syndrome, typically in the range of 100 to 350 micromol/L.
    According to some sources, ammonia levels usually peak during the 2 to 3 days following the onset of vomiting and then decline rapidly. Levels may be normal if taken too early or too late in the course of illness.
    Peak ammonia levels usually occur within 4 hours of admission and may be useful in assigning patients to treatment groups. Those with levels greater than 3 times normal usually require fluid restriction, controlled hyperventilation, and mannitol, while those with levels greater than 5 times normal should be placed in a barbiturate coma.
    Peak ammonia level is a good predictor of the severity of illness. A level greater than 300 mcg/dL indicates a poor prognosis. In one study, patients with an ammonia level greater than 45 mcg/dL had a significantly increased risk of neurologic complications and death.

Frequency of Monitoring
Ammonia levels should be obtained daily during acute Reye's syndrome.

ABNORMAL RESULTS
• Results increased in:
  • Exercise
  • Smoking
  • Some hematologic diseases (eg, acute leukemia, status post bone marrow transplantation)

COLLECTION/STORAGE INFORMATION
• Collect specimen in EDTA (lavender top) or heparin (green top) tube.
• Place specimen on ice and transport to lab immediately because levels increase on standing.
• Avoid having patient clench fist or using tight tourniquet during blood draw because muscle contraction and ischemia may cause ammonia to be released into venous blood.
• Avoid hemolysis.

Amniotic fluid lecithin/sphingomyelin ratio

TEST DEFINITION
Measurement of lecithin/sphingomyelin (L/S) ratio in amniotic fluid for evaluation and management of fetal lung immaturity

SYNONYMS
• Fetal lung maturity profile
• L/S ratio, amniotic fluid
• Phospholipid profile, amniotic fluid

INDICATIONS
Assessment of fetal lung immaturity during pregnancy
    Strength of Recommendation: Class IIa
    Strength of Evidence: Category B
Results Interpretation:
Fetal lung immaturity
The lecithin/sphingomyelin (L/S) ratio is used to detect fetal lung immaturity when delivery of the fetus is considered before 37 weeks gestation and the risk of respiratory distress syndrome (RDS) is elevated. The measurement compares the relative quantities of two phospholipids found in amniotic fluid. Lecithin is the primary component of surfactant with levels that increase around 32 to 33 weeks' gestation. Since sphingo-myelin levels remain relatively constant, lecithin can be measured against it to generate a ratio.
• Ratios of Fetal Lung Maturity Status:
  • <1.5: - Immature
  • 1.5-1.9: - Transitional or intermediate, with 50% risk of RDS
  • ≥2: - Mature
  • ≥3.5: - Mature for fetus of poorly-controlled diabetic mother, with 1% risk of RDS
The volume of amniotic fluid does not influence measurement of the L/S ratio, most likely because the two measurements remain constant in the ratio.
Fluid from both sacs should be analyzed for predicting fetal lung immaturity. In a study of 58 pairs of di-amniotic twins, the comparison of L/S ratios between twin A and twin B, at less than or equal to 32 weeks' gestation, showed a 25% discordancy in values, significantly greater than the percentage of discordancy found at greater than 32 weeks' gestation (15%)..

False Results
Contamination of an amniotic fluid specimen with blood can affect the results of the ratio. Data from such samples should be used to predict immaturity only when the results are either very high or very low.
The presence of meconium can also confound results; if procedures for centrifuging the specimen for removal of debris are not followed, the ratio will be decreased.

Timing of Monitoring
Lecithin/sphingomyelin ratio determination before 33 weeks gestation is not recommended since fetal maturity is unlikely. When gestational age is well-documented, there is no need for fetal lung immaturity testing after 37 weeks' gestation.

CLINICAL NOTES
Results may be altered by certain obstetric conditions, particularly diabetes. For nonsterile specimens, a phosphatidylglycerol (PG) level is preferable.
Although the L/S ratio is a widely accepted measure of fetal lung immaturity, its cumbersome requirements make it less desirable than some of the newer tests available.

COLLECTION/STORAGE INFORMATION
- Specimen Collection and Handling:
    - Obtain 3 to 4 mL of uncontaminated amniotic fluid
    - Transfer specimen into a plastic tube
    - Centrifuge specimen
    - Refrigerate specimen if unable to centrifuge
    - Freeze specimen after centrifugation if contaminated

LOINC CODES
- Code: 2557-7 (*Short Name* - L/S Amn-mRto)

Amniotic fluid methylmalonic acid level

TEST DEFINITION
Measurement of methylmalonic acid (MMA) in amniotic fluid as a prenatal diagnostic tool for methylmalonic aciduria

SYNONYMS
- Amniotic fluid methylmalonic acid measurement

INDICATIONS
Suspected fetal methylmalonic aciduria
    Results Interpretation:
    Amniotic fluid chemistry - finding
    Elevated amniotic fluid methylmalonic acid levels seem to be accurate for prenatal diagnosis of methylmalonic aciduria.

LOINC CODES
- Code: 34627-0 (*Short Name* - MMA Amn-sCnc)

Amoxapine measurement

TEST DEFINITION
Measurement of amoxapine in serum or plasma to facilitate therapeutic or toxicity monitoring

REFERENCE RANGE
- Therapeutic concentration (amoxapine + 8-hydroxyamoxapine): 200-600 ng/mL (200-600 mcg/L)
    Please refer to your institution's reference ranges as lab normals may vary.

INDICATIONS
Drug level monitoring during amoxapine therapy
    Strength of Recommendation: Class IIb
    Strength of Evidence: Category C

Results Interpretation:
Blood drug levels - finding
   The suggested therapeutic window for amoxapine plus 8-hydroxyamoxapine is 200 to 400 ng/mL, while the usual therapeutic concentration of amoxapine alone is less than 100 ng/mL.
   The serum concentration of the active metabolite 8-hydroxyamoxapine is much higher, and the half-life is much longer, than that of amoxapine.
   Interpretation of amoxapine serum levels is difficult because the therapeutic range is not clearly defined. In addition, serum levels fail to correlate with therapeutic response, and wide variations in serum concentrations occur.

Suspected amoxapine toxicity
   Strength of Recommendation: Class IIb
   Strength of Evidence: Category C
   Results Interpretation:
   Increased level (laboratory finding)
   Toxic concentration thresholds are not well defined.
   Fatalities have been reported with serum amoxapine levels between 261 and 7,160 ng/mL.
   Serious toxicity with eventual recovery has been reported with amoxapine levels between 1,820 and 2,114 ng/mL. Serum amoxapine concentrations of 648 to 2,509 ng/mL have been associated with persistent neurologic deficits.

COLLECTION/STORAGE INFORMATION
· Collect plasma in a tube containing EDTA.

LOINC CODES
· Code: 3343-1 (*Short Name* - Amoxapine Ur-mCnc)
· Code: 3341-5 (*Short Name* - Amoxapine SerPl-mCnc)
· Code: 3340-7 (*Short Name* - Amoxapine SerPl Ql)
· Code: 3342-3 (*Short Name* - Amoxapine Ur Ql)

Amphetamine measurement, Blood

TEST DEFINITION
   Measurement of amphetamine in serum or plasma for drug level monitoring or suspected abuse

SYNONYMS
· Amphetamine level

REFERENCE RANGE
· Adult, therapeutic level: 20-30 ng/mL (148-222 nmol/L)
· Adult, toxic level: >200 ng/mL (>1480 nmol/L)
   Please refer to your institution's reference ranges as lab normals may vary.

INDICATIONS
Suspected amphetamine abuse
   Strength of Recommendation: Class IIa
   Strength of Evidence: Category C
   Results Interpretation:
   Blood drug levels - finding
   Patients receiving amphetamines for legitimate indications will generally have plasma levels of 30 to 40 ng/mL. Patients receiving therapeutic doses of 10 to 12.5 mg have had peak blood levels of 20 to 30 ng/mL. Hyperactive children receiving a single sustained-release dose of 0.5 mg/kg had a mean peak plasma level of 70 ng/mL. Adults receiving 30 mg orally had a mean peak level of 111 ng/mL. Chronic abusers have been reported to have plasma levels of up to 3,000 ng/mL.
   The duration of detectability in plasma depends on the dose and the half-life, which is dependent on urine pH. In a normal individual with a slightly acid urine pH and a maximal half-life of 14 hours, the plasma may contain measurable amphetamine for up to 70 hours.

Longer plasma elimination half-life has been observed in drug-dependent users (21.8 ± 1.4 hours) as compared to non-users (13.9 ± 3.4 hours) at the same 25 mg oral dose. Metabolism was not different in these two groups, indicating higher distribution volume with resultant higher tissue affinity in tolerant amphetamine abusers.

Blood levels of methylenedioxymethamphetamine (MDMA, ecstacy) have not correlated with toxicity, but may confirm the intoxicant.

COLLECTION/STORAGE INFORMATION

- Collect specimen in an EDTA (lavender top) tube.
- Follow chain of custody if indicated.

LOINC CODES

- Code: 26895-3 (*Short Name* - Amphets Mec-mCnt)
- Code: 20525-2 (*Short Name* - D-amphet Ur Cnfrn-mCnc)
- Code: 31025-0 (*Short Name* - D-amphet % Ur)
- Code: 18431-7 (*Short Name* - Amphets Stl Ql Scn)
- Code: 19421-7 (*Short Name* - D-amphet CtO Ur Scn-mCnc)
- Code: 15366-8 (*Short Name* - D-amphet Ur-mCnc)
- Code: 8142-2 (*Short Name* - Amphets Gast Ql Scn)
- Code: 27205-4 (*Short Name* - Amphets Vitf Ql)
- Code: 8149-7 (*Short Name* - Amphets SerPl Ql Scn)
- Code: 19420-9 (*Short Name* - D-amphet Ur Ql Cnfrn)
- Code: 19424-1 (*Short Name* - D-methamphet Ur Ql Cfm)
- Code: 26791-4 (*Short Name* - Amphet Stl-mCnt)
- Code: 8143-0 (*Short Name* - Amphets Mec-mCnc)
- Code: 29530-3 (*Short Name* - Amphets XXX Ql)
- Code: 8141-4 (*Short Name* - Amphets Gast Ql Cfm)
- Code: 13497-3 (*Short Name* - D-/L-amphet Ur-mRto)
- Code: 30112-7 (*Short Name* - Amphet SerPl-mCnc)
- Code: 12477-6 (*Short Name* - D-methamphet Ur-mCnc)
- Code: 3348-0 (*Short Name* - Amphets SerPl Ql)
- Code: 12350-5 (*Short Name* - Amphets Stl Ql)
- Code: 8148-9 (*Short Name* - Amphets SerPl Ql Cnfrn)
- Code: 13498-1 (*Short Name* - D-/L-methamphet Ur-mRto)
- Code: 19423-3 (*Short Name* - D-methamphet Ur Ql Scn)
- Code: 9814-5 (*Short Name* - D-amphet SerPl-mCnc)
- Code: 27263-3 (*Short Name* - Amphets Vitf-mCnc)
- Code: 29592-3 (*Short Name* - Amphet SerPl Cnfrn-mCnc)
- Code: 8140-6 (*Short Name* - Amphets Gast Ql)
- Code: 19422-5 (*Short Name* - D-amphet CtO Ur Cfm-mCnc)
- Code: 9352-6 (*Short Name* - Amphets Har-mCnt)
- Code: 31026-8 (*Short Name* - D-methamphet % Ur)
- Code: 26959-7 (*Short Name* - Amphet Mec-mCnt)

Amylase measurement, peritoneal fluid

TEST DEFINITION

Measurement of amylase in ascitic fluid

REFERENCE RANGE

Value identical to or slightly less than serum amylase level
Please refer to your institution's reference ranges as lab normals may vary.

INDICATIONS

Suspected and known pancreatitis
      Strength of Recommendation: Class IIb
      Strength of Evidence: Category B

Results Interpretation:
Increased amylase level
   Elevated ascitic fluid amylase levels have been observed in pancreatitis; a correlation between elevated ascitic amylase levels and patient prognosis has not been established.

COLLECTION/STORAGE INFORMATION
   Store at 4°C.

LOINC CODES
• Code: 1797-0 (*Short Name* - Amylase Prt-cCnc)

Amylase measurement, pleural fluid

TEST DEFINITION
   Measurement of amylase in pleural fluid

REFERENCE RANGE
   Value identical to or slightly less than serum amylase level
   Please refer to your institution's reference ranges as lab normals may vary.

INDICATIONS
Suspected pancreatitis in patients with pleural effusion
   Strength of Recommendation: Class IIb
   Strength of Evidence: Category B
   Results Interpretation:
   Increased amylase level
   High pleural fluid (PF) amylase levels in children may indicate pancreatitis.
   A PF amylase level above the upper limit of normal for serum amylase or a PF/serum ratio of greater than 1 may indicate pancreatitis. PF amylase levels may be over 100,000 units in some patients with pancreatic disease.

Suspected ruptured esophagus in patients with pleural effusion
   Strength of Recommendation: Class IIb
   Strength of Evidence: Category C
   Results Interpretation:
   Increased amylase level
   A high pleural fluid (PF) amylase level in children and adults is recognized as an indicator of possible esophageal rupture.
   PF amylase elevation of at least 1.5 to 2 times greater than serum amylase indicates esophageal rupture.
   A PF amylase level above the normal for serum amylase or a PF/serum ratio of greater than 1 indicates esophageal rupture.

COLLECTION/STORAGE INFORMATION
   Store sample at 4°C.

LOINC CODES
• Code: 1796-2 (*Short Name* - Amylase Plr-cCnc)

Amylase measurement, serum

TEST DEFINITION
   Measurement of amylase in serum to aid in the evaluation for disorders of the pancreas and gastrointestinal tract, autoimmune and viral illnesses, shock, trauma, and hypersensitivity reactions

Synonyms
- Amylase - serum
- Serum amylase

Reference Range
- Adults: 60 to 180 units/L (0.8-3.2 microkatal/L)
- Pediatrics: amylase level remains low for the first two months and increases to adult values by the end of the first year of life

  Please refer to your institution's reference ranges as lab normals may vary.

Indications
Suspected pancreatic injury in patients with blunt abdominal trauma
Strength of Recommendation: Class IIb
Strength of Evidence: Category B
Results Interpretation:
Serum amylase raised

Sporadic elevations in pancreatic amylase levels occur in blunt trauma patients with multiple injuries.

Persistently elevated or rising levels of serum amylase are suggestive of more severe pancreatic injury; however, the actual number is not useful as a marker for the degree of injury.

One study suggested that serial serum amylase measurements 3 hours after trauma may be helpful in diagnosing pancreatic injury.

Due to the lack of specificity and delayed elevation of serum amylase after pancreatic trauma, an elevated amylase suggests the possibility of pancreatic injury, which should then be further evaluated by abdominal imaging.

Hemolytic uremic syndrome
Results Interpretation:
Serum amylase raised

Elevated levels of serum amylase and lipase may aid in the diagnosis of pancreatitis in hemolytic uremic syndrome.

Pancreatitis is not considered to be present unless elevations are greater than four times the normal value, or other evidence of pancreatitis is present.

Hemorrhagic shock
Results Interpretation:
Serum amylase raised

Hyperamylasemia, often occurring with minimal signs and symptoms of pancreatitis, has been observed following prolonged hypotension. Concurrent elevations in serum lipase, amylase/creatinine clearance, and serum pancreatic isoamylase levels suggest this is due to ischemic pancreatic injury.

Human immunodeficiency virus (HIV) infection
Strength of Recommendation: Class IIa
Strength of Evidence: Category B
Results Interpretation:
Serum amylase raised

Asymptomatic pancreatic enzyme elevations (usually less than two fold) may occur in human immunodeficiency virus (HIV) patients and usually are associated with hepatitis B or C, or with certain medications, such as intravenous (IV) trimethoprim/sulfamethoxazole or antiretrovirals.

The salivary gland may be a source of mild hyperamylasemia (less than two times the upper limit of normal) in HIV infected patients.

Hypothermia
Strength of Recommendation: Class III
Strength of Evidence: Category C
Results Interpretation:
Serum amylase raised

Some authors conclude that due to lack of positive evidence and a predominance of negative evidence, hypothermia is not an important risk factor for the development of acute pancreatitis.

Known inflammatory bowel disease
> **Strength of Recommendation:** Class IIb
> **Strength of Evidence:** Category C
>
> **Results Interpretation:**
> **Serum amylase raised**

Serum amylase levels may be increased in a small percentage of patients with inflammatory bowel disease.

Mumps
> **Strength of Recommendation:** Class IIa
> **Strength of Evidence:** Category B
>
> **Results Interpretation:**
> **Serum amylase raised**

In mumps, pancreatitis and/or a recurrent attack of parotitis can occur anytime during the course of the illness. Therefore, even if the initial amylase activity is normal, serial amylase isoenzyme measurements of salivary (S-type) and pancreatic (P-type) may be useful.

The serum amylase level can be used to differentiate parotid from nonparotid swelling, but it cannot be relied upon to differentiate pancreatitis from parotitis. Differentiation of pancreatitis can be achieved through amylase isoenzyme analysis or measurement of serum lipase, as well as by clinical findings.

An elevated serum amylase level in a patient with aseptic meningitis should suggest mumps as the etiologic agent.

Peptic ulcer
> **Strength of Recommendation:** Class IIb
> **Strength of Evidence:** Category C
>
> **Results Interpretation:**
> **Serum amylase raised**

Serum amylase activity may be elevated in patients with peptic ulcer disease, especially in those with perforated ulcers.

Suspected acute mesenteric ischemia
> **Results Interpretation:**
> **Serum amylase raised**

Serum amylase levels greater than 600 units/L may indicate an extremely poor prognosis.

Suspected cholecystitis
> **Results Interpretation:**
> **Serum amylase raised**

Amylase levels are elevated in 15% to 30% of patients with cholecystitis. The value may occasionally be greater than 1,000 units/dL, with or without concomitant pancreatitis.

Suspected esophageal perforation
> **Results Interpretation:**
> **Serum amylase (pancreatic) normal**

Serum amylase level is generally normal in patients with esophageal perforation unless pancreatitis is the cause of vomiting. An elevated amylase level in the pleural fluid and normal serum amylase level is strong evidence for perforated esophagus.

Suspected gallstone pancreatitis
> **Results Interpretation:**
> **Serum amylase raised**

Serum amylase elevations are common in gallstone pancreatitis. In the presence of midepigastric pain radiating through to the back, an elevated serum amylase obtained within 24 hours of pain onset suggests gallstone pancreatitis.

Suspected pancreatitis
> **Strength of Recommendation:** Class IIa
> **Strength of Evidence:** Category C
>
> **Results Interpretation:**
> **Serum amylase raised**

The diagnosis of acute pancreatitis is confirmed in a patient with characteristic clinical presentation by an amylase level greater than 4 times the upper limit of normal within 48 hours of onset of symptoms. Amylase levels peak within 24 to 36 hours and fall within 48 hours of illness onset. While both amylase and lipase are simulataneously elevated during pancreatic inflammation, amylase levels often return to normal just before lipase levels as the illness resolves.

Serum amylase levels are often elevated in the early stages of chronic pancreatitis and during acute exacerbations but are of little value between acute exacerbations.

Neither serum amylase or lipase has value in predicting disease severity.

Patients with gallstone pancreatitis tend to have higher amylase levels than patients with alcoholic pancreatitis, but there is no distinct cutoff between the two.

Pancreatitis occurs following cholangiopancreatography (ERCP) in 5.4% to 6.7% of patients. An elevation in serum amylase level greater than 4 times the upper limit of normal in a patient with symptoms (especially pain) following ERCP (usually within the first postoperative day) is diagnostic of post-ERCP pancreatitis.

Isoenzyme evaluation of the serum amylase may help differentiate other sources of amylase (salivary gland, prostate, breast, lung, fallopian tubes, ovaries, and endometrium) from the pancreatic source and thus rule out pancreatitis.

Normal laboratory findings

Up to one-third of patients with acute pancreatitis, especially those with acute alcoholic pancreatitis, have normal amylase levels. Normal amylase levels also occur in up to 50% of patients with acute pancreatitis and hypertriglyceridemia and normal amylase levels may be found in patients with long-standing pancreatitis.

A normal amylase level does not exclude the diagnosis of acute pancreatitis.

Toxic epidermal necrolysis
  Results Interpretation:
  Serum amylase raised

Hyperamylasemia (primarily salivary) is prominent in toxic epidermal necrolysis (TEN) and is associated with an increased risk of ocular sequelae. It may reflect the importance of mucous membrane involvement and could have predictive value of post-TEN Sjogren-like sicca syndrome.

COMMON PANELS
- Pancreatic panel

CLINICAL NOTES
Amylase activity is the same in males and females and is not affected by meals or time of day.

COLLECTION/STORAGE INFORMATION
- Collect venous blood in marble top tube.
- Store at room temperature for 7 days or at 4°C for 1 month.

LOINC CODES
- Code: 1802-8 (*Short Name* - Amylase P1 Ser-cCnc)
- Code: 1804-4 (*Short Name* - Amylase P3 Ser-cCnc)
- Code: 1803-6 (*Short Name* - Amylase P2 Ser-cCnc)
- Code: 15025-0 (*Short Name* - Amylase S3 % Ser)
- Code: 1798-8 (*Short Name* - Amylase SerPl-cCnc)

Amylase measurement, urine

TEST DEFINITION
Measurement of amylase in urine for evaluation of acute abdominal pain

SYNONYMS
- Urine amylase
- Urine amylase level

REFERENCE RANGE
- Adults: 4-400 units/L (0.07-7.67 nkat/L)
  Please refer to your institution's reference ranges as lab normals may vary.

INDICATIONS

Suspected acute pancreatitis
> **Strength of Recommendation:** Class IIb
> **Strength of Evidence:** Category B
Results Interpretation:
Increased amylase level
   The urinary amylase dipstick test has poor sensitivity but is moderately specific and therefore may be a helpful test in ruling in the diagnosis of acute pancreatitis.
   An elevation of urine amylase is seen several hours after the rise of serum amylase levels and may persist even after serum amylase levels return to normal.

ABNORMAL RESULTS

- Results decreased in
  - Lipemia

COLLECTION/STORAGE INFORMATION

- Specimen Collection and Handling:
  - Collect 1-hour or 24-hour urine sample
  - Adjust urine pH to alkaline range before storage
  - Store at 4° C

LOINC CODES

- Code: 15350-2 (*Short Name* - Amylase 2H Ur-cRate)
- Code: 1799-6 (*Short Name* - Amylase Ur-cCnc)
- Code: 30124-2 (*Short Name* - Amylase 1H Ur-cRate)

Amylase/creatinine clearance ratio measurement

TEST DEFINITION

   Measurement of amylase clearance, expressed as a percentage of the creatinine clearance, for the evaluation of pancreatic disease and macroamylasemia screening.

SYNONYMS

- Amylase/creatinine clearance ratio

REFERENCE RANGE

- Adults (conventional and standard international units): 1-5 (calculated as amylase clearance divided by creatinine clearance times 100).
  Please refer to your institution's reference ranges as lab normals may vary.

INDICATIONS

Suspected pancreatitis
> **Strength of Recommendation:** Class IIb
> **Strength of Evidence:** Category C
Results Interpretation:
Raised biochemistry findings
   An increased amylase/creatinine clearance measurement ratio may indicate pancreatitis; however, the persistence of symptoms (eg, abdominal pain, nausea, vomiting) greater than or equal to 48 hours duration is more specific for pancreatitis.

Suspected post-biliary surgery pancreatitis
> **Strength of Recommendation:** Class IIb
> **Strength of Evidence:** Category C

Results Interpretation:
Raised biochemistry findings
   Postoperative elevation of amylase/creatinine clearance ratio (ACCR) is nonspecific. Successive daily normal ACCRs, however, can help to exclude the diagnosis of postoperative pancreatitis.

Suspected post-gastric surgery pancreatitis
   Strength of Recommendation: Class IIb
   Strength of Evidence: Category C
Results Interpretation:
Raised biochemistry findings
   Postoperative elevation of amylase/creatinine clearance ratio (ACCR) is nonspecific.

ABNORMAL RESULTS
- Results increased in:
  - Burns
  - Diabetic ketoacidosis
  - Renal insufficiency
  - Duodenal perforation
  - Post-extracorporeal circulation
  - Hyperemesis of pregnancy
  - Post-abdominal surgery
  - Pancreatic cancer
  - Myeloma and light-chain disease
  - Marked hemoglobinuria
- Results decreased in
  - Persons under 30 years of age

CLINICAL NOTES
   The amylase creatinine clearance ratio (ACCR) is technique-dependent; reference range is correlated to the particular amylase assay method.
   Serial ACCR measurements do not add more significant diagnostic information than that offered by serum pancreatic enzyme levels. A very low ratio, however, can indicate macroamylasemia.
   ACCR may not be a useful test. It can be falsely raised due to a reduction in amylase reabsorption if the proximal tubule is dysfunctional. Also, if the amylase concentration is elevated in both urine and blood, the ratio may or may not be increased by the calculation.

COLLECTION/STORAGE INFORMATION
- Specimen Collection and Handling:
  - Serum:
    - Collect serum in red or marble top tube.
    - Store at 4°C or -20°C.
  - Urine:
    - Collect random urine.
    - Store at 4°C.

LOINC CODES
- Code: 30077-2 (*Short Name* - Amylase/CrCl Ur-Rto)
- Code: 13706-7 (*Short Name* - Amylase/creat Ur-mRto)
- Code: 1810-1 (*Short Name* - Amylase/creat SerPl-mRto)
- Code: 1811-9 (*Short Name* - Amylase/CrCl 24H Ur-Rto)

Anaerobic microbial culture

TEST DEFINITION
   Isolation and identification of microorganisms using anaerobic culture based on the appropriate specimen (eg, body fluids, deep aspirates of wounds, specimens collected by special techniques including transtracheal aspirates)

REFERENCE RANGE
- Adults and Children: Negative
  Please refer to your institution's reference ranges as lab normals may vary.

INDICATIONS
Suspected anaerobic infection
Results Interpretation:
Positive microbiology findings

Expected anaerobic bacteria isolates differ qualitatively and quantitatively depending on the anatomical site (eg, gastric contents, colon, oral cavity) to another. Overgrowth of normal flora or organisms that have spread into sterile tissue or body cavities may be an indicator of anaerobic infection.

Most anaerobic infections are polymicrobial (anaerobic and aerobic) with multiple species present on culture.

In healthy individuals, more than 500 anaerobic species are thought to be present in fecal flora and over 200 in oral flora. Normal counts vary by anatomical site as follows: 10^5 /mL in saliva, 10^3 /mL in gastric contents, and 10^8 /g to 10^{11} /g in feces.

Suspected brain abscess
Strength of Recommendation: Class IIa
Strength of Evidence: Category B
Results Interpretation:
Positive microbiology findings

Brain abscess is primarily an anaerobic infection and *Bacteroides fragilis* is the most commonly encountered anaerobe. *Bacteroides spp* are isolated in up to 60% of brain abscesses, and are commonly associated with chronic lung infection, sinogenic abscesses, and odontogenic infections. *Peptostreptococcus spp* and *Fusobacterium nucleatum* have also been associated with anaerobic brain abscess infection.

Suspected lung infection secondary to aspiration pneumonia
Strength of Recommendation: Class IIa
Strength of Evidence: Category C
Results Interpretation:
Positive microbiology findings

Anaerobic lung infections are typically caused by aspiration of normal oral flora (ie, culture isolates are often oropharyngeal anaerobes). Pneumonitis, lung abscess, empyema, and necrotizing pneumonia may also produce positive anaerobic isolates. *Bacteroides fragilis* is a frequent (up to 15% of cases) isolate from patients with nosocomial aspiration pneumonia.

The three most common anaerobic pathogens associated with aspiration pneumonia are *B melaninogenicus-B asaccharolyticus* group, *Fusobacterium nucleatum*, and anaerobic cocci. Other pathogens may include *Eubacterium* and *Peptostreptococcus*.

CLINICAL NOTES
Anaerobic infection should be suspected if no growth occurs in aerobic cultures, gas or foul odor in specimen on bacterial culture, anaerobic growth on proper media, and characteristic colonies on anaerobic plates.

Common anaerobic bacteria found in normal flora of major body sites (ie, skin, upper respiratory tract, vagina, and colon) may include: *Bacteroides, Actinomyces, Bifidobacterium, Clostridium, Eubacterium, FusobacteriumPropionibacterium, Lactobacillus, Peptococcus, Propionibacterium*, and *Veillonella*.

Unsuitable specimens due to the risk of contamination with normal flora and have no diagnostic value include: coughed sputum, bronchoscopy aspirates, gingival and throat swabs, feces, gastric aspirates, voided urine, and vaginal swabs. Exceptions may include Clostridium difficile in stool that is obtained from a patient with colitis.

Surgical specimens obtained by aspiration or excision should be submitted for both routine and anaerobic culture; fungal and mycobacterial cultures should also be performed as clinically indicated.

COLLECTION/STORAGE INFORMATION
- Specimen Collection and Handling
  - Direct needle aspiration is the best method to obtain a culture; swab cultures are much less desirable.
  - Specimen collection should avoid normal flora to prevent contamination.
  - Collect specimens by syringe puncture directly into the focus of infection to isolate anaerobic bacteria by anatomical site:
    - Lungs, bronchi - transtracheal aspiration (TAA)
    - Pleural space - thoracentesis
    - Abscess, pus - aspiration by syringe (eg, CSF fluid, joint fluid, bile, middle ear, maxillary sinus)

- Fistula, endometrium - aspiration through catheter inserted into deep site
- Peritoneal cavity - transabdominal aspiration
- Salpingitis - aspiration of deep tissues
- Urinary tract - suprapubic percutaneous bladder aspiration
- Collect all specimens (eg, body fluids, wound tissue) in an anaerobic transport vial.
- Transport specimen immediately to lab; do not refrigerate.
- Carefully transport specimens to avoid changes in anaerobic population (ie, sensitivity to oxygen causes some obligate anaerobes to die rapidly upon exposure to air).
- All specimens should be processed as rapidly (less than 24 hours) as possible after collection to avoid loss of fastidious oxygen-sensitive anaerobes.

LOINC CODES

- Code: 17927-5 (*Short Name* - Deep Wnd Anaerobe Cult org #3)
- Code: 17958-0 (*Short Name* - Fld Anaerobe BFld Cult org #3)
- Code: 12281-2 (*Short Name* - Cvx Anaerobe Cult)
- Code: 635-3 (*Short Name* - XXX Anaerobe Cult)
- Code: 20878-5 (*Short Name* - Islt Anaerobe Cult)
- Code: 17921-8 (*Short Name* - Nose Anaerobe Cult org #2)
- Code: 17924-2 (*Short Name* - Tiss Anaerobe Cult org #3)
- Code: 598-3 (*Short Name* - Asp Anaerobe Cult)
- Code: 17925-9 (*Short Name* - Deep Wnd Anaerobe Cult)
- Code: 17923-4 (*Short Name* - Tiss Anaerobe Cult org #2)
- Code: 17956-4 (*Short Name* - Fld Anaerobe BFld Cult)
- Code: 17934-1 (*Short Name* - Bld Anaerobe Cult)
- Code: 17922-6 (*Short Name* - Nose Anaerobe Cult org #3)
- Code: 17936-6 (*Short Name* - Bld Anaerobe Cult org #3)
- Code: 628-8 (*Short Name* - Tiss Anaerobe Cult)
- Code: 17957-2 (*Short Name* - Fld Anaerobe Cult org #2)
- Code: 17935-8 (*Short Name* - Bld Anaerobe Cult org #2)
- Code: 17926-7 (*Short Name* - Deep Wnd Anaerobe Cult org #2)
- Code: 633-8 (*Short Name* - Wnd Anaerobe Cult)

Anion gap measurement

TEST DEFINITION

Measurement of the difference between anions and cations in plasma or serum for evaluation of acid-base disorders

SYNONYMS

- Ion gap measurement, serum

REFERENCE RANGE

- Adults and Children:
- Without calculating in potassium: 7-16 mEq/L (7-16 mmol/L)
- With calculating in potassium: 10-20 mEq/L (10-20 mmol/L)
  Please refer to your institution's reference ranges as lab normals may vary.

INDICATIONS

Initial evaluation and monitoring of diabetic ketoacidosis
    Strength of Recommendation: Class I
    Strength of Evidence: Category C
    Results Interpretation:
    Increased anion gap
        Accumulation of ketoacids usually results in an increased anion gap metabolic acidosis for patients with diabetic ketoacidosis (DKA). Anion gap is greater than 10 mEq/L in mild DKA and greater than 12 mEq/L in moderate to severe cases.
    Frequency of Monitoring
        Following initial evaluation, calculate the anion gap every 2 to 4 hours to monitor resolution of acidosis.

Initial evaluation of suspected hyperglycemic hyperosmolar state
> **Strength of Recommendation:** Class I
> **Strength of Evidence:** Category C
Results Interpretation:
Increased anion gap
> The anion gap is variable in hyperglycemic hyperosmolar state (HHS).
> Approximately 50% of patients with HHS have an increased anion gap metabolic acidosis due to concomitant ketoacidosis and/or an increase in serum lactate levels.

Suspected alcoholic ketoacidosis
> **Strength of Recommendation:** Class I
> **Strength of Evidence:** Category C
Results Interpretation:
Increased anion gap
> In alcoholic ketoacidosis, the anion gap may be elevated and typically averages 29 mEq/L.

Suspected hypermagnesemia
> **Strength of Recommendation:** Class I
> **Strength of Evidence:** Category C
Results Interpretation:
Reduced anion gap
> A sudden fall in the anion gap may be a clue to the presence of hypermagnesemia. Because magnesium is an unmeasured cation, an increase in the magnesium level will lower the measured anion gap.

Suspected lactic acidosis
> **Strength of Recommendation:** Class I
> **Strength of Evidence:** Category B
Results Interpretation:
Increased anion gap
> An anion gap greater than 30 mEq/L may indicate the presence of an organic acidosis, such as lactic acidosis. The decrement in bicarbonate is roughly equal to the increment in the anion gap. Thus, lactic acidosis typically results in an anion gap metabolic acidosis.
> The anion gap should be adjusted in the presence of hypoalbuminemia; however, while hypoalbuminemia will affect measured anion gap, hypoalbuminemia will not mask clinically significant gap acidosis.

Suspected metabolic acidosis
> **Strength of Recommendation:** Class I
> **Strength of Evidence:** Category C
Results Interpretation:
Increased anion gap
> An anion gap greater than 20 mEq/L is highly elevated. Very high anion gaps (greater than 30 mEq/L) are usually due to an identifiable organic acidosis (eg, lactic acidosis or ketoacidosis), ethylene glycol toxicity, methanol toxicity, or multifactorial causes usually involving renal insufficiency.
> - An elevated anion gap may be caused by conditions other than metabolic acidosis, including:
>   - Dehydration
>   - Treatment with sodium salts of strong acids
>   - Treatment with sodium salts of antibiotics (eg, penicillin, carbenicillin)
>   - Alkalosis
>   - Decreased unmeasured cation (eg, hypokalemia, hypocalcemia, hypomagnesemia)
>   - Hyperalbuminemia
>   - Increased inorganic anion (eg, phosphate, sulfate)
>   - Laboratory error (eg, falsely increased serum sodium, falsely decreased serum chloride or bicarbonate)

Reduced anion gap
> - The anion gap may be lowered by one of three mechanisms:
>   - Increased unmeasured cation (eg, hyperkalemia, hypercalcemia, hypermagnesemia), multiple myeloma, lithium intoxication, polymyxin B administration)
>   - Decreased unmeasured anion (eg, hypoalbuminemia or bromide intoxication). Bromide will be recorded as chloride in most determinations
>   - Laboratory error (eg, falsely decreased serum sodium, falsely increased serum chloride or bicarbonate, hyperviscosity, hyperlipidemia, dilutional studies)

Presence of hypoalbuminemia will lead to underestimation of the anion gap. Calculation of the anion gap should be adjusted for albumin. The anion gap falls by approximately 2.5 mEq/L for every 1 g/dL reduction in serum albumin concentration.

COMMON PANELS
- Diabetic management panel

ABNORMAL RESULTS
- Increased results will occur when the serum sample is exposed to air for excessive periods of time.
- The anion gap falls by approximately 2.5 mEq/L for every 1 g/dL reduction in serum albumin concentration.

CLINICAL NOTES
Although anion gap can be measured with or without potassium, the standard is to measure anion gap without potassium since its variation is clinically insignificant.

Anti DNase B test

TEST DEFINITION
Measurement of antideoxyribonuclease-B antibodies in serum to document exposure to group A beta-hemolytic streptococcus, particularly in acute rheumatic fever, acute glomerulonephritis, and pyoderma

REFERENCE RANGE
- Adults and Children: ≤170 units/mL
- Normal titers may vary with age and region of world. The upper limit of normal can be determined regionally by that antibody titer exceeded by a certain percent (generally 15%-20%) of the healthy population in a geographic area.
  Please refer to your institution's reference ranges as lab normals may vary.

INDICATIONS
Suspected group A beta-hemolytic streptococcal infection or post-streptococcal sequelae (rheumatic fever and acute glomerulonephritis)
  Strength of Recommendation: Class IIa
  Strength of Evidence: Category B
  Results Interpretation:
  Increased level (laboratory finding)
  Elevated ADNase B titers, associated with certain clinical signs and symptoms, suggests past or current group A beta-hemolytic streptococcal infection (GAS).
  An elevated or rising ADNase B titer is supporting evidence of antecedent GAS infection, required in the modified Jones Criteria for diagnosis of acute rheumatic fever.
  ADNase B is specific for group A beta-hemolytic streptococcal infections, and may be particularly useful in evaluation of streptococcal skin infections such as erysipelas.
  Confirmation of a preceding GAS infection is necessary in the diagnosis of post-streptococcal sequelae such as acute glomerulonephritis and rheumatic fever; elevated ADNase B titers provide this evidence.
  Children tend to have higher ADNase B titers than adults.
  Variations in ADNase B titers in different age groups and geographic areas, as well as the local background prevalence of streptococcal infections, should be considered when using this test to evaluate GAS infection or post-streptococcal sequelae.
  Antibody levels peak during the convalescent phase, which is 3 to 5 weeks after the onset (acute phase) of group A beta-hemolytic streptococcal infection.

COLLECTION/STORAGE INFORMATION
- Draw 5 mL of blood into a red-top or serum separator tube for serum collection.
- Serum may be stored at -20°C.

LOINC CODES
- Code: 14207-5 (*Short Name* - Strep DNAse B Titr Ser)
- Code: 5133-4 (*Short Name* - Strep DNAse B Ser-aCnc)

Anti factor Xa measurement

TEST DEFINITION
Measurement of anti-activated factor X (anti-Xa) heparin assay in plasma for the therapeutic monitoring of low-molecular-weight heparin or unfractionated heparin

SYNONYMS
- Anti factor Xa level

REFERENCE RANGE
- Adults, low molecular weight heparin: Therapeutic range 0.5-1 International Units/mL
- Adults, unfractionated heparin: Therapeutic range 0.3-0.7 International Units/mL
  Please refer to your institution's reference ranges as lab normals may vary.

INDICATIONS
Low-molecular-weight heparin (LMWH) therapy
      Strength of Recommendation: Class IIa
      Strength of Evidence: Category B
Results Interpretation:
Laboratory test finding
    Low-molecular-weight heparin (LMWH) has a highly-predictable dose-related therapeutic effect, which lessens the need for ongoing monitoring. Patients who may benefit from ongoing or intermittent LMWH anti-Xa therapy monitoring include those with decreased creatinine clearance (eg, renal insufficiency, acute coronary syndrome), patients on long-term LMWH therapy (eg long-term outpatients with malignancy), patients with thrombosis refractory to warfarin (eg antiphospholipid antibody syndrome, myeloproliferative disorders) or unable to take warfarin, those at high risk of a bleed, patients who are markedly obese or underweight, and newborn and pediatric patients. Some researchers have suggested that anti-Xa monitoring of LMWH is only necessary in patients with significant renal impairment, and not in those with less severe renal insufficiency. As studies have shown a fall in therapeutic heparin levels as measured by anti-Xa assay with subsequent trimesters of gestation, monitoring levels in pregnant patients receiving fixed-dose LMWH is recommended.
    Although therapeutic levels of LMWH have not been definitively established for patients with renal failure or morbid obesity, published guidelines recommended a peak therapeutic range of 0.6 to 1.0 International Units/mL with twice-daily dosing, and 1 to 2 International Units/mL for daily dosing.
    The recommended therapeutic peak range for twice-daily dosing in patients being treated for venous thromboembolism is 0.5 to 1.1 International Units/mL when measured by the anti-factor Xa method.
    Uncomplicated patients being treated for venous thromboembolism by weight-adjusted fixed-dose LMWH do not require laboratory monitoring. Clinically stable patients receiving prophylactic LMWH preoperatively or postoperatively for venous thromboembolism do not require laboratory monitoring.
    The predictability of the anticoagulant effect of weight-adjusted LMWH dosing may be altered in pediatric patients as compared to adults. As the efficacy of LMWH in children has not been established in many instances, therapeutic dosing in children has been extrapolated from adult studies. Infants less than 2 to 3 months of age or who weigh less than 5 kg have increased requirements per kg. Dosing requirements of LMWH in children to achieve adult anti-Xa levels have been established.
    Acute coronary syndrome patients with anti-Xa levels less than 0.5 International Units/mL may be at increased risk of recurrent ischemic events and mortality.
    There may be an increased risk of bleeding for patients receiving therapeutic doses of LMWH with anti-Xa levels greater than 0.8 Units/mL at steady state.
Timing of Monitoring
    Because peak heparin level measurement appears to be more strongly correlated with safety and efficacy than trough levels, samples for monitoring of low-molecular-weight heparin (LMWH) therapy should be drawn 4 hours after subcutaneous drug administration, the generally accepted time to peak concentration in non-pregnant patients. In pregnancy, earlier peak times of 2 hours and 3 hours have been observed. The timing of blood sampling as it relates to the dosing schedule is critical for accurate interpretation of pharmacokinetics.

Unfractionated heparin (UFH) therapy
      Strength of Recommendation: Class IIa
      Strength of Evidence: Category B

Results Interpretation:
Laboratory test finding

A therapeutic range for unfractionated heparin (UFH) by anti-Xa assay of approximately 0.25 to 0.5 International Units/mL corresponds to a comparable protamine titration range of 0.2 to 0.4 Units/mL.

The target anti-Xa assay level for patients with venous thrombosis or pulmonary embolus receiving UFH is 0.3 to 0.7 Units/mL when a nomogram is used. For patients with venous thromboembolism or unstable angina, the recommended activated partial thromboplastin time should correspond to a heparin level of 0.3 to 0.7 Units/mL by antifactor Xa heparin levels. When a nomogram is used for patients with acute myocardial infarction receiving UFH, a target therapeutic range corresponding to an anti-Xa range of 0.14 to 0.34 Units/mL has been proposed. When using nomograms, locally established therapeutic ranges based on laboratory reagents must be used with recommended dosages adjusted accordingly; failure to adapt nomograms to the therapeutic range can result in potentially serious errors in heparin therapy dosing.

For heparin-resistant patients receiving more than 35,000 Units of UFH per 24 hours, the target anti-Xa assay heparin level is 0.35 to 0.7 International Units/mL.

COLLECTION/STORAGE INFORMATION

- Collect blood in a blue-top sodium citrate tube.
- For low molecular weight heparin, centrifuge sample within 1 hour of sample collection; perform assay within 2 to 4 hours of sample collection or may be frozen at -20°C.

LOINC CODES

- Code: 31159-7 (*Short Name* - Heparin Anti Xa Fld.NB-aCnc)

Anti-IgA assay

TEST DEFINITION

Measurement of anti-IgA antibodies in serum for the identification and management of potential and recognized blood transfusion reactions

INDICATIONS

Suspected anaphylactic blood transfusion reaction
Strength of Recommendation: Class IIa
Strength of Evidence: Category B
Results Interpretation:
Abnormal immunology findings

Detection of anti-IgA antibodies in the serum of blood transfusion recipients suggests that a patient may be at risk for (or may have had) an anaphylactic reaction.

Patients with anti-IgA antibodies and little to no IgA tend to have more severe anaphylactic transfusion reactions, particularly those patients with antibody titers greater than 1:1,000. The severity of transfusion reaction also correlates with the amount of IgA infused.

Suspected anti-IgA antibodies in the presence of IgA deficiency
Strength of Recommendation: Class IIa
Strength of Evidence: Category B
Results Interpretation:
Abnormal immunology findings

Healthy patients with severe IgA deficiency may develop anti-IgA antibodies, the levels of which tend to remain unchanged with long-term follow-up.

Postpartum levels of anti-IgA1 antibodies in pregnant women tend to rise; in contrast, levels of anti-IgA2 antibodies tend to fall after delivery.

COLLECTION/STORAGE INFORMATION

- Draw pretransfusion serum sample, if possible.
- Store at -2°C to -8°C if tested within 48 hours or at -20°C if tested after 48 hours.

LOINC CODES

- Code: 13312-4 (*Short Name* - IgA IgG SerPl-aCnc)

Anti-cyclic citrullinated peptide antibody level

TEST DEFINITION

Measurement of anti-cyclic citrullinated peptide antibodies in serum for the evaluation and management of rheumatoid arthritis.

SYNONYMS

- Anti-cyclic citrullinated peptide antibody measurement

REFERENCE RANGE

- Adults: Negative
  Please refer to your institution's reference ranges as lab normals may vary.

INDICATIONS

Suspected and known rheumatoid arthritis (RA)
    Strength of Recommendation: Class IIb
    Strength of Evidence: Category B
    Results Interpretation:
    Positive immunology findings

Anti-cyclic citrullinated peptide (anti-CCP) antibodies are generally considered to be indicators of a less favorable outcome; however, the ability to use anti-CCP to predict a poorer outcome in any individual patient has not been achieved.

Anti-CCP antibodies may be useful in differentiating early onset RA from polymyalgia rheumatica.

COMMON PANELS

- Arthritis panel

Antibody to JO-1 measurement

TEST DEFINITION

Measurement of anti-Jo-1 antibody levels in serum for the evaluation and management of inflammatory muscle disease and interstitial lung disease

REFERENCE RANGE

- Negative
  Please refer to your institution's reference ranges as lab normals may vary.

INDICATIONS

Diagnosis or monitoring of interstitial lung disease in patients with polymyositis/dermatomyositis
    Strength of Recommendation: Class IIa
    Strength of Evidence: Category B
    Results Interpretation:
    Jo-1 antibody positive

Elevated anti-Jo-1 antibodies in adults with polymyositis (PM) may indicate the presence of interstitial lung disease (ILD) and a more aggressive disease course.

Although relatively insensitive for detecting PM, a positive anti-Jo-1 antibody test may identify a subgroup of PM patients at higher risk for ILD.

A positive anti-Jo-1 antibody test in polymyositis/dermatomyositis (PM/DM) is considered a marker for possible ILD, which may be subclinical. However, PM/DM patients should be routinely screened for ILD, regardless of presence or absence of anti-Jo-1 antibody, as a large percentage of ILD patients may be seronegative.

The anti-Jo-1 antibody assay may be useful in evaluating patients with ILD and undefined connective tissue disease.

Suspected and known idiopathic inflammatory myopathy associated with connective tissue disease
    Strength of Recommendation: Class IIa
    Strength of Evidence: Category B
    Results Interpretation:
    Jo-1 antibody positive
       Elevated anti-Jo-1 antibodies appear to be specific to polymyositis/dermatomyositis (PM/DM), and may be used to differentiate PM/DM from other connective tissue disorders.

       Antibody to Jo-1 is considered a myositis-specific antibody (MSA), and should be measured in patients with suspected idiopathic inflammatory myopathy. A positive test suggests the presence of PM/DM, and/or a more aggressive disease course.

       Anti-Jo-1 antibody is rarely seen in connective tissue disorders other than polymyositis and dermatomyositis, and rarely seen in children with polymyositis and dermatomyositis.

       Anti-Jo-1 antibody is more commonly seen in polymyositis than dermatomyositis, and particularly in association with interstitial lung disease.

       Anti-Jo-1 antibodies are mainly IgG1 isotype (94%), but also include IgG3 and IgM isotypes. Two or more techniques are recommended to detect anti-Jo-1 antibodies, especially in the case of low-titer positive results.

COLLECTION/STORAGE INFORMATION
- Specimen Collection and Handling:
  - Collect serum specimen.
  - May be stored at -70°C.

LOINC CODES
- Code: 17031-6 (*Short Name* - ENA Jo1 Ab Ser QI IF)
- Code: 8076-2 (*Short Name* - ENA Jo1 Ab Ser QI)
- Code: 5235-7 (*Short Name* - ENA Jo-1 Ab Ser QI ID)
- Code: 5234-0 (*Short Name* - ENA Jo1 Ab Ser QI EIA)
- Code: 17032-4 (*Short Name* - ENA Jo1 Ab Ser IF-aCnc)
- Code: 14235-6 (*Short Name* - ENA Jo1 Ab Titr Ser)
- Code: 11565-9 (*Short Name* - ENA Jo-1 Ab Ser-aCnc)

Antibody to SM measurement

TEST DEFINITION
    Measurement of antibodies to the Smith antigen for the diagnosis and management of systemic lupus erythematosus

SYNONYMS
- Anti-Smith antibody measurement

REFERENCE RANGE
- Adults: Negative
Please refer to your institution's reference ranges as lab normals may vary.

INDICATIONS
Suspected lupus nephritis
    Strength of Recommendation: Class IIb
    Strength of Evidence: Category A
    Results Interpretation:
    Positive laboratory findings
       A positive result on an anti-Smith antibody assay is a questionable predictor of lupus nephritis.

Suspected systemic lupus erythematosus (SLE)
    Strength of Recommendation: Class IIa
    Strength of Evidence: Category A

Results Interpretation:
Positive laboratory findings
    A positive result on a Smith antibody assay usually confirms diagnosis of systemic lupus erythematosus (SLE). However, a negative result on a Smith antibody assay does not necessarily exclude a diagnosis of SLE. It is also of note that anti-Smith antibodies occur more frequently in SLE patients of African descent and may be a predictor of developing lupus nephritis.

CLINICAL NOTES
    Anti-Smith antibodies are more prevalent in African-Americans and other individuals of African descent.

COLLECTION/STORAGE INFORMATION
• Draw serum sample using a marbled tube.

LOINC CODES
• Code: 21523-6 (*Short Name* - ENA SM IgG Ser QI)
• Code: 5355-3 (*Short Name* - ENA SM Ab Ser QI CIE)
• Code: 17592-7 (*Short Name* - ENA SM Ab Ser IF-aCnc)
• Code: 31627-3 (*Short Name* - ENA SM Ab Ser QI)
• Code: 5357-9 (*Short Name* - ENA SM Ab Ser QI ID)
• Code: 18323-6 (*Short Name* - ENA SM IgG Ser-aCnc)
• Code: 17590-1 (*Short Name* - ENA SM Ab Titr Ser EIA)
• Code: 5356-1 (*Short Name* - ENA SM Ab Ser QI EIA)
• Code: 9722-0 (*Short Name* - ENA SM Ab Titr Ser)
• Code: 11090-8 (*Short Name* - ENA SM Ab Ser-aCnc)
• Code: 17591-9 (*Short Name* - ENA SM Ab Ser QI IF)
• Code: 17589-3 (*Short Name* - ENA SM Ab Titr Ser ID)

Antibody to SS-A measurement

TEST DEFINITION
    Detection of SS-A (anti-Ro) antibodies in serum or ocular fluid for the evaluation of immunological disorders

SYNONYMS
• Anti-Ro/SSA antibody measurement

REFERENCE RANGE
• Adults: Negative
    Please refer to your institution's reference ranges as lab normals may vary.

INDICATIONS
Suspected neonatal systemic lupus erythematosus
        Strength of Recommendation: Class IIa
        Strength of Evidence: Category B
    Results Interpretation:
    Serology positive
        The presence of SS-A (anti-Ro) antibodies at birth is the strongest indicator of neonatal lupus erythematosus (NLE).

Suspected Sj|f-gren's syndrome
        Strength of Recommendation: Class IIa
        Strength of Evidence: Category B
    Results Interpretation:
    Serology positive
        The presence of SS-A (anti-Ro) antibodies may be predictive of primary Sj|f-gren's syndrome, but the association is not as strong as that for SS-B (anti-La).
        In a study of 62 patients with primary Sj|f-gren's syndrome, the presence of SS-A (anti-Ro) antibodies was associated with kidney involvement and vasculitis.

In a study of 40 patients with autoimmune disease who tested positive for SS-A antibodies, those with primary Sj|f-gren's syndrome had higher SS-A antibody levels than patients with systemic lupus erythematosus.

Suspected systemic lupus erythematosus
    Strength of Recommendation: Class IIa
    Strength of Evidence: Category B
    Results Interpretation:
    Abnormal laboratory findings
       A positive anti-Ro/SSA antibody test is highly indicative of SLE and may be clinically useful when antinuclear antibody (ANA) and anti-dsDNA are absent in a patient with suspected SLE.
       A positive result by anti-SS-A (anti-Ro) antibody test prior to the onset of clinical symptoms indicates that a patient may be 40 times more likely than normal patients to develop systemic lupus erythematosus (SLE); nevertheless, antibody positivity does not imply that onset of clinical disease is imminent.
       SLE patients who have both anti-SS-A and anti-SS-B (anti-La) antibodies are less likely to have renal disease than patients with only anti-SS-A antibodies.

COLLECTION/STORAGE INFORMATION
- Draw serum sample in a red marbled tube.
- Store sample at -20°C or -30°C.

LOINC CODES
- Code: 17585-1 (*Short Name* - ENA SS-A IgG Ser Ql EIA)
- Code: 17792-3 (*Short Name* - ENA SS-A Ab Ser-aCnc)
- Code: 5352-0 (*Short Name* - ENA SS-A Ab Ser Ql ID)
- Code: 8093-7 (*Short Name* - ENA SS-A Ab Ser Ql)
- Code: 17583-6 (*Short Name* - ENA SS-A Ab Ser Ql IF)
- Code: 17584-4 (*Short Name* - ENA SS-A Ab Ser IF-aCnc)
- Code: 31625-7 (*Short Name* - ENA SS-A IgG Ser Ql)
- Code: 29964-4 (*Short Name* - ENA SS-A IgG Ser EIA-aCnc)
- Code: 5351-2 (*Short Name* - ENA SS-A Ab Ser Ql EIA)

Antibody to SS-B measurement

TEST DEFINITION
Detection of SS-B (anti-La) antibodies in serum for the evaluation of autoimmune disorders

SYNONYMS
- Anti-SS-B/La antibody measurement

REFERENCE RANGE
- Adults: Negative
Please refer to your institution's reference ranges as lab normals may vary.

INDICATIONS
Suspected Sj|f-gren syndrome
    Strength of Recommendation: Class IIa
    Strength of Evidence: Category B
    Results Interpretation:
    Abnormal laboratory findings
       A positive result on an SS-B (anti-La) antibody test may be diagnostically useful or be predictive of the development of Sj|f-gren syndrome.
       Positive serum samples for SS-B antibodies typically report 1,000 or more antibody units and are at least 50% inhibited by 10 mcg/mL of SS-B antibody.
       Patients with purpura tend to have more than a 1,000-fold higher level of SS-B binding than healthy patients.

Suspected systemic lupus erythematosus
>   **Strength of Recommendation:** Class IIa
>   **Strength of Evidence:** Category B
>   **Results Interpretation:**
>   **Abnormal laboratory findings**

A positive anti-SS-B (anti-La) antibody titer indicates that a patient may be 40 times more likely than normal patients to develop systemic lupus erythematosus (SLE).

Patients with late-onset systemic lupus erythematosus (SLE) are more likely than early-onset patients to have anti-SS-B (anti-La) antibodies in their serum. SLE patients who have both anti-SS-B and anti-SS-A antibodies are less likely to have renal disease than patients with only anti-SS-A antibodies.

In a patient with suspected systemic lupus erythematosus (SLE) but a negative antinuclear antibody (ANA) test, a positive anti-La/SSB antibody test supports the diagnosis of SLE. However, Sj|f-gren syndrome must be excluded, because a positive anti-La/SSB antibody test is also common in that disorder.

COLLECTION/STORAGE INFORMATION
- Draw serum sample in a red marbled tube.
- Store sample at -20°C or -30°C.

LOINC CODES
- Code: 29965-1 (*Short Name* - ENA SS-B IgG Ser EIA-aCnc)
- Code: 5354-6 (*Short Name* - ENA SS-B Ab Ser QI ID)
- Code: 5353-8 (*Short Name* - ENA SS-B Ab Ser QI EIA)
- Code: 17586-9 (*Short Name* - ENA SS-B Ab Ser QI IF)
- Code: 17588-5 (*Short Name* - ENA SS-B IgG Ser QI EIA)
- Code: 17791-5 (*Short Name* - ENA SS-B Ab Ser-aCnc)
- Code: 17587-7 (*Short Name* - ENA SS-B Ab Ser IF-aCnc)
- Code: 8094-5 (*Short Name* - ENA SS-B Ab Ser QI)
- Code: 31626-5 (*Short Name* - ENA SS-B IgG Ser QI)
- Code: 29949-5 (*Short Name* - ENA SS-B Ab Titr Ser ID)

Antibody to Scl-70 measurement

TEST DEFINITION
Detection of anti-Scl-70 antibodies in serum for the evaluation of immunological disorders

SYNONYMS
- Topoisomerase I antibody measurement

REFERENCE RANGE
- Adults: Negative
  Please refer to your institution's reference ranges as lab normals may vary.

INDICATIONS
Suspected systemic lupus erythematosus
>   **Strength of Recommendation:** Class IIa
>   **Strength of Evidence:** Category B
>   **Results Interpretation:**
>   **Serology positive**

A positive result on an anti-Scl-70 antibody test may indicate systemic lupus erythematosus (SLE).

In SLE patients, levels of anti-Scl-70 antibodies fluctuate widely but are highly correlated to manifestations of disease activity, particularly pulmonary hypertension and renal involvement. In general, levels of anti-Scl-70 antibodies in patients with SLE are lower than levels in patients with systemic sclerosis.

Suspected systemic sclerosis (scleroderma)
>   **Strength of Recommendation:** Class IIa
>   **Strength of Evidence:** Category A

Results Interpretation:
Serology positive

A positive result on an anti-Scl-70 antibody test may aid in the diagnosis of systemic sclerosis.

In general, levels of anti-Scl-70 antibodies in patients with systemic sclerosis tend to be higher than levels in patients with systemic lupus erythematosus.

The presence of anti-Scl-70 antibodies in patients with systemic sclerosis is associated with higher mortality and clinical manifestations such as pulmonary fibrosis and diffuse cutaneous involvement.

Anti-Scl-70 antibodies are rare in healthy individuals. Patients with systemic sclerosis who are anti-Scl-70 antibody positive tend to have a worse prognosis that systemic sclerotic patients who are positive for other autoantibodies.

COLLECTION/STORAGE INFORMATION

- Draw serum sample in a red marbled tube.
- Store sample at -20°C.

LOINC CODES

- Code: 8092-9 (*Short Name* - ENA Scl70 Ab Ser QI)
- Code: 17570-3 (*Short Name* - ENA Scl70 IgG Ser QI EIA)
- Code: 5348-8 (*Short Name* - ENA Scl70 Ab Ser QI EIA)
- Code: 5349-6 (*Short Name* - ENA Scl70 Ab Ser QI ID)
- Code: 27416-7 (*Short Name* - ENA Scl70 Ab Ser-aCnc)
- Code: 21518-6 (*Short Name* - ENA Scl-70 IgG Ser QI)
- Code: 26975-3 (*Short Name* - ENA Scl70 Ab Ser EIA-aCnc)
- Code: 17569-5 (*Short Name* - ENA Scl70 Ab Ser QI IF)

Antibody to centromere measurement

TEST DEFINITION

Detection of anti-centromere (kinetochore) antibodies in serum for the evaluation of immunological disorders.

REFERENCE RANGE

- Adults: Negative
Please refer to your institution's reference ranges as lab normals may vary.

INDICATIONS

Raynaud phenomenon (RP)
> **Strength of Recommendation:** Class IIa
> **Strength of Evidence:** Category B

Results Interpretation:
Serology positive

A positive anti-centromere antibody (ACA) may suggest Raynaud phenomenon (RP).

Positive ACA may be predictive of scleroderma in patients with RP.

Frequency of Monitoring

Once patients are seropositive for anti-centromere antibodies they remain so over time, making serial measurements unnecessary.

Suspected and known CREST syndrome (calcinosis, Raynaud phenomenon, esophageal dysmotility, sclerodactyly, and telangiectasia)
> **Strength of Recommendation:** Class IIa
> **Strength of Evidence:** Category B

Results Interpretation:
Serology positive

A positive anti-centromere antibody finding is suggestive of CREST syndrome.

Frequency of Monitoring

Once patients are seropositive for anti-centromere antibodies they remain so over time, making serial measurements unnecessary.

Suspected and known systemic sclerosis (scleroderma)
    Strength of Recommendation: Class IIa
    Strength of Evidence: Category B
Results Interpretation:
Serology positive
    A positive anti-centromere antibody (ACA) finding by immunofluorescence is associated with systemic sclerosis (SSc). ACA are more commonly found in Caucasian SSc patients than in SSc patients of Hispanic, Asian, African-American, or Thai origin. ACA are uncommon in healthy individuals or in patients with other connective tissues diseases.
Frequency of Monitoring
    Once patients are seropositive for anti-centromere antibodies they remain so over time, making serial measurements unnecessary.

COLLECTION/STORAGE INFORMATION
- Draw serum specimen in red-top or serum separator tube.
- Store specimen at -20°C.

LOINC CODES
- Code: 31290-0 (*Short Name* - Centromere IgG Ser-aCnc)
- Code: 5077-3 (*Short Name* - Centromere Ab Titr Ser IF)
- Code: 16570-4 (*Short Name* - Centromere Ab Ser Ql IF)
- Code: 17830-1 (*Short Name* - Centromere Ab Fld-aCnc)
- Code: 16137-2 (*Short Name* - Centromere Ab Ser Ql)
- Code: 29966-9 (*Short Name* - Centromere IgG Titr Ser IF)

Antibody to double stranded DNA measurement

TEST DEFINITION
    Serologic test that detects or distinguishes native (double-stranded) DNA IgG or IgM autoantibodies (anti-dsDNA) that are highly specific for systemic lupus erythematosus (SLE)

SYNONYMS
- Antibody to native DNA measurement

REFERENCE RANGE
- Adults and Children: Negative at 1:10 dilution
  Please refer to your institution's reference ranges as lab normals may vary.

INDICATIONS
Suspected systemic lupus erythematosus (SLE)
    Strength of Recommendation: Class I
    Strength of Evidence: Category B
Results Interpretation:
Serology positive
    High-titer IgG antibodies against dsDNA (anti-dsDNA) and/or against Smith antigen (Anti-Sm) are usually specific for SLE. However, because of the almost 100% sensitivity, anti-nuclear antibodies (ANA) tests using Hep-2 cells are the screening method of choice.
    Patients with negative ANA studies are unlikely to have SLE. If the ANA test is positive, anti-dsDNA, anti-ENAs, and antiphospholipid antibody studies are necessary to confirm the diagnosis and define the patient subset.
    An increase followed by a decrease in anti-dsDNA antibody titers is statistically associated with a flare of SLE, but the clinical utility of using anti-dsDNA antibody titers as biomarkers for flares appears to be limited.

COMMON PANELS
- Collagen/Lupus panel

CLINICAL NOTES

Anti-dsDNA antibodies are a principal marker in the American College of Rheumatology diagnostic criteria for SLE.

A quantitative determination of anti-dsDNA (ELISA or Farr assay) is preferable for monitoring SLE disease activity, particularly nephritis.

COLLECTION/STORAGE INFORMATION

- Specimen Collection and Handling:
  - Collect a 7-mL venous blood sample in a red- or marble-topped tube
  - Store serum at -30° C

LOINC CODES

- Code: 6457-6 (*Short Name* - dsDNA Ab Ser Ql CLIF)
- Code: 31348-6 (*Short Name* - dsDNA Ab Ser Ql)
- Code: 5130-0 (*Short Name* - dsDNA Ab Ser-aCnc)
- Code: 12277-0 (*Short Name* - dsDNA Ab Ser Ql Farr)
- Code: 15177-9 (*Short Name* - dsDNA Ab Fld-aCnc)
- Code: 11013-0 (*Short Name* - dsDNA Ab Titr Ser)
- Code: 5131-8 (*Short Name* - dsDNA Ab Ser Ql IF)

Antibody to gastric parietal cell measurement

TEST DEFINITION

Detection of parietal cell antibodies in blood for the evaluation and management of chronic atrophic type A (autoimmune) gastritis and related pernicious anemia

SYNONYMS

- Parietal cell autoantibodies
- Parietal cell autoantibody level

REFERENCE RANGE

- Adults: Negative at 1:20 dilution
  Please refer to your institution's reference ranges as lab normals may vary.

INDICATIONS

Suspected pernicious anemia secondary to chronic atrophic gastritis
  Strength of Recommendation: Class IIb
  Strength of Evidence: Category C
  Results Interpretation:
  Autoantibody titer positive
    The presence of parietal cell antibodies is predictive of the presence of autoimmune gastritis, which may progress to pernicious anemia over 20 to 30 years.
    Parietal cell antibodies are also found in 30% of asymptomatic first degree relatives of patients with pernicious anemia and in patients with autoimmune endocrinopathies.

COLLECTION/STORAGE INFORMATION

- Specimen Collection and Handling:
  - Collect the serum sample in a red top tube.
  - Serum is stable for 12 months at $-20°C$.

LOINC CODES

- Code: 31556-4 (*Short Name* - PCA IgG Ser Ql)
- Code: 5271-2 (*Short Name* - PCA Ab Titr Ser IF)
- Code: 8087-9 (*Short Name* - PCA Ab Ser-aCnc)
- Code: 27320-1 (*Short Name* - PCA Ab Titr Ser)
- Code: 14241-4 (*Short Name* - PCA Ab Ser Ql)
- Code: 29963-6 (*Short Name* - PCA IgG Ser Ql IF)

• Code: 26969-6 (*Short Name* - PCA Ab Ser QI IF)

Antibody to mitochondria measurement

TEST DEFINITION
Detection of antimitochondrial antibodies in serum for evaluation of primary biliary cirrhosis

SYNONYMS
• Antimitochondrial autoantibod.
• Antimitochondrial autoantibody level
• Mitochondrial antibody level

REFERENCE RANGE
• Negative
Please refer to your institution's reference ranges as lab normals may vary.

INDICATIONS
Suspected primary biliary cirrhosis
    Strength of Recommendation: Class I
    Strength of Evidence: Category C
    Results Interpretation:
    Antibody titer - finding
    An antimitochondrial antibody (AMA) titer of 1:40 or greater by immunofluorescence, along with an elevated serum alkaline phosphatase level, is characteristic of primary biliary cirrhosis.
    An AMA titer of 1:40 or greater with a normal alkaline phosphatase level should be be evaluated annually for biochemical alterations.

    False Results
    In approximately 5% to 10% of patients with clinical and biochemical evidence of primary biliary cirrhosis (PBC), antimitochondrial antibody titers remain consistently negative. The absence of seropositivity in patients with PBC has been referred to as 'autoimmune cholangitis' or 'immune cholangitis'.

COLLECTION/STORAGE INFORMATION
• Store serum at -20°C

LOINC CODES
• Code: 8077-0 (*Short Name* - Mitochondria Ab Ser-aCnc)
• Code: 14236-4 (*Short Name* - Mitochondria Ab Ser QI)
• Code: 17284-1 (*Short Name* - Mitochondria Ab Ser QI IF)
• Code: 5247-2 (*Short Name* - Mitochondria Ab Titr Ser IF)
• Code: 17285-8 (*Short Name* - Mitochondria Ab Ser IF-aCnc)

Antidiuretic hormone measurement

TEST DEFINITION
Measurement of antidiuretic hormone (vasopressin) in serum for the evaluation of body water balance disorders

SYNONYMS
• Arginine vasopressin measurement

REFERENCE RANGE
• Normal range is dependent on serum osmolality:
• Serum osmolality 270-280 mOsm/kg: <1.5 pg/mL (<1.4 pmol/L)
• Serum osmolality 280-285 mOsm/kg: <2.5 pg/mL (<2.3 pmol/L)

- Serum osmolality 285-290 mOsm/kg: 1-5 pg/mL (0.9-4.6 pmol/L)
- Serum osmolality 290-295 mOsm/kg: 2-7 pg/mL (1.9-6.5 pmol/L)
- Serum osmolality 295-300 mOsm/kg: 4-12 pg/mL (3.7-11.1 pmol/L)
  Please refer to your institution's reference ranges as lab normals may vary.

INDICATIONS

Suspected diabetes insipidus
> **Strength of Recommendation:** Class IIb
> **Strength of Evidence:** Category C
> **Results Interpretation:**
> **Abnormal laboratory findings**
>> Differential diagnosis of both neurogenic and nephrogenic diabetes insipidus (DI) requires simultaneous evaluation of urine and serum sodium and osmolality, and serum antidiuretic hormone (ADH).
>> In neurogenic DI, ADH levels decrease as plasma osmolality increases. In nephrogenic DI, plasma ADH levels are often elevated in relation to plasma osmolality.
>> In congenital DI, family members who are heterozygous carriers of the ADH gene mutation may present with decreased ADH levels, which may be the sole subclinical manifestation of ADH deficiency observed in these patients.

Suspected syndrome of inappropriate antidiuretic hormone secretion (SIADH)
> **Strength of Recommendation:** Class IIa
> **Strength of Evidence:** Category C
> **Results Interpretation:**
> **Abnormal laboratory findings**
>> Elevated serum ADH levels out of proportion to serum osmolality changes are often seen in patients with syndrome of inappropriate antidiuretic hormone (SIADH). For more than 80% of patients, absolute ADH levels will be normal, and must therefore be interpreted in conjunction with plasma osmolality levels.

CLINICAL NOTES

Antidiuretic hormone assay results must always be interpreted in conjunction with serum osmolality, urine osmolality, intravascular volume status, and blood pressure.

COLLECTION/STORAGE INFORMATION

- Specimen Collection and Handling:
    - Collect specimen in EDTA (lavender) tube.
    - Separate specimen immediately in refrigerated centrifuge.
    - Freeze specimen at −20°C.

LOINC CODES

- Code: 26928-2 (*Short Name* - Vasopressin 24H Ur Ql)
- Code: 12982-5 (*Short Name* - Vasopressin sp2 p chal Plas-mCnc)
- Code: 13903-0 (*Short Name* - Vasopressin Ur-mCnc)

Antineuronal nuclear antibody type 2 measurement

TEST DEFINITION

Measurement of antineuronal nuclear antibodies type 2 (anti-Ri) in serum for the identification and management of paraneoplastic cerebellar disorders

SYNONYMS

- ANNA-2 measurement
- Anti-Ri measurement
- Neuronal nuclear type 2 antibody assay

REFERENCE RANGE
- Negative
  Please refer to your institution's reference ranges as lab normals may vary.

INDICATIONS
Suspected paraneoplastic cerebellar degeneration (cerebellar ataxia)
    Strength of Recommendation: Class IIa
    Strength of Evidence: Category B
  Results Interpretation:
  Abnormal immunology findings
    In the presence of CNS clinical signs and symptoms, a positive antineuronal nuclear antibody type 2 (anti-Ri) assay may indicate paraneoplastic cerebellar degeneration (cerebellar ataxia), and may initiate clinical investigation into a possible neoplasm, if not already identified.
    Not all patients with paraneoplastic cerebellar degeneration have antineuronal autoantibodies. A minority of patients with high titers of anti-Ri antibodies do not develop tumors.

Suspected paraneoplastic opsoclonus-myoclonus syndrome
    Strength of Recommendation: Class IIa
    Strength of Evidence: Category B
  Results Interpretation:
  Abnormal immunology findings
    In the presence of relevant CNS clinical signs and symptoms, a positive result on an antineuronal nuclear antibodies type 2 (anti-Ri) antibody assay may indicate paraneoplastic opsoclonus-myoclonus syndrome, and may initiate clinical investigation into a possible neoplasm, if not already identified.
    Anti-Ri antibodies are not observed in patients with nonparaneoplastic opsoclonus. Not all patients with paraneoplastic syndromes have antineuronal antibodies.
    Titers of anti-Ri antibody were higher in serum than in cerebrospinal fluid (CSF), although relative amounts were found to be higher in CSF.

LOINC CODES
- Code: 17344-3 (*Short Name* - Hu2 Ab Ser IF-aCnc)
- Code: 13998-0 (*Short Name* - Hu 2 Ab Titr Ser)
- Code: 17343-5 (*Short Name* - Hu2 Ab CSF QI)
- Code: 17342-7 (*Short Name* - Hu2 Ab Ser-aCnc)
- Code: 24401-2 (*Short Name* - Hu 2 Ab Titr CSF IF)
- Code: 24404-6 (*Short Name* - Hu2 Ab Titr CSF IB)
- Code: 31539-0 (*Short Name* - Hu2 Ab Ser QI)
- Code: 31538-2 (*Short Name* - Hu2 Ab CSF-aCnc)

Antineuronal nuclear antibody-type I measurement

TEST DEFINITION
    Measurement of antineuronal nuclear antibody type 1 (anti-Hu) in serum for the identification and management of paraneoplastic disorders

SYNONYMS
- ANNA-I measurement

REFERENCE RANGE
- Negative
  Please refer to your institution's reference ranges as lab normals may vary.

INDICATIONS

Suspected or known paraneoplastic sensory neuropathy
   Strength of Recommendation: Class IIa
   Strength of Evidence: Category B
   Results Interpretation:
   Abnormal immunology findings
      In the presence of clinical signs and symptoms not attributable to other pathology, a positive result for type 1 antineuronal nuclear antibodies (anti-Hu) may be indicative of paraneoplastic sensory neuropathy.
      High titers of anti-Hu antibodies in the presence of either subacute sensory neuropathy and/or encephalomyelopathy is diagnostic for anti-Hu syndrome.
      Anti-Hu antibodies are not found in normal subjects.

Suspected paraneoplastic encephalomyelitis syndrome
   Strength of Recommendation: Class IIa
   Strength of Evidence: Category B
   Results Interpretation:
   Abnormal immunology findings
      In the presence of relevant clinical signs and symptoms not attributable to other pathologies, a positive result on an assay for antineuronal nuclear antibodies type 1 (anti-Hu) may be indicative of paraneoplastic encephalomyelitis.
      High titers of anti-Hu antibodies in the presence of either subacute sensory neuropathy and/or encephalomyelopathy is diagnostic for anti-Hu syndrome
      Anti-Hu antibodies are very seldom identified in normal subjects.

LOINC CODES

- Code: 12854-6 (*Short Name* - Hu 1 Ab Ser-aCnc)
- Code: 13115-1 (*Short Name* - Hu 1 Ab Ser)
- Code: 24400-4 (*Short Name* - Hu 1 Ab Titr CSF IF)
- Code: 24403-8 (*Short Name* - Hu1 Ab Titr CSF IB)
- Code: 13997-2 (*Short Name* - Hu1 Ab Titr Ser)
- Code: 31537-4 (*Short Name* - Hu1 Ab CSF-aCnc)
- Code: 33615-6 (*Short Name* - Hu1 Ab Ser QI)

Antiphospholipid antibody measurement

TEST DEFINITION
   Measurement of a heterogeneous population of immunoglobulin in serum for evaluation of antiphospholipid syndrome (APS)

REFERENCE RANGE
- Adults:
- Anti-beta$_2$ -glycoprotein I antibody assay:
- IgG: 0-15 units/mL
- Anticardiolipin antibody assay:
- IgG: 0-15 GPL units (0-15 arbitrary units)
- IgM: 0-15 MPL units (0-15 arbitrary units)
- Lupus anticoagulant screen: Negative
   Please refer to your institution's reference ranges as lab normals may vary.

INDICATIONS

Patients with systemic lupus erythematosus and suspected antiphospholipid syndrome.
   Strength of Recommendation: Class IIa
   Strength of Evidence: Category B
   Results Interpretation:
   Autoantibody titer positive
      Elevated antiphospholipid antibody titers identify systemic lupus erythematosus (SLE) patients who are at increased risk for subsequent thromboembolic complications. Approximately 10% of SLE patients have lupus anticoagulant antibodies.

Suspected antiphospholipid syndrome
> **Strength of Recommendation:** Class IIa
> **Strength of Evidence:** Category B
> **Results Interpretation:**
> **Autoantibody titer positive**
> The diagnosis of antiphospholipid syndrome (APS) requires both a history of thrombotic event (or presumptive evidence of placental insufficiency) and the identification of at least one antiphospholipid antibody. The identification of multiple antiphospholipid markers strongly supports the diagnosis of antiphospholipid syndrome; no single antibody is diagnostic.
> Antibodies to beta$_2$ -glycoprotein I appear to be more closely associated with APS (76%) versus systemic lupus erythematosus (15%).
> Presence of multiple antiphospholipid antibodies increases the risk of thrombotic events.

COMMON PANELS
- Antiphospholipid antibody panel

ABNORMAL RESULTS
- Results increased in:
  - HIV-1 infection
  - Hepatitis C
  - Syphilis

CLINICAL NOTES
To optimize disease diagnosis, patients should be screened for more multiple antiphospholipid antibodies (eg, anticardiolipin antibody, beta$_2$ -glycoprotein I antibody).

Laboratory concordance for IgG, IgM, and IgA antibodies to phospholipids has been reported at 55%, based upon a 20-patient sample tested at 10 centers. Clinical correlation and repeated testing is recommended.

COLLECTION/STORAGE INFORMATION
- Specimen Collection and Handling:
  - Lupus anticoagulant test:
    - Collect blood in citrate containing (blue-top) tube and place on ice
    - Stable at 4°C up to 4 hours and at -20°C for 2 months
  - Anticardiolipin antibody assay:
    - Collect blood in red-top tube for serum separation.
    - Store at -20°C.

LOINC CODES
- Code: 17459-9 (*Short Name* - Phospholipid IgA Ser EIA-aCnc)
- Code: 3285-4 (*Short Name* - Phospholipid Ab Ser EIA-aCnc)
- Code: 19140-3 (*Short Name* - Phospholipid Ab Ser QI)
- Code: 3286-2 (*Short Name* - Phospholipid IgG Ser EIA-aCnc)
- Code: 3287-0 (*Short Name* - Phospholipid IgM Ser EIA-aCnc)
- Code: 20429-7 (*Short Name* - Phospholipid IgM Ser QI)
- Code: 20428-9 (*Short Name* - Phospholipid IgG Ser QI)
- Code: 31561-4 (*Short Name* - Phospholipid IgA Ser-aCnc)
- Code: 7800-6 (*Short Name* - Phospholipid Ab Ser-aCnc)

Antithrombin III assay

TEST DEFINITION
Measurement of antithrombin III in plasma for the evaluation and management of coagulation disorders

REFERENCE RANGE
- Adults:
- Antigenic: 22-39 mg/dL (220-390 mg/L)
- Functional: 80%-130% (0.8-1.3 units/L)
  Please refer to your institution's reference ranges as lab normals may vary.

INDICATIONS

Sepsis
Strength of Recommendation: Class IIb
Strength of Evidence: Category C
Results Interpretation:
Antithrombin III deficiency
Decreased antithrombin levels may be a manifestation of septic physiology.
A decrease of antithrombin III (AT-III) to a value below 50% may predict mortality. Plasma levels of AT-III in sepsis were significantly lower in patients who died compared with those who survived.

Suspected antithrombin deficiency in venous thromboembolism
Strength of Recommendation: Class IIb
Strength of Evidence: Category B
Results Interpretation:
Antithrombin III deficiency
An antithrombin III level less than 75% of normal activity increases risk of thrombotic or thromboembolic disease. About 70% of persons with a venous thromboembolism have decreased antithrombin III levels prior to initiation of anticoagulation therapy; However, in over 90% of cases of venous thromboembolism associated with decreased levels of antithrombin III, low antithrombin levels are secondary to consumption following the development of clot as opposed to a hereditary disorder. In general, the larger the clot burden, the greater the decrease in antithrombin levels.
Patients with lower antithrombin III levels may have a suboptimal response to heparin therapy. Those with a level of less than 40% usually will not respond to heparin therapy at all.

Suspected DIC
Strength of Recommendation: Class IIb
Strength of Evidence: Category B
Results Interpretation:
Antithrombin III deficiency
Decreased antithrombin levels are indicative of a poor prognosis in DIC.

Suspected heparin resistance
Strength of Recommendation: Class IIa
Strength of Evidence: Category B
Results Interpretation:
Antithrombin III deficiency
Antithrombin III activity may be decreased in patients with heparin resistance.

Suspected hereditary antithrombin III (AT-III) deficiency
Strength of Recommendation: Class I
Strength of Evidence: Category C
Results Interpretation:
Antithrombin III deficiency
Risk for thrombosis is higher in patients with antithrombin deficiency than in other inherited thrombophilic states; approximately 60% will have an episode of venous thrombosis by age 60.
Antithrombin III (AT-III) deficiency, when inherited, may be type I or type II. Type I deficiency is associated with a quantitative deficit of AT-III that is approximately 50% of normal. In type II deficiency, the total antigen level is near normal but there is a reduction in functional activity.

Suspected preeclampsia
Results Interpretation:
Antithrombin III deficiency
Antithrombin III levels are lower in preeclamptic patients with more than or equal to 5 g/L of proteinuria than in women with normal pregnancies.

COMMON PANELS
• Hypercoagulation panel

ABNORMAL RESULTS
• Results increased in:
  • Menstruation

CLINICAL NOTES

Functional assays measure protein activity, while antigenic assays (immunoassays) simply measure the presence of protein.

COLLECTION/STORAGE INFORMATION

- Specimen Collection and Handling:
    - Collect venous blood in light blue tube (sodium citrate).
    - Specimen stable for 2 weeks at -25°C

LOINC CODES

- Code: 20991-6 (*Short Name* - AT III PPP-Imp)

Apolipoproteins E measurement

TEST DEFINITION

Measurement of apolipoprotein E in plasma for evaluation of a possible genetic component to lipid abnormalities, coronary disease, and/or cognitive decline

REFERENCE RANGE

- Adults: 3-6 mg/dL (0.8-1.6 micromol/L)
- Adults: 35 to 65 years: 28% higher than values at 20 to 30 years
- Adults over 60 years: 80% higher than values at 20 to 30 years
- Neonates: 62% higher than values at 20 to 30 years (may vary with gender)
- Children: 5 to 9 years: 15% -39% higher than values at 20 to 30 years
- Females: 0%-19% higher than males (may vary with age)
    Please refer to your institution's reference ranges as lab normals may vary.

INDICATIONS

Suspected Alzheimer's disease
    Strength of Recommendation: Class IIb
    Strength of Evidence: Category B
    Results Interpretation:
    Apolipoprotein E phenotype - finding
    An association has been established between apolipoprotein E (APOE) e4 allele and Alzheimer's disease (AD). The APOE e4 allele is present in 34% to 65% of patients with AD, and its presence increases risk for AD 2-fold.
    Conclusive diagnosis of AD can only be made at autopsy through identification of neuronal loss, senile plaques, and neurofibrillary tangles.

Suspected coronary atherosclerosis and known hyperlipidemia
    Strength of Recommendation: Class IIb
    Strength of Evidence: Category B
    Results Interpretation:
    Apolipoprotein E phenotype - finding
    The apolipoprotein E (APOE) e4 allele has been associated with elevated plasma total cholesterol, while the e2 allele has been associated with decreased plasma total cholesterol. APOE e2 and e4 alleles may be associated with elevated plasma triglyceride. The levels and allele isoforms seen in cardiovascular disease are highly variable.

CLINICAL NOTES

Apolipoprotein E presents as 3 major isoforms: E-2, E-3, and E-4.

COLLECTION/STORAGE INFORMATION

- Have patient fast overnight.
- Collect blood in purple top (EDTA) tube.

LOINC CODES
- Code: 15351-0 (*Short Name* - Apo E-II Bld Ql)
- Code: 15352-8 (*Short Name* - Apo E-III Bld Ql)
- Code: 1886-1 (*Short Name* - Apo E SerPl-mCnc)
- Code: 1879-6 (*Short Name* - Apo E-II SerPl-mCnc)

Apt-Downey test

TEST DEFINITION
Evaluation of bloody stools or hematemesis in neonates to differentiate fetal from maternal blood

INDICATIONS
Suspected gastrointestinal tract bleeding in neonates
   Strength of Recommendation: Class IIb
   Strength of Evidence: Category B
   Results Interpretation:
   Finding of body product
      Bloody stool or emesis, when mixed with water and 1% sodium hydroxide solution, will turn yellow-brown after several minutes if the blood is of maternal origin; fetal blood will remain pink. If the test is positive for fetal hemoglobin, a gastrointestinal bleed work-up should follow.
      Subjective visual determination of color change can lead to misinterpretation of results or inconclusive findings.
      A time lapse of greater than 30 minutes from the origin of the stain to the time of testing will decrease the accuracy of the results.

COLLECTION/STORAGE INFORMATION
- Stool or emesis sample should be as fresh as possible; test within 30 minutes.
- Stool sample should be grossly bloody but not tarry.
- A small stool sample size increases the risk of inconclusive or misinterpreted results.
- If the only available sample is a bloody diaper, water and sodium hydroxide can be added directly to the stain with results apparent in several minutes

LOINC CODES
- Code: 4631-8 (*Short Name* - Hgb Apt Stl Ql)

Arginine measurement

TEST DEFINITION
Measurement of arginine in plasma for detection of acquired and hereditary amino acid disorders

REFERENCE RANGE
- Premature neonate, 1 day: 0.87 ± 0.35 mg/dL (50 ± 20 micromol/L)
- Neonate, 1 day: 0.38-1.53 mg/dL (22-88 micromol/L)
- Infants 1 to 3 months: 0.84 ± 0.23 mg/dL (48 ± 13 micromol/L)
- Infants 2 to 6 months: 0.98-2.47 mg/dL (56-142 micromol/L)
- Infants 9 to 24 months: 0.19-1.13 mg/dL (11-65 micromol/L)
- Children 3 to 10 years: 0.4-1.5 mg/dL (23-86 micromol/L)
- Children 6 to 18 years: 0.77-2.26 mg/dL (44-130 micromol/L)
- Adults: 0.37-2.4 mg/dL (21-138 micromol/L)
   Please refer to your institution's reference ranges as lab normals may vary.

INDICATIONS
Suspected inborn error of metabolism
   Strength of Recommendation: Class IIa
   Strength of Evidence: Category C

Results Interpretation:
Increased amino acid

Inherited amino acid disorders are directly related to the absence of an enzyme involved in the metabolism of one or more amino acids; therefore, an elevated plasma level of a particular amino acid is highly suggestive of an inherited metabolic defect. In the majority of cases amino acid and organic acid analysis together permit diagnostic confirmation in infants. Immediate treatment should be initiated when an inborn error of metabolism is suspected, even if a definitive diagnosis has not yet been determined.

Arginase deficiency is associated with an elevated serum arginine level. Carbamoyl phosphate synthetase deficiency is associated with increased blood levels of alanine, glutamine, glycine and lysine, as well as low or undetectable arginine and citrulline levels.

COLLECTION/STORAGE INFORMATION

- Specimen Collection and Handling:
  - Immediately place sample in ice water.
  - Isolate plasma sample and freeze it within 1 hour; sample stable for 1 week at -20°C.
  - Sample should be deproteinized and stored at -70°C for protracted periods of usage.

LOINC CODES

- Code: 27296-3 (*Short Name* - Arginine Ur-sCnc)
- Code: 1895-2 (*Short Name* - Arginine 24H Ur-mRate)
- Code: 1891-1 (*Short Name* - Arginine CSF-mCnc)
- Code: 16401-2 (*Short Name* - Arginine Ur Ql)
- Code: 26985-2 (*Short Name* - Arginine Amn-sCnc)
- Code: 13708-3 (*Short Name* - Arginine/creat Ur-mRto)
- Code: 22727-2 (*Short Name* - Arginine XXX-sCnc)
- Code: 25860-8 (*Short Name* - Arginine 24H Ur-sCnc)
- Code: 25322-9 (*Short Name* - Arginine 24H Ur-sRate)
- Code: 22697-7 (*Short Name* - Arginine/creat Ur-sRto)
- Code: 25861-6 (*Short Name* - Arginine/creat 24H Ur-sRto)
- Code: 32226-3 (*Short Name* - Arginine Vitf-sCnc)
- Code: 30062-4 (*Short Name* - Arginine/creat Ur-Rto)
- Code: 1894-5 (*Short Name* - Arginine Ur-mCnc)
- Code: 13387-6 (*Short Name* - Arginine Amn-mCnc)
- Code: 22656-3 (*Short Name* - Arginine CSF-sCnc)

Arsenic measurement

TEST DEFINITION

Measurement of arsenic in hair and nails can be used as a biomarker of environmental burden, or as an indicator of arsenic poisoning

REFERENCE RANGE

- Normal Concentration:
- Adults: Hair <1 mcg/g dry weight
- Acceptable Range for Industrial Exposure:
- Adults: Hair <65 mcg/100 g dry weight (<8.65 nmol/g dry weight)
- Adults: Nail <180 mcg/100 g dry weight (<23.94 nmol/g dry weight)
  Please refer to your institution's reference ranges as lab normals may vary.

INDICATIONS

Suspected acute or chronic arsenic exposure (ie, occupational, environmental) or poisoning
    Strength of Recommendation: Class IIa
    Strength of Evidence: Category C
Results Interpretation:
Increased level (laboratory finding)

Acute poisoning is defined as hair arsenic levels of 20,000 mcg/100 g dry weight (2,660 nmol/g dry weight)

Chronic poisoning is defined as hair arsenic levels of 100 to 4,700 mcg/100 g dry weight (13.3 to 625.1 nmol/g dry weight)

Arsenic has been demonstrated in hair and nails within hours of exposure and following chronic arsenic poisoning. Hair and nail samples have been used as biomarkers of environmental arsenic exposure (ie, drinking water, food).

The relationship between hair analysis and severity of arsenic poisoning can be misleading, because hair analysis is only an approximation of arsenic exposure. Data on nail arsenic analysis is even more limited.

CLINICAL NOTES

Individual hair strand analyses should be avoided because they are unreliable.

Many commercial laboratories performing hair analyses for consumers have not been shown to yield consistent and reliable results.
.

COLLECTION/STORAGE INFORMATION

- Specimen Collection and Handling :
  - Hair Sampling:
    - Do not obtain samples from chemically (dyed, tinted, permanently waved) processed hair
    - Obtain at least 1 g hair cutting close to scalp from several areas at the nape of neck
    - Wash hair to remove surface contamination prior to analysis
  - Nail Sampling:
    - Wash nails to remove surface contamination
    - Collect clippings from all fingers and toes

LOINC CODES

- Code: 9366-6 (*Short Name* - Arsenic XXX-mCnt)
- Code: 8158-8 (*Short Name* - Arsenic Tiss-mCnt)
- Code: 9489-6 (*Short Name* - Arsenic Fld-mCnc)

Arylsulfatase A measurement

TEST DEFINITION

Measurement of arylsulfatase A in amniotic fluid and body fluids to aid in the diagnosis of metachromatic leukodystrophy

SYNONYMS

- Arylsulphatase A measurement

REFERENCE RANGE

- Serum:
- Adults and Children: 32.0 to 129.6 nanomoles of 4-nitrocatchechol/ml of serum/4 hours
  Please refer to your institution's reference ranges as lab normals may vary.

INDICATIONS

Suspected metachromatic leukodystrophy
  Strength of Recommendation: Class IIb
  Strength of Evidence: Category C
  Results Interpretation:
  Abnormal laboratory findings
    Deficiency of arylsulfatase A (atsA) in serum is characteristic of metachromatic leukodystrophy (MLD) patients, though it is not a definitive test for MLD heterozygous individuals. Serum samples are preferred because peripheral leukocytes and cultured skin fibroblasts require special, time-consuming techniques. Urinary atsA is only beneficial as a semiquantitative screening test.

CLINICAL NOTES

Arylsulfatase A in amniotic fluid and body fluids is useful in the diagnosis of metachromatic leukodystrophy.

Asparagine measurement

Test Definition
Measurement of asparagine in plasma for detection of acquired and hereditary amino acid disorders

Reference Range
- Infants 1 to 3 months: 0.08 ± 0.44 mg/dL (6-33 micromol/L)
- Infants 3 months to 6 years: 0.95-1.9 mg/dL (72-144 micromol/L)
- Children 6 to 18 years: 0.42-0.82 mg/dL (32-62 micromol/L)
- Adults: 0.4-0.91 mg/dL (30-69 micromol/L)
  Please refer to your institution's reference ranges as lab normals may vary.

Indications
Suspected inborn error of metabolism
　　Strength of Recommendation: Class IIa
　　Strength of Evidence: Category C
Results Interpretation:
Increased amino acid
　　Inherited amino acid disorders are directly related to the absence of an enzyme involved in the metabolism of one or more amino acids; therefore, an elevated plasma level of a particular amino acid is highly suggestive of an inherited metabolic defect. In the majority of cases amino acid and organic acid analysis together permit diagnostic confirmation in infants. Immediate treatment should be initiated when an inborn error of metabolism is suspected, even if a definitive diagnosis has not yet been determined.

Collection/Storage Information
- Specimen Collection and Handling:
  - Immediately place sample in ice water.
  - Isolate plasma sample and freeze it within 1 hour; sample stable for 1 week at -20°C.
  - Sample should be deproteinized and stored at -70°C for protracted periods of usage.

Aspartate aminotransferase measurement

TEST DEFINITION

Measurement of aspartate aminotransferase in serum for the evaluation of liver, heart, and other systemic diseases

SYNONYMS

- AST measurement
- Glutamic oxaloacetic transaminase measurement
- GOT measurement
- SGOT measurement

REFERENCE RANGE

- Adults: 0-35 units/L (0-0.58 microkat/L)
- Strenuous exercise: up to 25% increase of normal value
  Please refer to your institution's reference ranges as lab normals may vary.

INDICATIONS

Hantavirus pulmonary syndrome
   Results Interpretation:
   AST/SGOT level raised
      AST is often mildly elevated at the time of admission and increases during the hospital course. Levels rise to 2 to 5 times the upper limit of normal as the clinical picture worsens.

Indicator of pancreatic necrosis in acute pancreatitis
   Results Interpretation:
   Increased liver aminotransferase level
      AST levels greater than 250 IU/L reflect a high degree of pancreatic necrosis and signal a poor prognosis.

Sickle cell disease
   Results Interpretation:
   AST/SGOT level raised
      Aspartate aminotransferase is increased in certain complications of sickle cell disease such as obstructive cholelithiasis, transfusion hepatitis, acute hepatic crisis, and transfusion hemosiderosis.

Suspected blunt abdominal trauma
   Results Interpretation:
   AST/SGOT level raised
      An aspartate aminotransferase (AST) level greater than 450 units/L is associated with liver injury in children with blunt abdominal trauma (BAT).
      Elevation of serum AST and alanine aminotransferase (ALT) levels is a marker for intra-abdominal injury in BAT patients and an indication for obtaining an abdominal CT.
      An excessive and rapid increase of total bilirubin level after liver trauma with only moderately elevated liver enzymes is indicative of bilhemia (biliovenous fistula).

Suspected cholecystitis
   Results Interpretation:
   AST/SGOT level raised
      Increased serum aspartate aminotransferase levels, typically less than 5 times the normal value, are commonly seen in cholecystitis.
   Timing of Monitoring
      Aspartate aminotransferase levels should be drawn during the acute phase of the illness as values typically return to normal within one week after symptoms resolve, unless suppuration ensues.

Suspected drug-induced liver disease
      Strength of Recommendation: Class I
      Strength of Evidence: Category C
   Results Interpretation:
   Abnormal hematology findings
      Hepatocellular or cytolytic injury is characterized by elevations to marked elevations in AST levels.

In alcoholic liver injury, the AST stays below 300 IU/L, the ALT is less than 100 IU/L, and a 2:1 or 3:1 ratio is maintained. Liver injury attributable to alcohol should be suspected if the AST level is greater than the ALT level by a ratio of 2:1.

Viral hepatitis and many drug-related causes of injury involve elevations in AST and ALT that are several times higher than what is seen with alcohol-induced injury or in a reverse ratio.

Biochemically, acetaminophen toxicity is associated with levels of AST and ALT often exceeding 10,000 IU/L.

Suspected ehrlichiosis
Results Interpretation:
AST/SGOT level raised
Mild to moderate increases in aspartate aminotransferase levels can indicate focal hepatocellular necrosis in patients with ehrlichiosis.
Timing of Monitoring
Aspartate aminotransferase levels should be drawn during the first week of the acute illness as mild to moderate elevations are noted in about 85% of patients.

Suspected inflammatory liver disease or hepatitis
Strength of Recommendation: Class IIa
Strength of Evidence: Category C
Results Interpretation:
AST/SGOT level raised
Increased serum aminotransferase levels are suggestive of acute viral hepatitis.

Markedly increased serum aminotransferase levels suggest hepatocellular necrosis in acute and chronic liver disease.

Suspected Reye's syndrome
Results Interpretation:
AST/SGOT level raised
Aspartate aminotransferase is typically elevated 1.5 to 2 times normal in Reye's syndrome. Markedly elevated aspartate aminotransferase levels indicate fulminant hepatic failure in Reye's syndrome and suggest a poor prognosis.

COMMON PANELS
- Comprehensive metabolic panel
- Hepatic function panel
- Transplant panel

ABNORMAL RESULTS
- Results increased in:
  - Hypothyroidism
  - Celiac sprue

CLINICAL NOTES
Individual aminotransferase assays, used in isolation, do not discriminate well among the various diseases affecting the liver and biliary tree. The magnitude of elevation and rate of change of aminotransferase alteration may aid in the differential diagnosis.

COLLECTION/STORAGE INFORMATION
- Collect sample in a red top tube.

LOINC CODES
- Code: 1918-2 (*Short Name* - AST CSF-cCnc)
- Code: 14410-5 (*Short Name* - AST Prt-cCnc)
- Code: 1917-4 (*Short Name* - AST Amn-cCnc)
- Code: 14414-7 (*Short Name* - AST Diaf-cCnc)
- Code: 1919-0 (*Short Name* - AST Fld-cCnc)
- Code: 14409-7 (*Short Name* - AST Plr-cCnc)
- Code: 14411-3 (*Short Name* - AST Snv-cCnc)
- Code: 14412-1 (*Short Name* - AST Gast-cCnc)

- Code: 14413-9 (*Short Name* - AST Ur-cCnc)
- Code: 16412-9 (*Short Name* - AST RBC-cCnc)

Avian influenza virus antibody assay

TEST DEFINITION
Detection of antibodies to avian influenza A virus in serum for the diagnosis of avian influenza A.

REFERENCE RANGE
- Adults and children: negative
  Please refer to your institution's reference ranges as lab normals may vary.

INDICATIONS
Suspected avian influenza A
> **Strength of Recommendation:** Class IIb
> **Strength of Evidence:** Category C
> **Results Interpretation:**
> **Viral antibody level - finding**
> A four-fold or greater rise in antibody titer using paired acute and convalescent serum samples indicates recent infection and is required for serologic diagnosis. Because hemagglutination inhibition (HAI) titers are often undetectable or very low in patients with avian influenza virus, a more sensitive serologic test such as microneutralization may be necessary. An immune response can be detected in influenza A H5N1 survivors by microneutralization assay 10 to 14 days after illness onset.
> **Timing of Monitoring**
> Paired serum specimens from the same patient are required in order to diagnose H5N1 influenza. Acute-phase sera should be collected within one week of the onset of symptoms; convalescent sera should be obtained 2 to 4 weeks later.

CLINICAL NOTES
Clinicians should contact their local or state health departments in all cases of suspected infection with any novel influenza A virus; state and local health departments should in turn contact the Centers for Disease Control (CDC) Emergency Response Hotline.

COLLECTION/STORAGE INFORMATION
Collect both acute and convalescent sera for antibody testing. Collect 5 to 10 ml of whole blood in a serum separator tube. After allowing the blood to clot, briefly centrifuge, collecting resulting sera in vials with external caps and internal O-ring seals. If no O-ring is available, seal tightly with cap provided and secure with Parafilm®. For pediatric patients, collect 1 cc whole blood in an EDTA tube and 1 cc in a clotting tube. If only 1 cc can be obtained, collect in a clotting tube. Label all samples with patient's ID and collection date. If unfrozen and transported domestically, ship with cold packs to keep sample at -4°C. Frozen or internationally transported specimens must be shipped on dry ice. Contact the Centers for Disease Control (CDC) Emergency Response Hotline before shipping influenza A specimens. Specimens should be sent Priority Overnight Shipping for receipt within 24 hours. CDC protocols for standard interstate shipping of etiologic agents must be adhered to.
All commercial antigen detection testing of specimens suspicious for avian influenza should be performed under standard BSL 2 conditions.

LOINC CODES
- Code: 22823-9 (*Short Name* - Avian FLU Ab Titr Ser Aggl)
- Code: 15444-3 (*Short Name* - Avian FLU Ab Ser QI ID)
- Code: 31241-3 (*Short Name* - Avian FLU Ab Ser-aCnc)
- Code: 22096-2 (*Short Name* - Avian FLU Ab Ser QI)
- Code: 22821-3 (*Short Name* - Avian FLU Ab Titr Ser)
- Code: 22822-1 (*Short Name* - Avian FLU Ab Ser QI EIA)
- Code: 22824-7 (*Short Name* - Avian FLU Ab Titr Ser HAI)

Babesia species antibody assay

TEST DEFINITION
Measurement of circulating antibody to the intraerythrocytic parasite *Babesia microti* in the diagnosis of babesiosis

REFERENCE RANGE
- Adults and children:
- Negative antibody titer (cut-off titer of 1:64 [IFAT, ELISA])
- Cut-off for negative antibody titer of 1:128 yields lower false-positive rate (IFAT, ELISA)
- Negative test: less than 2 reactive bands (immunoblot test)
  Please refer to your institution's reference ranges as lab normals may vary.

INDICATIONS
Suspected babesiosis
> **Strength of Recommendation:** Class IIa
> **Strength of Evidence:** Category B
> **Results Interpretation:**
> **Serology positive**
>> The presence of serum antibody to *Babesia microti* in serological testing is diagnostic of babesiosis.
>> Indirect immunofluorescent antibody testing has been useful in the the diagnosis of *Babesia microti* infection. Whereas the cutoff titer for positive diagnosis has been variable among laboratories, cutoff titers of 1:128 to 1:256 are considered to be more accurate than a lower titer of 1:64. Antibody titers have remained elevated for up to 6 years after initial infection.
>> Coinfection with *Babesia microti* and *Borrelia burgdorferi*, as suggested by serologic data, frequently occurs in areas endemic for both organisms. Clinical manifestations of babesiosis may or may not be present, as the majority of babesiosis infections are subclinical in nature.
>> Coinfection with babesiosis and human granulocytic ehrlichiosis (HGE) has been documented. In one study, 5% of patients with HGE had immunoserologic evidence of coinfection with *Babesia microti* and one patient diagnosed with *B microti* was also seropositive for HGE.
>> Coinfection with a second tick-borne agent may explain why tick-borne diseases vary in severity from patient to patient. Because of the high risk of coinfection, testing for both HGE and babesiosis should be considered in febrile patients presenting with a history of tick bite or in patients who experience a prolonged flu-like illness that fails to respond to appropriate antiborrelial therapy.

ABNORMAL RESULTS
- Results increased in::
  - Connective tissue (autoimmune) disorders such as lupus erythematosus, rheumatoid arthritis
  - Coinfection with other protozoal parasites
- Results decreased in::
  - HIV-infected patients
  - Immunosuppressed patients
  - Splenectomized patients

CLINICAL NOTES
Indirect immunofluorescent antibody testing (IFAT) is currently the preferred method for serological detection of *Babesia microti* infection. The enzyme-linked immunosorbent assay (ELISA) and the immunoblot serologic test may both serve as less labor-intensive testing alternatives to IFAT.

Production of specific anti-*B microti* antibody generally occurs within 2 weeks of the onset of babesiosis symptoms. The antibody titer may decline below the level of detection at 18 months postinfection, yet detectable antibody levels may persist for as long as 6 years.

COLLECTION/STORAGE INFORMATION
- Specimen Collection and Handling:
  - Separate serum from whole blood within one hour of collection (immunoblot test)
  - Store sample at −80°F until testing (immunoblot test)

LOINC CODES

- Code: 23663-8 (*Short Name* - Bab bovis Ab Ser QI CF)
- Code: 22108-5 (*Short Name* - Babesia IgM Ser-aCnc)
- Code: 9584-4 (*Short Name* - Babesia IgG Titr Ser IF)
- Code: 7813-9 (*Short Name* - Babesia Ab Ser-aCnc)
- Code: 23665-3 (*Short Name* - Bab divergens Ab Ser QI CF)
- Code: 22107-7 (*Short Name* - Babesia IgG Titr Ser)
- Code: 23662-0 (*Short Name* - Bab bigemina Ab Ser QI CF)
- Code: 5054-2 (*Short Name* - Babesia Ab Titr Ser IF)
- Code: 22846-0 (*Short Name* - Bab bigemina Ab Ser QI EIA)
- Code: 22848-6 (*Short Name* - Bab bovis Ab Ser QI EIA)
- Code: 22855-1 (*Short Name* - Bab divergens Ab Ser QI)
- Code: 31246-2 (*Short Name* - Babesia IgG Ser-aCnc)
- Code: 22106-9 (*Short Name* - Babesia Ab Titr Ser)
- Code: 22854-4 (*Short Name* - Bab divergens Ab Ser QI IF)
- Code: 22845-2 (*Short Name* - Bab bigemina Ab Ser QI IF)
- Code: 23666-1 (*Short Name* - Babesia Ab Titr Ser CF)
- Code: 22844-5 (*Short Name* - Bab bigemina Ab Ser QI)
- Code: 9585-1 (*Short Name* - Babesia IgM Titr Ser IF)
- Code: 22849-4 (*Short Name* - Bab bovis Ab Ser QI IF)
- Code: 22847-8 (*Short Name* - Bab bovis Ab Ser QI)

Bacterial culture, bronchial specimen

TEST DEFINITION

Detection of pulmonary pathogens obtained by bronchoalveolar lavage or bronchial brushings for evaluation of respiratory infections

REFERENCE RANGE

- Adults and Children:
- Bronchial brush: Colony counts of <1000 organisms/mL of broth
- Bronchoalveolar lavage: Colony counts of <10,000 colonies/mL of fluid
  Please refer to your institution's reference ranges as lab normals may vary.

INDICATIONS

Suspected bronchopneumonia in severely ill or immunocompromised patients
    Strength of Recommendation: Class IIb
    Strength of Evidence: Category B
    Results Interpretation:
    Positive microbiology findings
        Culture growth exceeding the values for normal flora is indicative of pneumonia. The pathogenic threshold level is determined by which specimen retrieval technique is utilized.
        For protected specimen brushing, greater than 1,000 colony-forming units/mL and greater than 10,000 colony-forming units/mL for bronchoalveolar lavage are necessary for reliable microscopic detection of specific organisms causing pneumonia.

COLLECTION/STORAGE INFORMATION

- Specimen Collection and Handling:
  - For bronchial brushings, place brush in 1 mL sterile saline or broth
  - For bronchoalveolar lavage, place fluid in sterile container
  - Transport specimen to lab and process as soon as possible
  - If unable to process specimen immediately, store in refrigerator

Bacterial culture, conjunctiva

TEST DEFINITION

Detection and identification by ocular culture of potential causes of severe conjunctivitis or if the suspected organism includes chlamydia, gonococcal or meningococcal organisms

REFERENCE RANGE

· Adults and Children: Negative or no growth
Please refer to your institution's reference ranges as lab normals may vary.

INDICATIONS

Suspected and known severe bacterial conjunctivitis
Results Interpretation:
Positive microbiology findings
Bacterial cultures are only required for severe forms of conjunctivitis that have not responded to initial therapy, because most cases of bacterial infection are diagnosed and treated based on clinical evaluation. Culture and sensitivity are performed to identify the organism and determine targeted therapy.

A positive culture may be due to any of the following organisms and can produce conjunctivitis or acute dacryocystitis which can spread to the conjunctiva: *S aureus, Pneumococcus, Streptococcus, Pseudomonas, Klebsiella, Candida, Aspergillus, N gonorrhoeae, N meningitidis, Moraxella catarrhalis, Corynebacterium, Proteus,* and *Vibrio*.

CLINICAL NOTES

Cultures and antibiotic sensitivity testing are required in all cases in which Gram stain show gram-negative diplococci to differentiate among gonococcal, meningococcal and *Branhamella* infection

B catarrhalis may easily be confused with *N gonorrhoeae* on the basis of the Gram stain and is identified by the lack of acid production from glucose and maltose.

Sugar fermentation reactions will usually differentiate *N gonorrhoeae* from *N meningitidis*. Some strains of meningococcus do not ferment maltose and may be misidentified as gonococci; meningococci that do not ferment maltose initially may do so after additional subcultures.

All gonococcal isolates should be tested for beta-lactamase production and antimicrobial susceptibility.

COLLECTION/STORAGE INFORMATION

· Specimen Collection and Handling:
  · Obtain specimens without a topical anesthetic (preservatives may markedly reduce the recovery of some bacterial pathogens).
  · Obtain specimens from both eyes, using a moistened cotton tip applicator or Calgiswab (a dry swab may not collect enough organisms or they will be killed by desiccation).
  · Wipe the applicator along the entire cul-de-sac with the lower lid everted (do not touch the lid margins as this may cause contamination by staphylococci).
  · Apply specimen to glass slide.

Bacterial culture, middle ear fluid

TEST DEFINITION

Detection of bacteria by culture in middle ear fluid for evaluation and managment of acute otitis media or chronic suppurative otitis media

REFERENCE RANGE

· No growth of pathogenic organisms
Please refer to your institution's reference ranges as lab normals may vary.

INDICATIONS

Acute otitis media
    Strength of Recommendation: Class IIa
    Strength of Evidence: Category B

Results Interpretation:
Positive microbiology findings

The most frequent organisms associated with acute otitis media (AOM) are *Streptococcus pneumoniae* (25%-50%), followed by *Haemophilus influenzae* (15% to 30%) and *Moraxella catarrhalis* (3% to 20%). Between 20% to 30% of middle ear fluid cultures for AOM do not identify an organism.

Timing of Monitoring

A culture of middle ear fluid should be performed after failure of antibiotic therapy.

Chronic purulent otitis media
　　Strength of Recommendation: Class IIa
　　Strength of Evidence: Category B
Results Interpretation:
Positive microbiology findings

Organisms most commonly associated with chronic suppurative otitis media include: *Pseudomonas aeruginosa* (29% to 98%), *Staphylococcus aureus* (18% to 43%), *Klebsiella* (10% to 27%), and diphtheroids. The external auditory canal normal flora includes *S aureus*, *S epidermidis* and diphtheroids.

Suspected mastoiditis
　　Results Interpretation:
　　Positive microbiology findings
- Findings depend on the technique used to obtain the culture specimen, whether mastoiditis is acute or chronic, presence of antecedent ear disease, and prior antibiotic therapy. The distribution of causative organisms in acute mastoiditis differs from that seen in acute otitis media. The following organisms are isolated most frequently:
  - *Streptococcus pneumoniae*, 20% to 30% of the time
  - *Streptococcus pyogenes*
  - *Staphylococcus aureus*
  - Nontypable *Haemophilus influenzae*
  - *Pseudomonas aeruginosa*
  - *P aeruginosa* is the most prevalent in children with recurrent acute otitis media. The cultures are often negative or may yield mixed flora.
- In chronic mastoiditis the most commonly seen bacteria are:
  - *S aureus*
  - *Enterobacteriaceae*
  - *P aeruginosa*
  - Anaerobes
- Immunocompromised patients are subject to mastoiditis due to unusual pathogens, such as *Nocardia*, tuberculosis, or *Actinomyces*.

CLINICAL NOTES

Viruses are found in up to 25% of middle ear fluid specimens. The presence of viruses in the middle ear is strongly associated with bacterial infections.

COLLECTION/STORAGE INFORMATION
- Use a sterile culture swab for obtaining external auditory canal specimen

Barbiturates measurement, quantitative

TEST DEFINITION

Quantitative measurement of barbiturate level in serum for drug level monitoring

REFERENCE RANGE

Adults and Children: Negative
- Therapeutic range:
- Short-acting (secobarbital): 1-2 mcg/mL (4.2-8.4 micromol/L)
- Intermediate-acting (amobarbital): 1-5 mcg/mL (4-22 micromol/L)
- Long-acting (phenobarbital): 15-40 mcg/mL (65-172 micromol/L)
- **Please refer to your institution's reference ranges as lab normals may vary.**

INDICATIONS

Monitoring of barbiturate level in barbiturate induced coma
> **Strength of Recommendation:** Class IIa
> **Strength of Evidence:** Category B

Results Interpretation:
Blood drug levels - finding

> For patients in a barbiturate-induced coma for treatment of increased intracranial pressure, the therapeutic range for pentobarbital levels appears to be 15-40 mcg/mL. Levels above this range can lead to toxicity. As the levels needed to achieve effect may vary, it is critical to monitor other neurological and cardiac parameters.

> For patients with increased intracranial pressure in barbiturate-induced coma, serum thiopental levels needed to induce the burst-suppression pattern in EEG are greater than 40 mcg/mL. Serum thiopental levels greater than 70 mcg/mL may totally suppress cerebral activity.

> Therapeutic ranges are considered to be 1-2 mcg/mL for secobarbital, 1-5 mcg/mL for amobarbital, and 15-40 mcg/mL for phenobarbital. These ranges are guidelines; since levels to achieve the desired effect may vary; other parameters must also be monitored.

Suspected barbiturate overdose
> **Strength of Recommendation:** Class IIa
> **Strength of Evidence:** Category C

Results Interpretation:
Blood drug levels - finding

> An increased blood barbiturate level indicates that an excess of barbiturate has been injected or ingested. There is little correlation between serum barbiturate levels and level of consciousness or length of coma. Specific identification of the drug involved is indicated in order to direct treatment.

> The toxic level of most short-acting barbiturates is greater than 5 mcg/mL, intermediate-acting is greater than 10 mcg/mL, and long-acting is greater than 35 mcg/mL.

> If the serum barbiturate level is much higher than would be expected for a given degree of intoxication, then it should be suspected that the patient has a sedative-hypnotic habit or has a seizure disorder and is on phenobarbital.

> If the serum short-acting barbiturate level is lower than expected, then other medical complications or the presence of multiple intoxications should be suspected.

COLLECTION/STORAGE INFORMATION
- Specimen Collection and Handling:
  - Collect specimen in a red top tube.
  - Follow chain of custody, if indicated.

LOINC CODES
- Code: 10338-2 (*Short Name* - Barbiturates SerPl-mCnc)
- Code: 11022-1 (*Short Name* - Barbiturates Mec-mCnc)
- Code: 12490-9 (*Short Name* - Talbutal SerPl-mCnc)
- Code: 29161-7 (*Short Name* - Barbiturates Mec-mCnt)
- Code: 9427-6 (*Short Name* - Barbiturates Gast-mCnc)
- Code: 11092-4 (*Short Name* - Barbiturates Har-mCnt)

Bartonella antibody level

TEST DEFINITION
Measurement of host antibody response to suspected *Bartonella* infection.

REFERENCE RANGE
- Adults and children: Negative
  Please refer to your institution's reference ranges as lab normals may vary.

INDICATIONS

Suspected bacillary angiomatosis in immunocompromised persons
Strength of Recommendation: Class IIb
Strength of Evidence: Category B
Results Interpretation:
Bacterial antibody titer - finding
Bacillary angiomatosis (BA) caused by both *B quintana* and *B henselae* is a disease affecting immunocompromised persons and thus does not mount a predictable antibody response to infection; serology has limited utility in the diagnosis of acute bacillary angiomatosis in the immunocompromised patient.

Suspected blood culture-negative endocarditis (BCNE)
Strength of Recommendation: Class IIa
Strength of Evidence: Category B
Results Interpretation:
Bacterial antibody titer - finding
Serologic testing for antibodies to *Bartonella sp* (*B quintana* and *B henselae*), provides a rapid diagnostic tool for blood culture-negative endocarditis and should be considered, in addition to blood cultures and DNA amplification, in all patients with endocarditis.

Suspected cat scratch disease (CSD)
Strength of Recommendation: Class IIb
Strength of Evidence: Category B
Results Interpretation:
Bacterial antibody titer - finding
Serologic testing for the presence of antibody to *Bartonella* may be useful in the diagnosis of cat scratch disease (CSD). Positive titer is consistent with infection. However, there does not appear to be correlation between antibody titer and disease severity and/or duration. Using the IFA assay, IgG antibodies greater than or equal to 64 may be indicative of early acute infection, past infection, or simply organism exposure. Serologic diagnosis of acute *B henselae* infection requires a single titer of 512 or higher, a four-fold rise in titer, or seroconversion.

Suspected urban trench fever
Strength of Recommendation: Class IIb
Strength of Evidence: Category B
Results Interpretation:
Bacterial antibody titer - finding
In at risk patients, serologic testing for antibodies to *Bartonella quintana* may aid in the diagnosis of suspected urban trench fever.

CLINICAL NOTES

The cut-off titer at which antibody levels become diagnostic for disease has yet to be determined. An IgG titer of >100 has been proposed.

In most patients, IgM titers begin to rise within 1 to 2 weeks of *Bartonella* infection. IgM levels peak within 4 weeks and decrease to undetectable levels within 100 days of the onset of clinical symptoms. However, some patients have no detectable IgM response at the time of onset of clinical symptoms and may not manifest a response during the entire infectious process. IgG titers increase after the IgM response, peak at 7 weeks, and may persist or slowly decline over a more protracted period.

There are seven species of *Bartonella* that have been identified as causing human disease.

Results interpretation can be difficult because considerable cross reactivity has been observed between *B henselae* and *B quintana*, and between *Bartonella* species and other organisms, such as *Coxiella burnetii* and *Chlamydia* spp. Further, the point at which titer is detected is dependent upon the assay preparation method used, and can even vary with different batches of the same antigen preparation. There is also a substantial variability in the prevalence of antibodies to different *Bartonella* species among asymptomatic individuals in different geographic and social populations.

LOINC CODES
- Code: 26678-3 (*Short Name* - B elizabethae Ab Ser QI)

Bartonella culture

TEST DEFINITION
Culture of *Bartonella* from blood or tissue for diagnosis of suspected infectious pathology

REFERENCE RANGE
• Adults and children: no growth
Please refer to your institution's reference ranges as lab normals may vary.

INDICATIONS
Suspected bacillary angiomatosis in immunocompromised persons
    Strength of Recommendation: Class IIb
    Strength of Evidence: Category B
Results Interpretation:
Sample: organism cultured
    Bartonella is difficult to culture from immunocompromised patients with bacillary angiomatosis. Primary *Bartonella* isolates take 12 to 14 days to incubate but may require up to 45 days before results can be determined.

Suspected blood culture-negative endocarditis (BCNE)
    Strength of Recommendation: Class IIb
    Strength of Evidence: Category B
Results Interpretation:
Sample: organism cultured
    Bartonella sp culture yields low sensitivity for the diagnosis of endocarditis; valvular tissue may be preferred over blood. In suspected *Bartonella* endocarditis, serologic, histologic, and/or nucleic acid testing should be considered to expedite diagnosis and treatment.

Suspected cat scratch disease
    Strength of Recommendation: Class IIb
    Strength of Evidence: Category B
Results Interpretation:
Sample: organism cultured
    Blood cultures for *B henselae* are rarely positive in cat scratch disease, possibly due to organism intraerythrocytic sequestration or limitation to affected lymph nodes. Diagnostic sensitivity may be improved by employing serologic or nucleic acid testing.

Suspected urban trench fever
    Strength of Recommendation: Class IIb
    Strength of Evidence: Category B
Results Interpretation:
Sample: organism cultured
    A positive blood culture for *Bartonella sp* is diagnostic of trench fever; however, a negative culture does not exclude the diagnosis. Diagnostic sensitivity may be improved by combining culture techniques.

CLINICAL NOTES
There are seven species of *Bartonella* that have been identified as causing human disease. These species are responsible for numerous infections with unique epidemiologies and clinical presentations. All species are fastidious, slow-growing and difficult to culture. Primary isolates can often be obtained in 12 to 14 days using blood agar, but incubation periods of up to 45 days may be required. Standardization of laboratory culture methods and procedures is lacking.

Bartonella species DNA assay

TEST DEFINITION
Amplification of *Bartonella* sp DNA, by polymerase chain reaction (PCR), for diagnosis of disease

INDICATIONS

Suspected bacillary angiomatosis in immunocompromised persons
Strength of Recommendation: Class IIa
Strength of Evidence: Category B
Results Interpretation:
Nucleic acid sequence homology

The antibody response to *Bartonella* infection is unpredictable, and culture has limited sensitivity in immunocompromised persons with bacillary angiomatosis. Using genus-specific primers, DNA amplification by polymerase chain reaction has demonstrated the ability to detect *Bartonella* infection to the species level in this patient population.

Suspected blood culture-negative endocarditis (BCNE)
Strength of Recommendation: Class IIb
Strength of Evidence: Category B
Results Interpretation:
Nucleic acid sequence homology

DNA amplification by polymerase chain reaction (PCR) has diagnostic value in the evaluation of blood culture-negative endocarditis (BCNE). PCR may have particular usefulness in evaluating patients with BCNE caused by antibiotic therapy, and when the identification of less common *Bartonella* species is desired. Further studies are needed to identify the optimal gene targets, primer sets, and detection techniques.

Suspected cat scratch disease (CSD)
Strength of Recommendation: Class IIb
Strength of Evidence: Category B
Results Interpretation:
Nucleic acid sequence homology

DNA amplification by polymerase chain reaction is correlated with the diagnosis of cat scratch disease secondary to infection with *Bartonella henselae*. PCR is not generally recommended for routine diagnosis of CSD but may be used as a confirmatory test or as a diagnostic test when CSD is highly suspected in the presence of negative or conflicting clinical and serological findings.

Suspected peliosis hepatis in immunocompromised persons
Strength of Recommendation: Class IIb
Strength of Evidence: Category B
Results Interpretation:
Nucleic acid sequence homology

DNA amplification by polymerase chain reaction (PCR) in blood and tissue samples may offer value for a rapid, conclusive diagnosis of the causative organism in patients with disseminated *Bartonella* infections such as peliosis. Further studies are needed to identify the optimal gene targets, primer sets, and detection techniques.

Suspected urban trench fever
Strength of Recommendation: Class IIb
Strength of Evidence: Category C
Results Interpretation:
Nucleic acid sequence homology

DNA amplification by polymerase chain reaction (PCR) has had limited use in the diagnosis of trench fever. It may hold clinical utility as a confirmatory test for *B. quintana* infection.

CLINICAL NOTES

- Test limitations include:
- Presence of DNA sequences in non peer-reviewed databases
- Incomplete or fragmented DNA sequences of unclear attribute in GenBank and EMBL databases
- Possibility of contamination with interfering substances such as blood or microbial DNA

COLLECTION/STORAGE INFORMATION

- Specimen Collection and Handling:
  - Cell lysates, serum, and whole blood may be used.
  - Avoid anticoagulants. Heparin and heme inhibit polymerase chain reaction (PCR). Citrate and EDTA are acceptable.
  - Store nucleic acids at $\leq$ -20°C.

LOINC CODES
- Code: 16275-0 (*Short Name* - Bartonella DNA Bld Ql PCR)

Basophil count

TEST DEFINITION
Measurement of basophils in whole blood for the evaluation and management of allergic, hematologic, and neoplastic disorders, as well as parasitic infections

REFERENCE RANGE
- Adults:
- Relative: 0%-3%
- Absolute: 0-0.19 x 10^3 cells/microL
- Adults, 21 years:
- Relative: 0.5%
- Absolute: 0-0.2 x 10^3 cells/microL
- Children, 1 year:
- Relative: 0.4%
- Children, 2 to 10 years:
- Relative: 0.5%-0.6%
- Absolute: 0.02 x 10^3 cells/microL
- **Please refer to your institution's reference ranges as lab normals may vary.**

INDICATIONS
Chronic myeloid leukemia
    Strength of Recommendation: Class IIb
    Strength of Evidence: Category B
Results Interpretation:
Basophilia
    In chronic myeloid leukemia (CML), a higher basophil percentage at diagnosis is associated with a significantly decreased probability of survival. The New CML score, used for the prognostic stratification of newly diagnosed patients, identifies a basophil percentage greater than or equal to 3% (along with increased age, greater spleen size, higher eosinophil percentage and platelet count) as predicting decreased survival among patients treated with interferon alpha.

Myelodysplastic syndrome.
    Strength of Recommendation: Class IIb
    Strength of Evidence: Category B
Results Interpretation:
Abnormal basophil production
    In patients with myelodysplastic syndrome (MDS), blood basophil counts reflect bone marrow basophilia, and low circulating basophil counts are associated with longer survival rates. Bone marrow basophilia, however, is a more significant prognostic factor for MDS disease course

Suspected allergic rhinitis
    Strength of Recommendation: Class IIb
    Strength of Evidence: Category C
Results Interpretation:
Basophilia
    Allergic reactions are frequently associated with elevated differential blood basophil counts.
    In patients with allergic rhinitis, an elevated basophil blood count may occur during seasonal pollenosis and correlate with degree of symptom severity.

Suspected parasitic infection
    Strength of Recommendation: Class IIb
    Strength of Evidence: Category B

Results Interpretation:
Basophilia
The basophil differential blood count does not have clinical utility as a marker for suspected parasitic infection. In helminth parasitic infections, however, the number of basophil high-affinity IgE receptors may increase in response to parasitic infection without an associated increase in the absolute basophil cell count.

COMMON PANELS
- Complete blood count with automated differential

ABNORMAL RESULTS
- Results increased in:
  - Ulcerative colitis
  - Hypothyroidism
  - Postsplenectomy
  - Nephrosis
- Results decreased in:
  - Ovulation
  - Pregnancy
  - Hyperthyroidism (50% of patients)

CLINICAL NOTES
Basophil blood concentration is lowest in the morning and highest at night.

COLLECTION/STORAGE INFORMATION
- Specimen Collection and Handling:
  - Collect whole blood in lavender top tube (EDTA)
  - Specimen stable for 24 hours at 23°C, or 48 hours at 4°C
  - Heparin should not be used

bcl-2 gene rearrangement test

TEST DEFINITION
Identification of bcl-2 translocation in body fluids and tissue for diagnosis and monitoring of lymphoid malignancies

SYNONYMS
- bcl-2 gene analysis

INDICATIONS
Evaluation and management of diffuse large B-cell lymphoma (DLBCL)
    Strength of Recommendation: Class IIb
    Strength of Evidence: Category B
Results Interpretation:
Nucleic acid sequence homology
The Bcl-2 (14;18) translocation is significantly associated with germinal center (GC) diffuse large B-cell lymphoma (DLBCL). A significantly poorer prognosis has been observed in Bcl-2 positive patients with both GC and non-GC DLBCL.

Evaluation and post-treatment monitoring of follicular lymphoma
    Strength of Recommendation: Class IIa
    Strength of Evidence: Category B
Results Interpretation:
Nucleic acid sequence homology
The Bcl-2 (14;18) translocation is useful as a tumor-specific marker for minimal residual disease evaluation in follicular lymphoma. The persistence of translocation, typically defined as 2 or more positive PCR findings in repeated post-treatment follow up, may have clinical significance as a poor prognostic indicator.

CLINICAL NOTES

Bcl-2 translocation testing can be useful in a number of clinical situations including post-treatment monitoring and determination of molecular remission or early relapse, detection of minimal residual disease, evaluation of bone marrow involvement and monitoring of patients undergoing bone marrow transplantation, determination of metastatic sites, and identification of patients who may require different treatment management - such as additional chemotherapy - when remission is not confirmed at the molecular level. It has been suggested that initial diagnosis be performed using both polymerase chain reaction (PCR) and Southern blot analysis while PCR alone can be used for monitoring response to therapy. PCR methods have identified residual Bcl-2 positive cells for over 5 years in the presence of negative Southern blot results and complete remission by clinical, morphologic, and cytogenetic criteria.

Because PCR methods have higher specificities and sensitivities than Southern blot analysis, PCR is useful for specimens containing small numbers of Bcl-2 positive lymphoma cells such as in bone marrow aspirate collected during or after chemotherapy, fine-needle aspirate, and cerebrospinal fluid. In addition, PCR turnaround time is typically less than 24 hours, as compared to 1 to 2 weeks for Southern blot, and does not require radioisotopically labeled probes, as some Southern blot protocols do. PCR can detect one bcl-2 positive lymphoma cell in 10^5 to 10^6 normal cells; this high sensitivity also carries a risk for false-positive results requiring meticulous PCR assay quality control. PCR limitations include use of inadequate control sequences resulting in inadequate quantification, and possible contamination with interfering substances such as blood or microbial DNA.

Specimens appropriate for use with Southern blot analysis include lymph node biopsies, fine-needle aspirate, extranodal mass biopsies, bone marrow aspirate, body fluids and peripheral blood in leukemic-phase lymphoma patients.

LOINC CODES
- Code: 21095-5 (*Short Name* - BCL2 Gene Rear Ql)

Benzodiazepine measurement, serum/plasma

TEST DEFINITION
Measurement of benzodiazepine in serum or plasma for therapeutic monitoring and detection and evaluation of suspected toxicity

REFERENCE RANGE
- Therapeutic ranges of selected benzodiazepines are as follows. Therapeutic and/or toxic ranges have not been established for all benzodiazepines:
- Diazepam: 100-1,000 ng/mL (0.35-3.51 micromol/L)
- Clonazepam: 15-60 ng/mL (48-190 nmol/L)
- Alprazolam: 10-50 ng/mL (32-162 nmol/L)
- Chlordiazepoxide: 700-1,000 ng/mL (2.34-3.34 micromol/L)
- Lorazepam: 50-240 ng/mL
- Oxazepam: 0.2-1.4 mcg/mL
  Please refer to your institution's reference ranges as lab normals may vary.

INDICATIONS
Therapeutic benzodiazepine monitoring and suspected toxicity
   Strength of Recommendation: Class IIa
   Strength of Evidence: Category B
   Results Interpretation:
   Abnormal laboratory findings
   When benzodiazepine concentration is measured in terms of binding activity, serum dose-levels up to 1,000 ng/mL can be considered therapeutic under normal conditions. Toxic effects may occur at diazepam equivalents as low as 1,000 ng/mL and include muscle weakness and decreased consciousness. Ingestion of large amounts of diazepam alone, resulting in high blood concentrations, are not necessarily life-threatening and are not likely to results in coma.
   Urine benzodiazepine results may be less informative than serum when quantitative differentiation between therapeutic and toxic levels is desired.
- Toxic levels of selected benzodiazepines:
  - Diazepam: >5,000 ng/mL (>17.55 micromol/L)
  - Clonazepam: >80 ng/mL (>254 nmol/L)

- Alprazolam: >75 ng/mL (>243 nmol/L)
- Chlordiazepoxide: >5,000 ng/mL (>16.7 micromol/L)

COLLECTION/STORAGE INFORMATION
- Collect serum or plasma in lavender EDTA tube.

LOINC CODES
- Code: 11024-7 (*Short Name* - Benzodiazepines SerPl-mCnc)
- Code: 3389-4 (*Short Name* - Benzodiaz SerPl Ql)
- Code: 32052-3 (*Short Name* - Benzodiazepines SerPl-sCnc)
- Code: 27197-3 (*Short Name* - Benzodiaz Vitf Ql)
- Code: 12359-6 (*Short Name* - Benzodiazepines Stl Ql)
- Code: 31081-3 (*Short Name* - Benzodiazepines Mec Ql Scn)
- Code: 29209-4 (*Short Name* - Benzodiazepines Fld-mCnc)
- Code: 13933-7 (*Short Name* - Benzodiazepines Har-mCnt)
- Code: 11023-9 (*Short Name* - Benzodiaz Mec-mCnc)
- Code: 12364-6 (*Short Name* - Benzodiazepines Gast Ql)
- Code: 29160-9 (*Short Name* - Benzodiazepines Mec-mCnt)

Benzodiazepine measurement, urine

TEST DEFINITION
Detection of benzodiazepine and metabolite levels in urine

SYNONYMS
- Urine benzodiazepine level

INDICATIONS
Urine drug screening for suspected benzodiazepine use or abuse
   Strength of Recommendation: Class IIa
   Strength of Evidence: Category B
   Results Interpretation:
   Urine drug levels - finding
   Immunoassays predict the presence of benzodiazepines based on a preset cutoff value. Results are presumptive; if confirmation is needed, a non-immunoassay test is indicated. With a confirmed overdose, an immunoassay value that falls below the cutoff may be due to the inability of the assay to detect the multiple metabolites generated from benzodiazepines.

COMMON PANELS
- Drugs of abuse testing, urine

CLINICAL NOTES
Several factors such as the dose, the drug, and the time of sample collection may change the concentration of benzodiazepine metabolites in urine.

Urine testing of benzodiazepines for abuse is preferred over blood testing because of its less invasive nature, ease of analysis, and longer time scale for detection.

COLLECTION/STORAGE INFORMATION
- Specimen Collection and Handling:
  - Obtain a random urine sample in a 20 mL container
  - Note indication for testing (if known), including whether there is suspected abuse, and suspected drug or drugs

LOINC CODES
- Code: 9428-4 (*Short Name* - Benzodiazepines Ur-mCnc)
- Code: 14316-4 (*Short Name* - Benzodiaz Ur Ql Scn)
- Code: 19279-9 (*Short Name* - Benzodiazepines Tested Ur Scn)

- Code: 3390-2 (*Short Name* - Benzodiazepines Ur Ql)
- Code: 19286-4 (*Short Name* - Benzodiaz Cfm Meth Ur)
- Code: 19284-9 (*Short Name* - Benzodiaz CtO Ur Cfm-mCnc)
- Code: 19064-5 (*Short Name* - Benzodiaz CtO Ur-mCnc)
- Code: 20412-3 (*Short Name* - Benzodiazepines Ur Cnfrn-mCnc)
- Code: 19285-6 (*Short Name* - Benzodiaz Scn Meth Ur)
- Code: 19280-7 (*Short Name* - Benzodiazepines Tested Ur Scn)

Beta-2-microglobulin measurement

TEST DEFINITION
Measurement of beta-2-microglobulin in serum for the evaluation and management of renal failure, multiple myeloma and other neoplasms, and as a prognostic indicator in lymphoid malignancies

REFERENCE RANGE
- Adults: <0.27 mg/dL (<2.7 mg/L)
  Please refer to your institution's reference ranges as lab normals may vary.

INDICATIONS
Hodgkin's disease and non-Hodgkin's lymphoma
　　Results Interpretation:
　　Finding of serum tumor marker level
　　　　Beta 2-microglobulin (beta-2-M) has been used as an indicator and serological staging agent to predict freedom from relapse and survival time with some lymphomas. Patients at low risk for disease recurrence have normal serum levels, whereas elevation predicts shortened remission and survival.

Multiple myeloma
　　Strength of Recommendation: Class IIa
　　Strength of Evidence: Category B
　　Results Interpretation:
　　Increased level (laboratory finding)
　　　　An increased level of serum beta-2-microglobulin is significantly associated with poorer prognosis in multiple myeloma.

COLLECTION/STORAGE INFORMATION
- Specimen Collection and Handling:
  - Collect specimen in a red top tube.
  - Store specimen at 4°C for <72 hours.
  - Specimen is stable frozen at −20°C for 6 months, or indefinitely at −70°C.

LOINC CODES
- Code: 1951-3 (*Short Name* - B2 Microglob CSF-mCnc)

beta-Alanine measurement

TEST DEFINITION
Measurement of beta-alanine in plasma for detection of acquired and hereditary amino acid disorders.

REFERENCE RANGE
- Children 0 to 16 years: < 0.44 mg/dL (< 49 micromol/L)
- Adults: < 0.26 mg/dL (< 29 micromol/L)
  Please refer to your institution's reference ranges as lab normals may vary.

INDICATIONS

Suspected inborn error of metabolism
    Strength of Recommendation: Class IIa
    Strength of Evidence: Category C
Results Interpretation:
Increased amino acid
    Inherited amino acid disorders are directly related to the absence of an enzyme involved in the metabolism of one or more amino acids; therefore, an elevated plasma level of a particular amino acid is highly suggestive of an inherited metabolic defect. In the majority of cases amino acid and organic acid analysis together permit diagnostic confirmation in infants. Immediate treatment should be initiated when an inborn error of metabolism is suspected, even if a definitive diagnosis has not yet been determined.

COLLECTION/STORAGE INFORMATION

- Specimen Collection and Handling:
  - Immediately place sample in ice water.
  - Isolate plasma sample and freeze it within 1 hour; sample stable for 1 week at -20°C.
  - Sample should be deproteinized and stored at -70°C for protracted periods of usage.

LOINC CODES

- Code: 1933-1 (*Short Name* - B-Alanine Ur-mCnc)
- Code: 26604-9 (*Short Name* - B-Alanine SerPl-sCnc)
- Code: 25346-8 (*Short Name* - B-Alanine 24H Ur-sRate)
- Code: 13714-1 (*Short Name* - B-Alanine/creat Ur-mRto)
- Code: 25868-1 (*Short Name* - B-Alanine 24H Ur-sCnc)
- Code: 25869-9 (*Short Name* - B-Alanine/creat 24H Ur-sRto)
- Code: 1932-3 (*Short Name* - B-Alanine SerPl-mCnc)
- Code: 13368-6 (*Short Name* - B-Alanine CSF-mCnc)
- Code: 13390-0 (*Short Name* - B-Alanine Amn-mCnc)
- Code: 6872-6 (*Short Name* - B-Alanine 24H Ur-mRate)
- Code: 26578-5 (*Short Name* - B-Alanine/creat Ur-sRto)
- Code: 16452-5 (*Short Name* - B-Alanine Ur QI)
- Code: 26589-2 (*Short Name* - B-Alanine CSF-sCnc)
- Code: 26968-8 (*Short Name* - B-Alanine Ur-sCnc)
- Code: 1931-5 (*Short Name* - B-Alanine SerPl QI)
- Code: 28588-2 (*Short Name* - B-Alanine/creat Ur-Rto)

Beta-hydroxybutyrate measurement, Blood

TEST DEFINITION

Measurement of beta-hydroxybutyrate in whole blood, serum, or plasma to evaluate ketone-producing glycogenolytic metabolic energy deficits

REFERENCE RANGE

- Whole blood, serum or plasma: 0.21 to 2.81 mg/dL (20-270 micromol/L)
- Serum (enzymatic-kinetic technique): <3.02 mg/dL (290 micromol/L)
  Please refer to your institution's reference ranges as lab normals may vary.

INDICATIONS

Suspected alcoholic ketoacidosis
    Strength of Recommendation: Class IIa
    Strength of Evidence: Category C
Results Interpretation:
Increased level (laboratory finding)
    An elevated beta-hydroxybutyrate level is diagnostic of ketoacidosis. The absence of hyperglycemia supports the diagnosis of alcoholic ketoacidosis (AKA). However, many patients may present with hyperglycemia, making differentiation between AKA and diabetic ketoacidosis (DKA) more difficult.

Suspected diabetic ketoacidosis (DKA)
>   **Strength of Recommendation:** Class I
>   **Strength of Evidence:** Category C
>   **Results Interpretation:**
>   **Increased level (laboratory finding)**
>   Beta-hydroxybutyrate levels 3 mmol/L or greater are indicative of ketoacidosis. In very severe diabetic ketoacidosis (DKA), the beta-hydroxybutyrate serum concentration may exceed 25 mmol/L.

CLINICAL NOTES
Common tests for ketone bodies, such as Acetest, Chemstrip, and Ketostix, do not detect beta-hydroxybutyrate. A handheld meter sensor system is available to monitor beta-hydroxybutyrate and glucose levels.

COLLECTION/STORAGE INFORMATION
- Specimen Collection and Handling:
  - Plasma (lithium-heparin or fluoride-oxalate), serum, or perchloric acid (PCA) extracts can be analyzed.
  - EDTA-plasma samples will produce values that are 60% lower than specimens preserved with fluoride-oxalate or PCA.
  - Whole blood specimens are stable at room temperature up to 48 hours.
  - Plasma samples are stable at room temperature up to 7 days, 14 days at 4°C, and 6 months at -20°C.
  - PCA extracts are stable at -20°C up to 1 year.
  - Repeated freeze-thaw cycling has no detrimental effect.

LOINC CODES
- Code: 29509-7 (*Short Name* - B-OH-Butyr/creat Ur-sRto)
- Code: 29512-1 (*Short Name* - B-OH-Butyr SerPl-mCnc)
- Code: 1946-3 (*Short Name* - B-OH-Butyr CSF-mCnc)
- Code: 16455-8 (*Short Name* - B-OH-Butyr CSF-sCnc)
- Code: 1947-1 (*Short Name* - B-OH-Butyr Ur-mCnc)
- Code: 6873-4 (*Short Name* - B-OH-Butyr SerPl-sCnc)
- Code: 13684-6 (*Short Name* - B-OH-Butyr/creat Ur-mRto)
- Code: 16456-6 (*Short Name* - B-OH-Butyr Ur-sCnc)
- Code: 29622-8 (*Short Name* - B-OH-Butyr Ur Ql)

Bilirubin, direct measurement

TEST DEFINITION
Measurement of direct (conjugated) bilirubin in serum to evaluate liver function and bilirubin metabolism

SYNONYMS
- Bilirubin, conjugated measurement, serum

REFERENCE RANGE
- Adults: 0.1-0.3 mg/dL (1.7-5.1 micromol/ L)
- Neonates: <1 mg/dL with normal total bilirubin
  Please refer to your institution's reference ranges as lab normals may vary.

INDICATIONS
Suspected abnormal liver function in sickle cell (Hb S) disease
>   **Results Interpretation:**
>   **Increased level (laboratory finding)**
- Effect on direct bilirubin due (due to chronic hemolysis) with common liver function abnormalities associated with sickle cell disease include:
  - Markedly increased:
    - Obstructive cholelithiasis
    - Transfusion hepatitis
    - Acute hepatic cirrhosis
  - Slightly increased: Transfusion hemosiderosis

Suspected hepatitis
Results Interpretation:
Increased level (laboratory finding)
   In hepatitis, the total bilirubin level is divided between conjugated (direct) and unconjugated (indirect) studies. A marked increase in the bilirubin level ranging from 5 to 20 mg/dL may occur 3.5 to 5.5 months after exposure; an elevation of greater than 20 mg/dL suggests severe disease. Conjugated and unconjugated levels usually parallel each other, except in the rare complication of aplastic anemia when unconjugated bilirubin prevails.

Suspected neonatal hyperbilirubinemia
   Strength of Recommendation: Class I
   Strength of Evidence: Category C
Results Interpretation:
Increased level (laboratory finding)
   Conjugated hyperbilirubinemia is defined as a direct (conjugated) serum bilirubin level greater than 1 mg/dL if the total bilirubin is less than 5 mg/dL or as a direct bilirubin level more than 20% of total bilirubin if the total bilirubin level is greater than 5 mg/dL. If conjugated serum bilirubin is elevated, cholestasis is present and prompt stepwise clinical evaluation is necessary.
Timing of Monitoring
   Infants that are jaundiced beyond the second or third week of life should be evaluated for cholestasis by total and direct serum bilirubin measurements. In breast-fed infants who have a normal history (no dark urine or light stools), laboratory evaluation can be postponed until 3 weeks of age if evidence of jaundice persists.

Suspected obstructive jaundice
   Results Interpretation:
   Increased level (laboratory finding)
   Elevated direct bilirubin levels may occur in choledocholithiasis or gallstone pancreatitis but are not reliable for diagnosing choledocholithiasis. History and physical exam may be the only indicator of common bile duct stones
   If one value of the liver profile is elevated (alkaline phosphatase, AST, lactate dehydrogenase, or bilirubin), common bile duct stones will be found in 20% of cases. With two elevated values, the risk of common bile duct stones doubles, and with three elevated values, more than half of the patients will have choledocholithiasis.

COMMON PANELS
- Comprehensive metabolic panel
- Hemolysis panel
- Hepatic function panel
- Transfusion reaction workup
- Transplant panel

COLLECTION/STORAGE INFORMATION
- Specimen Collection and Handling:
   - Protect specimen from light to avoid formation of photobilirubin.
   - Serum or heparinized plasma may be used for Ektachem 700 method.

LOINC CODES
- Code: 33458-1 (*Short Name* - Bilirub Conj Fld-mCnc)

Bilirubin, total measurement

TEST DEFINITION
   Measurement of total bilirubin in serum to evaluate liver function and bilirubin metabolism

SYNONYMS
- Total bilirubin
- Total bilirubin level

Reference Range

- Adults: 0.3-1 mg/dL (5.1-17 micromole/L)
- Premature infants, cord blood: <2 mg/dL (<34 micromole/L)
- Premature infants. 0 to 1 day: <8 mg/dL (<137 micromole/L):
- Premature infants. 1 to 2 days: <12 mg/dL (<205 micromole/L):
- Premature infants. 3 to 5 days: <16 mg/dL (<274 micromole/L):
- Neonates, cord blood: <2 mg/dL (<34 micromole/L):
- Neonates, 0 to 1 day: 1.4-8.7 mg/dL (24-149 micromole/L):
- Neonates, 1 to 2 days: 3.4-11.5 mg/dL (58-197 micromole/L):
- Neonates, 3 to 5 days: 1.5-12 mg/dL (26-205 micromole/L):
- Children 6 days to 18 years: 0.3-1.2 mg/dL (5-21 micromole/L)
  Please refer to your institution's reference ranges as lab normals may vary.

Indications

Suspected biliary calculi in acute cholecystitis
> **Strength of Recommendation:** Class I
> **Strength of Evidence:** Category B
> **Results Interpretation:**
> **Increased bilirubin level**
> The serum bilirubin level is elevated (usually to less than 5 mg/dL) in up to one third of patients with cho-lelithiasis, and may indicate the presence of biliary calculi.
> The bilirubin values typically return to normal within one week after symptoms resolve, unless suppuration ensues. As a rule, direct hyperbilirubinemia predominates.

Suspected biliary cause of pancreatitis
> **Strength of Recommendation:** Class IIb
> **Strength of Evidence:** Category C
> **Results Interpretation:**
> **Increased bilirubin level**
> Although an elevated serum total bilirubin level suggests a biliary cause, levels are raised in only 10% of patients with acute pancreatitis. The increase is usually transient and without major clinical significance.
> In chronic pancreatitis, elevated total bilirubin levels may be caused by coexisting liver disease or cholestasis due to compression of the distal common bile duct by an inflamed pancreatic head.

Suspected bilovenous fistula in blunt abdominal trauma
> **Strength of Recommendation:** Class I
> **Strength of Evidence:** Category C
> **Results Interpretation:**
> **Hyperbilirubinemia**
> Following abdominal trauma, an excessively high serum total bilirubin, associated with only moderately elevated liver enzymes, may be seen in traumatic bilovenous fistula. Endoscopic retrograde cholangiopancreatography (ERCP) is the most reliable method to localize the fistula, whereas CT or ultrasonography help localize and assess the extent of parenchymal injury.

Suspected hepatic dysfunction in rhabdomyolysis
> **Strength of Recommendation:** Class IIa
> **Strength of Evidence:** Category C
> **Results Interpretation:**
> **Increased bilirubin level**
> About 25% of patients with rhabdomyolysis have reversible hepatic dysfunction. In a study of 34 patients with nontraumatic rhabdomyolysis, 60% of patients with and 41% without acute renal failure had transient hyperbilirubinemia (2.6 to 14.3 mg/dL); however, all the patients had marked elevations of LDH, AST, and ALT.
> Hyperbilirubinemia secondary to rhabdomyolysis associated with intravenous drug abuse and shock may be a consequence of hemolysis or hepatic underperfusion.

Suspected liver disease
> **Strength of Recommendation:** Class I
> **Strength of Evidence:** Category C

Results Interpretation:
Increased bilirubin level

A marked increase in the serum total bilirubin level ranging up to 20 mg/dL or higher may occur 3-5 months after viral exposure. Jaundice or icterus is usually evident when the serum bilirubin level exceeds 2.5 mg/dL. An elevation greater than 20 mg/dL suggests severe liver disease.

In patients with hepatitis-induced acute liver failure, a serum total bilirubin level greater than 17.5 mg/dL (300 mmol/L) is a criterion for predicting death and the need for liver transplantation. A low transaminase level associated with a high bilirubin level in the presence of chronic liver disease also indicates a poor prognosis.

Suspected liver dysfunction in ehrlichiosis
Strength of Recommendation: Class IIa
Strength of Evidence: Category C
Results Interpretation:
Increased bilirubin level

Abnormal liver profiles and cytopenias are important clues to diagnosis of ehrlichiosis, but the contribution of total bilirubin levels to diagnosis appears limited. Only about 25% of ehrlichiosis patients have elevated serum total bilirubin levels. In contrast, focal hepatocellular necrosis typically induces mild to moderate elevations of AST (about 85% of patients), ALT (75% to 80%), and LDH in the first week of illness.

Suspected liver dysfunction in Hb S (sickle cell) disease
Strength of Recommendation: Class I
Strength of Evidence: Category C
Results Interpretation:
Increased bilirubin level

- Sickle cell (SS) disease patients have baseline elevated levels of serum total (mean 2.5 mg/dL; range 1.5 to 4 mg/dL) and indirect (unconjugated) bilirubin. Increased hyperbilirubinemia above baseline without accompanying increased liver enzyme or direct (conjugated) bilirubin levels indicates marked hemolysis. Hyperhemolytic crises typically occur following exposure to oxidant drugs or chemicals in patients with associated G-6-PD deficiency, but it also may occur during vaso-occlusive crises.
- Serum total bilirubin levels (vs baseline) in sickle cell disease-associated hepatobiliary disorders include:
  - Nonobstructive cholelithiasis: Stable (at baseline)
  - Obstructive cholelithiasis: Markedly increased
  - Transfusion hepatitis: Increased
  - Acute hepatic crisis: Markedly increased
  - Transfusion hemosiderosis: Stable or slightly increased

Suspected liver dysfunction in HIV infection
Strength of Recommendation: Class IIa
Strength of Evidence: Category C
Results Interpretation:
Increased bilirubin level

Potential causes of increased bilirubin levels in HIV/AIDS include intrahepatic or extrahepatic malignancy, sclerosing cholangitis, papillary stenosis, and drug-induced hepatitis.

Suspected or known bacterial septicemia
Strength of Recommendation: Class I
Strength of Evidence: Category B
Results Interpretation:
Increased bilirubin level

Both hepatocellular dysfunction and increased red blood cell destruction may account for elevated serum total bilirubin levels in septic patients.

Hyperbilirubinemia (total bilirubin greater than 4 mg/dL) may be associated with organ dysfunction in severe sepsis.

Elevated bilirubin levels suggest bacteremia with *Bacteroides* infection, hemolysis secondary to clostridial infection, or DIC.

Hyperbilirubinemia in patients with *Staphylococcus aureus* sepsis may portend a high risk of death from overwhelming sepsis. In a study of 47 patients with *S aureus* endocarditis, 11 patients had hyperbilirubinemia (serum total bilirubin 2 mg/dL or greater). Although none were hypotensive on admission, 4 of the 11 patients with hyperbilirubinemia (vs 2 of 36 without) died of overwhelming sepsis.

Timing of Monitoring
Liver function tests should be obtained at baseline, because septic patients may subsequently develop hepatic dysfunction secondary to hypoperfusion (ie, shock liver).

Suspected Reye's syndrome
Strength of Recommendation: Class IIa
Strength of Evidence: Category C
Results Interpretation:
Increased bilirubin level
In Reye's syndrome, the total bilirubin level is usually normal but may be mildly elevated. If the total bilirubin level is greater than 5 mg/dL, other diagnostic possibilities should be considered.

Suspected toxic shock syndrome
Strength of Recommendation: Class IIb
Strength of Evidence: Category C
Results Interpretation:
Increased bilirubin level
Modest elevations of serum total bilirubin levels occur in toxic shock syndrome, but are transient and non-specific. The hyperbilirubinemia usually resolves within 1 to 2 weeks.

COMMON PANELS
- Comprehensive metabolic panel
- Hemolysis panel
- Hepatic function panel
- Transfusion reaction workup
- Transplant panel

CLINICAL NOTES
Total bilirubin measurement includes unconjugated (indirect), conjugated (direct), and delta (albumin-bound conjugated) bilirubin and usually are sufficient for clinical purposes (ie, fractionated bilirubins measurements are less accurate and unnecessary).

COLLECTION/STORAGE INFORMATION
- Specimen Collection and Handling:
  - Collect venous blood specimen in marble top tube.
  - Avoid exposing specimen to light.

LOINC CODES
- Code: 25564-6 (*Short Name* - Bilirubin Direct Fld-sCnc)
- Code: 14152-3 (*Short Name* - Bilirubin Direct Fld-mCnc)

Biopsy of muscle

TEST DEFINITION
Histologic exam of muscle tissue for evaluation and management of neuromuscular disease

REFERENCE RANGE
- Normal muscle morphology
Please refer to your institution's reference ranges as lab normals may vary.

INDICATIONS
Suspected congenital myopathy
Strength of Recommendation: Class I
Strength of Evidence: Category C
Results Interpretation:
Abnormal histology findings
- Findings suggesting congenital myopathies include:

- Predominant type 1 fibers with selected atrophy and numerous clustered nemaline (threadlike) rods suggest nemaline myopathy, which has a higher incidence in females than in males
- Abundance of fibers with a single, centrally located core primarily in type 1 fibers suggests central core disease
- Multiple fibers with a central (or near central) nucleus, fibers resembling those seen in fetal development, and an abundance of type 1 fibers with atrophy suggest centronuclear myopathy
- Few type 2 fibers accompanied by an abundance of type 1 fibers suggests congenital fiber-type disproportion

Conclusive diagnosis of congenital myopathy should incorporate clinical data and laboratory results (creatine kinase and electromyography), as well as histologic exam of muscle tissue.

Suspected inflammatory myopathy
Strength of Recommendation: Class IIa
Strength of Evidence: Category C
Results Interpretation:
Abnormal histology findings
- Findings associated with inflammatory myopathies include:
  - Rimmed vacuoles and nuclear inclusions: Inclusion-body myositis
  - Multinucleated giant cells: Inflammatory myopathy as a direct result of HIV infection
  - Inflammatory cells (typically lymphocytes) infiltrating the endomysium, fiber atrophy, interstitial fibrosis, and widespread necrosis: Polymyositis/dermatomyositis complex (higher incidence in males over age of 50 years)
- Polymyositis is one of the most common myopathies associated with HIV infection. It may be difficult to distinguish it, or other HIV-related myopathies, from myopathy associated with antiretroviral therapy.
- Conclusive diagnosis of an inflammatory myopathy should incorporate clinical data and laboratory results (creatine kinase and electromyography), as well as histologic exam of muscle tissue.

Suspected metabolic myopathy
Strength of Recommendation: Class IIa
Strength of Evidence: Category C
Results Interpretation:
Abnormal histology findings
Metabolic myopathies typically involve alterations in the storage of glycogen. Marked accumulation of glycogen, vacuoles of varying size, or crescentic vacuoles, and blebs protruding above fibers may all indicate a form of metabolic myopathy (eg, acid-maltase deficiency, McArdle's disease).

Confirmed diagnosis should incorporate evaluation of clinical data, serum creatine levels, and electromyography.

COLLECTION/STORAGE INFORMATION
- Specimen Collection and Handling:
  - Remove two sections of tissue, each 1 to 2 mm in diameter
  - Orient and stretch sections on filter paper prior to fixation
  - Fixate specimens in 4% buffered glutaraldehyde or Karnovsky's fixative
  - If specimen is adequate, preserve an additional sample in formalin
  - If examination is completed within 24 hours, keep specimen in saline-soaked gauze
  - If examination is not completed within 24 hours, freeze specimen at 4°C
  - Do not allow specimen to thaw and refreeze

Bite wound culture for bacteria

TEST DEFINITION
Detection and identification of bacteria by culture for evaluation of bite wounds

REFERENCE RANGE
- Adults and children: No growth
  Please refer to your institution's reference ranges as lab normals may vary.

INDICATIONS
Infected human bites
> **Results Interpretation:**
> **Wound swab culture positive**
>> A positive wound culture from an infected human bite may help direct antibiotic therapy.
>> In a study that sent wound culture specimens from 23 patients to both a research and local laboratory, few organisms were isolated in the local laboratory, with 2 cultures demonstrating no growth (all wound cultures were positive in the research laboratory) and fastidious organisms, *Eikenella corrodens,* and anaerobes rarely isolated despite being among the most common organisms isolated in the research laboratory.
>
> **Timing of Monitoring**
>> Prior to the initiation of antibiotic therapy, aerobic and anaerobic cultures should be obtained from the infected wound as both types of bacteria have been isolated from human bite wounds. Sensitivity testing should follow culture. Wound cultures should be obtained during wound exploration and should not delay antibiotic therapy.

Infected cat and dog bites
> **Results Interpretation:**
> **Wound swab culture positive**
>> A positive wound culture from an infected cat or dog bite may help direct antibiotic therapy.

COLLECTION/STORAGE INFORMATION
- Specimen Collection and Handling:
  - Aspirate abscess with a needle
  - Sample open lacerations using standard cotton or rayon swab
  - Sample puncture wounds using calcium alginate miniswabs
  - Place specimen in tube containing anaerobic transport medium

Bleeding time

TEST DEFINITION
Measurement of time for bleeding to stop following a standardized cut to the skin to evaluate primary hemostasis

SYNONYMS
- Bleeding time - observation

REFERENCE RANGE
- Adults:
- Simplate (template) method: 2-9.5 minutes
- Mielke (template) method: <10 minutes
- Duke (ear lobe) method: 1-3 minutes
- Newborn to 8 years (Mielke [modified] method): 3.4 +/- 1.3 minutes
- Children 8 to 18 years (Mielke [modified] method): 2.8 +/- 1.6 minutes
-

Please refer to your institution's reference ranges as lab normals may vary.

INDICATIONS
Suspected and known preeclampsia
> **Results Interpretation:**
> **Blood coagulation disorder with prolonged bleeding time**
>> Bleeding times may be prolonged in women with preeclampsia and may occur even in the presence of a normal platelet count. Though additional research is needed, prophylactic magnesium sulfate administration may be associated with prolonged bleeding times in preeclamptic patients.

Suspected von Willebrand disease
> **Strength of Recommendation:** Class IIb
> **Strength of Evidence:** Category C

Results Interpretation:
Increased level (laboratory finding)

Prolonged bleeding time is one of the diagnostic criteria widely associated with von Willebrand disease, although inter-user reliability varies and bleeding time may be normal in mild disease; additional laboratory studies are recommended to confirm the diagnosis.

Frequency of Monitoring

Repeat evaluation may be necessary in patients with mild von Willebrand disease and normal bleeding time.

ABNORMAL RESULTS

- Results increased in:
  - Anxiety
  - Females
  - Improper technique/operator error (eg, increased cuff pressure, increased length or depth of cut, antecubital fossa cut instead of volar surface of the arm)
- Results decreased in:
  - Advancing age
  - Repeating the test within 4 hours of first bleeding time
- Other factors affecting the results:
  - Handedness
  - Ethnicity
  - Serum triglycerides
  - Skin fold thickness
  - Social class
  - Weight to height ratio

CLINICAL NOTES

Preoperative bleeding time is no longer recommended because it is not a reliable predictor of perioperative bleeding risk.

In a review of 640 articles, the authors concluded that the value of the bleeding time test in diagnosis of disease is unclear; no evidence was found to support its use in prognosis or for monitoring of therapy.

COLLECTION/STORAGE INFORMATION

- Specimen Collection and Handling:
  - Perform test at bedside
  - Apply blood pressure cuff to upper arm and inflate to 40 mm Hg to increase capillary pressure in forearm; use a pediatric cuff for children
  - Make small standardized incision horizontally onto the volar aspect of forearm; begin timer
  - Remove blood from surface of the wound with filter paper every 30 seconds until blood no longer stains the paper (avoiding the wound edges); stop timer
  - Record time required for bleeding to stop after skin puncture

Blood alcohol level

TEST DEFINITION

Quantitative measurement of ethanol in blood for the assessment of recent ethanol intake

SYNONYMS

- Blood ethanol level
- Blood ethanol measurement

REFERENCE RANGE

Negative
Please refer to your institution's reference ranges as lab normals may vary.

INDICATIONS

Submersion
   Results Interpretation:
   Raised biochemistry findings
      Blood ethanol levels greater than 100 mg/100 dL have been reported in about one third of adolescent and adult submersion victims. Others have reported that 30% to 70% of submersion victims aged 15 years or older have alcohol in their blood.

Suspected alcohol intoxication
   Strength of Recommendation: Class IIa
   Strength of Evidence: Category C
   Results Interpretation:
   Finding of alcohol in blood
      The blood ethanol level is typically elevated to 100 to 300 mg/dL (32.6 to 65.2 millimol/L) in acute intoxication. Most fatalities occur with levels greater than 400 mg/dL (86.8 millimol/L). The lethal dose is variable, depending in part on chronic versus sporadic ethanol use. Minimal lethal exposure in a nontolerant adult is 5 to 6 g/kg of body weight taken orally. In the pediatric population, minimum lethal exposure is 3 g/kg of body weight taken orally.
      - Physiologic effects at specific ethanol concentrations:
         - Slowing of reflexes, impaired visual activity: 50 to 100 mg/dL (10.9 to 21.7 mmol/L)
         - CNS depression: greater than 100 mg/dL (greater than 21.7 mmol/L)
         - Potentially fatal: greater than 400 mg/dL (greater than 86.8 mmol/L)
      The rate, but not extent, of alcohol absorption is affected by several factors including the presence of food (particularly high-fat foods), amount of alcohol ingested, time frame of consumption, and metabolic differences among individuals. On an empty stomach, peak blood ethanol level may occur in 30 to 75 minutes; on a full stomach or when large amounts of food have been consumed, peak level may not occur until 3 hours after ethanol ingestion.
      The universally accepted blood alcohol concentration results for legal purposes are reported in percent weight/volume units or g/dL truncated to 2 decimal places.
      The level of ethanol in blood equating to intoxication differs by state and country statute.

COMMON PANELS
- Volatile alcohol screen, serum

COLLECTION/STORAGE INFORMATION
- Specimen Collection and Handling:
   - Use alcohol-free swabs or betadine when collecting the specimen.
   - Collect sample from an arm vein of a living person.
   - Collect sample from the aorta of a dead person.
   - Collect serum or whole blood sample (statutes defining BAC limits usually refer to whole blood as the biologic specimen).
   - Preserve with 1% sodium fluoride (weight/volume).
   - Store specimen with sodium fluoride at 25°C up to 2 weeks, at 5°C up to 3 months, and at -15°C up to 6 months.
   - Store specimen without sodium fluoride at 25°C up to 2 days, 5°C up to 2 weeks, and at -15°C up to 4 weeks.

LOINC CODES
- Code: 5640-8 (*Short Name* - Ethanol Bld-mCnc)
- Code: 15120-9 (*Short Name* - Ethanol Bld-sCnc)
- Code: 5639-0 (*Short Name* - Ethanol Bld Ql)

Blood cadmium measurement

TEST DEFINITION
   Measurement of cadmium in blood for the evaluation and management of cadmium exposure

SYNONYMS
- Blood cadmium level

REFERENCE RANGE
- Smokers: 0.6-3.9 mcg/L (5.3-34.7 nmol/L)
- Nonsmokers: 0.3-1.2 mcg/L (2.7-10.7 nmol/L)
  Please refer to your institution's reference ranges as lab normals may vary.

INDICATIONS
Cadmium poisoning
> **Strength of Recommendation:** Class IIa
> **Strength of Evidence:** Category B
> **Results Interpretation:**
> **Increased level (laboratory finding)**
> Blood cadmium levels rise and fall rapidly in response to exposure, with an initial half-time of 2 to 3 months. While elevated blood cadmium concentrations primarily reflect recent exposure they are also influenced by a patient's accumulated body burden, particularly with prolonged or heavy exposure. In those newly exposed, blood cadmium levels increase gradually over 4 to 6 months, then level off in proportion to the average intensity of exposure. Since blood cadmium is a reflection of accumulated cadmium in the body, concentrations rarely return to pre-exposure levels.
> Cadmium levels of 100 to 1,000 micrograms/L (0.9 to 26.7 micromol/L) are considered toxic. Patients whose cadmium levels exceed 7 nanomols/L have an increased risk for tubular proteinuria.
> Smokers have higher blood cadmium levels than non-smokers. Ex-smokers have higher blood cadmium levels than non-smokers, but lower blood cadmium levels than current smokers.
> In general, women have higher blood cadmium levels than men.
> While substantial individual variability in blood levels has been observed in people of the same age group and geographic area, average blood cadmium levels may be population-specific.

COLLECTION/STORAGE INFORMATION
- Draw whole blood in heparin or EDTA tube.
- Collect sample in metal-free container.

LOINC CODES
- Code: 15117-5 (*Short Name* - Cadmium Bld-sCnc)
- Code: 21129-2 (*Short Name* - Cadmium SerPl-mCnc)
- Code: 5609-3 (*Short Name* - Cadmium Bld-mCnc)
- Code: 12505-4 (*Short Name* - Cadmium RBC-mCnc)
- Code: 27117-1 (*Short Name* - Cadmium RBC-mCnt)
- Code: 25359-1 (*Short Name* - Cadmium SerPl-sCnc)

Blood culture

TEST DEFINITION
Measurement of aerobic and anaerobic microorganism growth in blood for evaluation of infection

SYNONYMS
- BC - Blood culture

REFERENCE RANGE
- Adults and children: No growth
  Please refer to your institution's reference ranges as lab normals may vary.

INDICATIONS
Hospitalized patients with community-acquired pneumonia
> **Strength of Recommendation:** Class I
> **Strength of Evidence:** Category B
> **Results Interpretation:**
> **Positive microbiology findings**
> Etiologic diagnosis is established with recovery of a probable causative agent. Blood cultures may help to identify the presence of bacteremia or a resistant pathogen.

Timing of Monitoring
Two sets of blood cultures should be drawn prior to the initiation of antimicrobial therapy.

Suspected staphylococcal scalded skin syndrome with possible sepsis
Results Interpretation:
Positive microbiology findings
Staphylococcus aureus is isolated from the blood of most adults with staphylococcal scalded skin syndrome as they usually are septic and have a definable source of bacteremia.
Negative microbiology findings
In children, *Staphylococcus aureus* endotoxin is produced at a distal site resulting in negative blood cultures over 97% of the time.

Febrile seizure
Results Interpretation:
Positive microbiology findings
Blood cultures are positive in up to 5% of patients with febrile seizures.

Obtain in patients with epiglottitis after the airway is secured
Results Interpretation:
Positive microbiology findings
Bacteremia is associated with a high risk of airway obstruction.
Throat and blood cultures may yield different pathogens.
No definable pathogen is isolated in the majority of patients with mild disease.

Sickle cell disease
Results Interpretation:
Abnormal laboratory findings
In young children with sickle cell disease, most bacteremias are caused by Streptococcus pneumoniae (S pneumoniae) and Haemophilus influenzae (H influenzae), with occasional cases due to Salmonella species.
In older sickle cell patients, gram-negative enterics, Staphylococcus aureus (S aureus), and Salmonella deserve greater consideration as causative organisms of sepsis.

Suspected acute hematogenous osteomyelitis
Results Interpretation:
Positive microbiology findings
Approximately 25% of cases of vertebral osteomyelitis yield positive blood culture results.

Suspected bacterial endocarditis
    Strength of Recommendation: Class I
    Strength of Evidence: Category A
Results Interpretation:
Positive microbiology findings
Positive cultures occur in about 95% of cases when 3 sets of cultures are obtained. Community-acquired bacteremia without evidence of localized infection signals high risk of endocarditis.

    False Results
    Use meticulous skin preparation technique to avoid contamination with skin flora (S epidermidis and diptheroids).
Negative microbiology findings
- Negative cultures may occur in 3% to 5% of cases. Possible causes of a negative culture include:
  -
    - Fastidious organisms: *Coxiella burnetii*, Haemophilus sp, anaerobes, fungi, coryneforms, Chlamydia, Rickettsia, Bartonella, and HACEK organisms (*Haemophilus parainfluenzae, Haemophilus aphrophilus, Actinobacillus actinomycetemcomitans, Cardiobacterium hominis, Eikenella corrodens, Kingella kingae*). Further investigation for fastidious organisms recommended in patients with culture-negative infective endocarditis.
    - Prior antibiotic therapy
- Although the cause is unknown, patients with a culture-negative infective endocarditis have a worse prognosis and higher rate of complications than those with positive blood cultures

False Results

Use meticulous skin preparation technique to avoid contamination with skin flora (S epidermidis and diptheroids).

Frequency of Monitoring

Obtain at least 3 sets of venous samples for suspected native valve endocarditis and at least 4 sets for patients with prosthetic valves or who are IV drug abusers.

Obtain 10 to 20 mL of blood for each culture, to be divided equally for anaerobic and aerobic cultures.

In acutely ill patients, obtain cultures are at 5- to 10-minute intervals from different peripheral venous sites before initiating empiric antibiotic therapy; do not initiate antibiotic therapy until adequate blood has been drawn for multiple cultures.

In non-acutely ill patients, obtain blood samples for culture at 20- to 30-minute intervals from different peripheral venous sites.

Suspected cellulitis

Strength of Recommendation: Class IIb
Strength of Evidence: Category C
Results Interpretation:
Positive microbiology findings

Blood cultures are nondiagnostic in patients with suspected cellulitis.

Suspected disseminated gonococcal infection (DGI or gonococcemia)

Results Interpretation:
Positive microbiology findings

The blood culture is positive in 10% to 30% of patients with disseminated gonococcal infection (DGI). Blood cultures are rarely positive when the synovial fluid cultures are positive.

Suspected erysipelas

Strength of Recommendation: Class IIb
Strength of Evidence: Category C
Results Interpretation:
Positive microbiology findings

Blood culture results are positive in 3% to 6% of cases. Contaminants may be more common than true pathogens.

Suspected infective endocarditis

Results Interpretation:
Positive microbiology findings

In infective endocarditis, blood cultures are positive in 95% of the cases when 3 sets of cultures are obtained.

A thorough search for fastidious organisms is indicated in culture-negative infective endocarditis, which occurs in about 3% to 5% of the patients with infective endocarditis, and may be caused by *Coxiella burnetii, Haemophilus spp.*, anaerobes, fungi, coryneforms, *Chlamydia spp., Rickettsia spp., Bartonella spp.*, and HACEK organisms (*Haemophilus parainfluenzae, Haemophilus aphrophilus, Actinobacillus actinomycetemcomitans, Cardiobacterium hominis, Eikenella corrodens*, and *Kingella kingae*).

Patients who received prior antibiotic therapy may also develop a culture-negative infective endocarditis, which is associated with a worse prognosis and a higher rate of complications than those with positive blood cultures.

Negative microbiology findings

A thorough search for fastidious organisms is indicated in culture-negative infective endocarditis, which occurs in 3% to 5% of the patients with infective endocarditis, and may be caused by *Coxiella burnetii*, Haemophilus, anaerobes, fungi, coryneforms, chlamydia, rickettsia, bartonella (rochalimaea), and HACEK organisms (*Haemophilus parainfluenzae, Haemophilus aphrophilus, Actinobacillus actinomycetemcomitans, Cardiobacterium hominis, Eikenella corrodens*, and *Kingella kingae*).

Patients who received prior antibiotic therapy may also have culture negative infective endocarditis, which is associated with a worse prognosis and a higher rate of complications than those with positive blood cultures.

Community-acquired bacteremia without evidence of localized infection indicates a high risk of endocarditis.

Timing of Monitoring

In acutely ill patients, blood samples for culture should be obtained at 5- to 10-minute intervals from different peripheral venous sites before initiating empiric antibiotic therapy. Antibiotic therapy should not be initiated prior to blood drawing for multiple cultures.

In patients who are not acutely ill, blood samples for culture should be obtained at different peripheral venous sites at 20- to 30-minute intervals.

Suspected Ludwig's angina
Results Interpretation:
Positive microbiology findings
Blood cultures are positive in 10% to 15% of cases. The yield of blood cultures is lower than that of surgical pus aspirate.

Pseudomonas aeruginosa and *Haemophilus influenzae* are isolated most frequently.

Suspected meningococcal disease
Strength of Recommendation: Class IIa
Strength of Evidence: Category C
Results Interpretation:
Positive microbiology findings
Cultures may or may not be positive for gram-negative diplococcus depending on the degree of septicemia. Preadmission antibiotics reduce the rate of positive blood cultures.
Timing of Monitoring
Blood cultures should be obtained before the start of antibiotic therapy, unless it delays treatment.

Suspected or known gastroenteritis with possible bacteremia
Results Interpretation:
Sample: salmonella cultured
Salmonellosis is associated with bacteremia in children who are in a toxic condition, particularly those under 1 year of age or who are immunocompromised; salmonellosis may occur in older children who do not appear to be toxic.

AIDS patients with salmonellosis often present with bacteremia.
Positive microbiology findings
Campylobacter jejuni may be present and complicate gastroenteritis, particularly in infants and patients more than 50 years.

Shigellosis is rarely associated with bacteremia. It occurs primarily in young children; however, cases have been reported in adults, particularly in elderly and immunocompromised patients.

In bacteremic children, *Shigella dysenteriae* is the primary causative species, whereas in adults, *Shigella flexneri* and *Shigella sonnei* are isolated most frequently. *Shigella* bacteremia is associated with a relatively high mortality, particularly if the organism is isolated from blood only, rather than from both blood and stool.

Suspected plague
Results Interpretation:
Positive microbiology findings
Organisms may be seen in blood smears if the patient is septicemic, while blood smears taken from suspected bubonic plague patients are usually negative for bacteria. Bacteria may be intermittently released from affected lymph nodes into the bloodstream; therefore, a series of blood specimens taken 10 to 30 minutes apart may be productive in the isolation of *Yersinia pestis*.

Plague bacilli are both aerobic and facultatively anaerobic.

It takes about 48 hours before colonies can be seen on plain agar.

The colonies are small and grayish.

Suspected sepsis
Strength of Recommendation: Class I
Strength of Evidence: Category B
Results Interpretation:
Positive microbiology findings
Blood cultures are usually positive, but negative cultures do not rule out sepsis. In septic patients, 70% of blood cultures ultimately are positive. In 10% to 30% of patients, causative organisms may not be isolated.
Frequency of Monitoring
All patients with suspected sepsis should receive at least 3 (preferably 4 to 6) sets of blood cultures (anaerobic and aerobic) obtained 15 minutes apart, with a minimum of 3 sets of cultures obtained in a 24-hour period. Additional cultures may be needed, if the patient is receiving antibiotics.
Timing of Monitoring
Blood cultures should be obtained prior to initiation of antibiotic therapy. Two sets of blood cultures should be obtained at the initial evaluation of each episode of suspected bacteremia.

Suspected septic arthritis
  Results Interpretation:
  Positive microbiology findings
    Blood cultures are positive at the time of positive synovial fluid cultures in one third to one half of cases. Positive blood cultures are relatively common in patients with joints infected with gram-negative bacilli. In 1 series, 50% to 70% of patients with nongonococcal bacterial arthritis had positive blood cultures. In another series, blood cultures were positive in 40% of patients with staphylococcal arthritis and in almost 60% of patients with proven streptococcal arthritis.

    Blood cultures are often positive in IV drug abusers, particularly those with staphylococcal arthritis.

    Cultures are positive in approximately 50% of children with staphylococcal septic arthritis of the hip.

    In a study of 147 children, blood cultures were positive in about 10% when synovial fluid cultures were negative.

    Blood cultures are positive in only about 20% of patients with gonococcal arthritis and in less than 10% of those with disseminated gonococcal infection (DGI). Patients with DGI almost never have simultaneously positive blood and synovial fluid cultures.

CLINICAL NOTES
  Blood cultures are incubated for 5 to 7 days before the final results are available. Aerobic cultures are initially examined 18 to 24 hours after start of incubation; anaerobic cultures should be examined after 48 hours. Preliminary results are usually available after 24 to 48 hours and are update as indicated.

COLLECTION/STORAGE INFORMATION
- Specimen Collection and Handling:
  - Obtain up to three to four sets of blood cultures to detect the causative agent
  - Collect 20 mL blood (adults and children); divide equally between two 100 mL blood culture bottles or between a 100 mL blood culture bottle and a lysis centrifugation tube
  - Collect 1 to 5 mL blood (infants) per 100-mL blood culture bottle containing sodium polyanetholsulfonate (SPS) or 0.5 to 1 mL blood per lysis centrifugation tube (eg, pediatric isolator tube, Wampole Isolator™)
  - Collect one culture from each lumen of indwelling vascular access devices that have been in place for at least 48 hours and one peripheral site
  - To maximize overall organism recovery, blood drawn for culture should be processed in two different systems (eg, Septi-Chek™ and isolator systems useful in suspected staphylococci; isolator recovers more fungal organisms; broth more likely to recover pneumococci).
  - Anaerobic cultures should be placed in an anaerobic environment as soon as possible.

LOINC CODES
- Code: 600-7 (*Short Name* - Bld Cult)

Blood methanol measurement

TEST DEFINITION
  Detection and measurement of methanol in serum or plasma to evaluate poisoning

SYNONYMS
- Blood methanol level

REFERENCE RANGE
  Normal methanol blood concentration from endogenous production and dietary sources is up to 1.5 mg/L.
  Please refer to your institution's reference ranges as lab normals may vary.

INDICATIONS
Suspected methanol poisoning
    Strength of Recommendation: Class IIa
    Strength of Evidence: Category C
  Results Interpretation:
  Methanol toxicity
    Blood methanol concentration greater than 200 mg/L (greater than 6.24 millimol/L) is considered toxic.

Plasma methanol concentration of about 40 mg/100mL (12 millimol/L) is typically fatal, but individual sensitivity varies. Deaths have been reported with blood methanol levels of 19.4 mg/100mL (6 millimol/L), 27.7 mg/100mL (8.6 millimol/L), and 27.5 mg/100mL (8.6 millimol/L) at 48, 50 and 50 hours, respectively, postingestion. In most of these cases, true peak methanol levels were unknown.

Ingestion of 60 to 240 mL of methanol is typically fatal. However, the smallest amount of methanol reported to cause death is 15 mL of 40% methanol.

One of the highest reported cases of patient survival noted methanol ingestion of 500 to 600 mL. Methanol is rapidly absorbed; peak values can be obtained within 30 to 60 minutes. However, onset of toxicity is delayed by 12 to 24 hours as methanol is metabolized to formate. As an example, a methanol level of 20 mg/dL 1 hour post ingestion will correspond to peak levels of 113 mg/dL, 215 mg/dL and 420 mg/dL, respectively, at 12, 24 and 48 hours postingestion.

Most cases of severe poisoning occur by ingestion, although poisoning has occurred with skin contact and inhalation. The range of methanol toxicity is variable; blindness has followed ingestion of about 4 mL.

Blood methanol concentration is not predictive of poisoning leading to permanent organ damage. Extremely high exposures (greater than 25,000 ppm) are necessary to produce sensory irritation.

COMMON PANELS
- Volatile alcohol screen, serum

CLINICAL NOTES
Methanol, or wood alcohol, is used as a solvent, denaturing agent, antifreeze constituent, and a fuel in internal combustion engines or cooking appliances. Methanol can be absorbed by inhalation, through skin contact, intravenous injection, and most commonly, by ingestion of contaminated drinks.

LOINC CODES
- Code: 5690-3 (*Short Name* - Methanol Bld Ql)
- Code: 5692-9 (*Short Name* - Methanol SerPl Ql)
- Code: 20579-9 (*Short Name* - Methanol SerPl Ql Scn)
- Code: 9334-4 (*Short Name* - Methanol Bld-mCnc)
- Code: 14835-3 (*Short Name* - Methanol SerPl-sCnc)
- Code: 5693-7 (*Short Name* - Methanol SerPl-mCnc)

Blood spot TSH level

TEST DEFINITION
Measurement of thyroid stimulating hormone (TSH) in newborns to screen for thyroid dysfunction

REFERENCE RANGE
- Neonates: <20 microInternational Units/mL
  Please refer to your institution's reference ranges as lab normals may vary.

INDICATIONS
Suspected congenital hypothyroidism
    Strength of Recommendation: Class I
    Strength of Evidence: Category B
    Results Interpretation:
    Raised TSH level

Primary screening with thyroid stimulating hormone (TSH) may be more accurate for the diagnosis of congenital hypothyroidism than an initial screen of T_4 followed by TSH when T_4 values fall below a preset cutoff. TSH testing should be done after 48 hours of life.

Some experts have suggested using a cutoff of 50 microunits/mL for TSH when used as a primary screen, or a T_4 cutoff of 64 nmol/L in conjunction with a TSH range of 20 to 50 microunits/mL.

A positive TSH screen for hypothyroidism should be followed up by a radioisotope scan to identify the etiology.

Timing of Monitoring

Timing of the newborn screen is critical. A well-documented thyroid stimulating hormone (TSH) surge is seen in many neonates soon after birth, stabilizing between 24 and 48 hours post-delivery when hypothyroidism is not present.

A study of 161,244 neonates found that TSH levels had a very wide range until after 48 hours of life, suggesting that TSH testing before 24 hours would be unreliable. For infants of unknown age, a conservative TSH cutoff of 20 microInternational Units/mL was recommended.

Suspected neonatal iodine deficiency
Strength of Recommendation: Class I
Strength of Evidence: Category B
Results Interpretation:
Raised TSH level
Iodine deficiency is often associated with transient hypothyroidism and a transient elevation in thyroid stimulating hormone (TSH) levels.

COLLECTION/STORAGE INFORMATION
- Specimen Collection and Handling:
  - Collect whole blood from heel stick on filter paper 3 to 7 days after birth.
  - May refrigerate specimen with desiccant for many months

Blood urea nitrogen measurement

TEST DEFINITION
Measurement of serum or plasma blood urea nitrogen (BUN) for the evaluation and management of volume status and renal disorders

SYNONYMS
- BUN measurement

REFERENCE RANGE
- Adults: 10-20 mg/dL (3.6-7.1 mmol/L)
- Children: 5-18 mg/dL (1.8-6.4 mmol/L)
Please refer to your institution's reference ranges as lab normals may vary.

INDICATIONS
Adrenal insufficiency
Results Interpretation:
Serum blood urea nitrogen raised
Moderate elevations in blood urea nitrogen (BUN) levels are consistent with both acute and chronic adrenal insufficiency. The increased BUN is largely due to dehydration secondary to aldosterone deficiency, which leads to excretion of sodium in excess of intake and results in azotemia. Patients with secondary adrenal insufficiency are less affected because of intact aldosterone secretion.
Elevation of the BUN level is usually reversible with restoration of normal renal hemodynamics and circulating blood volume.

Community-acquired pneumonia
Strength of Recommendation: Class IIa
Strength of Evidence: Category B
Results Interpretation:
Serum blood urea nitrogen raised
In one study, an elevated blood urea nitrogen (BUN), along with increased respiratory rate and decreased diastolic blood pressure, was predictive of mortality in patients with community-acquired pneumonia.

Hemolytic uremic syndrome (HUS)
Results Interpretation:
Serum blood urea nitrogen raised
In hemolytic uremic syndrome (HUS), blood urea nitrogen (BUN) level is consistently increased, with the elevation usually occurring very rapidly. The combination of renal insufficiency, a catabolic state, and reabsorption of blood from the GI tract can cause BUN levels to increase as much as 50 mg/dL/day.
In children with uncomplicated dehydration and diarrhea, the BUN level should fall to one half the admission level within 24 hours; if this does not occur, renal disease should be suspected.

Hemorrhagic shock
Results Interpretation:
Serum blood urea nitrogen raised
In hemorrhagic shock, acute tubular necrosis (ATN) from prolonged hypotension results in renal failure. Blood urea nitrogen (BUN) and creatinine levels typically rise over the first few postshock days in a fixed ratio of 10:1.

Increased BUN levels also occur secondary to the breakdown of blood in the gastrointestinal tract, as seen in gastrointestinal tract hemorrhage, and as a result of prerenal azotemia.

Initial evaluation and monitoring of hyperosmolar hyperglycemic state
Strength of Recommendation: Class I
Strength of Evidence: Category C
Results Interpretation:
Serum blood urea nitrogen raised
Blood urea nitrogen (BUN) is almost always increased in hyperglycemic hyperosmolar state (HHS) secondary to dehydration and renal damage, even in the absence of significant diabetic nephropathy. The mean level of BUN is 61 mg/dL in patients presenting with HHS.
Frequency of Monitoring
During treatment for HHS, check blood urea nitrogen (BUN) every 2 to 4 hours until the patient is stable.

Initial evaluation and monitoring of suspected diabetic ketoacidosis
Strength of Recommendation: Class I
Strength of Evidence: Category B
Results Interpretation:
Serum blood urea nitrogen raised
Blood urea nitrogen (BUN) level is usually mildly to moderately elevated (mean 32 mg/dL) in diabetic ketoacidosis (DKA), attributable to significant volume loss rather than diabetic nephropathy.
Frequency of Monitoring
During treatment of diabetic ketoacidosis (DKA), check blood urea nitrogen (BUN) every 2 to 4 hours until the patient is stable.

Metabolic acidosis
Results Interpretation:
Abnormal laboratory findings
Anion gap metabolic acidosis develops when the glomerular filtration rate is less than 20 mL/min (BUN level greater than 40 mg/dL).

An elevation of BUN may be seen in volume-depleted patients with metabolic acidosis, and in patients with metabolic acidosis secondary to chronic renal failure.

Sickle cell disease
Results Interpretation:
Serum blood urea nitrogen raised
A chronically elevated BUN level in conjunction with an elevated serum creatinine, even if only mildly increased, indicates renal insufficiency.

Acute increases in BUN are seen in severe urinary tract infection.

Suspected cardiogenic shock
Results Interpretation:
Serum blood urea nitrogen raised
In the setting of cardiogenic shock, elevated BUN may occur secondary to preexisting renal disease or poor renal perfusion; poor renal perfusion may lead to eventual prerenal azotemia or frank acute tubular necrosis (ATN) from renal ischemia.

Suspected dehydration in children with acute gastroenteritis
Strength of Recommendation: Class IIb
Strength of Evidence: Category B
Results Interpretation:
Decreased blood urea nitrogen level
In a study of young children with acute gastroenteritis, a BUN level below 40 mg/dL was associated with mild to moderate dehydration.

Serum blood urea nitrogen raised

In a study of young children with acute gastroenteritis, a BUN level above 100 mg/dL was associated with moderate to severe dehydration.

Suspected hypertensive crisis
Results Interpretation:
Serum blood urea nitrogen raised

In hypertensive crisis, the BUN and creatinine levels tend to rise at the onset of therapy but eventually improve as the renal arterioles recover from the effects of the high pressure. The rise in BUN, and thus the progression of renal failure, may be faster in patients with essential hypertension in the malignant phase than in patients with other underlying primary renal disease.

Suspected necrotizing soft tissue infection
Results Interpretation:
Serum blood urea nitrogen raised

In one study, a BUN greater than 51 mg/dL was reported in 60% of cases of synergistic necrotizing cellulitis. This reflects intravascular fluid volume loss into tissues that occurs with the massive edema seen with synergistic necrotizing cellulitis, streptococcal gangrene, and necrotizing fasciitis.

Suspected or known acute renal failure
Strength of Recommendation: Class I
Strength of Evidence: Category C
Results Interpretation:
Serum blood urea nitrogen raised

The blood urea nitrogen (BUN) level increases progressively at a rate of at least 10 mg/dL/day in the setting of clinically significant renal failure. In patients with extensive tissue necrosis, it can rise at a rate of 50 to 100 mg/dL/day.

A BUN of 50 to 150 mg/100mL suggests serious renal impairment, and a BUN of 150 to 250 mg/100 mL is virtually diagnostic of severe glomerular dysfunction. In a steady state, a 50% decrease in the glomerular filtration rate (GFR) will result in a doubling of the BUN.

Suspected or known renal failure
Strength of Recommendation: Class I
Strength of Evidence: Category C
Results Interpretation:
Serum blood urea nitrogen raised

In patients with chronic renal insufficiency, an acute increase in serum creatinine or BUN, or a decrease in GFR, should trigger a rapid search for reversible causes of acute (ie, acute-on-chronic) renal dysfunction.

In patients with no history of renal disease, acute renal failure may be defined either by a BUN level of at least 40 mg/dL (14.3 mmol/L) or a serum creatinine level of at least 2 mg/dL (177 micromoles/L).

If the GFR falls to less than 10 mL/min, serum creatinine should increase by 0.5 to 1.5 mg/dL (44 to 133 micromol/L) per day, depending on age, muscle mass, and muscle injury. The BUN level should increase by 10 to 20 mg/dL (3.6 to 7.1 mmol/L) per day, but the rate of increase can be higher in hypercatabolic states like sepsis, gastrointestinal bleeding, or with corticosteroid use.

- Causes of rapid serial increases in BUN levels:
  - Clinically significant renal failure (eg, GFR <10 mL/minute): increases 10 to 20 mg/dL/day
  - Extensive tissue necrosis: increases 50 to 100 mg/dL/day
  - Hypercatabolic states (eg, sepsis, gastrointestinal hemorrhage, corticosteroid use)

Suspected post-streptococcal glomerulonephritis
Strength of Recommendation: Class I
Strength of Evidence: Category C
Results Interpretation:
Increased level (laboratory finding)

BUN is elevated to some extent in 60% to 75% of post-streptococcal glomerulonephritis patients, which may result from a reduction in glomerular filtration rate, as well as from prerenal factors (eg, cardiac decompensation and continued dietary intake of protein).

Suspected sepsis
Strength of Recommendation: Class I
Strength of Evidence: Category C

Results Interpretation:
Serum blood urea nitrogen raised
   Blood urea nitrogen (BUN) levels may be elevated in sepsis due to prerenal azotemia, gastrointestinal bleeding, drug toxicity or acute tubular necrosis (ATN).
Timing of Monitoring
   The Infectious Disease Society of America recommends BUN and serum creatinine be done at baseline and at least every 3 days during the course of intensive antibiotic therapy. The use of renal toxic drugs such as Amphotericin B require more frequent monitoring.

Suspected toxic shock syndrome
   Results Interpretation:
   Abnormal laboratory findings
      BUN may be elevated in toxic shock syndrome secondary to myoglobinemia or shock.

To differentiate between upper and lower acute gastrointestinal bleeding
   Results Interpretation:
   Serum blood urea nitrogen raised
   - In patients with acute gastrointestinal (GI) bleeding, a BUN:creatinine ratio of 36 or greater suggests an upper GI bleeding site.
   - In patients with GI bleeding and no renal disease, a BUN level over 40 mg/dL with a normal creatinine level suggests significant GI blood loss.
   - A BUN level greater than 85 mg/dL with a normal creatinine level may indicate a loss of 2 or more units of blood into the GI tract.
   - In patients with normal renal function, a mild BUN elevation (4 to 7 mg/dL above baseline) secondary to hemorrhage should return to normal within 24 hours. In patients with GI bleeding, persistent BUN elevations greater than 7mg/dL above baseline values suggest hypovolemia, renal insufficiency, or continued hemorrhage.
   - In patients with acute GI bleeding, the absence of a rise in BUN does not rule out an upper GI source of bleeding.

COMMON PANELS
- Basic metabolic panel
- Comprehensive metabolic panel
- Enteral/Parenteral nutritional management panel
- General health panel
- Hypertension panel
- Prenatal screening panel
- Renal panel
- Transplant panel

ABNORMAL RESULTS
- Results increased in:
   - Febrile illness
   - High protein diet
- Results decreased in:
   - Low protein diet
   - High carbohydrate diet

COLLECTION/STORAGE INFORMATION
- Sample is stable for 24 hours at room temperature, for several days at 4°C to 6°C, and for 2 to 3 months when frozen.

LOINC CODES
- Code: 12963-5 (*Short Name* - BUN BldP-mCnc)
- Code: 6299-2 (*Short Name* - BUN Bld-mCnc)
- Code: 12961-9 (*Short Name* - BUN BldA-mCnc)
- Code: 17759-2 (*Short Name* - BUN p dialysis BldA-mCnc)
- Code: 12964-3 (*Short Name* - BUN BS Bld-mCnc)
- Code: 12962-7 (*Short Name* - Urea Nit BldV-mCnc)
- Code: 3094-0 (*Short Name* - BUN SerPl-mCnc)
- Code: 12966-8 (*Short Name* - BUN 2H spec SerPl-mCnc)

- Code: 14937-7 (*Short Name* - BUN SerPl-sCnc)

Bone histomorphometry, aluminum stain

TEST DEFINITION
The measurement of aluminum in bone for the diagnosis and management of complications associated with aluminum overload

SYNONYMS
- Bone histomorphometry, aluminium stain

REFERENCE RANGE
Bone aluminum level: 1 microgram/g wet weight
Please refer to your institution's reference ranges as lab normals may vary.

INDICATIONS
Suspected aluminum intoxication
> **Strength of Recommendation:** Class IIa
> **Strength of Evidence:** Category B
> **Results Interpretation:**
> **Biopsy finding**
> A bone aluminum level of at least 10 mcg/g wet tissue weight and a positive aluminum stain in the appropriate clinical setting indicates aluminum toxicity.
> Histologic examination of bone biopsy specimens is employed in the diagnosis of aluminum toxicity; and may be the most effective method to diagnose such toxicity.
> Plasma aluminum concentration should be measured for patients with a high index of suspicion for aluminum overload; nevertheless, aluminum bone disease or osteomalacia should always be confirmed by bone biopsy.
> Aluminum toxicity is linked to development of osteomalacic osteodystrophy and dialysis encephalopathy syndrome (DES).

Suspected and known aluminum bone disease
> **Strength of Recommendation:** Class IIa
> **Strength of Evidence:** Category B
> **Results Interpretation:**
> **Biopsy finding**
> A bone aluminum level of at least 10 mcg/g wet tissue weight, positive aluminum staining at the osteoid/calcified-bone boundary, and the presence of histologic osteomalacia are strongly indicate aluminum bone disease.
> Positive aluminum staining of cement lines and of osteoid/calcified bone interfaces are indicative of adynamic bone disease and osteomalacia. Bone biopsy showing aluminum present at the mineral front, at cement lines, and near osteocytes is indicative of osteomalacic osteodystrophy.
> Histologic examination of a bone biopsy specimen is the most reliable test to diagnose aluminum-related osteomalacia.
> Bone biopsy can differentiate aluminum bone disease from severe hyperparathyroidism in patients with symptomatic bone disease.
> Type 1 osteomalacia seen in patients with chronic renal failure on long-term hemodialysis is characterized by high bone content of aluminum, low plasma calcium and phosphorus, and wide osteoid seams. Type 2 osteomalacia is characterized by moderate bone aluminum content and thin, extensive, inactive osteoid.
> Increased bone aluminum content may be present in patients receiving dialysis, total parenteral nutrition, therapeutic plasma exchange, and long-term oral intake of aluminum-containing phosphate binders, aluminum hydroxide, or aluminum salts.
> Patients with chronic renal failure may have bone aluminum content ten times greater than those without renal disease. Bone aluminum levels increase the longer a patient undergoes hemodialysis.
> Bone biopsies are of greater diagnostic value for aluminum bone disease than bone x-rays.
> Heavy aluminum burden evidenced by bone biopsy with histological staining and aluminum concentration measurement, plus a positive desferroxamine test, support initiation of long-term desferroxamine treatment.

Frequency of Monitoring
Obtain two or more bone biopsy specimens at the beginning of and during therapy for bone disease to monitor therapeutic effect. Additional samples may be collected yearly or less frequently. Patients in severe chronic renal failure should have routine aluminum staining of bone biopsy specimens.

COLLECTION/STORAGE INFORMATION
- Use local anesthesia for procedure.
- Collect specimen by bone biopsy taken from trans-iliac site using trocars.

LOINC CODES
- Code: 10740-9 (*Short Name* - Aluminum Bone Histomorph Stn)

Bone marrow culture

TEST DEFINITION
Detection of bacterial or mycobacterial infection in bone marrow in susceptible individuals (eg, immunocompromised patients {HIV infection, AIDS})

REFERENCE RANGE
- Adults and Children: Negative or No Growth
  Please refer to your institution's reference ranges as lab normals may vary.

INDICATIONS
Suspected microbial infection disseminated to bone marrow
  Strength of Recommendation: Class IIb
  Strength of Evidence: Category B
  Results Interpretation:
  Positive microbiology findings
  A positive bone marrow culture can be useful in immunocompromised patients (ie, HIV infection or AIDS) with disseminated mycobacterial or fungal infections that present with prolonged fever. Bone marrow examination in febrile patients with HIV infection is a high-yield procedure, particularly because mycobacterial infection is a common cause of fever of unknown origin in these patients.
  Acid-fast bacteria bone marrow cultures are often positive in patients with mycobacterial infection. However, mycobacterial blood cultures have a sensitivity comparable to bone marrow cultures in detecting disseminated mycobacterial infections and are less invasive and less costly to perform. Routine bone marrow culture and histopathologic review in AIDS patients was also not found to be useful in the evaluation of common opportunistic infections and less-invasive tests were suggested as first line diagnostic procedures.
  Bone marrow culture has not been found to be useful in the initial evaluation of fever of unknown (FUO) origin; culture may be of use when blood cultures are negative.

CLINICAL NOTES
A complete blood count, including platelet count and reticulocyte count, should be obtained and analyzed at the time of bone marrow examination.
Routine bone marrow cultures do not appear diagnostically useful in patients with fever of unknown origin (FUO).
In a systematic review of FUO, the diagnostic yield of bone marrow cultures in immunocompetent individuals was found to be 0% to 2% and; therefore, bone marrow cultures are not recommended in these patients as part of a diagnostic workup.

COLLECTION/STORAGE INFORMATION
- Specimen Collection and Handling:
  - Collect bone marrow aspirate with aseptic technique.
  - Transport to lab as soon as possible.

Bordetella antibody assay

TEST DEFINITION
Detection of antibodies to *Bordetella pertussis* in serum for surveillance of pertussis

SYNONYMS
• Serologic test for Bordetella

REFERENCE RANGE
• Adults and Children: Negative
Please refer to your institution's reference ranges as lab normals may vary.

INDICATIONS
Suspected pertussis
> **Strength of Recommendation:** Class IIa
> **Strength of Evidence:** Category B
Results Interpretation:
Serology positive
> A substantial increase in antibody levels between acute and convalescent sera diagnoses pertussis. Serologic testing is more helpful in diagnosing pertussis than culture in the later stages of disease. Detection of IgA can aid in the diagnosis of pertussis.
Timing of Monitoring
> Maximum IgM titers appear within 2 to 3 weeks after primary infection with pertussis, therefore, it is recommended to perform a follow up serology 2 weeks after onset of infection.

CLINICAL NOTES
Serologic tests for *Bordetella pertussis* are used in epidemiologic investigations and in pertussis vaccine trials. They are not widely available for diagnosis in a clinical setting.

COLLECTION/STORAGE INFORMATION
• Collect sample in a red top tube.

LOINC CODES
• Code: 22886-6 (*Short Name* - B bronch Ab Ser Ql)
• Code: 22887-4 (*Short Name* - B bronch Ab Ser Ql Aggl)

Bordetella pertussis culture

TEST DEFINITION
Detection of *Bordetella pertussis* or *B parapertussis* by culture of nasopharyngeal aspirate or swab

REFERENCE RANGE
• Negative
Please refer to your institution's reference ranges as lab normals may vary.

INDICATIONS
Suspected pertussis of less than 3 weeks duration
> **Strength of Recommendation:** Class IIa
> **Strength of Evidence:** Category B
Results Interpretation:
Nose swab culture positive
> For diagnosis, a positive culture in a symptomatic patient is specific for pertussis. Positive culture results have the highest predictive value when the age of the patient is less than 5 years and acute symptoms of spasmodic cough plus lymphocytosis are present.

The rate of recovery of *B pertussis* from culture varies, depending on when cultures are obtained as well as on the vaccination status and the age of the patient. The highest yields are obtained when cultures are done during an interval starting at the end the incubation period, through the catarrhal stage, and into the early paroxysmal stage. Unfortunately, except during epidemics, pertussis is usually not suspected at these stages of illness.

Cultures are more likely to be positive in patients who have had less than 3 doses of pertussis vaccine.

Failure to isolate *B pertussis* does not exclude the diagnosis. It can take 4 to 5 days for culture results to become positive. Because the bacteria is slow growing, extending the incubation period to 12 days improves recovery of both *B pertussis* and *B parapertussis* .

Timing of Monitoring

Cultures are positive in 50% to 60% of patients during the first 2 weeks of illness, decreasing to 30% to 40% in the following 2 weeks. Cultures are not positive after 6 weeks.

CLINICAL NOTES

Although culture test for *Bordetella pertussis* is specific and has been regarded as a 'gold-standard' method for diagnosis, its sensitivity may be influenced by various factors such as duration of symptoms prior to sample collection, patient age, transport conditions of the sample, and immunization status.

COLLECTION/STORAGE INFORMATION

* Specimen Collection and Handling:
  * Immediate plating of specimen onto agar medium is preferred to insure loss of bordetellae.
  * Nasopharyngeal aspirate (preferred method):
    * Use a size 6 or 8 French DeeLee suction catheter with mucous trap connected to vacuum pump or syringe with tubing that includes an in-line filter. Carefully insert end of catheter along floor of nasopharynx.
    * When posterior pharynx has been reached, apply suction while catheter is withdrawn to mid nasal cavity. Stop suctioning and remove catheter.
    * Apply some of aspirated material to a primary culture plate with a sterile swab or bacteriological loop. Seal ends of trap, label specimen and primary plate with accession number and patient identifier. Refrigerate specimen if not transported immediately.
  * Nasopharyngeal swab:
    * After immobilizing patient's head, insert Dacron (not cotton) nasopharyngeal swab into nostril to posterior nares. Leave in place for 15 to 30 seconds, then slowly remove.
    * Streak primary culture plate. Insert swab into transport medium. Cap tube and label both tube and plate with accession number and patient identifier.
* For both methods of collection, transport sample in sterile, room temperature casamino broth if transported within 2 hours and in Amies medium with charcoal if transported within 24 hours. Use Regan-Lowe semisolid transport medium if longer transport time is expected.

LOINC CODES

* Code: 548-8 (*Short Name* - B pert Thrt Ql Cult)
* Code: 549-6 (*Short Name* - B pert XXX Ql Cult)

Bordetella pertussis direct fluorescent antibody measurement

TEST DEFINITION

Detection of *Bordetella pertussis* and *Bordetella parapertussis* by direct fluorescent antibody (DFA) staining of nasopharyngeal secretions

REFERENCE RANGE

* Negative
  Please refer to your institution's reference ranges as lab normals may vary.

INDICATIONS
Suspected pertussis
> **Strength of Recommendation:** Class IIb
> **Strength of Evidence:** Category B
Results Interpretation:
Positive microbiology findings
> A positive direct fluorescent antibody assay provides a rapid presumptive diagnosis of pertussis.. Test results must be confirmed by culture.

False Results
> Healthcare workers must weigh the benefit of presumptive diagnosis of pertussis based on the direct fluorescent antibody (DFA) test with the disadvantage of a high proportion of false-positive and false-negative results. Cross-reactions with normal nasopharyngeal flora account for false-positive results in up to 85% of tests and may lead to substantial unnecessary testing. False-negative DFA test results may delay treatment in infants (pending culture results) and thereby increase morbidity.

COLLECTION/STORAGE INFORMATION
- Specimen Collection and Handling:
  - Nasopharyngeal aspirate (preferred method):
    - Use a size 6 or 8 French DeeLee suction catheter with a mucous trap connected to a vacuum pump or syringe with tubing that includes an in-line filter. Carefully insert end of catheter along floor of nasopharynx.
    - When the posterior pharynx has been reached, apply suction while catheter is withdrawn to mid nasal cavity. Stop suctioning and remove catheter.
    - Seal ends of trap. Refrigerate specimen if not transported immediately.
  - Nasopharyngeal swab:
    - After immobilizing patient's head, insert a Dacron (not cotton) nasopharyngeal swab into nostril to posterior nares. Leave swab in place for 15 to 30 seconds, then remove slowly.
    - Insert swab into transport medium and cap tube.
  - For both methods of collection, transport sample in sterile, room temperature casamino broth if transported within 2 hours and in Amies medium with charcoal if transported within 24 hours. Use Regan-Lowe semisolid transport medium if longer transport time is expected.

Borrelia burgdorferi DNA assay

TEST DEFINITION
> Detection of *Borrelia burgdorferi* -specific nucleic acid in cerebrospinal fluid, blood, skin biopsy specimen, synovial fluid, or urine

SYNONYMS
- Borrelia burgdorferi PCR
- Lyme disease DNA detection

REFERENCE RANGE
- Negative
Please refer to your institution's reference ranges as lab normals may vary.

INDICATIONS
Suspected Lyme disease
> **Strength of Recommendation:** Class IIb
> **Strength of Evidence:** Category B
Results Interpretation:
Polymerase chain reaction observation
> Polymerase chain reaction (PCR) of skin biopsy specimens is more sensitive and specific for the diagnosis of erythema migrans than either culture or serological testing.
> In patients with neuroborreliosis, specific intrathecal antibody synthesis is better than PCR; however, in patients who have been ill less than 14 days, PCR sensitivities are higher and therefore, it may be a diagnostic adjunct.

PCR of urine samples has a very low sensitivity and is not useful in the diagnosis of erythema migrans or neuroborreliosis.

Shedding of the DNA of dead organisms can cause a PCR to be positive after curative antimicrobial therapy and therefore, does not prove active disease.

CLINICAL NOTES

Urine specimens may have polymerase chain reaction (PCR) inhibitors that can interfere with the amplification process. Also, the amount of specific DNA present in urine and cerebrospinal fluid (CSF) is near the detectable limit with PCR. Using multiple CSF or urine samples or amplification of two different target genes in parallel may be necessary to get an adequate diagnostic sensitivity.

COLLECTION/STORAGE INFORMATION

* Specimen Collection and Handling:
  * Collect specimen (crude cell lysates, serum, or whole blood may be used directly)
  * Avoid heparin and heme; citrate and EDTA are acceptable anticoagulants
  * Store nucleic acids frozen at -20°C or below

LOINC CODES

* Code: 11551-9 (*Short Name* - B burgdorf DNA CSF QI Amp Prb)
* Code: 10846-4 (*Short Name* - B burgdor DNA Bld QI Amp Prb)
* Code: 4991-6 (*Short Name* - B burgdor DNA XXX QI PCR)
* Code: 10847-2 (*Short Name* - B burgdorf DNA Fld QI Amp Prb)
* Code: 21120-1 (*Short Name* - B burgdor DNA Ur QI PCR)

Borrelia burgdorferi antibody assay

TEST DEFINITION

Detection of antibodies to *Borrelia burgdorferi* in serum for the serologic evaluation of Lyme disease

SYNONYMS

* Serologic test for Borrelia burgdorferi

REFERENCE RANGE

* Adults and children: Seronegative
Please refer to your institution's reference ranges as lab normals may vary.

INDICATIONS

Suspected Lyme disease
> **Strength of Recommendation:** Class IIb
> **Strength of Evidence:** Category B
> **Results Interpretation:**
> **Serology: organism - finding**
>> In the United States, a two-tiered approach is typically used for serologic testing, whereby a positive screening test for Lyme borreliosis (usually immunofluorescence, hemagglutination, or enzyme-linked immunosorbent assay [ELISA]) is followed by immunoblot testing to increase specificity. A significant change in IgM or IgG antibody response to *Borrelia burgdorferi* in paired acute- and convalescent-phase serum samples also may be used for the laboratory diagnosis of Lyme disease.
>> IgM levels usually peak 3 to 6 weeks after infection; IgG antibodies become detectable several weeks after infection, may continue to rise for several months, and generally persist for years.
>> The diagnosis of Lyme disease is based on clinical criteria assisted by serologic testing in patients with characteristic manifestations; in most cases, Lyme disease can be diagnosed on clinical grounds. Serologic tests are of questionable diagnostic value.
> **Negative laboratory findings**
>> Serologic testing for Lyme disease may be negative in the first several weeks of infection.
>> A negative serologic test is helpful in predicting the absence of disease in both endemic and non-endemic areas, though the negative predictive value is higher in non-endemic areas.

A negative serologic test result does not exclude the diagnosis of Lyme disease early in the course of illness, nor can the presence of chronic Lyme disease be excluded by the absence of antibodies against *Borrelia burgdorferi*.

A negative ELISA result indicates only that there was no serologic evidence of infection with *B burgdorferi* and should not be used as the basis for excluding *B burgdorferi* as the cause of illness, especially if the blood was collected within 2 weeks of symptom onset. A negative Western blot indicates that no reliable serologic evidence of *B burgdorferi* infection was present and should not be used as the sole basis for excluding *B burgdorferi* as the cause of illness. If Lyme disease is suspected, a second specimen should be collected 2 to 4 weeks after the first and retested; if the ELISA is positive or equivocal, a Western blot should be repeated.

A negative serologic assay for Lyme disease can be found, even on repeat testing, if antibiotics are administered during the first several weeks of infection, as such treatment can affect antibody response to *Borrelia burgdorferi*.

Serology positive

A positive serologic test is helpful primarily in areas where Lyme disease is endemic. A positive test result does not necessarily indicate current infection with *B burgdorferi*. A positive serologic result in certain patients is more likely to represent a false positive than proof of infection, with increasing uncertainty as one goes from an area of high to low endemicity. In most cases, a positive serologic test will only provide laboratory confirmation of a clinical diagnosis.

Because antibodies to *B burgdorferi* may remain at detectable levels for years, a positive result cannot distinguish between active and prior infection, indicating that serology should not be used to assess treatment response. Serial determinations of serum antibodies appear to be of little value in monitoring the effectiveness of antibiotic therapy for Lyme disease or in predicting persistent or recurrent disease.

A positive or equivocal ELISA result yields presumptive evidence of the presence of antibodies to *Borrelia burgdorferi* but should be followed by second-step (ie, Western blot) testing. A positive Western blot provides serologic evidence of past or current infection with *B burgdorferi*.

Timing of Monitoring

Serologic testing is unlikely to be helpful at the time that the tick bite is discovered. Serologies should be drawn at this point only if antibiotics are to be withheld and repeat testing is planned several weeks later.

CLINICAL NOTES

Laboratories do not use a standard method for *Borrelia burgdorferi* antigen preparation or for reporting results.

COLLECTION/STORAGE INFORMATION

- Collect serum in red top tube.

LOINC CODES

- Code: 22118-4 (*Short Name* - B burgdor Ab CSF QI)
- Code: 22122-6 (*Short Name* - B burgdor Ab Titr Ser)
- Code: 22124-2 (*Short Name* - B burgdorf IgA Ser QI)
- Code: 16475-6 (*Short Name* - B burgdor Ab CSF QI EIA)
- Code: 22120-0 (*Short Name* - B burgdor Ab Fld-aCnc)
- Code: 9586-9 (*Short Name* - B burgdor Ab Ser-Imp)
- Code: 16476-4 (*Short Name* - B burgdor Ab Fld QI EIA)
- Code: 31155-5 (*Short Name* - B burgdor Ab XXX EIA-aCnc)
- Code: 5061-7 (*Short Name* - B burgdor Ab Titr Ser IF)
- Code: 22119-2 (*Short Name* - B burgdor Ab CSF-aCnc)
- Code: 30128-3 (*Short Name* - B burgdor Ab #2 Ser-aCnc)
- Code: 23833-7 (*Short Name* - B burgdor Ab Indx Ser+CSF QI)
- Code: 6319-8 (*Short Name* - B burgdorf Ab Fld EIA-aCnc)
- Code: 16477-2 (*Short Name* - B burgdor Ab Fld QI)
- Code: 26006-7 (*Short Name* - B burgdor Ab Ser QI IHA)
- Code: 23676-0 (*Short Name* - B burgdor Ab Ser QI IF)
- Code: 6318-0 (*Short Name* - B burgdorf Ab CSF EIA-aCnc)
- Code: 11006-4 (*Short Name* - B burgdor Ab Ser QI)
- Code: 20449-5 (*Short Name* - B burgdor Ab Ser QI EIA)
- Code: 5060-9 (*Short Name* - B burgdor Ab Ser EIA-aCnc)
- Code: 22121-8 (*Short Name* - B burgdor Ab Ser-aCnc)
- Code: 16478-0 (*Short Name* - B burgdorf IgA Ser QI EIA)

Borrelia burgdorferi culture

TEST DEFINITION
Isolation of *Borrelia burgdorferi* by culture of skin lesion biopsy specimens, blood, or cerebrospinal fluid

REFERENCE RANGE
• Negative
Please refer to your institution's reference ranges as lab normals may vary.

INDICATIONS
Suspected Lyme disease (LD)
    Strength of Recommendation: Class IIb
    Strength of Evidence: Category B
    Results Interpretation:
    Positive microbiology findings
        Patients with positive blood cultures for *B burgdorferi* do not appear to be at greater risk for an unfavorable course and outcome than patients with negative cultures.

CLINICAL NOTES
    Culture of *Borrelia burgdorferi* is not feasible in most practice settings. Although the organism grows well in the laboratory, it is not easily recovered from clinical specimens other than biopsy samples of skin lesions. Saline-lavage needle aspiration and 2-mm punch biopsies of the leading edge of suspected lesions successfully obtain organisms in 50% to 80% of cases.
    Yield of blood cultures from plasma is higher than from serum cultures. Rate of recovery is low from cerebro-spinal fluid and almost negligible from synovial fluid.

COLLECTION/STORAGE INFORMATION
• Specimen Collection and Handling:
    • Collect blood in EDTA or serum tubes
    • Transport specimens directly to the laboratory

LOINC CODES
• Code: 11550-1 (*Short Name* - B burgdorf XXX Ql Cult)

Brain natriuretic peptide level

TEST DEFINITION
Measurement of brain-type natriuretic peptide (BNP) in plasma for the evaluation and management of ventricular dysfunction

SYNONYMS
• BNP level

REFERENCE RANGE
• Adults: <167 pg/mL (<167 ng/L)
Please refer to your institution's reference ranges as lab normals may vary.

INDICATIONS
Pulmonary embolism
    Strength of Recommendation: Class IIb
    Strength of Evidence: Category B
    Results Interpretation:
    Normal laboratory findings
        With pulmonary embolism, a brain natriuretic peptide (BNP) level less than 50 pg/mL may suggest a benign clinical course.

Suspected heart failure
    Strength of Recommendation: Class IIa
    Strength of Evidence: Category A
    Results Interpretation:
    Increased level (laboratory finding)
        A brain-type natriuretic peptide (BNP) level above 100 pg/mL is suggestive of a diagnosis of symptomatic heart failure, and a BNP greater than 400 pg/mL is strongly suggestive of congestive heart failure (CHF), although the average BNP level in patients with CHF is greater than 600 pg/mL. An elevated BNP may not correlate with chest X-ray findings of CHF. BNP is particularly influential in affecting the post-test probability of CHF in those patients with an intermediate pre-test probability.

        BNP may be helpful in deciding the disposition of patients presenting with acute dyspnea. An elevated BNP may also be helpful in predicting a deterioration in functional status and in identifying those at increased risk of mortality.

        Because BNP increases with age and is affected by gender, comorbidity, and drug therapy, it should not be used in isolation from the clinical context. BNP may be moderately elevated (from 100 to 500 pg/mL) in the absence of CHF in those patients with a history of atrial fibrillation, cardiomegaly on chest X-ray, increased age, decreased body mass index (BMI), or a low Hgb.
    Normal laboratory findings
        A BNP less than 50 pg/mL indicates the absence of CHF.

        BNP is particularly influential in affecting the post-test probability of CHF in those patients with an intermediate pre-test probability. BNP may be helpful in deciding the disposition of patients presenting with acute dyspnea.

CLINICAL NOTES

    The criteria for defining normal and abnormal ranges in brain-type natriuretic peptide (BNP) are largely lab- and test-specific. The described significant interassay variability depends on the specific peptide fragment being quantified and the specific immunoassay being used.

COLLECTION/STORAGE INFORMATION

- Collect 5 mL of blood in EDTA (lavender-top) tube.

Bromides measurement, blood

TEST DEFINITION

    The measurement of bromides in blood for evaluation of toxicity and therapeutic monitoring.

REFERENCE RANGE

- Blood (therapeutic): 500-1000 mcg/mL
  Please refer to your institution's reference ranges as lab normals may vary.

INDICATIONS

Drug level monitoring during bromide therapy
    Strength of Recommendation: Class I
    Strength of Evidence: Category B
    Results Interpretation:
    Therapeutic drug level - finding
        Bromide dose should be adjusted to avoid toxic serum levels (greater than 1250 mcg/mL), while maintaining serum levels up to 500 to 1000 mcg/mL.

Suspected bromide toxicity
    Strength of Recommendation: Class I
    Strength of Evidence: Category B
    Results Interpretation:
    Increased level (laboratory finding)
        Serum levels of 500 to 1000 mcg/mL may be associated with symptoms.
        Serum levels greater than 1250 mcg/mL are considered toxic.
        Serum levels greater than 3000 mcg/mL may be fatal.
        Urinary bromide levels are unreliable for assessing toxicity.

CLINICAL NOTES
Urinary bromide levels are unreliable for treatment monitoring

COLLECTION/STORAGE INFORMATION
• Collect blood in red marbled top tube for serum

LOINC CODES
• Code: 25171-0 (*Short Name* - Bromide Bld-sCnc)

Brucella antibody assay

TEST DEFINITION
Detection and measurement of *Brucella* species antibodies in serum

SYNONYMS
• Serologic test for Brucella

REFERENCE RANGE
• Adults and Children: Negative
Please refer to your institution's reference ranges as lab normals may vary.

INDICATIONS
Suspected acute, chronic or relapsing brucellosis
      Strength of Recommendation: Class IIa
      Strength of Evidence: Category B
      Results Interpretation:
      Serology positive

Brucellosis is diagnosed when there is 4-fold or greater rise in *Brucella* agglutination titers between acute- and convalescent-phase serum, in specimens obtained at least 2 weeks apart and tested at the same laboratory, according to the Centers for Disease Control and Prevention (CDC) case definition. A diagnosis of brucellosis can also be made upon a positive immunofluorescence finding for any *Brucella* species in a clinical specimen.

A single serum agglutination test titer greater than or equal to 160 is presumptive evidence of brucellosis. In endemic areas, a titer greater than or equal to 320 may be more accurate.

Test results may vary with disease state (acute, subacute, chronic, relapsing) and by the immunoglobulin type assessed and the antigen used (eg, *B canis* is very difficult to detect).

Elevated levels of anti-*Brucella* IgM antibodies are consistent with acute illness; IgM may be present in serum alone or together with IgG and IgA; elevated titers of IgE, IgG1 and IgG3 may also be present.

Patients who experience a return of disease signs or symptoms, or have a positive blood culture may be defined as having a brucellosis relapse. Increasing levels of IgG and IgA may be indicators of relapse.

Patients with brucellosis symptoms lasting more than 12 months from the time of diagnosis may be categorized as having chronic brucellosis. While elevated levels of anti-*Brucella* IgG antibodies are consistent with chronic illness, the persistence of IgG alone does not indicate chronic infection, as it, together with IgA, may persist for a long period despite satisfactory treatment. Patients with chronic brucellosis may also have elevated titers of IgE, IgG1 and IgG3.
      Negative laboratory findings

In cases of chronic brucellosis, agglutination tests may give false-negative results.

Serology testing for brucellosis may fail to identify infections caused by *B canis*, as the antibodies present may not cross-react to the antigens of other *Brucella* species.
      Timing of Monitoring

Serum sample collection is done during the first week of illness ('acute phase') and after a period of 3 to 4 weeks ('convalescent phase') to detect diagnostic titer changes.

CLINICAL NOTES
Brucellosis is tracked by local and national public health entities in the US, as *Brucella* is a potential bioterrorism agent.

In humans, brucellosis may be caused by 4 species: *B melitensis*, *B suis*, *B abortus*, and *B canis*.

Tube agglutination and slide agglutination are the test methods most commonly used for brucellosis detection.

COLLECTION/STORAGE INFORMATION
- Collect blood specimen in a marbled-top serum-separator tube (SST).
- Collect two specimens: one in the first week of illness ('acute phase') and the second 3 weeks to 4 weeks later ('convalescent phase').

LOINC CODES
- Code: 6328-9 (*Short Name* - Brucella Ab Titr Ser IF)
- Code: 29250-8 (*Short Name* - Brucella Ab sp1 Titr Ser)
- Code: 13210-0 (*Short Name* - Brucella IgG Ser-aCnc)
- Code: 24397-2 (*Short Name* - Brucella IgM Ser QI)
- Code: 30129-1 (*Short Name* - Brucella Ab sp1 Ser QI)
- Code: 24387-3 (*Short Name* - Brucella IgG Ser QI EIA)
- Code: 24396-4 (*Short Name* - Brucella IgG Ser QI)
- Code: 13211-8 (*Short Name* - Brucella IgA Ser-aCnc)
- Code: 24388-1 (*Short Name* - Brucella IgM Ser QI EIA)
- Code: 22159-8 (*Short Name* - Brucella Ab Titr Ser)
- Code: 10349-9 (*Short Name* - Brucella Ab Ser-aCnc)
- Code: 30202-6 (*Short Name* - Brucella Ab Ser QI)

Brucella species culture

TEST DEFINITION
Detection of *Brucella* species by culture of blood, bone marrow, sterile body fluids, and other tissue

REFERENCE RANGE
- Negative
  Please refer to your institution's reference ranges as lab normals may vary.

INDICATIONS
Suspected brucella arthritis
    Strength of Recommendation: Class IIa
    Strength of Evidence: Category B
Results Interpretation:
Positive microbiology findings
    Isolation of *Brucella* species in synovial fluid culture is diagnostically definitive for brucellosis infection. Recovery of *Brucella* species varies depending on the phase of illness.
    In patients treated with antimicrobial agents, a culture incubation time of 4 to 6 weeks is recommended; if there is a high suspicion of bacterial exposure, blind subcultures on negative culture bottles should be performed.

    False Results
    Brucellar bacteremia detection is dependent on the specimen volume. Small specimen volume and the associated low bacterial count can result in false negatives.

Suspected Brucellosis
    Strength of Recommendation: Class IIa
    Strength of Evidence: Category B
Results Interpretation:
Positive microbiology findings
    Isolation of *Brucella* species from culture is diagnostically definitive for brucellosis.
    Diagnosis of suspected brucellosis in patients treated with antimicrobial agents requires an incubation period of 4 to 6 weeks.
    In suspected brucella endocarditis, cardiac vegetation specimens frequently yield *Brucella* species regardless of prior antimicrobial therapy.

Negative microbiology findings

Negative cultures should undergo blind subcultures for a minimum of 4 weeks regardless of culture method utilized.

CLINICAL NOTES

Standard culture methods are incubated for 4 to 6 weeks. Blind terminal subcultures are recommended.

New culture instrumentation (continuous-monitoring automated blood culture systems) has been shown to provide accurate results in under 10 days.

COLLECTION/STORAGE INFORMATION

- Specimen Collection and Handling:
  - Obtain 10 mL to 20 mL blood and inoculate specimen in a lysis centrifugation tube or in a blood culture bottle
  - Apply strict safety precautions when handling suspected positive *Brucella* species specimens
  - Inform lab personnel of suspected positive *Brucella* species specimens

LOINC CODES

- Code: 24003-6 (*Short Name* - Brucella Mar Cult)
- Code: 20734-0 (*Short Name* - Brucella Tiss Cult)
- Code: 552-0 (*Short Name* - Brucella XXX Cult)
- Code: 551-2 (*Short Name* - Brucella Bld Cult)

C-ANCA measurement

TEST DEFINITION

Measurement of antineutrophil cytoplasmic antibodies found in cytoplasmic granules (C-ANCA) of neutrophils and monocytes that are associated with small-vessel vasculitides, such as Wegener's granulomatosis and microscopic polyangiitis

REFERENCE RANGE

- Adults, Qualitative method: Negative
- Adults, Quantitative method (antibodies to proteinase 3): <2.8 units/mL (<2.8 kU/L)
  Please refer to your institution's reference ranges as lab normals may vary.

INDICATIONS

Suspected microscopic polyangiitis
    Strength of Recommendation: Class IIa
    Strength of Evidence: Category B
    Results Interpretation:
    c-Antineutrophil cytoplasmic antibody positive

In microscopic polyangiitis, 30% of the patients have a positive cytoplasmic antineutrophil cytoplasmic antibody (C-ANCA) with proteinase 3 (PR3) specificity. Occasionally C-ANCA with myeloperoxidase (MPO) specificity will be detected.

    False Results

In a study of 166 patients that were C-ANCA positive, 27 had active pulmonary disease and underwent lung biopsy. Of those patients, 8 (30%) were found to have disease (ie, various connective tissue disorders, chronic hypersensitivity pneumonia, postinfectious bronchitis and ulcerative colitis-related lung disease) other than Wegener's granulomatosis or microscopic polyangiitis. Findings indicate that ANCA positivity in the absence of appropriate clinical and pathologic findings may result.

CLINICAL NOTES

The combined use of immunofluorescence and ELISA testing that detects anti-neutrophil cytoplasmic antibodies (ANCA) specific for proteinase 3 (PR3) and myeloperoxidase (MPO) is recommended to diagnose small vessel vasculitides, because many other antigens can be recognized by ANCAs that are clinically irrelevant to the diagnosis.

COLLECTION/STORAGE INFORMATION
• Store sample at -20°C.

LOINC CODES
• Code: 14277-8 (*Short Name* - C-ANCA Titr Ser IF)
• Code: 17353-4 (*Short Name* - C-ANCA Ser QI IF)
• Code: 8084-6 (*Short Name* - C-ANCA Ser-aCnc)

C3 complement assay

TEST DEFINITION
Measurement of complement C3 in serum for the evaluation and management of immune complex diseases

SYNONYMS
• C>3< complement assay
• Complement component 3 test

REFERENCE RANGE
• Adult: 86-184 mg/dL (0.86-1.84 g/L)
• Since C3 levels vary, use of multiple of age- and gender-specific medians as reference ranges enhances clinical utility of measurements and simplifies interpretation.
  Please refer to your institution's reference ranges as lab normals may vary.

INDICATIONS
Suspected C3 deficiency
  Strength of Recommendation: Class IIa
  Strength of Evidence: Category B
  Results Interpretation:
  Complement 3 deficiency
  Immune complex diseases, such as systemic lupus erythematosus (SLE), subacute bacterial endocarditis, parasitemias, rheumatoid arthritis, bacterial sepsis, and viremias, have been associated with decreased levels of complement C3. C3 deficiency may predispose to SLE, and decreased C3 levels in a patient with SLE can indicate active disease.

  Absence of the central complement component, C3, results in failure to generate an appropriate response to pyogenic infections by disrupting the integrity of both the classical and alternative pathways. This disruption may occur through the absence of normal chemotactic factor (C5a) and leukocytosis promoting factor (C3e). The increased susceptibility to bacterial infections is manifested primarily as pneumonia, meningitis, otitis, and pharyngitis.

  Deficiencies of the components of the alternative pathway of complement result in increased susceptibility to various pyogenic infections, probably as a result of failure in the generation of C3-dependent opsonization.

COMMON PANELS
• Collagen/Lupus panel

ABNORMAL RESULTS
• Results increased in females

COLLECTION/STORAGE INFORMATION
• Collect blood in tube containing EDTA, EGTA, heparin, or citrate, or in marbled tube.
• Store at -70°C if unable to process sample immediately

LOINC CODES
• Code: 6801-5 (*Short Name* - C3 Fld-mCnc)
• Code: 15164-7 (*Short Name* - C3 Snv-mCnc)
• Code: 4485-9 (*Short Name* - C3 SerPl-mCnc)

C4 complement assay

TEST DEFINITION
Measurement of complement C4 (one of 9 major components in the complement cascade) in serum for the evaluation and management of immunologic and inflammatory conditions

SYNONYMS
- C>4< complement assay
- Complement C4 measurement
- Complement component 4 test

REFERENCE RANGE
- Adults: 20-58 mg/dL (0.2-0.58 g/L)
- Infants, 1 month: 27.5-47.3 mg/dL (275-473 mg/L)
- Infants, 6 months: 30.5-58.7 mg/dL (305-587 mg/L)
Please refer to your institution's reference ranges as lab normals may vary.

INDICATIONS
Suspected C4 deficiency
    Results Interpretation:
    Complement 4 deficiency
        Autoimmune diseases that present as glomerulonephritis, rheumatoid arthritis, or systemic lupus-like syndromes are seen in more than half of patients with complement C2 or C4 deficiencies.
        C4 deficiency may predispose to SLE, and decreased C4 levels in patients with SLE can indicate active disease

Suspected hereditary angioedema
    Results Interpretation:
    Complement 4 deficiency
        In hereditary angioedema (HAE), the lack of complement 1 esterase inhibitor (C1NH) results in activation of complement C4 by activated C1, with subsequent depletion of C4.
        Eighty percent to 85% of patients with HAE have a decreased amount of functionally normal C1NH (quantitative deficiency). The diagnosis is made by decreased C4 and C1NH levels.
        Fifteen percent to 20% of patients with HAE have a normal amount of functionally abnormal C1NH (qualitative deficiency). Standard quantitative assays for C1NH level will be normal in these patients. If the C4 level is low and HAE is still suspected, a functional assay for C1NH should be done.
        C4 plasma levels should show decreased values in patients with either type of hereditary angioedema.

COMMON PANELS
- Collagen/Lupus panel

ABNORMAL RESULTS
- Results increased in:
  - Increasing body mass index (BMI)
  - Females
  - Increasing age (from age 24 to 55 years)
- Results decreased in:
  - Increasing age (after age 55 years, levels drop to those seen in third decade of life)

COLLECTION/STORAGE INFORMATION
- Collect blood in tube containing EDTA, EGTA, heparin, or citrate, or in marbled tube.
- Store at -70°C.

LOINC CODES
- Code: 4498-2 (*Short Name* - C4 SerPl-mCnc)
- Code: 6908-8 (*Short Name* - C4 Fld-mCnc)
- Code: 26931-6 (*Short Name* - C4 SerPl-aCnc)
- Code: 13085-6 (*Short Name* - C4 Nephritic SerPl-mCnc)

CA 125 measurement

TEST DEFINITION
Serologic tumor marker for monitoring clinical course of endometrial and ovarian cancer

REFERENCE RANGE
• Adults: 0-35 units/mL (0-35 kilounits)/L
Please refer to your institution's reference ranges as lab normals may vary.

INDICATIONS
Assessment of stage in endometrial cancer
    Strength of Recommendation: Class IIa
    Strength of Evidence: Category C
Results Interpretation:
Increased level (laboratory finding)
    In a retrospective study of 65 patients, using the International Federation of Gynecologists and Obstetricians (FIGO) staging, the mean CA-125 value found in early stage endometrial cancer (I and II) was 42.7 International Units/mL and 346.9 International Units/mL in advanced stage (III and IV). When measured against grade, a similar correlation existed; CA-125 levels, in International Units/mL, were 21.02 for grade 1, 82.35 for grade 2, and 245 for grade 3.

Evaluation of response to ovarian cancer treatment and assessment for recurrence
    Strength of Recommendation: Class IIb
    Strength of Evidence: Category B
Results Interpretation:
Increased level (laboratory finding)
    CA-125 can be used as an aid in following ovarian cancer. A falling level can be associated with a positive response to treatment, whereas a rising level can indicate progressive disease or treatment failure.
    A false decrease in the level is possible while undergoing therapy, as is a negative result with tumor recurrence.

    False Results
    Because CA-125 will be normal in 50% of early-stage ovarian cancers and 20% to 25% of advanced cancers, a normal level is inadequate for ruling out disease.

DRUG/LAB INTERACTIONS
• Bexarotene - elevated CA 125 assay values
• Satumomab Pendetide - falsely elevated levels of CA 125
• Technetium Tc 99m Nofetumomab Merpentan - interference with murine antibody-based immunoassays

ABNORMAL RESULTS
• Results increased in:
    • Endometriosis
    • Menses
    • Pelvic inflammatory disease
    • Pregnancy

LOINC CODES
• Code: 19165-0 (*Short Name* - Cancer Ag125 Plr-aCnc)
• Code: 15156-3 (*Short Name* - Cancer Ag125 Fld Dil-aCnc)
• Code: 2006-5 (*Short Name* - Cancer Ag125 SerPl Ql)
• Code: 11210-2 (*Short Name* - Cancer Ag 125 Fld-aCnc)
• Code: 15157-1 (*Short Name* - Cancer Ag125 SerPl Dil-aCnc)

CA 15-3 measurement

TEST DEFINITION
Measurement of cancer antigen CA 15-3 in serum, plasma, or other body fluids; used as a tumor marker but elevated in a variety of conditions

REFERENCE RANGE
- Adults (serum): 0-30 units/mL (0-30 kilounits/L)
  Please refer to your institution's reference ranges as lab normals may vary.

INDICATIONS
Breast cancer
> **Strength of Recommendation:** Class IIb
> **Strength of Evidence:** Category B
> **Results Interpretation:**
> **Increased level (laboratory finding)**
> An elevated preoperative serum CA 15-3 concentration is associated with a lower overall and disease-free survival in patients with breast cancer, independent of lymph node status. There is conflicting data as to whether CA 15-3 has prognostic value in patients with negative lymph nodes or estrogen receptor negative status.
> CA 15-3 immunostaining appears to have a high sensitivity and moderately high specificity for detecting the presence of breast cancer in body cavity effusions.
> According to the American Society for Clinical Oncology Recommendations 2000 Update, CA 15-3 should not be used routinely to monitor response to breast cancer treatment. Although a rising CA 15-3 may suggest disease recurrence, CA 15-3 cannot be used for staging disease.
> **Decreased level (laboratory finding)**
> According to the American Society for Clinical Oncology Recommendations 2000 Update, a low CA 15-3 concentration does not exclude metastases.

COLLECTION/STORAGE INFORMATION
- Specimen Collection and Handling:
  - Collect serum or plasma specimen.
  - May keep for up to 5 days at 2°C to 8°C.
  - After 5 days, freeze at −20°C or colder.

LOINC CODES
- Code: 6875-9 (*Short Name* - Cancer Ag15-3 SerPl-aCnc)
- Code: 2007-3 (*Short Name* - Cancer Ag15-3 SerPl Ql)
- Code: 19186-6 (*Short Name* - Cancer Ag15-3 Plr-aCnc)
- Code: 29153-4 (*Short Name* - Cancer Ag 15-3 Fld-aCnc)

CA 19-9 measurement

TEST DEFINITION
Measurement of carbohydrate antigen 19-9 in serum for the evaluation and treatment of malignant disease

REFERENCE RANGE
Adults: 0-37 units/mL (0-37 kunits/L)
Please refer to your institution's reference ranges as lab normals may vary.

INDICATIONS
Suspected malignant tumor of ampulla of Vater
> **Strength of Recommendation:** Class IIb
> **Strength of Evidence:** Category B

Results Interpretation:
Finding of serum tumor marker level
Elevated CA 19-9 levels can be associated with periampullary tumors, but should not be used as a diagnostic indicator. Serum CA 19-9 measurement can be used as an adjunct in detecting periampullary cancers, evaluating resectability and monitoring tumor recurrence. CA 19-9 levels can correlate with tumor size and can help predict prognosis.

Suspected malignant tumor of biliary tract
Strength of Recommendation: Class IIb
Strength of Evidence: Category B
Results Interpretation:
Finding of serum tumor marker level
Elevated carbohydrate antigen 19-9 levels may be found in both malignant and benign biliary disease, and are not useful for screening or diagnosing biliary cancer.

Suspected malignant tumor of colon
Strength of Recommendation: Class IIb
Strength of Evidence: Category B
Results Interpretation:
Finding of serum tumor marker level
An elevated CA 19-9 may be associated with colorectal cancer, but currently is not recommended for evaluation, diagnosis, or monitoring of this condition

Suspected malignant tumor of pancreas
Strength of Recommendation: Class IIa
Strength of Evidence: Category B
Results Interpretation:
Finding of serum tumor marker level
Elevated carbohydrate antigen (CA) 19-9 can be found in patients with pancreatic carcinoma as well as other pancreatic diseases.
Elevated CA 19-9 levels following resection would indicate incomplete tumor removal, recurrence, or metastasis. Elevated CA 19-9 levels during chemotherapy can determine efficacy of antitumor drugs.
CA 19-9 may best be used as a diagnostic adjunct in the monitoring of disease in patients with pancreatic cancer.

COLLECTION/STORAGE INFORMATION
- Specimen Collection and Handling:
  - Serum is stable at 2 to 8°C for up to 24 hours; for longer periods, freeze serum at −20°C.
  - Plasma should be fresh, not frozen or thawed.

LOINC CODES
- Code: 19163-5 (*Short Name* - Cancer Ag19-9 Plr-aCnc)
- Code: 24108-3 (*Short Name* - Cancer Ag19-9 SerPl-aCnc)
- Code: 26924-1 (*Short Name* - Cancer Ag 19-9 Fld-aCnc)
- Code: 2009-9 (*Short Name* - Cancer Ag19-9 SerPl Ql)

CA 27.29 measurement

TEST DEFINITION
Serologic tumor marker for monitoring clinical course of breast cancer

SYNONYMS
- CA 27-29 measurement

REFERENCE RANGE
- Adults: <38 units/mL
  Please refer to your institution's reference ranges as lab normals may vary.

INDICATIONS

Evaluation of treatment and recurrence risk for breast cancer
>**Strength of Recommendation:** Class IIb
>**Strength of Evidence:** Category B

Results Interpretation:

Raised biochemistry findings

CA 27.29 is a tumor marker that may be useful in conjunction with other clinical parameters in the management of breast cancer.

CA 27.29 levels can be elevated with certain other conditions, though when levels are more than 100 units per mL, benign breast disease is considered unlikely.

Frequency of Monitoring

In patients at high risk for breast cancer recurrence, a repeat CA 27.29 every 4 to 6 months may be useful in guiding treatment

ABNORMAL RESULTS

- Results increased in:
  - Colon carcinoma
  - Hepatocellular carcinoma
  - Lung carcinoma
  - Ovarian carcinoma
  - Pancreatic carcinoma
- Results increased in:
  - Benign disorders of:
    - Breast
    - Kidney
    - Liver
    - Ovary

LOINC CODES

- Code: 2012-3 (*Short Name* - Cancer Ag27-29 SerPl Ql)
- Code: 19187-4 (*Short Name* - Cancer Ag27-29 Plr-aCnc)
- Code: 17842-6 (*Short Name* - Cancer Ag27-29 SerPl-aCnc)

CMV rapid culture

TEST DEFINITION

Culture of saliva and urine for rapid detection of cytomegalovirus

SYNONYMS

- Cytomegalovirus rapid culture

REFERENCE RANGE

- Negative growth

Please refer to your institution's reference ranges as lab normals may vary.

INDICATIONS

Suspected cytomegalovirus infection
>**Strength of Recommendation:** Class IIb
>**Strength of Evidence:** Category B

Results Interpretation:

Positive microbiology findings

The cytomegalovirus rapid culture test provides results in 24 to 72 hours with sensitivities and specificities similar to the tissue culture method.

CLINICAL NOTES

Urine is the optimum specimen for recovery of cytomegalovirus (CMV). Collecting 2 to 3 specimens over successive days maximizes recovery of CMV.

COLLECTION/STORAGE INFORMATION
- Obtain culture specimen during acute phase of illness.
- Transport specimen in viral transport medium and process immediately.
- Obtain mid-void urine specimen.
- Store urine at 4°C for up to 5 days, but do not freeze.
- Freeze viral suspension specimen at −70°C if processing will be delayed more than 5 days.

CSF albumin/plasma albumin ratio measurement

TEST DEFINITION
The ratio of albumin in cerebrospinal fluid to serum albumin for the evaluation of the blood-cerebrospinal fluid barrier function

REFERENCE RANGE
- Pediatric and Adolescents, 15 years of age and under: 5
- Adolescents and Adults, 16 to 40 years of age: 6.5
- Adults, 60 to 65 years of age: 8-9
- Adults, >65 years of age: 8-9
  Please refer to your institution's reference ranges as lab normals may vary.

INDICATIONS
Suspected multiple sclerosis
> **Strength of Recommendation:** Class IIb
> **Strength of Evidence:** Category C
> **Results Interpretation:**
> **Increased level (laboratory finding)**
> A cerebrospinal fluid (CSF)/serum albumin ratio level of less than 9 indicates no significant impairment of CSF-blood barrier, a level of 9 to 14.3 indicates slight impairment, a level of 14.3 to 33.3 indicates moderate impairment, a level of 33.3 to 100 indicates severe impairment and a level greater than 100 indicates total breakdown.
> A CSF albumin/serum albumin ratio of greater than 7 suggests an abnormal blood-CSF barrier function and is seen in 12% of patients with clinically definite multiple sclerosis.
> An increased CSF albumin/serum albumin ratio is one of the main signs of an acute, active central nervous system disease.
> An elevated CSF albumin level in the presence of a normal serum albumin level can indicate a change in the permeability of the blood-CSF barrier, which can affect CSF IgG measurements used in the diagnosis of multiple sclerosis.
> CSF albumin/serum albumin ratio is used in calculation of IgG index.

CLINICAL NOTES
Cerebrospinal fluid albumin and serum albumin concentrations should be analyzed by the same method and within the same analytical series.

COLLECTION/STORAGE INFORMATION
- Specimen Collection and Handling:
  - Collect serum specimen in a red top tube.
  - Store serum at 4°C for up to 72 hours, frozen at −20°C for 6 months, or at −70°C indefinitely.
  - Collect 10 mL of cerebrospinal fluid (CSF).
  - Transport CSF specimen to laboratory as soon as possible.

LOINC CODES
- Code: 1756-6 (*Short Name* - Alb SerPl/CSF-mRto)

CSF gram stain method

TEST DEFINITION
Detection of bacterial microorganisms or inflammatory cells in cerebrospinal fluid for presumptive evidence of infection (bacterial or fungal)

SYNONYMS
- CSF gram stain
- Gram stain, CSF

REFERENCE RANGE
- Adults and Children: Negative
Please refer to your institution's reference ranges as lab normals may vary.

INDICATIONS
Suspected bacterial meningitis
  Strength of Recommendation: Class I
  Strength of Evidence: Category B
  Results Interpretation:
  Positive microbiology findings
    Detection of bacterial pathogens on Gram stain of cerebrospinal fluid (CSF) is considered diagnostic of bacterial meningitis; however, the diagnostic accuracy of the Gram stain will vary in accordance with both the causative agent and the number of colony-forming units per mL that are present.
    Gram-positive diplococci indicative of *Streptococcus pneumoniae* most commonly cause meningitis. Occasionally, *Haemophilus influenzae* (gram-negative pleomorphic rods) are seen and Salmonella species are isolated in children with sickle cell disease.
    Rare cases of meningitis caused by gram-negative enteric organisms and meningococcus (gram-negative single or diplococci) have been reported among patients with sickle cell disease.

  False Results
- False-negative results are observed when Gram-negative cerebrospinal fluid (CSF) organism count is less than 1,000 microorganisms per mL.
- Prior antimicrobial treatment can reduce the effective diagnostic yield of CSF Gram stain by approximately 20%, as compared to a 30% reduction for culture.

Suspected fungal (mycotic) meningitis
  Strength of Recommendation: Class IIa
  Strength of Evidence: Category B
  Results Interpretation:
  Positive microbiology findings
    Detection of fungal microorganisms and other mycoses on Gram stain of cerebrospinal fluid (CSF) is considered diagnostic of fungal (mycotic) meningitis. Centrifuged Gram stained preparations of CSF may serve as an effective and rapid test alternative to the commonly used India ink stain technique.

  False Results
    False-positive: Cerebrospinal fluid (CSF) artifacts that resemble yeast cells have been observed in CSF specimens from patients who have recently undergone myelography.

CLINICAL NOTES
A negative Gram stain finding cannot definitively exclude the presence of bacteria, yeast cells, or leukocytes.
Gram stain of cerebrospinal fluid (CSF) generally requires a minimum bacterial load greater than or equal to 10^5 colony-forming units per milliliter of CSF to be accurate.

COLLECTION/STORAGE INFORMATION
- Specimen Collection and Handling:
  - Collect cerebrospinal fluid in a sterile, screw-capped tube.
  - Immediately transport specimen to lab.
  - Do not refrigerate specimen; if delay in processing may incubate specimen at 37°C.

CSF: angiotensin-converting enzyme level

TEST DEFINITION
Measurement of angiotensin-converting enzyme in cerebrospinal fluid for the evaluation of neurosarcoidosis

INDICATIONS
Suspected central nervous system neurosarcoidosis
>**Strength of Recommendation:** Class IIb
>**Strength of Evidence:** Category B
>**Results Interpretation:**
>**Increased level (laboratory finding)**
>>An elevated angiotensin-converting enzyme level in cerebrospinal fluid may be helpful in supporting the clinical diagnosis of neurosarcoidosis in patients who have brain and/or spinal cord diffuse contrast enhancing MRI lesions. Meningeal biopsy is required to confirm the diagnosis.

CLINICAL NOTES
Cerebrospinal fluid measurements of angiotensin-converting enzyme can be elevated in diseases other than neurosarcoidosis including CNS syphilis, multiple sclerosis, and viral encephalitis.

Cadmium measurement, urine

TEST DEFINITION
Detection of cadmium in urine for the evaluation and management of cadmium exposure

REFERENCE RANGE
· Unexposed to cadmium: 0.5-4.7 mcg/L (4.4-41.8 nmol/L)
Please refer to your institution's reference ranges as lab normals may vary.

INDICATIONS
Cadmium exposure
>**Strength of Recommendation:** Class IIa
>**Strength of Evidence:** Category B
>**Results Interpretation:**
>**Increased level (laboratory finding)**
>>At low exposure to cadmium, urinary cadmium levels primarily reflect the amount of cadmium stored in the body and the kidneys. At moderate exposure, urinary cadmium concentration increases proportionately to the rate of exposure and is significantly correlated with kidney cadmium concentrations. Once the cadmium binding sites become saturated, due to excessive exposure, cadmium is rapidly excreted in the urine in the short-term, while in the long-term urine cadmium levels decrease in the presence of persistent tubular damage, due to the kidney's inability to reabsorb cadmium.
>>Low level cadmium exposure is associated with an increase in proximal renal tubular dysfunction; the long-term health impact of these renal changes seen at low urine cadmium levels remains to be determined. The appropriate urinary biomarker cut-off values for identifying tubular proteinuria are variable depending upon individual physiological factors and associated disease states, although renal tubular dysfunction is not likely with urine cadmium levels below 2.5 mcg/g creatinine.
>>Urinary cadmium concentrations reflect chronic exposure and accumulated total body cadmium burden while blood cadmium levels are more indicative of recent exposure. Urine cadmium levels increase with age indicating accumulated body burden over time. Urine cadmium levels of 0.02 to 0.7 mcg/g creatinine are generally found in nonsmokers, with levels increasing slowly over time as cadmium accumulates in the

kidneys. Urinary cadmium levels above 2 nmols/mmol creatinine are uncommon in the non-occupationally exposed population. Urine cadmium levels are higher in women than men, particularly in women with low iron reserves, and are twice as high in smokers as in nonsmokers. Urine cadmium levels in the exposed population range from 10 to 580 mcg/L (0.09-5.16 mmol/L).

Urine cadmium levels above 2.5 mcg/g creatinine are associated with a 4% higher incidence of renal tubular damage. Early signs of kidney damage have been observed in patients with urine cadmium levels as low as 0.5 mcg/g creatinine.

Urinary cadmium levels above 2 mcg/g creatinine may lead to biochemical alterations, levels above 4 mcg/g creatinine may lead to cytotoxic effects and glomerular barrier dysfunction, and levels above 10 mcg/g creatinine may lead to tubular reabsorption dysfunction, including microproteinuria. Urinary cadmium levels above 2.5 mcg/g creatinine correspond to a cadmium concentration of 50 mcg/g in the renal cortex.

The recommended provisional tolerable weekly intake (PTWI) of cadmium is 7 mcg/kg body weight, with no tubular dysfunction likely at this PTWI.

COLLECTION/STORAGE INFORMATION
- Collect sample in metal-free container without preservatives.
- May store sample at room temperature for 7 days or freeze at -70°C for up to one month.

LOINC CODES
- Code: 5611-9 (*Short Name* - Cadmium Ur-mCnc)
- Code: 25360-9 (*Short Name* - Cadmium Ur-sCnc)
- Code: 13828-9 (*Short Name* - Cadmium/creat 24H Ur-mRto)
- Code: 5612-7 (*Short Name* - Cadmium 24H Ur-mRate)
- Code: 13471-8 (*Short Name* - Cadmium/creat Ur-mRto)
- Code: 22696-9 (*Short Name* - Cadmium/creat Ur-sRto)

Calcium, serum, ionized measurement

TEST DEFINITION
Detection of ionized calcium in serum, plasma or whole blood for the evaluation and management of metabolic and endocrine disorders

SYNONYMS
- Calcium, serum, ionised measurement

REFERENCE RANGE
- Adults (whole blood): 4.5-5.6 mg/dL (1.1-1.4 mmol/L)
- Adults (plasma): 4.12-4.92 mg/dL (1.03-1.23 mmol/L)
- Adults (serum): 4.64-5.28 mg/dL (1.16-1.32 mmol/L)
- Adults, 60-90 years (whole blood): 4.64-5.16 mg/dL (1.16-1.29 mmol/L)
- Adults, >90 years (whole blood): 4.48-5.28 mg/dL (1.12-1.32 mmol/L)
- Neonates, cord blood (serum): 5.2-6.4 mg/dL (1.3-1.6 mmol/L)
- Neonates, 2 hours (serum): 4.84-5.84 mg/dL (1.21-1.46 mmol/L)
- Neonates, 24 hours (serum): 4.4-5.44 mg/dL (1.1-1.36 mmol/L)
- Neonates, 6 to 36 hours (capillary blood): 4.2-5.48 mg/dL (1.05-1.37 mmol/L)
- Neonates, 60 to 84 hours (capillary blood): 4.4-5.68 mg/dL (1.1-1.42 mmol/L)
- Neonates, 3 days (serum): 4.6-5.68 mg/dL (1.15-1.42 mmol/L)
- Neonates, 5 days (serum): 4.88-5.92 mg/dL (1.22-1.48 mmol/L)
- Neonates, 108 to 132 hours (capillary blood): 4.8-5.92 mg/dL (1.2-1.48 mmol/L)
- Children (serum): 4.8-5.52 mg/dL (1.2-1.38 mmol/L)
  Please refer to your institution's reference ranges as lab normals may vary.

INDICATIONS
Ionized calcium monitoring in critically ill patients
    Strength of Recommendation: Class I
    Strength of Evidence: Category B

Results Interpretation:
Abnormal laboratory findings

Ionized calcium measurement provides the most accurate assessment of calcium status in the critically ill patient.

An ionized calcium level lower than 1.15 mmols/L is indicative of hypocalcemia.

Low critical limits for ionized calcium range from 2 to 4.29 mg/dL (0.5 to 1.07 mmols/L) in US medical centers and from 2.4 to 4.33 mg/dL (0.6 to 1.08 mmols/L) in US children's hospitals.

Measurement of ionized calcium detects true hypocalcemia that may otherwise go unrecognized in the critically ill patient.

Neurological and cardiac symptoms often appear when ionized calcium levels decrease below 1 mmol/L. Hypotension, sepsis, and cardiac dysrhythmias may be associated with low ionized calcium. Progressively lower levels may signify increased morbidity and mortality in critically ill patients.

When the reduction of ionized calcium is acute, tetany may occur.

High critical limits for ionized calcium range from 5.21 to 8.02 mg/dL (1.3 to 2 mmols/L) in US medical centers and from 5.41 to 7.01 mg/dL (1.35 to 1.75 mmols/L) in US children's hospitals.

Symptoms of hypercalcemia usually occur once ionized calcium levels are above 1.5 mmols/L.

Frequency of Monitoring

Critical care patients undergoing calcium resuscitation may require ionized calcium measurements every 1 to 4 hours. During transplantation, ionized calcium measurements may need to be drawn every 5 to 10 minutes.

Suspected hyperparathyroidism

Strength of Recommendation: Class IIa
Strength of Evidence: Category B
Results Interpretation:
Increased level (laboratory finding)

Elevated serum ionized calcium in association with raised parathyroid hormone (PTH) levels strongly suggests hyperparathyroidism.

Measurement of ionized calcium levels may detect hyperparathyroidism in symptomatic patients whose total calcium levels are normal.

Normal ionized calcium levels may occur in approximately 20% of patients with primary hyperparathyroidism.

Ionized calcium is the primary element influencing PTH secretion; normocalcemic hyperparathyroidism may be diagnosed when a calcium challenge increases ionized calcium levels with minimal reduction of serum PTH.

Suspected hypoparathyroidism

Strength of Recommendation: Class IIa
Strength of Evidence: Category C
Results Interpretation:
Decreased level (laboratory finding)

Decreased serum ionized calcium associated with low parathyroid hormone (PTH) and high serum phosphate levels suggests hypoparathyroidism.

Ionized calcium levels should be maintained at the lower limit of normal (about 1.15 mmol/L) in patients with surgical hypoparathyroidism to reduce risk of hypercalcemic episodes, as residual parathyroid tissue may still be present.

A decreased ionized calcium level in a patient who has had thyroid resection may indicate hypoparathyroidism.

Frequency of Monitoring

Ionized calcium levels should be assessed every 4 hours in hypocalcemic post parathyroidectomy patients being treated with IV calcium, to maintain levels greater than 0.8 mmol/L.

COLLECTION/STORAGE INFORMATION

- Collect anaerobic sample.
- Use heparinized tube for whole blood sample collection.
- Draw sample from non-static limb.
- Put sample on ice and deliver to laboratory promptly.
- Draw whole blood for emergent care samples, anticoagulate with less than 15 international units/mL of calcium-titrated heparinate, and process within 15 minutes.
- Store plasma or serum at -20°C for up to 6 months.

LOINC CODES

- Code: 12180-6 (*Short Name* - Ca-I SerPl ISE-sCnc)
- Code: 1995-0 (*Short Name* - Calcium Ion SerPl-sCnc)
- Code: 17864-0 (*Short Name* - Ca-I SerPl ISE-mCnc)
- Code: 17863-2 (*Short Name* - Ca-I SerPl-mCnc)
- Code: 13959-2 (*Short Name* - Calcium Ion SerPl Calc-sCnc)

California Encephalitis Virus antibody assay

TEST DEFINITION

Measurement of California encephalitis virus serology in serum for evaluation of viral infection

SYNONYMS

- Serologic test for California encephalitis virus

REFERENCE RANGE

- Negative
Please refer to your institution's reference ranges as lab normals may vary.

INDICATIONS

Suspected California encephalitis
    Results Interpretation:
    Serology positive
        A 4-fold increase in titer from the acute and convalescent sera or specific IgM detected in cerebrospinal fluid (CSF) is diagnostic of California encephalitis.
        A specimen (collected within 45 days of the onset of the symptoms) that is positive for IgG but negative for IgM, may indicate a past infection. Conversely, a positive IgM is suggestive of recent infection.
    Timing of Monitoring
        Test acute (onset of symptoms) and convalescent (2 to 4 weeks later) sera.

COLLECTION/STORAGE INFORMATION

- Collect serum at onset of symptoms and 2 to 4 weeks later.
- Freeze samples if testing is delayed.

Candida antigen assay

TEST DEFINITION

Serologic measurement of *Candida* antigen for detection of disseminated candidiasis

SYNONYMS

- Candida antigen level

REFERENCE RANGE

- Negative
Please refer to your institution's reference ranges as lab normals may vary.

INDICATIONS

Suspected disseminated candidiasis
      Strength of Recommendation: Class IIb
      Strength of Evidence: Category B
    Results Interpretation:
    Presence of microbial antigen - finding
        A positive *Candida* antigen assay may occur with disseminated candidiasis in immunosuppressed or other severely ill patients.

Although immunosuppressed patients may have candidiasis in normally colonized sites, this is not a definitive indication of infection. Because interpretation of antigen assays is difficult, these assays alone are inadequate for diagnosing disseminated candidiasis. Biopsy, histology and multiple-site cultures are important confirmatory tests.

Frequency of Monitoring

The likelihood of detecting disseminated candidiasis is increased when serum is assayed weekly or semiweekly for *Candida* species. Weekly serial determinations increase sensitivity for detection of the mannan antigen, which is specific for disseminated candidiasis.

LOINC Codes
- Code: 27440-7 (*Short Name* - Candida Ag SerPl EIA-aCnc)
- Code: 16539-9 (*Short Name* - Candida Ag Ser Ql)
- Code: 9501-8 (*Short Name* - Candida Ag Titr Ser)
- Code: 31760-2 (*Short Name* - Candida Ag Ser-aCnc)

Capillary blood glucose measurement

Test Definition
Measurement of capillary plasma glucose for the therapeutic management of diabetes.

Synonyms
- Capillary blood glucose level

Reference Range
- Adults preprandial: 90-130 mg/dL (5-7.2 mmol/L)
- Adults peak postprandial: <180 mg/dL (<10 mmol/L)
  Please refer to your institution's reference ranges as lab normals may vary.

Indications
Initial evaluation and monitoring of diabetic ketoacidosis
> **Strength of Recommendation:** Class IIa
> **Strength of Evidence:** Category C
> **Results Interpretation:**
> **Hyperglycemia, acute**
> Capillary blood glucose testing can measure glucose levels up to 600 mg/dL. A reading of HI on the monitor indicates a result above 600 mg/dL. Capillary glucose greater than 250 mg/dL meets diagnostic criteria for diabetic ketoacidosis (DKA), but should be confirmed with plasma glucose results.
> **Frequency of Monitoring**
> Capillary blood glucose may be used for hourly monitoring during the treatment period.
> **Timing of Monitoring**
> Capillary blood (finger-stick) glucose determination should be performed while awaiting results of the serum chemistry panel in patients with suspected diabetic ketoacidosis (DKA).

Initial evaluation of suspected hyperglycemic hyperosmolar state
> **Strength of Recommendation:** Class I
> **Strength of Evidence:** Category C
> **Results Interpretation:**
> **Hyperglycemia, acute**
> In hyperglycemic hyperosmolar state (HHS), plasma glucose is greater than 600 mg/dL.
> Capillary glucose measurement may be inaccurate in the presence of acidosis and poor peripheral circulation.
> **Timing of Monitoring**
> Capillary blood (finger-stick) glucose determination should be performed while awaiting results of the serum chemistry panel in patients with suspected hyperosmolar hyperglycemic state.

Self-monitoring of blood glucose in known diabetes
> **Strength of Recommendation:** Class I
> **Strength of Evidence:** Category C

Results Interpretation:
Normal range

The recommended preprandial capillary plasma glucose range in adult diabetics is 90 to 130 mg/dL (5 to 7.2 mmol/L). The recommended peak postprandial capillary plasma glucose level in adult diabetics is less than 180 mg/dL (less than 10 mmol/L). Peak levels generally occur 1 to 2 hours after the beginning of the meal. Healthcare providers are responsible for assisting the patient in making treatment modification decisions vis a vis diet, exercise, and medication, based on appropriate interpretation of test results.

The accuracy of test results is technique and instrument dependent. Elevated hematocrit causes low glucose readings and low hematocrit causes high glucose results. Results may also be affected by altitude, temperature, humidity, hypotension, hypoxia, triglycerides and the quality of test strips. Either very high or very low readings should be confirmed with an alternate glucose testing method.

Frequency of Monitoring

The frequency and timing of self-monitoring blood glucose (SMBG) should be individualized based on each patient's needs and goals. SMBG should be performed 3 or more times per day for type 1 diabetics taking multiple insulin injections and for pregnant women taking insulin. Generally, type 1 diabetics require more frequent monitoring than patients not taking insulin. Additions or modifications to therapy require more frequent monitoring in all patients. The optimal frequency and timing of SMBG for patients with type 2 diabetes on oral agents, or diet-managed patients only, is not known. Postprandial monitoring using SMBG may be appropriate to achieve postprandial glucose goals.

Suspected hypoglycemia
Results Interpretation:
Decreased glucose level

A blood glucose level less than 40 mg/dL associated with symptoms of hypoglycemia generally is required to diagnose hypoglycemia in either a newborn or an adult. However, there is no absolute blood glucose level that will allow the diagnosis to be made, as patients with a glucose level less than 40 mg/dL may be asymptomatic, while others with a higher level may be symptomatic, particularly when the decline in blood glucose is rapid

Timing of Monitoring

Capillary blood (finger-stick) glucose determination should be performed while awaiting results of the serum chemistry panel in patients with suspected hypoglycemia.

LOINC CODES
• Code: 32016-8 (*Short Name* - Glucose BldC-mCnc)

Carbamazepine blood measurement

TEST DEFINITION
Measurement of carbamazepine levels in serum or plasma to facilitate therapeutic or toxicity monitoring

SYNONYMS
• Carbamazepine: blood level

REFERENCE RANGE
• 4-12 mcg/mL (17-51 micromol/L)
Please refer to your institution's reference ranges as lab normals may vary.

INDICATIONS
Drug level monitoring during carbamazepine therapy
    Strength of Recommendation: Class I
    Strength of Evidence: Category C
Results Interpretation:
Carbamazepine level - finding

Carbamazepine blood levels are only meaningful in the context of clinical findings, such as a change in seizure frequency.

The effects of antiepileptic medication may correlate better with the serum concentration than with the dose.

Serum concentrations of carbamazepine may be affected by the coadministration of other antiepileptic drugs and by the patient's age.

Seizure protection is best assessed at trough levels, and toxicity potential is best assessed by peak levels.

At the onset of treatment, carbamazepine levels initially rise, followed by a slow decrease over the next 3 to 4 weeks.

Carbamazepine level high

Although monitoring blood concentrations can reduce the toxic effects of carbamazepine, the evaluation of therapeutic efficacy should be based on the patient's clinical response.

Carbamazepine level low

Subtherapeutic carbamazepine levels may indicate patient noncompliance or an interaction with another substance in the serum sample.

Timing of Monitoring

Carbamazepine levels should be drawn several days (about 4 to 5 half-lives) after initiating therapy and immediately before the next dose is due. Levels should be obtained approximately 3 weeks later at the same time of day to ensure that concentrations have stabilized. Concentrations should be measured following any change in medication (including a switch from the brand name to the generic formulation), any change in liver, cardiac, or gastrointestinal tract function, or any change in seizure frequency.

Suspected carbamazepine toxicity

Strength of Recommendation: Class I
Strength of Evidence: Category B
Results Interpretation:
Carbamazepine level therapeutic

Due to pharmacokinetic variability, toxic effects may occur with blood concentrations in the therapeutic range.

Carbamazepine level high

- Toxic level (adults): >15 mcg/mL (>63 micromol/L)
- Cardiac toxic effects (eg, dysrhythmias and conduction defects) may occur at levels as low as 3.2 mg/L.
- Neurologic toxic effects may occur at concentrations of 4 to 5 times the upper therapeutic limit and include:
  - Nystagmus
  - Ataxia
  - Gross intention tremor
  - Dysarthria
  - Respiratory depression
  - Drowsiness, stupor, or coma

COLLECTION/STORAGE INFORMATION

- Draw serum or plasma in heparin or EDTA tube.
- If using serum separator tube, fill tube completely and process promptly.
- Collect trough sample.
- Collect at a consistent time of day.
- Avoid hemolysis.
- May store at room temperature for several hours
- May store at -20°C for up to 1 year

Carbamazepine-10,11-epoxide measurement

TEST DEFINITION

Measurement of carbamazepine-10,11 epoxide levels in serum or plasma to facilitate therapeutic or toxicity monitoring

REFERENCE RANGE

- Carbamazepine: 4-12 mcg/mL (17-51 micromol/L)
  Please refer to your institution's reference ranges as lab normals may vary.

INDICATIONS

Monitoring of the metabolite carbamazepine-10,11-epoxide level during carbamazepine therapy

Strength of Recommendation: Class IIb
Strength of Evidence: Category B
Results Interpretation:
Carbamazepine level - finding

In patients prescribed carbamazepine only, trough concentrations of carbamazepine-10,11-epoxide are roughly 15% to 20% of carbamazepine concentrations.

Carbamazepine-10,11-epoxide is not routinely measured for therapeutic monitoring, as its significance is not well known, although the simultaneous measurement of carbamazepine and its metabolite carbamazepine-10,11-epoxide may give a more accurate measure of total concentration of active drug.

The protein binding of carbamazepine-10,11-epoxide may show dose-dependent variability among patients taking carbamazepine, which may account for toxicity present despite a therapeutic carbamazepine level.

In immunoassays to measure carbamazepine alone, some antibodies may cross-react up to 90% with carbamazepine-10,11-epoxide, giving an apparent elevated carbamazepine level.

High concentrations of carbamazepine-10,11-epoxide may weaken seizure control.

Suspected carbamazepine-10,11-epoxide toxicity as a result of carbamazepine poisoning

Strength of Recommendation: Class IIb
Strength of Evidence: Category B
Results Interpretation:
Carbamazepine level - finding

In carbamazepine-poisoned patients, the level of carbamazepine-10,11-epoxide ranges from 0.8 to 3.2 mg/L.

Elevated levels of carbamazepine-10,11-epoxide may occur in carbamazepine poisoning and add to toxicity.

The protein binding of carbamazepine-10,11-epoxide may show dose-dependent variability among patients taking carbamazepine, which may account for toxicity present despite a therapeutic carbamazepine level.

High concentrations of carbamazepine-10,11-epoxide may weaken seizure control and have occurred in patients with massive carbamazepine overdose.

COLLECTION/STORAGE INFORMATION

- Specimen Collection and Handling:
  - Draw serum or plasma in heparin or EDTA tube.
  - May store at room temperature for several hours.
  - May store at -20°C for up to 1 year.

LOINC CODES

- Code: 14056-6 (*Short Name* - CBZ EP Free SerPl-mCnc)
- Code: 18270-9 (*Short Name* - CBZ EP SerPl-sCnc)
- Code: 9415-1 (*Short Name* - CBZ EP SerPl-mCnc)

Carbon dioxide content measurement

TEST DEFINITION

Total carbon dioxide content (TCO_2) measurement is the sum of the bicarbonate, carbonic acid, and dissolved carbon dioxide (CO_2) in plasma, serum, or whole blood

SYNONYMS

- CO>2< content measurement

REFERENCE RANGE

- Adults, plasma, at sea level: 21-30 mEq/L (21-30 mmol/L)
- Adults, capillary (heparin) plasma: 22-28 mEq/L (22-28 mmol/L)
- Adults, whole blood, arterial: 19-24 mEq/L (19-24 mmol/L)
- Adults, whole blood, venous: 22-26 mEq/L (22-26 mmol/L)

- Adults over 60 years, plasma or serum, venous: 23-31 mEq/L (23-31 mmol/L)
- Adults over 90 years, plasma or serum, venous: 20-29 mEq/L (20-29 mmol/L)
- Premature, 1 week, capillary (heparin) plasma: 14-27 mEq/L (14-27 mmol/L)
- Newborn, capillary (heparin) plasma: 13-22 mEq/L (13-22 mmol/L)
- Cord blood: 14-22 mEq/L (14-22 mmol/L)
- Infant, capillary (heparin) plasma: 20-28 mEq/L (20-28 mmol/L)
- Child, capillary (heparin) plasma: 20-28 mEq/L (20-28 mmol/L)
  Please refer to your institution's reference ranges as lab normals may vary.

INDICATIONS
Suspected metabolic acidosis
Results Interpretation:
Hypocapnia
The blood total carbon dioxide (TCO_2) concentration, a surrogate for bicarbonate (HCO_3^-), is reduced in both metabolic acidosis and respiratory alkalosis. A reduced blood pH measurement confirms the diagnosis of metabolic acidosis.

Suspected metabolic alkalosis
Results Interpretation:
Hypercapnia
The blood total carbon dioxide (TCO_2) concentration, a surrogate for bicarbonate (HCO_3^-), is elevated in both metabolic alkalosis and respiratory acidosis. An elevated blood pH measurement confirms the diagnosis of metabolic alkalosis.

The serum electrolyte pattern in metabolic alkalosis is characterized by an elevated total carbon dioxide level, hypochloremia, and hypokalemia. The plasma anion pattern is similar in all forms of metabolic alkalosis.

Primary metabolic alkalosis is the only acid-base disturbance associated with simultaneous elevation of all 3 of the following variables: pH, bicarbonate, and PCO_2.

Suspected respiratory acidosis
Results Interpretation:
Hypercapnia
The blood total carbon dioxide (TCO_2) concentration, a surrogate for bicarbonate (HCO_3^-), is increased in both respiratory acidosis and metabolic alkalosis. A reduced blood pH measurement confirms the diagnosis of respiratory acidosis

Acute primary respiratory acidosis (defective ventilation) elevates pCO_2, which causes acidemia. The acidemia is modulated by a compensatory increase in bicarbonate.

Suspected respiratory alkalosis
Results Interpretation:
Hypocapnia
The blood total carbon dioxide (TCO_2) concentration, a surrogate for bicarbonate (HCO_3^-), is reduced in both respiratory alkalosis and metabolic acidosis. An elevated blood pH measurement confirms the diagnosis of respiratory alkalosis.

In respiratory alkalosis, the decrease in pCO_2 is primary and the decrease in bicarbonate is secondary (compensatory), and pH is increased.

COMMON PANELS
- Arterial blood gases

CLINICAL NOTES
Full characterization of acid-base status requires arterial blood gas studies (ie, pH and pCO_2). Total carbon dioxide measurement is unnecessary if arterial blood gas studies are performed.

Arterial blood is often preferred, because arteriovenous differences reflect the metabolic activity of the organ or tissue source of venous blood.

Total carbon dioxide (TCO_2) may be a useful surrogate for plasma bicarbonate, because bicarbonate comprises 90% to 95% of TCO_2 content. The TCO_2 overestimates the plasma bicarbonate by 1-2 mmol/L..

COLLECTION/STORAGE INFORMATION
- Specimen Collection and Handling:
  - Collect blood sample in a heparinized syringe
  - Use minimum amount of liquid heparin, to avoid dilutional errors and pH changes

• Transfer blood sample anaerobically to a marbled top tube

LOINC CODES

• Code: 2024-8 (*Short Name* - dis CO2 Plas-sCnc)
• Code: 19223-7 (*Short Name* - CO2 BldMV-sCnc)
• Code: 2027-1 (*Short Name* - CO2 BldV-sCnc)
• Code: 2026-3 (*Short Name* - CO2 BldA-sCnc)
• Code: 20565-8 (*Short Name* - CO2 Bld-sCnc)
• Code: 2025-5 (*Short Name* - dis CO2 RBC-sCnc)
• Code: 2028-9 (*Short Name* - CO2 SerPl-sCnc)
• Code: 16551-4 (*Short Name* - CO2 BldC-sCnc)

Carboxyhemoglobin measurement

TEST DEFINITION

Measurement of carboxyhemoglobin levels in whole blood for the diagnosis and management of carbon monoxide poisoning

SYNONYMS

• Carbon monoxide measurement
• Carboxyhaemoglobin measurement
• COHb measurement

REFERENCE RANGE

• Adults: <2.3% (0.023)
• Adult smokers: 2.1%-4.2% (0.021-0.042)
• Adult heavy smokers (more than 2 packs/day): 8%-9% (0.08-0.09)
• Hemolytic anemia: Up to 4%
  Please refer to your institution's reference ranges as lab normals may vary.

INDICATIONS

Suspected carbon monoxide poisoning
    Strength of Recommendation: Class I
    Strength of Evidence: Category B
  Results Interpretation:
  Increased carboxyhemoglobin

Carboxyhemoglobin (COHb) levels higher than 5% in a nonsmoker and 10% in a smoker confirm the diagnosis, but correlate poorly with severity of Carbon monoxide (CO) poisoning.

• Potential associations between COHb levels and clinical findings include:
  • COHb 10%: Asymptomatic or headache
  • COHb 20%: Atypical dyspnea, throbbing headache, dizziness, nausea
  • COHb 30%: Severe headache, impaired thinking, disturbed vision
  • COHb 40%: Syncope, confusion
  • COHb 50%: Lethargy, seizures, coma
  • COHb 60% or higher: Cardiopulmonary failure, seizures, coma, death

However, in many patients with CO poisoning, COHb level and clinical manifestation associations are unreliable because of prehospital delay or oxygen therapy before blood sampling, and/or concomitant cyanide poisoning.

Even if asymptomatic, patients with COHb levels higher than 20% to 25% are candidates for further studies and hospital admission.

Fetal blood COHb levels are about 30% higher than maternal blood levels, because fetal hemoglobin has a higher affinity for CO than does adult hemoglobin.

ABGs will show a normal PaO_2 but a decreased oxygen saturation. In severe cases there may also be a metabolic acidosis. Pulse oximetry measures oxygen saturation inaccurately in the presence of CO poisoning/exposure, because oxyhemoglobin and COHb are absorbed at the same wavelength.

Frequency of Monitoring

Obtain the carboxyhemoglobin (COHb) level at presentation and repeat every two to four hours until the patient is asymptomatic or the level is normal.

CLINICAL NOTES

Carboxyhemoglobin (COHb) levels are best determined by a co-oximeter (dedicated spectrophotometer) that simultaneously measures total hemoglobin and fractional (%) values for COHb, oxyhemoglobin, deoxyhemoglobin, and methemoglobin. Carbon monoxide (CO)-oximeter measurements include calculation of the oxygen content and oxygen carrying capacity of the blood.

COHb levels in venous blood samples closely correlate with those in arterial blood samples.

COLLECTION/STORAGE INFORMATION

- Specimen Collection and Handling:
    - Collect arterial or venous blood in a lavender (EDTA) or green (heparin) top tube
    - Do not remove stopper
    - If possible, collect blood before or while starting oxygen
    - Specimen relatively stable for at least 2 weeks in filled well-capped (anaerobic) tube

Carcinoembryonic antigen measurement, pleural fluid

TEST DEFINITION

Measurement of carcinoembryonic antigen (CEA) in pleural fluid for the diagnosis of patients with malignant pleural disease

SYNONYMS

- CEA measurement, pleural fluid

REFERENCE RANGE

- Adults, pleural fluid: <3 ng/mL
    Please refer to your institution's reference ranges as lab normals may vary.

INDICATIONS

Suspected malignant pleural effusion
    Strength of Recommendation: Class IIa
    Strength of Evidence: Category B
Results Interpretation:
Increased carcinoembryonic antigen level
    CEA levels in pleural fluid may be higher in patients with pleural fluid malignancies than in patients with benign effusions; the magnitude of increase correlates with tumor type. The sensitivity of pleural fluid CEA in diagnosing pleural malignancies varies with tumor type. Sensitivity can be increased, albeit at the expense of specificity, when CEA is combined with other tumor markers. The combination of CYFRA 21-1, CEA and CA125 may be useful in addition to pleural fluid cytology when diagnosing pleural effusion malignancy.

LOINC CODES

- Code: 19168-4 (*Short Name* - CEA Plr-aCnc)
- Code: 19169-2 (*Short Name* - CEA Plr-mCnc)
- Code: 19170-0 (*Short Name* - CEA Plr-sCnc)

Carcinoembryonic antigen measurement, serum

TEST DEFINITION

Measurement of carcinoembryonic antigen (CEA) in serum for the diagnosis and management of malignant disease

REFERENCE RANGE

- Adults: 0-3.4 ng/mL (0-3.4 mcg/L)
  Please refer to your institution's reference ranges as lab normals may vary.

INDICATIONS

Colorectal cancer
Strength of Recommendation: Class IIa
Strength of Evidence: Category A
Results Interpretation:
Increased carcinoembryonic antigen level

Although preoperative carcinoembryonic antigen (CEA) levels greater than 5 ng/mL may correlate with poorer prognosis, data are insufficient to support the use of CEA to determine whether to treat a patient with adjuvant therapy. Two values above baseline are adequate to document progressive disease, even if corroborating radiographs are not performed.

Postoperatively, slowly rising serial CEA levels may indicate local recurrence, while a rapid rise in CEA values or a CEA level greater than 20 ng/mL has been associated with more extensive local reoccurrence or distant metastasis. In general, an elevated postoperative CEA level suggests a more advanced cancer and a decreased chance of survival and, when confirmed by retesting, necessitates further workup for metastatic disease.

Frequency of Monitoring

The routine use of serum carcinoembryonic antigen (CEA) alone is not recommended for monitoring treatment response. In the absence of another simple test to monitor treatment response, CEA should be measured at the beginning of metastatic disease treatment and every 2 to 3 months during active treatment. If resection of liver metastases is clinically indicated, postoperative serum CEA testing may be performed every 2 to 3 months for 2 or more years after diagnosis in patients with stage II or III disease. In patients with elevated CEA levels confirmed by retesting, further evaluation for metastatic disease is recommended but does not justify the institution of adjuvant or systemic therapy for presumed metastatic disease.

Gastric carcinoma
Strength of Recommendation: Class IIb
Strength of Evidence: Category B
Results Interpretation:
Increased carcinoembryonic antigen level

More advanced stages of gastric carcinoma are proportionately associated with increasing carcinoembryonic antigen (CEA) levels and decreasing rates of curative resection. In patients in stages 1, 2, and 3, CEA levels greater than 10 ng/mL may provide greater prognostic information than that obtained by conventional staging methods. Preoperative CEA levels are useful in predicting tumor progression and prognosis postoperatively.

Only 10% to 20% of patients with surgically resectable disease will have elevated CEA levels, limiting its usefulness as an early diagnostic marker.

Suspected malignant pleural effusion
Strength of Recommendation: Class IIb
Strength of Evidence: Category B
Results Interpretation:
Increased carcinoembryonic antigen level

With the exception of lung adenocarcinoma and breast cancer, pleural fluid CEA levels are substantially higher than serum CEA levels in patients with metastatic pleural effusions. The degree to which serum CEA levels are elevated is dependent upon the tumor type.

ABNORMAL RESULTS

Carcinoembryonic antigen values are an average of 1.5 times higher in healthy subjects who smoke than in nonsmokers.

COLLECTION/STORAGE INFORMATION

- Specimen Collection and Handling:
  - Specimen is stable up to 24 hours at 2°C to 8°C.
  - Beyond 24 hours, freeze the specimen to at least -20°C.
  - Do not use turbid samples.

LOINC CODES
- Code: 2039-6 (*Short Name* - CEA SerPl-mCnc)
- Code: 19167-6 (*Short Name* - CEA SerPl-sCnc)
- Code: 19166-8 (*Short Name* - CEA SerPl-aCnc)

Catecholamines, fractionation measurement, urine

TEST DEFINITION
Measurement of catecholamines in urine for detection of catecholamine-secreting neoplasms including pheochromocytoma and paraganglioma

SYNONYMS
- Free catecholamine fractionation measurement, urine

REFERENCE RANGE
- Adults:
- Epinephrine: 0-20 mcg/dL (0-109 nmol/dL)
- Norepinephrine: 15-80 mcg/dL (89-473 nmol/dL)
- Dopamine: 65-400 mcg/dL (424-2612 nmol/dL)
- Infant less than 1 year old:
- Epinephrine: 0-2.5 mcg/dL (0-14 nmol/dL)
- Norepinephrine: 0-10 mcg/dL (0-59 nmol/dL)
- Dopamine: 0-85 mcg/dL (0-555 nmol/dL)
- Children 1-2 years of age:
- Epinephrine: 0-3.5 mcg/dL (0-19 nmol/dL)
- Norepinephrine: 1-17 mcg/dL (6-100 nmol/dL)
- Dopamine: 10-140 mcg/dL (65-914 nmol/dL)
- Children 2-4 years of age:
- Epinephrine: 0-6.0 mcg/dL (0-33 nmol/dL)
- Norepinephrine: 4-29 mcg/dL (24-171 nmol/dL)
- Dopamine: 40-260 mcg/dL (261-1697 nmol/dL)
- Children 4-10 years of age – Epinephrine: 0.2-10 mcg/dL (1-55 nmol/dL)
- Children 4-7 years of age – Norepinephrine: 8-45 mcg/dL (47-266 nmol/dL)
- Children 7-10 years of age – Norepinephrine: 13-65 mcg/dL (77-384 nmol/dL)
- Children 10-15 years of age:
- Epinephrine: 0.5-20 mcg/dL (3-109 nmol/dL)
- Norepinephrine: 15-80 mcg/dL (89-473 nmol/dL)
- Children 4-15 years of age – Dopamine: 65-400 mcg/dL (424-2612 nmol/dL)
  Please refer to your institution's reference ranges as lab normals may vary.

INDICATIONS
Suspected pheochromocytoma
> **Strength of Recommendation:** Class IIa
> **Strength of Evidence:** Category B
> **Results Interpretation:**
> **Raised biochemistry findings**
> Elevated urine levels of free catecholamines is considered diagnostic of pheochromocytoma; however, the absence of elevated urine catecholamine concentrations does not automatically rule out the presence of the disease due to the episodic nature of catecholamine secretion from both pheochromocytomas and paragangliomas.
> Diagnostic sensitivity for pheochromocytoma may be increased by combining urine free catecholamine measurement with the measurement of conjugated urinary metanephrines.
> **Timing of Monitoring**
> In the event that repeated analysis of 24-hour urine collections are within the reference range, it may be helpful for the patient to collect a 'timed' urine specimen for analysis of catecholamine excretion immediately following a typical symptomatic episode.

COMMON PANELS
- Hypertension panel
- Metanephrine panel

ABNORMAL RESULTS
- Results increased in:
  - Diabetic ketoacidosis
  - Hypothyroidism
- Results decreased in:
  - Autonomic neuropathic conditions including diabetes, parkinsonism

CLINICAL NOTES
Epinephrine and norepinephrine excretion tends to increase during the luteal phase of the menstrual cycle prior to declining to minimum values during ovulation.

Measurement of urinary catecholamines is recommended as an initial screening test for pheochromocytoma.

COLLECTION/STORAGE INFORMATION
- Specimen Collection and Handling:
  - If possible, have patient discontinue all drugs at least 1 week prior to testing
  - Preserve specimen with 20 mL HCL (6 mol/L)
  - Refrigerate specimen
  - Preferred specimen: 24-hour urine collection

LOINC CODES
- Code: 27055-3 (*Short Name* - Catechol Free 24H Ur-mRate)
- Code: 11133-6 (*Short Name* - Catechol Free Ur-mCnc)
- Code: 14643-1 (*Short Name* - Catechol Free 24H Ur-sRate)

Cerebrospinal fluid IgG measurement, quantitative

TEST DEFINITION
Measurement of IgG in cerebrospinal fluid for evaluation of neurologic disease

SYNONYMS
- Cerebrospinal fluid IgG level
- Cerebrospinal fluid IgG measurement
- CSF IgG level

REFERENCE RANGE
- Adolescents, 15-20 years: 3.5 ± 2 mg/dL (35 ± 20 mg/L)
- Adults, 21-40 years: 4.2 ± 1.4 mg/dL (42 ± 14 mg/L)
- Adults, 41-60 years: 4.7 ± 1 mg/dL (47 ± 10 mg/L)
- Adults, 61-87 years: 5.8 ± 1.6 mg/dL (58 ± 16 mg/L)
  Please refer to your institution's reference ranges as lab normals may vary.

INDICATIONS
Suspected multiple sclerosis
> **Strength of Recommendation:** Class IIa
> **Strength of Evidence:** Category B
> **Results Interpretation:**
> **Increased immunoglobulin**
>> An elevated level of cerebrospinal fluid (CSF) IgG is a common finding in multiple sclerosis (MS) but may be present in other neurologic or inflammatory conditions.
>>
>> Quantitative IgG measurement includes calculation of the IgG index as follows: $(IgG_{CSF}/IgG_{serum})/(albumin_{CSF}/albumin_{serum})$, and may detect approximately 75% of patients with MS.

Quantitative IgG measurement also includes calculation of the CSF IgG synthesis rate, a more accurate indicator of MS than the IgG index.

Quantitative IgG analysis complements qualitative IgG in the diagnosis of MS, but qualitative (detection of oligoclonal bands in CSF) tests are considered the gold standard.

CLINICAL NOTES

Quantitative IgG measurements in both cerebrospinal fluid (CSF) and serum are usually used in conjunction with serum and CSF albumin levels to calculate the IgG index and IgG CSF synthesis rate. These derived values are helpful in differentiating neurologic diseases but are still less useful than qualitative CSF IgG evaluations.

COLLECTION/STORAGE INFORMATION

- Specimen Collection and Handling:
    - Collect atraumatic (no blood in specimen) cerebrospinal fluid in sterile tubes.
    - Analyze fresh or store at 4°C for up to 72 hours.
    - Freeze at -20°C for 6 months, or at -70°C indefinitely.

LOINC CODES

- Code: 2464-6 (*Short Name* - IgG CSF-mCnc)

Cerebrospinal fluid albumin measurement

TEST DEFINITION

Measurement of cerebrospinal fluid albumin concentration in patients with suspected bacterial meningitis, Guillain-Barre syndrome, CNS trauma, and other conditions that affect permeability of the blood-brain barrier

SYNONYMS

- Cerebrospinal fluid albumin level

REFERENCE RANGE

- Adults and Children: 0.066-0.442 g/L (6.6-44.2 mg/dL).
- Children 3 months to 4 years of age: <45 mg/dL (<450 mg/L)
- Children greater than 4 years of age: 10-30 mg/dL (100-300 mg/L)
    Please refer to your institution's reference ranges as lab normals may vary.

INDICATIONS

Patients with suspected or known multiple sclerosis
   Strength of Recommendation: Class IIb
   Strength of Evidence: Category C
Results Interpretation:
Raised biochemistry findings
   Elevations in cerebrospinal fluid (CSF) concentration of albumin may be predictive of multiple sclerosis; however, concurrent testing of albumin serum concentrations is recommended to account for fluctuations in serum/CSF equilibrium.

CLINICAL NOTES

Cerebrospinal fluid (CSF) concentration of albumin represents the equilibrium between serum and CSF concentration levels, rendering the test for CSF albumin concentration of marginal value when performed in isolation. Concurrent measurement of albumin in blood plasma is therefore recommended.

Albumin CSF concentrations are known to vary widely among individuals, even under normal conditions. Such disparity of values is determined by individual differences in blood protein concentrations, permeability of the CSF-blood barrier, CSF flow dynamics, and differences in CSF resorption.

COLLECTION/STORAGE INFORMATION

- Specimen Collection and Handling
    - Centrifuge specimen before analysis.
    - Analyze fresh, or store at 4°C for no more than 72 hours.
    - May store frozen at −20°C for 6 months, or at −70°C indefinitely.

• Avoid contaminating specimens with blood.

LOINC CODES
• Code: 2861-3 (*Short Name* - Alb CSF Elph-mCnc)
• Code: 1746-7 (*Short Name* - Alb CSF-mCnc)

Cerebrospinal fluid culture

TEST DEFINITION
Detection of organism(s) in cerebrospinal fluid to diagnose or rule out bacterial meningitis

REFERENCE RANGE
• Adults and Children: Negative or no growth
  Please refer to your institution's reference ranges as lab normals may vary.

INDICATIONS
Suspected bacterial meningitis
> **Strength of Recommendation:** Class IIa
> **Strength of Evidence:** Category B

Results Interpretation:
Positive microbiology findings
> Bacterial culture is considered the 'gold standard' for the diagnosis of bacterial meningitis.
> Bacterial concentrations in cerebrospinal fluid (CSF) greater than or equal to 10^7 colony forming units (CFU)/mL correlate with increased morbidity and mortality; however, quantitative culturing is usually not necessary or practical for diagnosis.
> Culture plates with no growth after 72 hours may be discarded, and negative enrichment broths may be discarded after 5 days.

Frequency of Monitoring
> Cultures should be obtained on cerebrospinal fluid (CSF) specimens whenever bacterial meningitis is suspected.

Timing of Monitoring
> CSF cultures may not be accurate if antibiotics are given first; however, antibiotics should be given without delay to obtain CSF for culture. CSF sterilization occurs rapidly after the administration of antibiotics, with complete sterilization of meningococcus within 2 hours and the beginning of sterilization of pneumococcus within 4 hours into therapy.

Suspected sepsis
> **Strength of Recommendation:** Class IIb
> **Strength of Evidence:** Category C

Results Interpretation:
Abnormal microbiology findings
> Cerebrospinal fluid cultures should be obtained in the presence of meningeal signs or mental status changes.

CLINICAL NOTES
Growth of normal skin flora on CSF culture is highly suggestive of contamination.
Quantitative cultures are usually not necessary or practical for CSF specimens.
Request culture for anaerobes or mycobacteria or fungi if clinically indicated.

COLLECTION/STORAGE INFORMATION
• Specimen Collection and Handling:
  • Collect cerebrospinal fluid in sterile, screw-capped tube.
  • Transport immediately to lab; do not refrigerate.
  • Incubate specimen to 37°C if delay in processing specimen.

LOINC CODES
• Code: 606-4 (*Short Name* - CSF Fld Cult)

Cerebrospinal fluid oligoclonal bands

TEST DEFINITION
Detection of protein components in cerebrospinal fluid for the evaluation of various central nervous system inflammatory disorders.

REFERENCE RANGE
- Oligoclonal banding (OGB): less than 2 discrete bands not present, or of lesser intensity, than the bands in a matched serum sample
- Prealbumin: 2%-7% of total cerebrospinal fluid (CSF) protein (0.02-0.07 mass fraction of total protein)
- Albumin: 56%-76% of total CSF protein (0.56-0.76 mass fraction of total protein) or 0.066-0.442 g/L (6.6-44.2 mg/dL)
- Alpha$_1$ globulin: 2%-7% of total CSF protein (0.02-0.07 mass fraction of total protein)
- Alpha$_2$ globulin: 4%-12% of total CSF protein (0.04-0.12 mass fraction of total protein)
- Beta globulin: 8%-18% of total CSF protein (0.08-0.18 mass fraction of total protein)
- Gamma globulin: 3%-12% of total CSF protein (0.03-0.12 mass fraction of total protein)
  Please refer to your institution's reference ranges as lab normals may vary.

INDICATIONS
Suspected multiple sclerosis
  Strength of Recommendation: Class IIa
  Strength of Evidence: Category C
  Results Interpretation:
  CSF protein electrophoretic profile - finding
  Cerebrospinal fluid (CSF) protein electrophoresis in patients with multiple sclerosis (MS) typically reveals two or more distinct oligoclonal bands (OB) as compared with serum protein electrophoresis, conforming with the underlying inflammatory pathology. The presence of OBs in monosymptomatic patients predicts a significantly higher rate of progression to MS than the absence of bands (42% versus 16% at 5-year follow-up). The combination of CSF OB and an elevated CSF IgG index may identify most patients with MS and exclude those without MS.
  The presence of OBs is not definitively diagnosis for MS due to the prevalence of false positives and the variability in technique and interpretation between laboratories.

COLLECTION/STORAGE INFORMATION
- Ensure that the CSF sample is not contaminated with blood.
- Analyze the CSF sample immediately or store at 4°C for up to 72 hours. Sample is stable frozen at 20°C for 6 months, or at 70°C indefinitely. Serum and CSF samples should be analyzed simultaneously.

Chlamydia antibody assay

TEST DEFINITION
Detection and measurement of the chlamydia-group, genus-specific antibody in serum to evaluate respiratory infection or lymphogranuloma venereum (LGV)

SYNONYMS
- Serologic test for Chlamydia

REFERENCE RANGE
- Adults and Children: Negative
  Please refer to your institution's reference ranges as lab normals may vary.

INDICATIONS
Pneumonia with suspected etiology of chlamydia
  Strength of Recommendation: Class IIb
  Strength of Evidence: Category B

Results Interpretation:
Serology positive

A positive chlamydia-group antibody result may indicate chlamydial respiratory disease.

A 4-fold increase between acute and convalescence titer levels is diagnostic for chlamydial infection.

Chlamydial respiratory disease identified by chlamydia-group antibody may be caused by *C trachomatis,C psittaci* or *C pneumoniae*. Additional testing confirms the finding of chlamydia and identifies the chlamydial species.

Timing of Monitoring

Specimens should be collected during acute illness and convalescence. A 4-fold or greater change in titer between the 2 specimens is considered diagnostic for infection.

Suspected lymphogranuloma venereum (LGV) due to *Chlamydia trachomatis* **infection**

Strength of Recommendation: Class IIa

Strength of Evidence: Category C

Results Interpretation:
Serology positive

For patients with symptoms of lymphogranuloma venereum (LGV), a 4-fold titer rise with microimmunofluorescence (MIF) antibody testing or a complement fixation (CF) titer of greater than or equal to 1:32 supports a presumptive diagnosis of LGV.

LGV is a more invasive type of *C. trachomatis* genital tract infection, leading to higher titer levels than seen with *C. trachomatis* serotypes D through K infections. A CF titer of greater than or equal to 1:256 is strongly presumptive for LGV while a titer of less than or equal to 1:32 rules out LGV except in the very initial stages.

A titer of greater than or equal to 1:128 with MIF testing is strongly suggestive for LGV.

Public health confirmation of LGV requires testing of rectal swabs for direct detection of *C trachomatis* and identification of LGV serotype L1, L2 or L3.

CLINICAL NOTES

Chlamydial tests that detect lipopolysaccharide (LPS) antibodies cannot distinguish between different species of chlamydia and are thus genus-specific tests.

Psittacosis and *C trachomatis* genital infections are monitored by state and federal public health offices in the US.

In 2004, the US Centers for Disease Control and Prevention (CDC) began requesting that clinicians who identify patients with possible lymphogranuloma venereum (LGV) contact the CDC and local public health entities.

Laboratories in the US capable of testing for LGV can be found at: http://www.cdc.gov/std/lgv-labs.htm .

COLLECTION/STORAGE INFORMATION

· Collect blood in a serum tube (marble-top/gold-top serum-separator tube [SST] or a red top tube).
· Label the specimen as 'acute phase' or 'convalescence phase'.

LOINC CODES

· Code: 5082-3 (*Short Name* - Chlamydia Ab Ser EIA-aCnc)
· Code: 27273-2 (*Short Name* - Chlamydia Ab Titr CSF IF)
· Code: 21185-4 (*Short Name* - Chlamydia IgG Ser QI)
· Code: 23990-5 (*Short Name* - Chlamydia Ab Titr CSF CF)
· Code: 16589-4 (*Short Name* - Chlamydia Ab Ser IF-aCnc)
· Code: 5084-9 (*Short Name* - Chlamydia Ab Titr Ser IF)
· Code: 10848-0 (*Short Name* - Chlamydia IgG Titr Ser IF)
· Code: 5083-1 (*Short Name* - Chlamydia Ab Titr Ser CF)
· Code: 31292-6 (*Short Name* - Chlamydia Ab CSF-aCnc)
· Code: 5085-6 (*Short Name* - Chlamydia IgG Ser-aCnc)
· Code: 22184-6 (*Short Name* - Chlamydia IgG Titr Ser)
· Code: 16591-0 (*Short Name* - Chlamydia IgG CSF IF-aCnc)
· Code: 22182-0 (*Short Name* - Chlamydia Ab Titr Ser)
· Code: 22183-8 (*Short Name* - Chlamydia IgG CSF-aCnc)
· Code: 16590-2 (*Short Name* - Chlamydia Ab Ser CF-aCnc)
· Code: 23967-3 (*Short Name* - Chlamydia Ab Titr CSF)
· Code: 7823-8 (*Short Name* - Chlamydia Ab Ser-aCnc)

Chlamydia psittaci antibody assay

TEST DEFINITION
Serologic detection of *Chlamydia psittaci* antibodies in serum to confirm diagnosis of psittacosis

REFERENCE RANGE
- Negative
Please refer to your institution's reference ranges as lab normals may vary.

INDICATIONS
Suspected psittacosis
    Strength of Recommendation: Class IIb
    Strength of Evidence: Category C
Results Interpretation:
Serology positive
    In a patient with clinical evidence of psittacosis, diagnosis is confirmed by a fourfold rise in antibody titer (typically greater than or equal to 32) between acute and convalescent phase paired sera or detection of *Chlamydia psittaci* immunoglobulin M antibody by microimmunofluorescence. A probable diagnosis of psittacosis is established with clinical evidence of illness and a single sera antibody titer, greater than or equal to 32, obtained in at least one specimen after symptom onset.

    False Results
    Although rare, elevated antibody titers can occur in patients with Legionnaires' disease, resulting in a false-positive test for psittacosis.
    Timing of Monitoring
    Serologic testing should be performed at onset of acute illness and during the convalescent phase of illness (eg, 2 weeks or more after initial symptom onset).

CLINICAL NOTES
All sera from one patient should be tested simultaneously at the same laboratory.

COLLECTION/STORAGE INFORMATION
- Collect serum in a marble top tube

LOINC CODES
- Code: 22994-8 (*Short Name* - C psittaci Ab Ser Ql Aggl)
- Code: 20754-8 (*Short Name* - C psittaci Ab Ser Ql CF)
- Code: 22996-3 (*Short Name* - C psittaci Ab Ser Ql EIA)
- Code: 22176-2 (*Short Name* - C psittaci Ab Titr Ser)
- Code: 22995-5 (*Short Name* - C psittaci Ab Ser Ql ID)
- Code: 22175-4 (*Short Name* - C psittaci Ab Ser Ql)
- Code: 14198-6 (*Short Name* - C psittaci Ab Titr Ser IF)
- Code: 5079-9 (*Short Name* - C psittaci Ab Titr Ser CF)
- Code: 7822-0 (*Short Name* - C psittaci Ab Ser-aCnc)

Chlamydia trachomatis antigen assay

TEST DEFINITION
Detection of *Chlamydia trachomatis* antigens in endocervical, conjunctival, rectal and pharyngeal specimens for the screening, diagnosis and management of chlamydial infections

REFERENCE RANGE
Adults and Children: negative
Please refer to your institution's reference ranges as lab normals may vary.

INDICATIONS

Suspected *Chlamydia trachomatis* **infection**
> **Strength of Recommendation:** Class IIa
> **Strength of Evidence:** Category B

Results Interpretation:

Presence of microbial antigen - finding
> Positive *Chlamydia trachomatis* screening tests should be considered presumptive evidence of infection. Additional testing is recommended after an initial positive screening test if a low positive predictive value can be expected, if a false positive result could have adverse medical, psychosocial or legal consequences, or if risk factors indicate low disease prevalence. Because serious side effects from treatment are infrequent, patient counseling for high risk patients may include the option of empiric therapy while awaiting confirmatory test results.

Timing of Monitoring
> Direct fluorescent antibody serial testing after treatment is useful in identifying women with persistent *Chlamydia trachomatis* infections in pelvic inflammatory disease, as well as those at high risk for tubal sequelae.

COLLECTION/STORAGE INFORMATION

- Specimen collection and handling for direct fluorescent antibody tests:
  - Prepare slides immediately after specimen collection.
  - Air dry and fix slides in alcohol or acetone for 10 minutes.
  - Maintain slides at room temperature or 4°C and transport to the lab within 7 days.
  - Fixed and unstained slides can be stored at -20°C for 2 years or longer.
- Specimen collection and handling for immunoassays:
  - Transport specimen to the lab within 24 hours if maintained at room temperature, or within 5 days if maintained at 2°C to 8°C.
  - Process specimens within 5 days of collection.
  - Do not freeze specimens.
- Endocervical specimen collection and handling:
  - Remove all secretions and discharge from the cervical os with a sponge or large swab prior to collecting specimen.
  - For specimen collection, use the swab or endocervical brush supplied or specified by the test manufacturer.
  - Insert the swab or brush 1 to 2 cm into the endocervical canal and rotate it 2 times or more against the wall of the endocervical canal.
  - Withdraw the swab or brush without touching any vaginal surfaces and place in the specified transport medium.
- Intraurethral specimen collection and handling:
  - Obtain specimen 1 hour or more after the patient has voided.
  - Use the swab specified or supplied by the test manufacturer.
  - Insert the swab gently into the urethra (1 to 2 cm in females, 2 to 4 cm in males).
  - Rotate the swab in one direction for 1 or more revolutions and remove.

LOINC CODES

- Code: 14513-6 (*Short Name* - C trach Ag UrnS QI IF)
- Code: 31770-1 (*Short Name* - C trach Ag CSF QI)
- Code: 31776-8 (*Short Name* - C trach Ag Urth QI)
- Code: 31777-6 (*Short Name* - C trach Ag XXX QI)
- Code: 14469-1 (*Short Name* - C trach Ag CSF QI EIA)
- Code: 31771-9 (*Short Name* - C trach Ag Cvx QI)
- Code: 6353-7 (*Short Name* - C trach Ag Tiss QI IF)
- Code: 14473-3 (*Short Name* - C trach Ag Pen QI EIA)
- Code: 14507-8 (*Short Name* - C trach Ag Bld QI IF)
- Code: 31772-7 (*Short Name* - C trach Ag GenV QI)
- Code: 6351-1 (*Short Name* - C trach Ag Cnjt QI IF)
- Code: 6355-2 (*Short Name* - C trach Ag XXX QI IF)
- Code: 31769-3 (*Short Name* - C trach Ag Cnjt QI)
- Code: 14470-9 (*Short Name* - C trach Ag Cvx QI EIA)
- Code: 6350-3 (*Short Name* - C trach Ag Cnjt QI EIA)
- Code: 31768-5 (*Short Name* - C trach Ag Bld QI)
- Code: 31773-5 (*Short Name* - C trach Ag Pen QI)

- Code: 14508-6 (*Short Name* - C trach Ag CSF QI IF)
- Code: 14474-1 (*Short Name* - C trach Ag UrnS QI EIA)
- Code: 14511-0 (*Short Name* - C trach Ag Urth QI IF)
- Code: 14472-5 (*Short Name* - C trach Ag Urth QI EIA)
- Code: 14471-7 (*Short Name* - C trach Ag GenV QI EIA)
- Code: 31774-3 (*Short Name* - C trach Ag Stl QI)
- Code: 14512-8 (*Short Name* - C trach Ag Pen QI IF)
- Code: 31775-0 (*Short Name* - C trach Ag UrnS QI)
- Code: 6352-9 (*Short Name* - C trach Ag Stl QI IF)
- Code: 14510-2 (*Short Name* - C trach Ag GenV QI IF)
- Code: 14468-3 (*Short Name* - C trach Ag Bld QI EIA)
- Code: 6354-5 (*Short Name* - C trach Ag XXX QI EIA)

Chlamydia trachomatis culture

TEST DEFINITION
Detection by culture of *Chlamydia trachomatis* from epithelial cells of mucous membranes

REFERENCE RANGE
No growth.
Please refer to your institution's reference ranges as lab normals may vary.

INDICATIONS
Suspected chlamydial conjunctivitis
   Results Interpretation:
   Eye swab culture negative
      Chlamydia culture may be negative in patients with a long standing infection.

Suspected *Chlamydia trachomatis* **infection**
      Strength of Recommendation: Class IIa
      Strength of Evidence: Category B
   Results Interpretation:
   Positive microbiology findings
      A positive *Chlamydia trachomatis* culture is diagnostic of chlamydial infection.
      Positive culture results are more likely to occur when the patient has been symptomatic for 7 to 8 days.
   Negative microbiology findings
      A negative *Chlamydia trachomatis* culture result may be found in patients treated with antibiotics effective against *Chlamydia trachomatis*, and in those with long-standing infection.
      A negative culture result for *Chlamydia trachomatis* may be caused by a variety of clinical and technical factors, and does not rule out the presence of infection.

COMMON PANELS
- Prenatal screening panel

CLINICAL NOTES
Culture is suggested to find *Chlamydia trachomatis* in conditions where nonculture methods are not developed, are not sufficiently evaluated, or perform badly.
Chlamydia trachomatis culture is an essential test in medicolegal situations.

COLLECTION/STORAGE INFORMATION
- Specimen Collection and Handling:
  - Utilize rayon or cotton swabs for collection, avoid wood and calcium alginate swabs.
  - Send the specimen to the laboratory in specified transport medium.
  - Mucous and secretions should be removed before retrieval of specimen in order to obtain an adequate sample of epithelial cells.

LOINC CODES

- Code: 6349-5 (*Short Name* - C trach XXX QI Cult)
- Code: 14467-5 (*Short Name* - C trach UrnS QI Cult)
- Code: 14466-7 (*Short Name* - C trach Pen QI Cult)
- Code: 14463-4 (*Short Name* - C trach Cvx QI Cult)
- Code: 14461-8 (*Short Name* - C trach Bld QI Cult)
- Code: 14464-2 (*Short Name* - C trach GenV QI Cult)
- Code: 14465-9 (*Short Name* - C trach Urth QI Cult)
- Code: 14462-6 (*Short Name* - C trach CSF QI Cult)

Chlamydia trachomatis nucleic acid amplification test

TEST DEFINITION

Amplification and detection of *Chlamydia trachomatis* -specific DNA or RNA sequences in clinical specimens

REFERENCE RANGE

- Negative
  Please refer to your institution's reference ranges as lab normals may vary.

INDICATIONS

Suspected chlamydial conjunctivitis
    Results Interpretation:
    Polymerase chain reaction observation
    Polymerase chain reaction has been successfully used to detect conjunctival chlamydia in ocular specimens.

Suspected urogenital *Chlamydia trachomatis* **infection**
    Strength of Recommendation: Class IIa
    Strength of Evidence: Category A
    Results Interpretation:
    Nucleic acid conformation
    Nucleic acid amplification testing has moderate sensitivity and high specificity for the detection of urogenital *Chlamydia trachomatis* infections.
    Additional testing should be considered in the absence of risk factors for disease or in a low prevalence setting.

CLINICAL NOTES

Nucleic acid amplification testing (NAAT) may yield a positive result in the presence of very little target DNA or RNA.
NAAT may be helpful in settings that are not conducive to culture.

COLLECTION/STORAGE INFORMATION

- Specimen Collection and Handling:
  - Urine specimen
    - Obtain first-catch urine (first 10 to 30 cc's voided after initiating stream) approximately 1 hour after last void.
    - Store urine for up to 24 hours at room temperature or at 2°C to 8°C for up to 5 days.
  - Endocervical or urethral specimen
    - Endocervical specimen: Remove all secretions and discharge from cervical os. Insert manufacturer-supplied swab 1 to 2 cm into endocervical canal, rotate 2 or more times, and withdraw swab without touching vaginal walls.
    - Urethral specimen: Insert urogenital swab gently into the urethra (females, 1 to 2 cm; males, 2 to 4 cm), rotate in one direction for one or more revolutions, and withdraw. Intraurethral specimens are required regardless of the presence of exudate at the meatus.
    - Immerse swab in manufacturer-supplied or isolation transport medium.
    - Store swab at 2°C to 27°C for up to 5 days or at 2°C to 8°C for up to 7 days.

Chlamydia trachomatis nucleic acid hybridization test

TEST DEFINITION
Detection of nucleotide sequences for the diagnosis of *Chlamydia trachomatis* infection

REFERENCE RANGE
• Negative
Please refer to your institution's reference ranges as lab normals may vary.

INDICATIONS
Suspected *Chlamydia trachomatis* **infection**
> **Strength of Recommendation:** Class IIa
> **Strength of Evidence:** Category C
> **Results Interpretation:**
> **Positive biochemistry findings**
> A positive nucleic acid hybridization test should be considered presumptive evidence of *Chlamydia trachomatis* infection. Additional testing may be indicated in low-prevalence populations.
> When using a nucleic acid hybridization test that will exhibit a positive result in the presence of either *Neisseria gonorrhoeae* or *Chlamydia trachomatis*, additional testing should be done to identify the causative organism(s).

COLLECTION/STORAGE INFORMATION
• Specimen Collection and Handling:
  • Endocervical specimen: Insert manufacturer-provided swab 1 to 2 cm into endocervical canal and rotate 2 or more times. Withdraw swab without touching any vaginal surface.
  • Urethral specimen: Insert manufacturer-provided swab into urethra (males, 2 to 4 cm; females, 1 to 2 cm) 1 or more hours after voiding. Rotate several times in one direction. An intraurethral specimen is required regardless of the presence of exudate at the urethral meatus.
  • Immerse swab in manufacturer-supplied medium.
  • Transport specimen within 7 days at 2°C to 25°C.
  • Freeze specimen at -20°C or below.
  • Specimen can be tested up to 60 days after collection.

Chloride measurement, urine

TEST DEFINITION
Measurement of chloride in urine for the evaluation and management of acid-base, fluid, and electrolyte imbalances

REFERENCE RANGE
• Adults, 18 to 60 years: 110-250 mEq/day (110-250 mmol/day)
• Adults, greater than 60 years: 95-195 mEq/day (95-195 mmol/day)
• Infants, 0 to 2 years: 2-10 mEq/day (2-10 mmol/day)
• Children, 2 to 6 years: 15-40 mEq/day (15-40 mmol/day)
• Male children, 6 to 10 years: 36-110 mEq/day (36-110 mmol/day)
• Female children, 6 to 10 years: 18-74 mEq/day (18-74 mmol/day)
• Male children and adolescents, 10 to 14 years: 64-176 mEq/day (64-176 mmol/day)
• Female children and adolescents, 10 to 14 years: 36-173 mEq/day (36-173 mmol/day)
• Adolescents, 14 to 18 years: 110-250 mEq/day (110-250 mmol/day)
Please refer to your institution's reference ranges as lab normals may vary.

INDICATIONS

Suspected fluid and electrolyte imbalance
Strength of Recommendation: Class IIa
Strength of Evidence: Category C
Results Interpretation:
Increased level (laboratory finding)

In salt-retaining renal states and in oliguria due to renal hypoperfusion, urine sodium and chloride levels are typically less than 20 mEq/L; however, the need for urine electroneutrality may result in abnormally high sodium or chloride levels. A urine chloride level greater than 20 mEq/L suggests an electrolyte imbalance due to severe potassium depletion, syndrome of inappropriate secretion of antidiuretic hormone, or hypo-thyroidism. High urine chloride levels and low urine sodium levels may occur with hyperchloremic metabolic acidosis and extracellular fluid (ECF) volume depletion.

Decreased level (laboratory finding)

Urine chloride levels reflect dietary intake, ECF volume, and renal health. In the absence of an acid-base or renal disorder, chloride excretion approximates sodium excretion, and a low urine sodium level due to ECF depletion is confirmed by a low urine chloride level (less than 10 mmol/L).

Low urine chloride levels occur in edematous states with hyponatremia and nonrenal ECF volume de-pletion (eg, dehydration due to severe diarrhea and vomiting), intestinal fistulas, excessive sweating with in-sufficient sodium chloride intake, and postoperative chloride retention.

Suspected metabolic alkalosis
Strength of Recommendation: Class I
Strength of Evidence: Category C
Results Interpretation:
Chloride level - finding

Chloride-responsive hypochloremia in metabolic alkalosis indicates a volume depleted state, and the urine chloride measurement is less than 10 mEq/L. The low urine chloride level reflects an excess in total body bicarbonate due to gastrointestinal (eg, nasogastric drainage and vomiting) or renal (eg, correction of chronic hypercapnia, alkali or diuretic therapy, and decreased dietary chloride intake) causes.

Sodium chloride-resistant metabolic alkalosis indicates a volume-expanded state due to renal-mediated alkalosis, and the urine chloride level is greater than 20 mEq/L.

In the absence of volume depletion, a high urinary chloride concentration in metabolic alkalosis suggests Cushing's syndrome, primary hyperaldosteronism, or surreptitious sodium bicarbonate ingestion.

CLINICAL NOTES

Dietary chloride intake can cause pronounced variations in urine chloride levels.

COLLECTION/STORAGE INFORMATION

- Specimen Collection and Handling:
  - Obtain a 24-hour urine sample.
  - Add 10g to 15g of boric acid to urine specimen as a preservative.

LOINC CODES

- Code: 2079-2 (*Short Name* - Chloride 24H Ur-sRate)
- Code: 26762-5 (*Short Name* - Chloride Ur-aCnc)
- Code: 32542-3 (*Short Name* - Chloride ?Tm sub Ur Qn)
- Code: 2078-4 (*Short Name* - Chloride Ur-sCnc)
- Code: 21194-6 (*Short Name* - Chloride 24H Ur-sCnc)

Chorionic gonadotropin measurement, qualitative

TEST DEFINITION

Qualitative measurement of human chorionic gonadotropin (hCG) in serum for the presumptive diagnosis of pregnancy..

SYNONYMS
- HCG serum, qualitative

REFERENCE RANGE
- Nonpregnant women: Negative
  Please refer to your institution's reference ranges as lab normals may vary.

INDICATIONS
Suspected pregnancy.
> **Strength of Recommendation:** Class IIa
> **Strength of Evidence:** Category B
> **Results Interpretation:**
> **Positive laboratory findings**
>> A positive qualitative serum human chorionic gonadotropin (hCG) finding is possible before the first missed menstrual period. Pregnancy tests at a sensitivity of 25 International Units/mL can detect hCG 8 to 10 days following ovulation in maternal serum, as compared to 14 to 18 days with urinary assays; however, due to the potential for false-positives, ultrasound confirmation of pregnancy is recommended.
>> Because of the long half-life of hCG in blood, sensitive pregnancy tests are likely to continue to be positive long after fetal demise as placental tissue can continue to produce hCG even if fetal loss has occurred.

> **False Results**
>> False positive human chorionic gonadotropin results occur in approximately 1 in 3,300 women due to high concentrations of heterophilic antibodies in human serum. False positives are possible in women with hyperlipidemia or elevated immunoglobulin levels or in women who have received hCG therapy.

COLLECTION/STORAGE INFORMATION
- Store specimen at 2°C to 8°C for up to 24 hours or freeze at −20°C

LOINC CODES
- Code: 2118-8 (*Short Name* - HCG Ser Ql)
- Code: 12184-8 (*Short Name* - HCG Fld Ql)

Chromium measurement

TEST DEFINITION
Measurement of chromium (Cr) levels in whole blood, plasma, or serum for the evaluation and management of Cr exposure/poisoning and Cr deficiency

REFERENCE RANGE
- Whole blood:
- Adults and Children: 0.7 to 28 mcg/L (13.4 to 538 micromol/L)
- Serum:
- Adults and Children: 0.05 to 0.5 mcg/L (1 to 10 micromol/L)
  Please refer to your institution's reference ranges as lab normals may vary.

INDICATIONS
Suspected chromium deficiency
> **Strength of Recommendation:** Class IIb
> **Strength of Evidence:** Category C
> **Results Interpretation:**
> **Decreased level (laboratory finding)**
>> Serum chromium (Cr) levels do not correlate with Cr deficiency states, as they do not reflect total body Cr stores.

Suspected chromium exposure/poisoning
> **Strength of Recommendation:** Class IIb
> **Strength of Evidence:** Category C

Results Interpretation:
Increased level (laboratory finding)

Elevated serum chromium (Cr) is a marker for Cr exposure/poisoning.

A whole blood level of 2 to 3 mg/L chromium is considered fatal.

Occupational exposure may increase serum Cr; for the purposes of monitoring Cr in the workplace, a plasma Cr level of 10 mcg/L appears to correspond to the short-term atmospheric exposure limit of 0.1 mg/m^3.

Recent exposure to chromium, both hexavalent and trivalent, is revealed by plasma Cr levels, whereas erythrocyte levels only reflect hexavalent exposure.

COLLECTION/STORAGE INFORMATION

- Collect in a container that is free of metal.

LOINC CODES

- Code: 8181-0 (*Short Name* - Chromium Sal-mCnc)
- Code: 5619-2 (*Short Name* - Chromium Bld-mCnc)
- Code: 15118-3 (*Short Name* - Chromium Bld-sCnc)
- Code: 9690-9 (*Short Name* - Chromium XXX-mCnc)
- Code: 5620-0 (*Short Name* - Chromium Har-mCnt)
- Code: 5621-8 (*Short Name* - Chromium RBC-mCnc)
- Code: 21200-1 (*Short Name* - Chromium Nail-mCnt)
- Code: 20759-7 (*Short Name* - Chromium Tiss-mCnt)

Chromium measurement, urine

TEST DEFINITION

Measurement of chromium (Cr) in urine for the evaluation and management of Cr exposure and deficiency

REFERENCE RANGE

- Adults and children: 0.1 to 2 mcg/L (1.9 to 38.4 nmol/L)
  Please refer to your institution's reference ranges as lab normals may vary.

INDICATIONS

Suspected chromium deficiency
   Strength of Recommendation: Class IIb
   Strength of Evidence: Category B
   Results Interpretation:
   Normal laboratory findings

Healthy adults consuming 30 to 100 mcg per day of dietary Cr will excrete 2 to 10 mcg Cr/L in their urine.

Although urinary chromium is a reasonable measure of Cr absorption, urinary Cr may be unaffected by chromium supplementation, particularly in the presence of low urinary excretion. Patients with impaired renal function will excrete larger amounts of urinary Cr. An abnormal glucose clearance in response to Cr supplementation may be indicative of Cr deficiency, as Cr deficiency leads to impaired glucose tolerance in patients with normal circulating insulin levels.

Suspected chromium exposure
   Strength of Recommendation: Class IIb
   Strength of Evidence: Category B
   Results Interpretation:
   Abnormal laboratory findings

Urine chromium (Cr) concentration reflects Cr absorption over the previous 1 to 2 days. The urinary half-life of hexavalent Cr is 15 to 41 hours. Urine chromium concentrations of less than 10 mcg Cr/L are typical in patients with normal Cr exposure.

Substantial variation in Cr levels among individuals exists. In a select subpopulation of 'strong reducers,' high Cr urine levels may not indicate toxicity but rather reflect the individual's ability to more efficiently eliminate hexavalent Cr.

COLLECTION/STORAGE INFORMATION
- Specimen Collection and Handling:
    - Collect in a metal-free container
    - Do not use preservatives

LOINC CODES
- Code: 21201-9 (*Short Name* - Chromium 24H Ur-mCnc)
- Code: 5623-4 (*Short Name* - Chromium Ur-mCnc)
- Code: 13464-3 (*Short Name* - Chromium/creat Ur-mRto)
- Code: 29919-8 (*Short Name* - Chromium/creat 24H Ur-mRto)
- Code: 5624-2 (*Short Name* - Chromium 24H Ur-mRate)

Chromosome breakage assay

TEST DEFINITION
Cytogenetic detection of chromosomal breakage for evaluation of genetically-linked diseases

SYNONYMS
- Fanconi anemia, chromosome breakage study

REFERENCE RANGE
- No chromosomal abnormalities detected
  Please refer to your institution's reference ranges as lab normals may vary.

INDICATIONS
Suspected Fanconi's anemia
   Strength of Recommendation: Class IIa
   Strength of Evidence: Category C
   Results Interpretation:
   Cell chromosome exam. abnormal
   The number of chromosome breaks are scored per the International System for Human Cytogenetic Nomenclature.

CLINICAL NOTES
Almost any cell specimen with nucleated, viable cells can be tested cytogenetically.

COLLECTION/STORAGE INFORMATION
- Specimen Collection and Handling:
    - Collect heparinized peripheral blood sample (least invasive), bone marrow, amniotic fluid, chorionic villus sampling, or fibroblast cultures from skin biopsies or skin punches.
    - Collect and handle sample in a sterile manner.
    - Maintain blood, bone marrow, amniotic fluid, and chorionic villi specimens at room temperature, and process as soon as possible after collection.
    - Transport solid tissue on wet ice.

LOINC CODES
- Code: 34742-7 (*Short Name* - Chrom Break DEB-aCnc)
- Code: 34730-2 (*Short Name* - Chrom Break-Imp)

Citrulline measurement

TEST DEFINITION
Measurement of citrulline in plasma for detection of acquired and hereditary amino acid disorders.

REFERENCE RANGE
- Neonate, 1 day: 0.16-0.51 mg/dL (9-29 micromol/L)
- Infants 1 to 3 months: 0.37 ± 0.19 mg/dL (21 ± 11 micromol/L)
- Infants 2 to 6 months: 0.54-0.88 mg/dL (31-50 micromol/L)
- Children 9 months to 10 years: 0.21-0.53 mg/dL (12-30 micromol/L)
- Children 6 years to 18 years: 0.33-0.91 mg/dL (19-52 micromol/L)
- Adults: 0.21-0.96 mg/dL (12-55 micromol/L)
  Please refer to your institution's reference ranges as lab normals may vary.

INDICATIONS
Suspected inborn error of metabolism
> **Strength of Recommendation:** Class IIa
> **Strength of Evidence:** Category C
> **Results Interpretation:**
> **Increased amino acid**
>
> Inherited amino acid disorders are directly related to the absence of an enzyme involved in the metabolism of one or more amino acids; therefore, an elevated plasma level of a particular amino acid is highly suggestive of an inherited metabolic defect. In the majority of cases amino acid and organic acid analysis together permit diagnostic confirmation in infants. Immediate treatment should be initiated when an inborn error of metabolism is suspected, even if a definitive diagnosis has not yet been determined.
>
> Argininosuccinic acid synthetase deficiency is associated with an elevated citrulline level. Carbamoyl phosphate synthetase deficiency is associated with increased alanine, glutamine, glycine and lysine, and low or undetectable arginine and citrulline. N-acetylglutamic acid synthetase deficiency is associated with increased glutamine as well as low or undetectable citrulline levels.

COLLECTION/STORAGE INFORMATION
- Specimen Collection and Handling:
  - Immediately place sample in ice water.
  - Isolate plasma sample and freeze it within 1 hour; sample stable for 1 week at -20°C.
  - Sample should be deproteinized and stored at -70°C for protracted periods of usage.

LOINC CODES
- Code: 6876-7 (*Short Name* - Citrulline 24H Ur-mRate)
- Code: 13392-6 (*Short Name* - Citrulline Amn-mCnc)
- Code: 30161-4 (*Short Name* - Citrulline/creat Ur-Rto)
- Code: 22722-3 (*Short Name* - Citrulline XXX-sCnc)
- Code: 22654-8 (*Short Name* - Citrulline CSF-sCnc)
- Code: 32235-4 (*Short Name* - Citrulline Fld-sCnc)
- Code: 25376-5 (*Short Name* - Citrulline 24H Ur-sRate)
- Code: 22694-4 (*Short Name* - Citrulline/creat Ur-sRto)
- Code: 25877-2 (*Short Name* - Citrulline 24H Ur-sCnc)
- Code: 2131-1 (*Short Name* - Citrulline Ur-mCnc)
- Code: 26745-0 (*Short Name* - Citrulline Amn-sCnc)
- Code: 27056-1 (*Short Name* - Citrulline Ur-sCnc)
- Code: 25878-0 (*Short Name* - Citrulline/creat 24H Ur-sRto)
- Code: 9511-7 (*Short Name* - Citrulline CSF-mCnc)
- Code: 32234-7 (*Short Name* - Citrulline Vitf-sCnc)

Clomiphene test

TEST DEFINITION
Measurement of follicle stimulating hormone levels following clomiphene challenge for evaluation of ovarian reserve.

SYNONYMS
- Clomid stimulation test
- Clomid test
- Clomiphene stimulation test

REFERENCE RANGE
- Women (follicular phase): 3-20 milliInternational Units/mL (3-20 International Units/L)
  Please refer to your institution's reference ranges as lab normals may vary.

INDICATIONS
Female infertility due to suspected ovulatory dysfunction
> **Strength of Recommendation:** Class IIb
> **Strength of Evidence:** Category B
> **Results Interpretation:**
> **Increased pituitary follicle stimulating hormone level**
>> An abnormal clomiphene challenge as defined by an elevated follicle stimulating hormone (FSH) level, either on day 3 or day 10 of the menstrual cycle, generally correlates with infertility secondary to diminished ovarian reserve.
>> The clomiphene challenge test may be particularly useful for prognosis in women older than 35 years, a single ovary or prior ovarian surgery, known poor response to exogenous gonadotropin stimulation, a family history of early menopause, poor response to infertility treatment, idiopathic infertility, or prior treatment with gonadotropic drugs.
>> The clomiphene challenge test appears to have a higher sensitivity than a baseline FSH for detecting decreased ovarian reserve.
> **Timing of Monitoring**
>> A baseline follicle stimulating hormone (FSH) level is obtained on day 3 of the menstrual cycle. A repeat FSH level is obtained on day 10, after 5 days of clomiphene administration (days 5 through 9).

ABNORMAL RESULTS
- Results increased in :
  - Alcoholism
- Results decreased in:
  - Hemochromatosis
  - Sickle cell anemia
  - Hyperprolactinemia

CLINICAL NOTES
- Follicle stimulating hormone levels may be variable due to interassay differences.

COLLECTION/STORAGE INFORMATION
- Specimen Collection and Handling :
  - Collect specimen in a red top tube.
  - May store at room temperature for 8 days or at 4°C for 14 days

Clostridium botulinum culture

TEST DEFINITION
Identification of *Clostridium botulinum* in stool, wound, or food samples.

REFERENCE RANGE
- No growth
  Please refer to your institution's reference ranges as lab normals may vary.

INDICATIONS
Suspected infant botulism in patients less than 12 months
> **Strength of Recommendation:** Class I
> **Strength of Evidence:** Category C
> **Results Interpretation:**
> **Positive microbiology findings**
>> Isolation of *Clostridium botulinum* in a stool culture is diagnostic. Stools collected a week or more after illness onset may be culture-positive but toxin negative.

The stool culture is the criteria for the confirmation of infant botulism as *C botulinum* is not a normal intestinal flora in humans. Because mild cases of infant botulism and possible asymptomatic carriers of the organism, diagnosis can not be made on culture results alone but it is considered confirmation in a patient with the appropriate clinical syndrome.

A patient can excrete *C botulinum* toxin and organisms for weeks to months during and following recovery; excretion of type A toxin occurs for up to several months.

Suspected wound botulism
  Strength of Recommendation: Class I
  Strength of Evidence: Category C
  Results Interpretation:
  Positive microbiology findings
  Detection of *Clostridium botulinum* organism in wound cultures confirms the suspicion of wound botulism. Toxigenicity can be confirmed by bioassay.

COLLECTION/STORAGE INFORMATION
- Specimen Collection and Handling:
  - Immediately contact the Centers for Disease Control (CDC) or a state public health laboratory to determine proper specimen collection and transport; most hospitals are not equipped to process samples.
  - Handle all materials suspected of containing botulinum toxin with extreme caution
  - Place wound specimens in an anaerobic transport device (eg, Port-A-Cul tubes or vials); ship as soon as possible without refrigeration
  - Collect 25 to 50 g of stool, if possible
  - Refrigerate (do not freeze) all samples except wound specimens
  - Obtain feces samples prior to antitoxin treatment, if possible
  - A sterile water enema may be necessary if the patient is constipated

LOINC CODES
- Code: 33695-8 (*Short Name* - C bot Islt Ql Cult)
- Code: 33694-1 (*Short Name* - C bot XXX Ql Cult)

Clostridium botulinum toxin assay

TEST DEFINITION
Identification of *Clostridium botulinum* toxin in serum, feces, vomitus, gastric contents, and/or suspected foods producing illness.

REFERENCE RANGE
- No toxin identified
  Please refer to your institution's reference ranges as lab normals may vary.

INDICATIONS
Suspected infant botulism in patients less than 12 months
  Results Interpretation:
  Laboratory test finding
  The diagnosis is confirmed when botulinum toxin is demonstrated in a sterile filtrate by mouse lethality and neutralization tests.

Suspected botulism
  Strength of Recommendation: Class I
  Strength of Evidence: Category C
  Results Interpretation:
  Positive laboratory findings
  The diagnosis of botulism is confirmed when *Clostridium botulinum* neurotoxin is demonstrated in a sterile filtrate by mouse lethality and neutralization tests.

COLLECTION/STORAGE INFORMATION
- Specimen Collection and Handling:

- Immediately contact the Centers for Disease Control or state health department laboratories for specific information regarding specimen collection and transport; most hospitals are not equipped to process the samples
- Handle all materials suspected of containing botulinum toxin with extreme caution
- Collect approximately 30 mL of serum in a 'tiger' or red-top tubes (allows for repeat testing); less for children. A minimum of 3 mL is recommended.
- Refrigerate (do not freeze) all samples except wound specimens
- Leave food samples in their original containers
- List any medications (eg, anticholinesterase) that might interfere with toxin assay

LOINC CODES
- Code: 11470-2 (*Short Name* - C bot Tox Stl-aCnc)

Clostridium difficile culture

TEST DEFINITION
Isolation of *Clostridium difficile* from stool for the evaluation of suspected clostridium infection

REFERENCE RANGE
- No growth
  Please refer to your institution's reference ranges as lab normals may vary.

INDICATIONS
Suspected *Clostridium difficile* **infection**
  Strength of Recommendation: Class IIb
  Strength of Evidence: Category C
  Results Interpretation:
  Positive microbiology findings
    Detection of *Clostridium difficile* by culture suggests the diagnosis of *Clostridium difficile* -associated diarrhea. Use of a cytotoxin assay is valuable in confirming the diagnosis. A positive culture is diagnostic in patients with no other cause of diarrhea (eg, cathartics, enteral feedings, inflammatory bowel disease).
    Since *Clostridium difficile* culture takes 2 to 3 days to provide results and does not distinguish between toxinogenic and nontoxinogenic strain, it is rarely used for the clinical diagnosis of *Clostridium difficile* -associated diarrhea.

  False Results
- Colonization of *Clostridium difficile* in stool may be seen in:
- 2% to 3% of healthy adults and children over 2 years of age
- 10% to 20% of adults with no gastrointestinal symptoms who have had recent exposure to antibiotics and in hospitalized patients with no recent exposure to antibiotics or gastrointestinal symptoms

COLLECTION/STORAGE INFORMATION
- Specimen Collection and Handling:
  - Collect fresh stool sample, if possible.
  - Rectal swabs may be used if fresh specimen is not available.
  - Transfer stool in a closed container to the laboratory immediately; do not refrigerate.
  - Place sample in a transport medium if there is a 2- to 3-hour delay in delivering sample to laboratory.

LOINC CODES
- Code: 20762-1 (*Short Name* - C dif Stl QI Aerobe Cult)
- Code: 563-7 (*Short Name* - C dif XXX QI Cult)
- Code: 562-9 (*Short Name* - C dif Stl QI Cult)

Clostridium difficile detection

TEST DEFINITION

Detection of *Clostridium difficile* A and B cytotoxin and associated cytotoxicity for the diagnosis of *C difficile* infection

REFERENCE RANGE

• Adults and children: Negative tissue culture and/or toxin assay
   Please refer to your institution's reference ranges as lab normals may vary.

INDICATIONS

Suspected *Clostridium difficile* **infection**
   Results Interpretation:
   Abnormal cytology findings
      The finding of toxin-mediated cytopathic effect (CPE) on tissue culture cytotoxic assay for toxin B has been considered the 'gold standard' for confirming a diagnosis of *Clostridium difficile* infection, and has historically been the most sensitive and specific among the tests available for the detection of *C difficile*. Due to the length of time required for test completion, the tissue culture cytoxicity assay is not useful as a rapid screening test for the presence of *C difficile*.
   Positive immunology findings
      A positive ELISA finding of *C difficile* toxin is suggestive of *C difficile* infection. The test is moderately sensitive; however, due to the high specificity, the immunoassay is considered useful for rapid screening of patients suspected of having *C difficile* infection. Sequential testing with enzyme immunoassay followed by cytotoxin tissue cell culture is suggested as the optimal approach for maximizing detection of infection by *C difficile*.

CLINICAL NOTES

Tissue culture assay is considered the most sensitive and specific test available for the diagnosis of *Clostridium difficile* infection and has been historically used as the standard method for detection of cytotoxicity due to cytotoxins A and B. However, due to the 1-to-3 day time frame required for tissue culture testing, enzyme-linked immunosorbent assays (ELISAs) are preferred by clinical laboratories for rapid detection of *C difficile* infection.

Immunoassays for *Clostridium difficile* toxin should not be used to monitor response to therapy, since results have remained positive for extended periods of time in 25% of patients treated successfully for the infection.

COLLECTION/STORAGE INFORMATION

• Specimen Collection and Handling
   • Collect stool specimen in clean, wide-mouth container and transport promptly to laboratory
   • Refrigerate sample if not processed within 2 hours

Clot retraction, screen

TEST DEFINITION

Measurement of clot retraction for evaluation and management of platelet disorders

REFERENCE RANGE

• Adults and Children: 50%-100%/2 hours
   Please refer to your institution's reference ranges as lab normals may vary.

INDICATIONS

Suspected Glanzmann's thrombasthenia
      Strength of Recommendation: Class IIb
      Strength of Evidence: Category B
   Results Interpretation:
   Coag./bleeding tests abnormal
      Glanzmann's thrombasthenia is the only platelet function disorder in which poor or absent clot retraction is found.

CLINICAL NOTES

Clot retraction has little value for the detection of mild to moderate bleeding disorders and is a poor test of clotting function.

COLLECTION/STORAGE INFORMATION

- Specimen Collection and Handling:
  - Obtain a 5-mL blood sample
  - Place in an anticoagulant-free red top tube, do not agitate tube
  - Allow to clot at 37°C
  - Send sample to lab as soon as possible

LOINC CODES

- Code: 3245-8 (*Short Name* - Clot Retract Bld Ql Coag)

Clotting factor V assay

TEST DEFINITION

Measurement of factor V in plasma for evaluation and management of coagulation and bleeding disorders

SYNONYMS

- Ac-Globulin assay
- Factor V assay
- Factor V level
- Labile factor assay
- Proaccelerin assay

REFERENCE RANGE

- Adults: 60%-140% of normal activity (0.6-1.4 units/mL of normal activity)
  Please refer to your institution's reference ranges as lab normals may vary.

INDICATIONS

Suspected hereditary factor V deficiency
  Strength of Recommendation: Class IIb
  Strength of Evidence: Category C
  Results Interpretation:
  Hereditary factor V deficiency disease
    The plasma level of factor V activity in in patients with factor V deficiency is usually less than 2% of that in normal plasma. While factor V antigen in the plasma usually corresponds to factor V activity, patients with factor V deficiency (parahemophilia) show variable bleeding tendencies. Plasma factor V levels correlate poorly with the clinical severity of disease (ie, risk of bleeding).

COMMON PANELS

- Coagulation factor assay

COLLECTION/STORAGE INFORMATION

- Specimen Collection and Handling:
  - Collect serum in tube containing plasma citrate.
  - Place specimen on ice immediately and send to lab as soon as possible.
  - Specimen is stable for 2 hours on ice.
  - Freeze specimen if assay is delayed for more 2 hours.

LOINC CODES

- Code: 3193-0 (*Short Name* - FV Act/Nor PPP Qn Coag)
- Code: 3192-2 (*Short Name* - FVa PPP-aCnc)

Clotting factor VII assay

TEST DEFINITION
Measurement of factor VII levels in plasma for the evaluation and management of coagulation disorders

SYNONYMS
- Autoprothrombin I assay
- Factor VII assay
- Proconvertin assay
- Stable factor assay

REFERENCE RANGE
- Percent of normal activity: 60% - 140%
  Please refer to your institution's reference ranges as lab normals may vary.

INDICATIONS
Elevated plasma factor VII levels as a risk factor for cardiovascular disease.
> **Strength of Recommendation:** Class IIb
> **Strength of Evidence:** Category B
> **Results Interpretation:**
> **Increased level (laboratory finding)**
> Increased factor VIIa levels may be a significant predictor of reinfarction or death in post-infarction women but not men.
> Patients with increased factor VIIc levels may be more likely to experience myocardial infarction than those with lower levels (OR=5.2).
> Factor VII assays differ considerably and problems with interlaboratory standardization exist.

Suspected factor VII deficiency
> **Strength of Recommendation:** Class I
> **Strength of Evidence:** Category C
> **Results Interpretation:**
> **Factor VII deficiency**
> Patients with heterozygous factor VII deficiencies are usually asymptomatic; patients with homozygous factor VII deficiencies have an increased incidence of bleeding symptoms. Factor VII levels do not always correlate with the severity of symptoms. Severe factor VII deficiency has been associated with intracranial hemorrhage and clinical presentations as severe as those of hemophilia A or B.
> Activated factor VII levels (FVIIa) were significantly lower in 13 hemophilia A patients and significantly lower in 7 hemophilia B patients than FVIIa levels in 20 controls.
> Factor VII assays differ considerably and there are problems with interlaboratory standardization.

ABNORMAL RESULTS
- Results decreased in:
  - Liver disease
  - Healthy newborns

CLINICAL NOTES
The various assays currently available measure either the concentration of activated factor VII (FVIIa), factor VII clotting activity (FVII:C), the ratio of FVII:C to FVIIa, or the ratio of FVII:C to FVII. The ratio of activated factor VII to factor VII clotting activity is expressed as FVII:C/FVII amidolytic activity (FVII:AM) or FVII:C/FVII antigen.

COLLECTION/STORAGE INFORMATION
- Draw 5 mL of blood by 2-tube method in a sodium citrate tube.
- Place specimen on ice; assay should be performed as soon as possible
- Specimen is stable on ice for 2 hours; freeze specimen if lab assay is delayed for 2 hours or more
- Storage at 4°C may activate factor VII

LOINC CODES
- Code: 3199-7 (*Short Name* - FVII PPP Chro-aCnc)
- Code: 3197-1 (*Short Name* - FVIIa PPP Coag-aCnc)

Clotting factor X assay

TEST DEFINITION
Measurement of factor X in plasma for the evaluation and management of factor X deficiency

SYNONYMS
- Factor X assay
- Stuart factor assay
- Stuart-Prower factor assay

REFERENCE RANGE
- Adults: 60%-140% (0.6-1.4) of normal plasma activity
  Please refer to your institution's reference ranges as lab normals may vary.

INDICATIONS
Suspected and known factor X deficiency
    Strength of Recommendation: Class I
    Strength of Evidence: Category C
Results Interpretation:
Coag./bleeding tests abnormal
- Factor X levels:
  - 5% to 10% of normal plasma concentration (0.05-0.1): minimal hemostatic level
  - 15% to 20% of normal plasma concentration (0.15 -0.2): minimal level for major surgery
- Factor X deficiency classifications:
  - Type I: Antigen level and functional activity decreased
  - Type II: Antigen level near normal; functional activity decreased

COMMON PANELS
- Coagulation factor assay

COLLECTION/STORAGE INFORMATION
- Collect 5 mL of plasma in blue top tube (citrate).
- Transport to lab for immediate analysis.
- Storing sample at 4°C may activate factor X.

LOINC CODES
- Code: 3218-5 (*Short Name* - FX Act/Nor PPP Qn)
- Code: 3219-3 (*Short Name* - FX PPP Chro-aCnc)
- Code: 3217-7 (*Short Name* - FXa PPP Coag-aCnc)

Clotting factor XI assay

TEST DEFINITION
Measurement of coagulation factor XI (plasma thromboplastin antecedent) in plasma for evaluation and management of clotting and thrombotic disorders,

SYNONYMS
- Factor XI assay
- Plasma thromboplastin antecedent assay
- PTA assay

REFERENCE RANGE
- Adults: 60%-140% of normal plasma activity (0.6 -1.4)
  Please refer to your institution's reference ranges as lab normals may vary.

INDICATIONS
Suspected coagulopathy due to coagulation factor XI deficiency
> **Strength of Recommendation:** Class IIa
> **Strength of Evidence:** Category B
> **Results Interpretation:**
> **Decreased level (laboratory finding)**

Heredity factor XI deficiency is rare in the general population, but is more prevalent in certain ethnic groups, especially in Ashkenazi Jews. Suspect this condition in patients with an isolated prolonged aPTT and a family history of mild to moderate bleeding tendency with an autosomal inheritance pattern. Confirmation of the diagnosis requires a specific factor XI assay. It is possible for a factor XI deficient patient to show a normal PTT, depending on the sensitivity of the PTT reagent.

Factor XI levels correlate poorly with bleeding severity. Patients with factor XI deficiency can experience mild to moderate bleeding when exposed to a hemostatic stress such as surgery, especially involving the urinary tract, nose, tonsils or oral cavity. Studies of heterozygous factor XI deficient persons suggest that 20% to 50% bleed excessively. At least 15 variant mutations of the factor XI gene have been identified, with higher rates of bleeding seen in the II/III genotype. Both homozygous and heterozygous forms of factor XI deficiency can be at risk for increased bleeding.

Suspected elevated level of coagulation factor XI in venous thromboembolism
> **Strength of Recommendation:** Class IIa
> **Strength of Evidence:** Category B
> **Results Interpretation:**
> **Increased level (laboratory finding)**

An elevated level of factor XI doubles the risk for experiencing a thrombotic event. Up to 10% of the general population may have elevated factor XI levels. There is a continuous dose-response relationship seen with higher levels of factor XI, where as the factor XI level increases so does the thrombotic risk.

An elevated factor XI level, together with an elevated factor VIII level and an elevated factor IX level, predisposes patients to a 40-fold increase for the risk of experiencing a thrombotic event. In such multi-elevated factor patients, up to half of them will have an initial thrombotic event by 32 years of age. High levels also predispose patients to recurrent thrombotic events with increasing age.
> **Timing of Monitoring**

Perform factor XI assay prior to starting the patient on oral anticoagulants to limit drug interference.

COMMON PANELS
- Coagulation factor assay

ABNORMAL RESULTS
- Results decreased in:
  - Proteinuria
  - Liver disease
  - Lupus anticoagulant

CLINICAL NOTES
Clotted or hemolyzed specimens will adversely affect results. At least 15 variant mutations have been identified in persons with functional factor XI deficiency.

COLLECTION/STORAGE INFORMATION
- Specimen Collection and Handling:
  - Collect 4.5 mL venous blood in a blue top sodium citrate tube.
  - Place specimen on ice immediately; freeze specimen if assay delayed by more than 2 hours.

LOINC CODES
- Code: 3227-6 (*Short Name* - FXI PPP Chro-aCnc)
- Code: 3225-0 (*Short Name* - FXIa % PPP)
- Code: 3226-8 (*Short Name* - FXI Act/Nor PPP Qn)

Clotting factor XII assay

TEST DEFINITION
Measurement of factor XII in blood for assessment of inherited and acquired bleeding disorders

SYNONYMS
- Factor XII assay
- Hageman factor assay

REFERENCE RANGE
- Adults and Children: 60%-140% (0.6 to 1.4)
  Please refer to your institution's reference ranges as lab normals may vary.

INDICATIONS
Suspected bacterial septicemia
    Strength of Recommendation: Class IIb
    Strength of Evidence: Category B
  Results Interpretation:
  Increased level (laboratory finding)
    An increased level of factor XII can help to identify the primary cause of a hypercoagulable state.

Suspected factor XII deficiency
  Results Interpretation:
  Decreased level (laboratory finding)
    Factor XII assay is useful in the evaluation of disorder coagulation, particularly in the setting of an unexplained prolongation of the PTT.
    Factor XII deficiency does not typically cause a hemorrhagic diathesis. Some evidence suggests that it can increase the risk of thrombosis.

COMMON PANELS
- Coagulation factor assay

COLLECTION/STORAGE INFORMATION
Specimen Collection and Handling:
- Collect 5 mL of venous blood in a blue top tube
- Transfer to laboratory immediately

LOINC CODES
- Code: 3233-4 (*Short Name* - FXII PPP Chro-aCnc)
- Code: 3231-8 (*Short Name* - FXIIa PPP-aCnc)
- Code: 3232-6 (*Short Name* - FXII Act/Nor PPP Qn)

Coagulation time, activated

TEST DEFINITION
Measurement of time until clot formation occurs in whole blood

SYNONYMS
- ACT
- Activated clotting time
- Ground glass clotting time
- Whole blood activated clotting time

REFERENCE RANGE
- Adults: 70-180 seconds
  Please refer to your institution's reference ranges as lab normals may vary.

INDICATIONS
Monitoring anticoagulation therapy with heparin
   Strength of Recommendation: Class IIa
   Strength of Evidence: Category C
   Results Interpretation:
   Increased level (laboratory finding)
      Results are not standardized among different techniques and the correlation between activated clotting time (ACT) and heparin levels is poor. ACT's wide dose-response range makes it useful for monitoring high-dose heparin (greater than 0.8 units/mL) concentrations.
   - Suggested parameters for heparin therapy:
     - Cardiopulmonary bypass: Achieve an ACT >480 seconds before initiation and maintenance of extracorporeal circulation
     - Vascular catheterization, hemodialysis, or extracorporeal membrane oxygenation (ECMO): Determine the heparin dose from a standard nomogram adjusted for the patient's baseline ACT
     - Hemodialysis: Therapeutic range of 132 to 234 seconds
     - PTCA: HemoTec >275 to 300 seconds, or Hemochron >350 to 400 seconds

CLINICAL NOTES
   The results of different activated clotting times (ACT) tests are not interchangeable because various instruments use different activators and mechanical techniques.

COLLECTION/STORAGE INFORMATION
- Specimen Collection and Handling:
- Collect sample in a special black top tube containing a particulate activator
- Immediately perform test
- Avoid traumatic venipuncture
- Do not collect specimen from the extremity used for the heparin infusion

LOINC CODES
- Code: 3184-9 (*Short Name* - ACT Bld Qn)

Cocaine measurement, Blood

TEST DEFINITION
   Measurement of cocaine or related metabolites in blood for detecting and monitoring abuse or toxicity

REFERENCE RANGE
- Negative screening test (immunoassay) for cocaine metabolite, benzoylecgonine: <300 ng/mL
- Negative confirmatory test (GC-MS) for cocaine metabolite, benzoylecgonine: <150 ng/mL
  Please refer to your institution's reference ranges as lab normals may vary.

INDICATIONS
Suspected cocaine overdose
   Strength of Recommendation: Class IIa
   Strength of Evidence: Category B
   Results Interpretation:
   Finding of cocaine in blood
      The presence of cocaine can be preliminarily identified in serum or urine by immunoassay. Either liquid chromatography-mass spectrometry (LC-MS) or gas chromatography-mass spectrometry (GC-MS) are reliable for confirmation.
      Positive screening and confirmatory tests for the cocaine metabolite benzoylecgonine are 300 ng/mL or greater and 150 ng/mL or greater, respectively.

Due to the rapid clearance of benzoylecgonine (BZE) from blood, its identification is consistent with acute cocaine exposure. Quantitative blood levels, however, may not correlate with severity of toxicity or contribute to patient management.

ABNORMAL RESULTS

Ecgonine methylester (EME) is a metabolite of cocaine produced by pseudocholinesterase. Qualitative or quantitative impairment in pseudocholinesterase will alter excretion of this metabolite.

CLINICAL NOTES

Cocaine and its 8 metabolites can be specifically assayed for detection. Benzoylecgonine (BZE) and ecgonine methylester (EME) are the primary metabolites, accounting for approximately 35% to 54% and 32% to 49% of excreted cocaine. Non-metabolized cocaine, BZE, and EME are the most common targets for analysis. Other metabolites include norcocaine, benzoylnorecgonine, m-hydroxy-BZE, p-hydroxy-BZE, m-hydroxy-cocaine, and p-hydroxy-cocaine.

BZE has a mean blood elimination half-life of 3.6 hours, and its identification indicates acute cocaine exposure.

COLLECTION/STORAGE INFORMATION

- Maintain chain of custody, as appropriate.
- Collect specimen in sodium fluoride and potassium oxalate containing (gray-top) tube.
- Immediately place specimen on ice and assay within one hour of collection.
- If not assayed immediately, adjust specimen to ph 5 with dilute acetic acid, and preserve with fluoride to maintain stability.
  - Preserved in this manner, specimens can be refrigerated at 4°C or frozen for several months.

LOINC CODES

- Code: 8190-1 (*Short Name* - Cocaine SerPl Ql Cnfrn)
- Code: 31137-3 (*Short Name* - Cocaine Bifl-mCnc)
- Code: 27204-7 (*Short Name* - Cocaine Vitf-mCnc)
- Code: 16633-0 (*Short Name* - Cocaine Bld Ql)
- Code: 18208-9 (*Short Name* - Cocaine XXX-mCnc)
- Code: 8191-9 (*Short Name* - Cocaine SerPl Ql Scn)
- Code: 26758-3 (*Short Name* - Cocaine Stl-mCnt)
- Code: 3396-9 (*Short Name* - Cocaine SerPl-mCnc)
- Code: 16447-5 (*Short Name* - Cocaine SerPl-aCnc)
- Code: 27114-8 (*Short Name* - Cocaine Har-mCnt)
- Code: 26956-3 (*Short Name* - Cocaine Mec-mCnt)
- Code: 3395-1 (*Short Name* - Cocaine SerPl Ql)
- Code: 29323-3 (*Short Name* - Cocaine Gast-mCnc)

Cocaine measurement, urine

TEST DEFINITION

Measurement of cocaine or related metabolites in blood for detecting and monitoring abuse or toxicity

REFERENCE RANGE

- Negative screening test (immunoassay) for cocaine metabolite, benzoylecgonine:<300 ng/mL
- Negative confirmatory test (GC-MS) for cocaine metabolite, benzoylecgonine: <150 ng/mL
  Please refer to your institution's reference ranges as lab normals may vary.

INDICATIONS

Suspected cocaine overdose
    Strength of Recommendation: Class I
    Strength of Evidence: Category B
    Results Interpretation:
    Urine drug levels - finding
        The presence of cocaine can be preliminarily identified in serum or urine by immunologic methods. Either liquid chromatography-mass spectrometry (LC-MS) or GC-MS are reliable and sensitive for drug confirmation.

Positive screening and confirmatory tests for the cocaine metabolite benzoylecgonine are 300 ng/mL or greater and 150 ng/mL or greater, respectively.

BZE is rapidly cleared from blood, but depending on chronicity and route of use, BZE can be detected in urine for 48 hours or longer after exposure.

Urine drug screening tests are generally qualitative, and intended only to verify exposure to the substance(s) being assayed. They do not provide information regarding degree of clinical impairment, or the timing, chronicity, route or quantity of exposure. Serum cocaine testing may provide advantages over urine testing in cases of suspected cocaine toxicity.

ABNORMAL RESULTS

Ecgonine methylester (EME) is a metabolite of cocaine produced by pseudocholinesterase. Qualitative or quantitative impairment in pseudocholinesterase will alter excretion of this metabolite.

CLINICAL NOTES

Cocaine and its 8 metabolites can be specifically assayed for detection. Benzoylecgonine (BZE) and ecgonine methylester (EME) are the primary metabolites, accounting for approximately 35% to 54% and 32% to 49% of excreted cocaine. Non metabolized cocaine, BZE, and EME are the most common targets for analysis. Other metabolites include norcocaine, benzoylnorecgonine, m-hydroxy-BZE, p-hydroxy-BZE, m-hydroxy-cocaine, and p-hydroxy-cocaine.

The traditional window for detecting the BZE metabolite in urine is approximately 48 hours. However, chronic use and route of administration may alter metabolic processes and result in variable prolongation of clearance.

COLLECTION/STORAGE INFORMATION

- Maintain chain of custody, as appropriate.
- If not assayed immediately, adjust specimen pH to between 3 and 5 with dilute acetic acid and refrigerate at 4°C to maintain stability.

LOINC CODES

- Code: 3398-5 (*Short Name* - Cocaine Ur-mCnc)
- Code: 20519-5 (*Short Name* - Cocaine Ur Cnfrn-mCnc)
- Code: 16448-3 (*Short Name* - Cocaine Ur-aCnc)
- Code: 19359-9 (*Short Name* - Cocaine Ur Ql Scn)
- Code: 3397-7 (*Short Name* - Cocaine Ur Ql)

Coccidioides immitis detection

TEST DEFINITION

Detection of *Coccidioides immitis* antibodies in various body fluids for the diagnosis, prognosis, and management of coccidioidomycosis

REFERENCE RANGE

- Adults and Children: Negative
Please refer to your institution's reference ranges as lab normals may vary.

INDICATIONS

Suspected coccidioidomycosis
    Strength of Recommendation: Class IIa
    Strength of Evidence: Category B
    Results Interpretation:
    Serology positive

Qualitative serologic detection of coccidioidal IgM antibodies is virtually diagnostic for recent primary coccidioidomycosis. 53% of patients have a positive test within 1 week and 91% within 2 weeks. Antibody levels increase rapidly during the early stages of disease, decrease rapidly after the fourth week, and are typically absent 4 to 6 months after initial infection. Serum IgM antibodies may reappear with extrapulmonary dissemination during the late stages of the disease.

A negative IgM serologic test does not rule out a diagnosis of coccidioidomycosis.

Coccidioidal IgG antibodies are detected later in disease progression than IgM antibodies, with 50% of patients positive at 4 weeks and greater than 90% positive at 8 weeks. A presumptive diagnosis of coccidioidomycosis is made with a fourfold increase in IgG titer. IgG serum titers usually correlate with disease severity. A serum titer of 2 to 8 is possible with limited disease, titers of 16 or more indicate disseminated infection, and titers can be greater than 256 with extensive dissemination of disease.

If there is evidence that specific anatomical sites are involved in coccidioidomycosis, serologic testing of the associated anatomical fluids is indicated.

Detection of coccidioidal IgG in cerebrospinal fluid (CSF) typically indicates meningeal coccidioidomycosis. A negative CSF IgG test, however, does not rule out meningeal involvement, and serum IgG tests may be negative in the presence of meningitis. In addition, false positive coccidioidal IgG serologic reactions are possible in the absence of meningeal involvement.

A good prognosis is associated with a positive coccidioidin skin test in the presence of an absent or decreasing IgG antibody titer, whereas a poor prognosis is indicated by a negative skin test in the presence of a rapidly increasing IgG titer.

Coccidioidal IgG titers of 1:2 to 1:8 may occur from cross-reactions with blastomycosis or histoplasmosis.

False Results

False negative IgG antibody reactions in cerebrospinal fluid (CSF) may occur in approximately 5% of patients with active meningeal coccidioidomycosis. One serologic method for detection of coccidioidal IgM antibodies (latex particle agglutination) had a reported false-positive rate ranging from 6% to 10% in both CSF and serum.

Frequency of Monitoring

Quantitative IgG antibody serologic testing should be performed at 3 to 4 week intervals. Positive specimens are initially frozen and when additional specimens from the same anatomical compartment are available, the paired sequential specimens should be tested at the same time to reduce possible test variability.

LOINC CODES

- Code: 20767-0 (*Short Name* - C immitis Islt QI)

Coccidioidin skin test

TEST DEFINITION

Measurement of reaction to intradermal coccidioidin antigen for the assessment of coccidioidomycosis exposure or illness

SYNONYMS

- Coccioidin skin test
- Delayed hypersensitivity skin test for coccidiodin
- Skin test for coccidioidomycosis

REFERENCE RANGE

Adults and Children: Negative (induration of less than 5 mm at 48 hours post-test)
Please refer to your institution's reference ranges as lab normals may vary.

INDICATIONS

Suspected coccidioidomycosis exposure or infection
 Strength of Recommendation: Class IIa
 Strength of Evidence: Category C
Results Interpretation:
Positive skin test reaction
 The coccidioidin skin test becomes positive within three weeks of initial infection.
 While a positive skin test reaction (induration of greater than 5 mm at 48 hours) suggests coccidioidomycosis, the test does not establish the diagnosis as the result may reflect past self-limited illness and not the cause of current illness.

Absent skin test reaction
A negative skin test does not exclude coccidioidomycosis. Negative skin tests are common in patients with severe or disseminated coccidioidomycosis. Use of lymphocyte transformation assays are helpful in guiding therapeutic decisions in these patients.

A negative serial coccidioidin skin test performed in conjunction with a peak complement fixation antibody titer (results greater than 1:256) is associated with an increased risk of relapse.

CLINICAL NOTES
The coccidioidal skin test is routinely done first to determine if further studies are needed.

Cold agglutinin titer

TEST DEFINITION
Detects antibodies that agglutinate red blood cells in cold temperatures

SYNONYMS
· Cold agglutinin titre

REFERENCE RANGE
· Titers less than 1:32 are nondiagnostic.
Please refer to your institution's reference ranges as lab normals may vary.

INDICATIONS
Cold autoimmune hemolytic anemia
> **Strength of Recommendation:** Class IIa
> **Strength of Evidence:** Category C
Results Interpretation:
Cold agglutinins present
Cold agglutinin titers are markedly elevated in cold autoimmune hemolytic anemia, usually in the range of 1:1,024 to 1:512,000. The titer decreases after treatment.

High titers and the presence of monoclonal IgM cryoglobulins distinguish cold autoimmune hemolytic anemia from other causes of increased cold agglutinins.

Suspected *Mycoplasma pneumoniae* **pneumonia**
> **Strength of Recommendation:** Class IIb
> **Strength of Evidence:** Category C
Results Interpretation:
Cold agglutinins present
An initial titer of 1:128, or a four-fold increase between the acute and convalescent sera, suggests myco-plasma pneumonia.

Elevated cold agglutinins are observed in 30% to 50% of patients with mycoplasma pneumonia; therefore, a negative titer does not exclude the diagnosis.
Timing of Monitoring
The original sample should be drawn in the early acute phase followed by a second sample within the following seven to ten days.

ABNORMAL RESULTS
· Results increased in:
  · Blood dyscrasias
  · Liver disease
  · Collagen vascular diseases

CLINICAL NOTES
Hemolysis occurs in association with very high cold agglutinin titers (greater than 1:500).

COLLECTION/STORAGE INFORMATION
- Collect blood sample in a lavender- or blue-top tube.
- Keep sample at 37°C.

LOINC CODES
- Code: 5098-9 (*Short Name* - CA Titr SerPl Aggl)
- Code: 30901-3 (*Short Name* - CA Titr SerPl Cord RBC Aggl)
- Code: 14658-9 (*Short Name* - CA Titr SerPl)

Complement C1 esterase inhibitor, total measurement

TEST DEFINITION
Quantitative and functional assay of C1 esterase inhibitor (C1NH) in serum to detect deficiency associated with hereditary angioedema, autoimmune, and low-grade proliferative disorders

REFERENCE RANGE
- Adults: 12.4-24.5 mg/dL (0.12-0.25 g/L)
  Please refer to your institution's reference ranges as lab normals may vary.

INDICATIONS
Suspected acquired C1 esterase inhibitor deficiency
　　　Strength of Recommendation: Class IIa
　　　Strength of Evidence: Category C
　　Results Interpretation:
　　Abnormal biochemistry findings
　　　Acquired C1 esterase inhibitor (C1NH) deficiency is characterized by low levels of serum C1NH and C4, recurrent angioedema, and absence of family history.
　　　With acquired C1NH deficiency type I, there is less than 50% of the C1NH concentration and low C1NH function. With acquired C1NH deficiency type II, the C1NH concentration is low or normal and the C1NH function is low.

Suspected hereditary angioedema
　　　Strength of Recommendation: Class IIa
　　　Strength of Evidence: Category B
　　Results Interpretation:
　　Abnormal laboratory findings
　　　Hereditary angioedema (HAE) is diagnosed using family history, clinical course, and analysis of C1 esterase inhibitor (C1NH) and complement component levels. In HAE type I (deficient), C1NH and C4 levels are decreased. In hereditary angioedema type II (defective), C1NH levels are normal or increased and C4 levels are decreased. In a possible third variant of hereditary angioedema, found only in women thus far, C1NH and C4 levels remain normal regardless of whether the patient has symptoms.
　　　In HAE type 1, C1NH concentration and function are less than 30%. In HAE type 2, C1NH concentration is normal or increased, and the function is less than 30%.
　　Frequency of Monitoring
　　　To confirm a diagnosis of any type of C1 esterase inhibitor deficiency or dysfunction, 2 separate measurements should be done 1 to 3 months apart.

CLINICAL NOTES
　　The nephelometric immunoassay is more cost-effective than radial immunoassay due to its high level of automation.

COLLECTION/STORAGE INFORMATION
- Specimen Collection and Handling:
  - Collect blood in EDTA, EGTA, or citrate tube.
  - Store specimen at -70°C.

LOINC Codes
- Code: 4476-8 (*Short Name* - C1INH Functional SerPl-mCnc)

Complement assay, total

Test Definition
Measurement of total activity of complement in serum for the evaluation of congenital and acquired complement deficiency diseases

Synonyms
- CH>50< assay

Reference Range
- Adults: 63-145 units/mL (63-145 kilounits/L) as measured by enzyme immunoassay
  Please refer to your institution's reference ranges as lab normals may vary.

Indications
Suspected complement deficiency disease
> **Strength of Recommendation:** Class IIa
> **Strength of Evidence:** Category C
> **Results Interpretation:**
> **Complement abnormality**
>> Decrease of total activity in the classic pathway or alternative pathway suggests a complement deficiency. Inherited complement deficiency is associated with poor immune response to bacterial infections, particularly Neisseria, and autoimmune conditions such as systemic lupus erythematosus (SLE).
>> Complement deficiency secondary to activation occurs with normal immune response and may also reflect the activity of inflammatory diseases such as SLE or rheumatoid arthritis.

Clinical Notes
Complement assays measure the functional integrity of the entire complement cascade, which includes more than 20 distinct proteins. These individual components also may be measured by functional hemolytic assays as well as immunochemical methods.

Collection/Storage Information
- Specimen Collection and Handling:
  - Use a plain red-top tube to collect blood sample
  - Allow the sample to clot for 30 minutes
  - Do not allow sample to stand at 37°C for more than 1 hour
  - Store sample at -70°C
  - Ship sample on dry ice

Complexed prostate specific antigen measurement

Test Definition
Measurement of complexed prostate specific antigen (cPSA) in serum for the assessment of prostate cancer

Synonyms
- Complexed PSA measurement

Reference Range
- Men ages 40-49: 1 ng/mL
- Men ages 50-59: 1.5 ng/mL

- Men ages 60-69: 2 ng/mL
- Men ages 70-79: 3 ng/mL
   Please refer to your institution's reference ranges as lab normals may vary.

INDICATIONS
Suspected prostate cancer
   Strength of Recommendation: Class IIa
   Strength of Evidence: Category B
   Results Interpretation:
   Increased level (laboratory finding)
      An elevated complexed prostate specific antigen level is suggestive of prostate cancer.

CLINICAL NOTES
   With the exception of free prostate specific antigen (fPSA), complexed PSA (cPSA) measures all immunoassay detectable PSA complexes including alpha-1-antichymotrypsin and alpha-1-antitrypsin.
   Different manufacturer's immunoassays may produce different results when run on the same sample.

COLLECTION/STORAGE INFORMATION
- Store up to 18 months at -80°C.

LOINC CODES
- Code: 33667-7 (*Short Name* - Complexed PSA SerPl-mCnc)

Copper measurement, serum

TEST DEFINITION
   Measurement of copper in serum for evaluation of copper deficiency, toxicity and disorders of copper metabolism

REFERENCE RANGE
- Adults: 70-140 mcg/dL (11-22 micromol/L)
- Infants, 0 to 6 months: 20-70 mcg/dL (3.1-11 micromol/L)
- Children, 6 years: 90-190 mcg/dL (14.1-29.8 micromol/L)
- Children, 12 years: 80-160 mcg/dL (12.6-25.1 micromol/L)
- Pregnancy (at term): 118-302 mcg/dL (18.5-47.4 micromol/L)
- Levels in African-Americans are 8% to 12% higher
   Please refer to your institution's reference ranges as lab normals may vary.

INDICATIONS
Pregnancy complications secondary to suspected copper deficiency
   Strength of Recommendation: Class III
   Strength of Evidence: Category C
   Results Interpretation:
   Serum copper level abnormal
      Severe maternal copper deficiency can result in embryonic and fetal abnormalities, although the underlying mechanism for this is poorly understood. Maternal hypocupremia has been observed in cases of spontaneous abortion, postmaturity and premature rupture of fetal and placental membranes. Hypocupremia in midgestation pregnant women has been associated with an increased risk of anencephaly.

Suspected idiopathic copper toxicosis
   Strength of Recommendation: Class IIa
   Strength of Evidence: Category C
   Results Interpretation:
   Serum copper level abnormal
      In idiopathic copper toxicosis (ICT), serum copper and ceruloplasmin levels are normal or slightly elevated. These values assist in excluding the diagnosis of Wilson disease, but are not diagnostic for ICT.

Suspected Indian childhood cirrhosis
    Strength of Recommendation: Class IIb
    Strength of Evidence: Category C
    Results Interpretation:
    Serum copper level abnormal
        Plasma copper concentration may be normal or elevated in patients with Indian childhood cirrhosis.

Suspected Menkes syndrome
    Strength of Recommendation: Class IIb
    Strength of Evidence: Category C
    Results Interpretation:
    Serum copper level abnormal
        Serum copper <11 micromoles/L (<70 micrograms/dL)

Suspected Wilson disease
    Strength of Recommendation: Class I
    Strength of Evidence: Category C
    Results Interpretation:
    Serum copper level abnormal
        Patients with Wilson disease (WD) typically present with hypocupremia (40 to 60 mcg/dL), low ceruloplasmin levels and an increase in urinary copper excretion.
        Hypocupremia is secondary to due to low serum ceruloplasmin levels; serum copper levels are decreased in proportion to decreased ceruloplasmin levels.
        Patients with WD and severe liver injury may present with normal serum copper levels, even in the presence of decreased serum ceruloplasmin levels. In WD patients with fulminant hepatic failure, substantially elevated serum copper levels may occur. The combination of normal or elevated serum copper levels and decreased ceruloplasmin levels suggest an increase in nonceruloplasmin-bound copper in the blood.

ABNORMAL RESULTS
- Results increased in:
  - Women
  - Patients with dilated cardiomyopathy
  - Immediately after myocardial infarction
- Diurnal variations occur with highest levels noted in the morning.

COLLECTION/STORAGE INFORMATION
- Specimen Collection and Handling:
  - Collect serum in a metal-free container or plastic syringe using a stainless steel needle.
  - Store sample in a plastic vial or metal-free container

LOINC CODES
- Code: 5631-7 (*Short Name* - Copper SerPl-mCnc)
- Code: 14665-4 (*Short Name* - Copper SerPl-sCnc)

Coproporphyrin I/coproporphyrin III fraction measurement

TEST DEFINITION
Measurement of specific intermediates of heme synthesis used to diagnose and distinguish among the different porphyrias

SYNONYMS
- Coproporphyrin I/coproporphyrin III fraction

REFERENCE RANGE
- Urine (coproporphyrins types I and III): 100-300 mcg/24 hours (150-460 micromol/24 hours)
- Feces for fluorometry/HPLC (coproporphyrins): <200 mcg/24 hours (<306 nmol/24 hours)

- Feces for screening spectrophotometry or fluorometry (total porphyrins): <200 nmol/g dry weight
- Whole blood (total porphyrins): <60 mcg/dL (<600 mcg/L)
  Please refer to your institution's reference ranges as lab normals may vary.

INDICATIONS

Differentiates among certain types of porphyria, including congenital erythropoietic porphyria (CEP), 5-aminolevulinate (ALA) dehydratase deficiency, hereditary coproporphyria, and variegate porphyria in patients with positive initial porphyrin screening
     Strength of Recommendation: Class IIa
     Strength of Evidence: Category C
  Results Interpretation:
  Increased coproporphyrin
- Acute intermittent porphyria (ALA dehydratase deficiency): Elevated coproporphyrin III is found in urine
- Congenital erythropoietic porphyria: Elevated coproporphyrin I is found in urine, stool, and erythrocytes
- Hereditary coproporphyria (porphyria cutanea tarda) and variegate porphyria: Elevated coproporphyrin III is found in urine and stool

COLLECTION/STORAGE INFORMATION

- Collect 24-hour urine in dark container with 5 g $Na_2 CO_3$ and refrigerate
- Collect fresh feces (should not be liquid); may keep at 25° C for up to 36 hours or freeze for up to several months
- Collect whole blood in tube with heparin or EDTA; may keep at 4° C for up to 5 days
- Samples from patients with suspected bullous porphyria may be at higher risk of containing hepatitis C

LOINC CODES

- Code: 33618-0 (*Short Name* - Copro3/Copro1 24H Stl-mRto)

Corticotropin-releasing hormone stimulation test

TEST DEFINITION

    Serum or plasma adrenocorticotropin (ACTH) determination, following the intravenous administration of corticotropin releasing hormone (CRH) in the differential diagnosis of ACTH-dependent Cushing's syndrome

SYNONYMS

- Corticotrophin releasing factor test
- Corticotrophin releasing hormone test
- CRF - Corticotrophin releasing factor test
- CRH - Corticotrophin releasing hormone test

REFERENCE RANGE

- Plasma adrenocorticotropin (ACTH), adults (intravenous): 6-76 pg/mL (1.3-16.7 pmol/L)
- 2 to 4-fold increase in mean baseline concentrations of ACTH or cortisol
- Blood for plasma ACTH from both inferior petrosal sinus (IPS) veins, adults: ratio of IPS to peripheral venous adrenocorticotropin hormone concentration, < 3 to 1
  Please refer to your institution's reference ranges as lab normals may vary.

INDICATIONS

Suspected ACTH-dependent Cushing's syndrome
     Strength of Recommendation: Class IIa
     Strength of Evidence: Category B
  Results Interpretation:
  Increased corticotropin releasing factor level
    Intermediate adrenocorticotropin (ACTH) levels between 5 and 15 pg/mL (1.1 to 3.3 pmol/L) are typically consistent with ACTH-dependent Cushing's syndrome. However, while ACTH levels will identify patients with ACTH-dependent disorders, they cannot reliably distinguish between Cushing's disease (Cushing's syndrome caused by an ACTH-secreting pituitary tumor) and ectopic ACTH secretion.

Plasma ACTH concentrations in the inferior petrosal sinuses (IPS) have been shown to be higher than in peripheral blood for patients with Cushing's disease (ie, pituitary corticotroph adenoma); in fact, ACTH levels in IPS and peripheral blood were found to be similar regardless of the cause of Cushing's syndrome.

False Results
Failure to keep blood samples for adrenocorticotropin (ACTH) measurement refrigerated may result in falsely lowered results.

COLLECTION/STORAGE INFORMATION
- Specimen Collection and Handling:
  - Intravenous: Obtain plasma (heparin) adrenocorticotropin (ACTH) sample 15 minutes and 1 minute before, and 5, 15, 30, 60, and 120 minutes after corticotropin-releasing hormone (CRH) injection.
  - Petrosal sinus technique: Obtain plasma (heparin) ACTH sample from both inferior petrosal sinus veins (IPS) and from a peripheral vein before, and 2, 5, 10, and 15 minutes after CRH injection
  - Collect sample in pre-chilled EDTA tubes and transport in ice bath; specimen should be centrifuged refrigerated, and plasma separated promptly
  - ACTH concentrations reach their peak approximately 10 to 15 minutes after CRH injection.

LOINC CODES
- Code: 12283-8 (*Short Name* - ACTH RH SerPl-aCnc)

Cortisol measurement, free, urine

TEST DEFINITION
Measurement of free cortisol in a 24-hour urine specimen for the evaluation of Cushing's syndrome and other disorders characterized by activation of the hypothalamic-pituitary-adrenal axis

SYNONYMS
- UFC - Urine free cortisol level
- Urine free cortisol level
- Urine free cortisol titer
- Urine free cortisol titre

REFERENCE RANGE
- Radioimmunoassay:
- Adults: 20-70 mcg/24 hours (55-193 nmol/24 hours)
- High-performance liquid chromatography:
- Adults: ≤50 mcg/24 hours (≤138 nmol/24 hours)
  Please refer to your institution's reference ranges as lab normals may vary.

INDICATIONS
Suspected Cushing syndrome
    Strength of Recommendation: Class I
    Strength of Evidence: Category C
Results Interpretation:
Increased cortisol level
A diagnosis of Cushing syndrome is almost always confirmed when 24-hour urinary free cortisol levels are greater than 4 times normal, or more than 300 mcg in 24 hours.

False Results
Pseudo-Cushing conditions (eg, psychological stress) may elevate levels up to 4 times normal.
Creatinine clearance levels of less than 20 cc/minute may affect the reliability of the test.
Frequency of Monitoring
One or two additional 24-hour urinary free cortisol tests should be done to confirm results.

ABNORMAL RESULTS
- Results increased in:
  - Obesity and eating disorders

- Chronic illness
- Chronic alcoholism
- Depression
- Results decreased in:
  - Chronic fatigue syndrome

COLLECTION/STORAGE INFORMATION

- Specimen Collection and Handling:
  - Collect urine over 24 hours in 1 g boric acid as preservative
  - Freeze specimen for long-term storage

LOINC CODES

- Code: 25885-5 (*Short Name* - Cortis Free 24H Ur HPLC-sRate)
- Code: 14043-4 (*Short Name* - Cortis Free 12H Ur-mRate)
- Code: 16667-8 (*Short Name* - Cortis Free 48H Ur-mRate)
- Code: 2147-7 (*Short Name* - Cortis Free 24H Ur-mRate)
- Code: 16668-6 (*Short Name* - Cortis Free 72H Ur-mRate)
- Code: 25882-2 (*Short Name* - Cortis Free 24H Ur RIA-sCnc)
- Code: 25883-0 (*Short Name* - Cortis Free 24H Ur HPLC-sCnc)
- Code: 25884-8 (*Short Name* - Cortis Free 24H Ur RIA-sRate)
- Code: 11040-3 (*Short Name* - Cortis Free Ur-mCnc)

Corynebacterium diphtheriae throat culture

TEST DEFINITION

Isolation of *Corynebacterium diphtheriae* in cultures from nasopharyngeal and throat specimens

REFERENCE RANGE

- No growth
  Please refer to your institution's reference ranges as lab normals may vary.

INDICATIONS

Suspected pharyngeal diphtheria
    Strength of Recommendation: Class I
    Strength of Evidence: Category C
    Results Interpretation:
    Throat swab culture positive
        A positive culture must be tested further before a definite diagnosis of diptheria is made. Minimum confirmatory laboratory studies include rapid screening tests for detection of toxigenic strains of corynebacteria: catalase positive, urea negative, nitrate positive (except for the biotype *belfanti*), pyrazinamidase negative, and cystinase positive. All biotypes will ferment glucose and maltose; in addition the biotype *gravis* will ferment starch. Testing for toxin is confirmatory, but isolates may require evaluation at a referral lab.

    False Results
        Direct microscopy of a smear is unreliable in the diagnosis of diphtheria due to the possibility of both false positive and false negative results.

CLINICAL NOTES

Since *Corynebacterium diphtheriae* is difficult to isolate on blood agar, a tellurite-containing medium is recommended.
Rapid inoculation of special culture media is necessary.

COLLECTION/STORAGE INFORMATION

- Specimen Collection and Handling:
  - Notify lab personnel before specimen collection so that the proper medium can be prepared.
  - Using a flexible alginate swab, obtain multiple specimens of throat or nasopharynx, including the membrane, if present.
  - Transport specimen to lab immediately.

- If the sample must be sent to a reference laboratory, send the specimen dry in a packet or in a tube containing silica gel or other desiccant..

Cotinine measurement

TEST DEFINITION
Measurement of cotinine (nicotine metabolite) in blood or plasma for the evaluation of nicotine exposure and use

REFERENCE RANGE
- Smokers: 16 ng/mL - 145 ng/mL
- Non-smokers: 1 ng/mL - 8 ng/mL
  Please refer to your institution's reference ranges as lab normals may vary.

INDICATIONS
Suspected nicotine use or exposure
> **Strength of Recommendation:** Class IIa
> **Strength of Evidence:** Category B
> **Results Interpretation:**
> **Increased level (laboratory finding)**
Cotinine is considered a useful marker for evaluating nicotine use and exposure. Higher levels of cotinine have been associated with higher tobacco use and greater exposure.

ABNORMAL RESULTS
Black smokers have higher serum cotinine levels than Mexican-American or white smokers.

LOINC CODES
- Code: 10364-8 (*Short Name* - Cotinine Har-mCnt)
- Code: 10365-5 (*Short Name* - Cotinine SerPl-mCnc)
- Code: 9372-4 (*Short Name* - Cotinine XXX-mCnc)

Coxsackievirus antibody level

TEST DEFINITION
Serologic assay for the diagnosis of coxsackie virus infection

REFERENCE RANGE
- Negative
  Please refer to your institution's reference ranges as lab normals may vary.

INDICATIONS
Suspected coxsackie virus infection
> **Strength of Recommendation:** Class IIb
> **Strength of Evidence:** Category C
> **Results Interpretation:**
> **Serology positive**
A 4-fold or greater rise in antibody titers in serum or cerebrospinal fluid (CSF) or identification of IgM coxsackievirus antibody in the serum suggests a recent coxsackievirus infection; however, IgM levels may be high in the general population, especially during epidemic seasons. Since group B coxsackie virus (CVB) infection is common and is often asymptomatic, positive serological tests for CVB indicate exposure to the virus but CVB may not be the actual cause of the presenting symptoms. However, identification of IgM coxsackievirus antibody in the CSF is more likely to indicate that CVB is the cause of the CNS symptoms.
IgG serologic testing has a limited role in the diagnosis of CVB but is helpful as a confirmatory test in community-wide outbreaks, when there is a rise in IgG from the acute to convalescent sera.

IgM antibodies to CVB may persist in patients with chronic relapsing pericarditis from a year and a half up to 10 years in patients with dilated cardiomyopathy.
Timing of Monitoring
Acute and convalescent serum samples should be tested (2 to 4 weeks later).

COLLECTION/STORAGE INFORMATION
- Specimen Collection and Handling:
  - Obtain a serum sample at the onset of the disease
  - Obtain a serum sample after 2 to 4 weeks to measure the convalescent titer
  - Freeze the sample if testing is delayed

Creatine kinase MB isoenzyme/total creatine kinase ratio measurement

TEST DEFINITION
The calculated measurement of CK-MB to total creatine kinase (CK-MB index) in serum to evaluate suspected acute myocardial infarction

SYNONYMS
- CK - Creatine kinase MB isoenzyme/total creatine kinase ratio
- CKMB - Creatine kinase MB isoenzyme/total creatine kinase ratio
- Creatine kinase MB isoenzyme/total creatine kinase ratio

REFERENCE RANGE
CK-MB (mass) index is a calculated number = [CK-MB (ng/mL) ÷ total CK (Units/L)] x 100. Normal range is method and lab specific.
Please refer to your institution's reference ranges as lab normals may vary.

INDICATIONS
Suspected acute myocardial infarction
    Strength of Recommendation: Class IIa
    Strength of Evidence: Category B
    Results Interpretation:
    Raised cardiac enzyme or marker
    The CK-MB index in the presence of an elevated CK may assist in differentiating skeletal muscle injury from myocardial injury. Any process causing skeletal muscle injury will release CK isozymes, including CK-MB.
    CK-MB index mass assay values greater than 2.5% are generally associated with a myocardial source of CK-MB.

COMMON PANELS
- Cardiac injury panel

COLLECTION/STORAGE INFORMATION
- Store at 4°C if assayed within 24 hours; otherwise store at -20°C.

LOINC CODES
- Code: 12187-1 (*Short Name* - CK MB % SerPl Elph)
- Code: 12189-7 (*Short Name* - CK MB % SerPl Calc)
- Code: 20569-0 (*Short Name* - CK MB % SerPl)
- Code: 12188-9 (*Short Name* - CK MB % SerPl EIA)

Creatine kinase MB measurement

TEST DEFINITION
Measurement of CK-MB isoenzyme in serum for evaluation of acute coronary syndrome.

REFERENCE RANGE
• CK-MB isoenzyme: 0-7 ng/mL (0-7 mcg/L)
Please refer to your institution's reference ranges as lab normals may vary.

INDICATIONS
Suspected acute coronary syndrome
    Strength of Recommendation: Class IIb
    Strength of Evidence: Category B
Results Interpretation:
Increased creatine kinase MB level
    Elevated biomarkers should be obtained from at least 2 successive blood samples in order to diagnose myocardial infarction (MI). An elevated CK-MB is defined as a value that exceeds the 99th percentile of CK-MB values in a reference control group.
    When evaluating suspected ongoing or reinfarction and the initial troponin level is high, sequential samples of a more rapidly appearing biomarker such as CK-MB or myoglobin may be employed to clarify the timing of the MI.
    Increased CK-MB usually appears at about 6 hours and peaks at 24 hours post-infarction. Persistent elevation beyond 96 hours may suggest ongoing myocardial necrosis. The reappearance of elevated CK-MB levels suggests extension of infarction.
• Diagnosing suspected recurrent MI after ST-segment elevation MI (STEMI) using CK-MB:
  • If initial CK-MB elevation was greater than upper limit of normal (ULN):
    • Within 18 hours of STEMI: use recurrent ST-segment elevation on ECG and at least one supportive finding: chest pain or hemodynamic compromise
    • More than 18 hours after STEMI: Increase in CK-MB by at least 50%
  • If initial CK-MB was less than ULN:
    • Increase in CK-MB
  • Within 24 hours of percutaneous coronary intervention (PCI), use either:
    • CK-MB more than 3 times ULN
    • New Q waves
  • Within 24 hours of CABG, use either:
    • CK-MB more than 10 times ULN
    • CK-MB 5 times ULN and new Q waves

False Results
    False-positive elevations are more commonly seen with total CK levels rather than CK-MB levels. Sources of CK-MB elevation include technical causes such as spillover of CK-MM and isoenzyme variants; other types of myocardial injury, including pericarditis or intracardiac injections; peripheral sources of CK-MB, including rhabdomyolysis and prostate surgery; systemic disease with cardiac involvement such as muscular dystrophy or hyperthermia; thermal or electrical burns; alcoholism, and many other causes.
Timing of Monitoring
    CK-MB should be obtained upon presentation in all patients with possible acute coronary syndrome and repeated 6 to 12 hours after symptom onset if required for diagnosis. Typically, CK-MB, as well as other cardiac biomarkers, including cardiac troponins, are measured on presentation and 2 additional times, such as every 8 hours.

Suspected myocardial contusion
    Strength of Recommendation: Class IIb
    Strength of Evidence: Category B
Results Interpretation:
Increased creatine kinase MB level
    With significant contusion, CK-MB elevation may be present on admission and may clear within 24 hours.
    Elevated values have been used as a means of diagnosis; however, their value as a screening test is highly questionable.
    A CK-MB ratio greater than 5% is consistent with myocardial injury.

Normal creatine kinase MB level

A blow to the chest may be strong enough to produce cardiac arrhythmias without actual myocardial cell necrosis (cardiac concussion or commotio cordis). Such patients will have ECG abnormalities with normal CK-MB values.

COMMON PANELS

- Cardiac injury panel

COLLECTION/STORAGE INFORMATION

- Store at 4°C if assayed within 24 hours; otherwise store at -20°C.

Creatinine measurement, 24 hour urine

TEST DEFINITION

Measurement of urine creatinine along with serum creatinine to determine glomerular filtration rate (GFR)

REFERENCE RANGE

- Males (20 to 29 years): 94-140 mL/min/1.73 m^2 (0.91-1.35 mL/s/m^2)
- Females (20 to 29 years): 72-110 mL/min/1.73 m^2 (0.69-1.06 mL/s/m^2)
- Males (30 to 39 years): 59-137 mL/min/1.73 m^2 (0.57-1.32 mL/s/m^2)
- Females (30 to 39 years): 71-121 mL/min/1.73 m^2 (0.68-1.17 mL/s/m^2)
- Note: For each decade after the fourth decade in both sexes, values decrease approximately 6.5 mL/min based on 1.73 m^2 body surface (0.06 mL/s per m^2)
- Infant (0 to 1 year): 72 mL/min/1.73 m^2 (0.69 mL/s/m^2)
- Infant (1 year): 45 mL/min/1.73 m^2 (0.43 mL/s/m^2)
- Infant (2 years): 55 mL/min/1.73 m^2 (0.53 mL/s/m^2)
- Children (3 years): 60 mL/min/1.73 m^2 (0.58 mL/s/m^2)
- Children (4 years): 71 mL/min/1.73 m^2 (0.68 mL/s/m^2)
- Children (5 years): 73 mL/min/1.73 m^2 (0.70 mL/s/m^2)
- Children (6 years): 64 mL/min/1.73 m^2 (0.62 mL/s/m^2)
- Children (7 years): 67 mL/min/1.73 m^2 (0.65 mL/s/m^2)
- Children (8 years): 72 mL/min/1.73 m^2 (0.69 mL/s/m^2)
- Children (9 years): 83 mL/min/1.73 m^2 (0.80 mL/s/m^2)
- Children (10 years): 89 mL/min/1.73 m^2 (0.86 mL/s/m^2)
- Children (11 years): 92 mL/min/1.73 m^2 (0.89 mL/s/m^2)
- Children (12 years): 109 mL/min/1.73 m^2 (1.05 mL/s/m^2)
- Children (13 to 14 years): 86 mL/min/1.73 m^2 (0.83 mL/s/m^2)

Please refer to your institution's reference ranges as lab normals may vary.

INDICATIONS

Suspected gout

Results Interpretation:

Increased level (laboratory finding)

Increased creatinine clearance may indicate an increased glomerular filtration rate, and may be seen with a high-protein diet and hypercatabolic states.

Decreased level (laboratory finding)

Decreased creatinine clearance is seen with decreased renal blood flow and decreased glomerular filtration rate; it may be associated with various renal diseases and other systemic conditions.

Suspected impaired renal function

Strength of Recommendation: Class IIa

Strength of Evidence: Category B

Results Interpretation:

Decreased level (laboratory finding)

The National Kidney Foundation has established guidelines to describe the stages of chronic renal failure.

- Stages of Chronic Kidney Disease and related glomerular filtration rates (GFR) expressed in mL/min/1.73 m^2:
  - Stage 1: Kidney damage evident with a normal or increased GFR - >90

- Stage 2: Kidney damage with a mild decrease in GFR - 60 to 89
- Stage 3: Moderate decrease - GFR 30 to 59
- Stage 4: Severe decrease - GFR 15 to 29
- Stage 5: Renal failure - GFR <15 or dialysis

The guidelines may have limited utility in patients of extreme age (ie, greater than 80 years), those experiencing dehydration, muscle wasting, vegetarians, or in cases of severe malnutrition or obesity. Creatinine clearance (CrCl) estimates GFR fairly closely except at high levels of creatinine; at high levels the GFR is overestimated by CrCl because of creatinine secretion by renal tubules. A single dose of cimetidine (1200 mg) prevents excretion and makes CrCl a good measure of GFR.

Adults: Moderate renal impairment is described as a glomerular filtration rate (GFR) of less than 60 mL/min/1.73 m^2.

A persistently decreased GFR (<60 mL/min/1.73 m^2) along with proteinuria are important criteria used in chronic kidney disease to predict end stage renal disease.

Suspected renal disease in patients with diabetes mellitus
    Strength of Recommendation: Class IIa
    Strength of Evidence: Category B
Results Interpretation:
Laboratory test finding

Creatinine clearance can detect a decline in GFR. Progressively decreasing GFR signifies the progression of kidney disease in diabetics.

In the early stages of Type 1 diabetes, the glomerular filtration rate can be increased (greater than 130 mL/min/1.73 m^2) and is followed by persistent microalbuminuria, which has been associated with a 400% to 500% increase in the risk of progression to overt proteinuria and eventual end stage renal disease (ESRD).

Patients with type II DM may present with evidence of a decreased GFR at the time of diagnosis. In the NHANES III study, 13% of adults with type 2 diabetes had a decreased GFR (less than 60 mL/min/1.73 m^2) with noromoalbuminuria.

In the NHANES III study, 20% of diabetics with severe chronic kidney disease (GFR of less than 30 mL/min/1.73 m^2) had no albuminuria.

Over a period of years, 25% to 45% of Type 1 diabetics will develop macroalbuminuria (clinical proteinuria) leading to a decline in GFR and potentially end stage renal disease.

Based on the National Kidney Foundation staging system to evaluate glomerular filtration rate in the assessment of chronic kidney disease, diabetic patients (type 1 or 2) that have a normal to moderately decreased GFR (between 30 to 59 mL/min/1.73 m^2 ; stages 1 through 3), should be routinely monitored and treated to slow the progression of disease. Renal replacement therapy is likely when the GFR is between 15 to 29 (stage 4). A GFR of less than 15 or requirement for dialysis indicates a need for renal replacement therapy once uremia is present (stage 5).

ABNORMAL RESULTS

- Results decreased in:
  - Advanced age (ie, greater than 80 years)
    - GFR can decrease at a rate of 13 mL/decade after ages 45 to 50 years
  - Acute and chronic renal failure
  - Inadequate urine flow rate (ie, due to dehydration or incomplete voiding).
  - Exercise
  - Muscle wasting
- Results increased in:
  - Creatinine clearance can overestimate GFR by 10% to 20% at all levels of renal function
  - Pregnancy (rises rapidly in early pregnancy and remains elevated until term; returns to normal quickly following delivery)
- Other:
  - Gender (males have higher GFR, as compared to females)
  - Diet can influence renal function
  - Diurnal variation (ie, GFR typically lower at night and highest in late morning)

CLINICAL NOTES

A 24-hour urine collection is more physiologically complete than a spot collection, because it accounts for the normal variations that can influence renal function. However, studies have compared short- (eg, 8 hour collections) and longer-duration urine creatinine clearance tests, and found similar results.

COLLECTION/STORAGE INFORMATION
- Specimen Collection and Handling:
    - Collect urine for 24 hours; store sample on ice or refrigerate during collection period
    - Refrigerate sample until laboratory analysis
    - Record patient's height and weight with urine sample
    - Collect serum/plasma at midpoint of urine collection period

LOINC CODES
- Code: 14684-5 (*Short Name* - Creat 24H Ur-sRate)
- Code: 2162-6 (*Short Name* - Creat 24H Ur-mRate)
- Code: 20624-3 (*Short Name* - Creat 24H Ur-mCnc)
- Code: 25886-3 (*Short Name* - Creat 24H Ur-sCnc)

Creatinine measurement, serum

TEST DEFINITION
Measurement of creatinine in serum or plasma to assess renal function

SYNONYMS
- Serum creatinine

REFERENCE RANGE
- Adults: <1.5 mg/dL (<133 mcmol/L)
- Adult women (18-60 years): 0.6-1.1 mg/dL (53-97 mcmol/L)
- Adult men (18-60 years): 0.9-1.3 mg/dL (80-115 mcmol/L)
- Men aged 60 to 90 years: 0.8-1.3 mg/dL (71-115 mcmol/L)
- Women aged 60 to 90 years: 0.6-1.2 mg/dL (53-106 mcmol/L)
- Men aged >90 years: 1-1.7 mg/dL (88-150 mcmol/L)
- Women aged >90 years: 0.6-1.3 mg/dL (53-115 mcmol/L)
- Neonates:
- Cord blood: 0.6-1.2 mg/dL (53-106 mcmol/L)
- Newborn aged 1-4 days: 0.3-1 mg/dL (27-88 mcmol/L)
- Infants: 0.2-0.4 mg/dL (18-35 mcmol/L)
- Children: 0.3-0.7 mg/dL (27-62 mcmol/L)
- Adolescents: 0.5-1 mg/dL (44-88 mcmol/L)
    Please refer to your institution's reference ranges as lab normals may vary.

INDICATIONS
Acute adrenal insufficiency
    Strength of Recommendation: Class IIa
    Strength of Evidence: Category C
Results Interpretation:
Serum creatinine raised
    The serum creatinine level is usually elevated in acute adrenal insufficiency. Aldosterone deficiency causes excretion of sodium in excess of intake, which leads to dehydration and azotemia.

Acute coronary syndrome
    Strength of Recommendation: Class IIa
    Strength of Evidence: Category B
Results Interpretation:
Serum creatinine raised
    An elevated serum creatinine on presentation with acute myocardial infarction is associated with a markedly increased 1-year mortality, especially if associated with congestive heart failure.

Cardiovascular system disease
    Strength of Recommendation: Class I
    Strength of Evidence: Category C

Results Interpretation:
Serum creatinine raised
- In a prospective population-based study of persons older than 65 years and followed for a median of 7.3 years, 11.2% (648/5,808) had an elevated baseline serum creatinine (SCr) level (greater than or equal to 1.5 mg/dL in men and 1.3 mg/dL in women). Persons with an elevated SCr level had a higher:
  - Overall mortality: 76.7 vs 29.5/1,000 years
  - Cardiovascular (CV) mortality: 35.8 vs 13/1,000 years
  - CV disease risk: 54 vs 31.8/1,000 years
  - Stroke risk: 21.1 vs 11.9/1,000 years
  - Congestive heart failure risk: 38.7 vs 17/1,000 years
  - Symptomatic peripheral vascular disease risk: 10.6 vs 3.5/1,000 years
- An elevated SCr was a significant risk factor of overall mortality, cardiovascular (CV) mortality, total CV disease, claudication, and congestive heart failure, even after CV risk factors were considered. The increased risk was apparent early in renal disease, and increasing SCr levels were associated with increased risk.

Heart failure
Strength of Recommendation: Class I
Strength of Evidence: Category B
Results Interpretation:
Serum creatinine raised
Increased serum creatinine levels have major implications for heart failure management.
Most patients with severe heart failure will have an increased blood urea nitrogen (BUN)-to-creatinine ratio greater than 20:1 (normal is 10:1).
The serum creatinine level should be obtained at baseline. If oliguria develops, serial measurements are indicated.

Hemorrhagic shock
Results Interpretation:
Serum creatinine raised
Hemorrhagic shock-related prolonged hypotension causes acute tubular necrosis (ATN). Increasing serum creatinine levels imply ATN.
Blood urea nitrogen (BUN) and creatinine levels rise over the first few post-shock days typically in a fixed ratio of approximately 10:1.

Hypothyroidism
Strength of Recommendation: Class IIa
Strength of Evidence: Category B
Results Interpretation:
Serum creatinine raised
Serum creatinine may be elevated in hypothyroidism, and return to normal with thyroid hormone replacement.

Initial evaluation and monitoring of diabetic ketoacidosis
Strength of Recommendation: Class I
Strength of Evidence: Category C
Results Interpretation:
Serum creatinine raised
Serum creatinine level may be increased in diabetic ketoacidosis due to renal failure.

False Results
A falsely elevated creatinine level may result when measured by the colormetric method due to interference with acetoacetate.
Frequency of Monitoring
In suspected DKA, serum creatinine levels should be checked every 2 to 4 hours until the patient is stable.

Initial evaluation and monitoring of hyperosmolar hyperglycemic state
Strength of Recommendation: Class I
Strength of Evidence: Category C

Results Interpretation:
Serum creatinine raised

Serum creatinine is elevated in hyperosmolar hyperglycemic state (HHS). Patients may initially be azotemic secondary to both prerenal and renal causes. The blood urea nitrogen (BUN) to creatinine ratio may be greater than 30:1 on presentation,.

False Results

Creatinine measured by a colorimetric method may be falsely elevated because of acetoacetate interference.

Frequency of Monitoring

Monitor serum creatinine every 2 to 4 hours in patients with hyperosmolar hyperglycemic state.

Metabolic acidosis
Results Interpretation:
Serum creatinine raised

Patients with metabolic acidosis secondary to chronic renal failure have elevated serum creatinine levels. Anion gap metabolic acidosis develops when the glomerular filtration rate is less than 20 mL/minute (serum creatinine 4 to 5 mg/dL).

False Results

Falsely elevated serum creatinine concentrations may be found in ketoacidosis because acetoacetate interferes with the chemical reaction (Jaffe reaction) used for measurement.

Submersion
Results Interpretation:
Serum creatinine raised

Serial measurements of serum creatinine are recommended in all submersion victims to monitor for the development of acute renal impairment. This is particularly important when there is an increase in the initial creatinine level, marked metabolic acidosis on admission ABG analysis, an initially abnormal urinalysis, or significant lymphocytosis. These factors have been found to have predictive value for acute renal failure.

Suspected acute renal failure
Strength of Recommendation: Class I
Strength of Evidence: Category C
Results Interpretation:
Serum creatinine raised

In well-managed patients with intrinsic causes of acute renal failure, especially acute tubular necrosis without major complication, the serum creatinine level rises at a rate of 0.5 to 1 mg/dL/day. Serum creatinine measurement is particularly useful in renal failure because it is minimally affected by protein intake, hydration, and protein metabolism.

Acute renal failure is characterized by a rapid drop in GFR and a progressive increase in BUN and creatinine levels.

Suspected and known ovarian hyperstimulation syndrome
Results Interpretation:
Serum creatinine raised

A creatinine level greater than 1.2 mg/dL indicates possible grade 5 OHSS and is an indication for hospital admission.

Suspected and known preeclampsia
Results Interpretation:
Serum creatinine level - finding

The finding of an elevated serum creatinine level (greater than 1.2 mg/dL) increases the certainty of a preeclampsia diagnosis, especially when it is associated with oliguria.

Suspected chronic renal failure
Strength of Recommendation: Class I
Strength of Evidence: Category A

Results Interpretation:
Serum creatinine raised

The evaluation of all patients diagnosed with, or at increased risk of, chronic renal disease should include measurement of serum creatinine (SCr) to estimate GFR from prediction equations that also consider some or all of the following: age, sex, race, and body size.

SCr alone should not be used to assess kidney function. Minor elevations of SCr may be consistent with substantial reduction in GFR. Because of the wide range of SCr in normal persons, GFR must decline to approximately half the normal level before the SCr rises above the upper limit of normal.

Estimates of GFR are not more accurate using timed (eg, 24-hour) urine collections than SCr.

Suspected disseminated intravascular coagulation
> **Strength of Recommendation:** Class IIa
> **Strength of Evidence:** Category B

Results Interpretation:
Serum creatinine raised

Increased serum creatinine levels suggest end-stage organ damage or renal failure in patients with disseminated intravascular coagulation (DIC).

A low grade disseminated intravascular coagulation disorder may be associated with a renovascular disorder.

Suspected ehrlichiosis
Results Interpretation:
High

A serum creatinine level greater than 1.2 mg/dl may be indicative of decreased renal function.

Suspected post-streptococcal glomerulonephritis
> **Strength of Recommendation:** Class I
> **Strength of Evidence:** Category C

Results Interpretation:
Increased level (laboratory finding)

Serum creatinine may be increased in patients with post-streptococcal glomerulonephritis (PSGN). The creatinine level is a more reliable indicator of renal function than BUN content, and can be abnormal in more than 50% of patients with PSGN.

Suspected renal manifestations of diabetes mellitus
Results Interpretation:
Serum creatinine raised

Serum creatinine levels may not be elevated until more than 50% of kidney function is lost (ie, a greater than 50% reduction in GFR).

The serum creatinine level is used in the Cockcroft and Gault equation to calculate the estimated GFR and to stage diabetic nephropathy.

The serum creatinine alone should not be used as a measure of kidney function.

Suspected rhabdomyolysis
> **Strength of Recommendation:** Class I
> **Strength of Evidence:** Category B

Results Interpretation:
Serum creatinine raised

Elevated serum creatinine levels may be caused both by release of muscle creatine, which is subsequently converted to creatinine, and by myoglobinuria-induced renal failure.

In myoglobinuria with renal failure, the serum creatinine rises greater than 2.5 mg/dL in 24 hours due to the increased creatinine load, whereas in renal failure without myoglobinuria, serum creatinine levels rise an average of 2 mg/dL in 24 hours.

The creatinine/blood urea nitrogen (BUN) ratio is greater than 1:10, whereas in pure renal causes of renal failure the ratio is typically less than 1:10.

Suspected sepsis
> **Strength of Recommendation:** Class I
> **Strength of Evidence:** Category C

Results Interpretation:
Serum creatinine raised

A creatinine increase greater than 0.5 mg/dL may be associated with renal dysfunction in severe sepsis.

Timing of Monitoring

The Infectious Disease Society of America (IDSA) recommends a serum creatinine at baseline and at least every three days during the course of intensive antibiotic therapy. Renal toxic drugs such as Amphotericin B, require more frequent monitoring.

Thromboembolic stroke
Strength of Recommendation: Class IIb
Strength of Evidence: Category B
Results Interpretation:
Serum creatinine raised

An elevated serum creatinine, in a patient presenting with stroke, may predict mortality.

COMMON PANELS

- Basic metabolic panel
- Comprehensive metabolic panel
- Parathyroid panel
- Prenatal screening panel
- Transplant panel

ABNORMAL RESULTS

- Results increased in:
  - Meat meals
- Results decreased in:
  - Decreased muscle mass (elderly, debilitation)
  - Pregnancy

COLLECTION/STORAGE INFORMATION

- Collect specimen in marble top tube.
- Sample is stable at 4°C for 24 hours; should be frozen for longer periods.

LOINC CODES

- Code: 2160-0 (*Short Name* - Creat SerPl-mCnc)
- Code: 11041-1 (*Short Name* - Creat p dialysis SerPl-mCnc)
- Code: 14682-9 (*Short Name* - Creat SerPl-sCnc)
- Code: 11042-9 (*Short Name* - Creat pre dial SerPl-mCnc)

Cryptococcus species antigen assay

TEST DEFINITION

Detection of *Cryptococcus neoformans* antigen in serum or cerebrospinal fluid for the evaluation and management of cryptococcal meningitis

REFERENCE RANGE

- Adult and Children: Negative
  Please refer to your institution's reference ranges as lab normals may vary.

INDICATIONS

Suspected cryptococcal meningitis
Strength of Recommendation: Class IIa
Strength of Evidence: Category C
Results Interpretation:
Serology positive

Latex agglutination (LA) tests having cryptococcal titers greater than 1:8 in undiluted cerebrospinal fluid (CSF) are indicative of *Cryptococcus neoformans* meningitic disease, while a CSF titer greater than 1:4 is suggestive of the disease.

A negative LA test result does not rule out cryptococcosis, particularly when only one serum sample is tested.

Positive latex agglutination tests should be confirmed with serum or CSF cultured on chocolate agar or chocolate agar with tryptic soy agar with 5% sheep blood, and grown at 30°C.

Heat inactivation or pretreatment of serum samples with pronase significantly increases the sensitivity of the tests. The use of pronase also reduces the occurrence of prozoning: negative tests at low dilution becoming positive at higher dilution. Pretreatment of serum by 2-beta-mercaptoethanol (0.01 M 2-ME) also reduces false-positive reactivity.

COLLECTION/STORAGE INFORMATION
- Collect serum in a marbled-top tube and CSF in a plastic or glass tube.

LOINC CODES
- Code: 9817-8 (*Short Name* - Cryptoc Ag Titr CSF EIA)
- Code: 16692-6 (*Short Name* - Cryptoc Ag Fld Ql)
- Code: 11473-6 (*Short Name* - Cryptoc Ag Titr XXX)
- Code: 9819-4 (*Short Name* - Cryptoc Ag Titr CSF LA)
- Code: 29903-2 (*Short Name* - Cryptoc Ag Ser Ql EIA)
- Code: 9818-6 (*Short Name* - Cryptoc Ag Titr Ser EIA)
- Code: 16693-4 (*Short Name* - Cryptoc Ag Ur Ql)
- Code: 31790-9 (*Short Name* - Cryptoc Ag Ser Ql)
- Code: 31792-5 (*Short Name* - Cryptoc Ag XXX-aCnc)
- Code: 31791-7 (*Short Name* - Cryptoc Ag Ser-aCnc)
- Code: 9820-2 (*Short Name* - Cryptoc Ag Titr Ser LA)
- Code: 29533-7 (*Short Name* - Cryptoc Ag XXX Ql)

Culture of intravascular catheter

TEST DEFINITION
Detection and identification of bacterial colonization and assessment of possible catheter-related bloodstream infection

REFERENCE RANGE
- Adults and Children: Negative or growth of less than 15 colony-forming units (CFU)
  Please refer to your institution's reference ranges as lab normals may vary.

INDICATIONS
Suspected or known febrile neutropenia in cancer patients
> **Strength of Recommendation:** Class I
> **Strength of Evidence:** Category C
Results Interpretation:
Positive microbiology findings
Early positivity of blood culture results drawn from a central catheter is predictive of a catheter related infection. *Staphylococcus aureus,* and coagulase-negative staphylococci are common causes of catheter related infections that often respond to pathogen-specific antimicrobial therapy without catheter removal. Immediate catheter removal is advised when bloodstream infections are recurrent or caused by fungi, nontuberculosis mycobacteria, *Pseudomonas Aeruginosa, Stenotrophomonas maltophilia,* and vancomycin-resistant enterococci.
Timing of Monitoring
The Infectious Disease Society (IDSA), Guidelines for the Management of Intravascular Catheter-Related Infections, recommends that immediate blood samples be obtained from each central catheter lumen, as well as from a peripheral vein when a catheter related infection is suspected.

Suspected infection of intravenous catheter with potential for bacteremia
> **Strength of Recommendation:** Class IIa
> **Strength of Evidence:** Category A
Results Interpretation:
Positive microbiology findings
For culture methods requiring removal of the line (non-sparing) a semiquantitative method with a growth of 15 or more colony-forming units (CFU) in the absence of clinical signs of infection at the catheter site is

indicative of catheter colonization. Growth of 15 or more CFU along with signs of local inflammation is indicative of local catheter-related infection. Growth of more than 1000 CFU from a line tip segment is associated with bacteremia. Routine culture of IVDs is not indicated, but should be done when catheter-related bloodstream infection is clinically suspected.

CLINICAL NOTES

Gram stain and culture of a potentially infected line can provide a more rapid diagnosis than blood culture.

Catheter-related infection in patients with long-term venous access (ie, Broviac, Hickman, etc) sometimes can be treated successfully without removal of the line.

Other methods to assess catheter-related systemic infections include potential catheter-sparing culture methods by obtaining quantitative blood cultures from a peripheral site and the central line with comparison of the colony counts. A five- to ten-fold or greater colony count of the same organism from the central-line culture is predictive of a catheter-related bloodstream infection.

COLLECTION/STORAGE INFORMATION

- Specimen Collection and Handling:
  - Nonsparing Method: Remove catheter by sterile forceps; roll tip back and forth onto blood agar plate. Incubate overnight at 37°C.
  - Intraluminal Method: Insert a sterile swab into the distal lumen of the catheter administration set; withdraw and roll swab on a blood agar plate for culture.

LOINC CODES

- Code: 17942-4 (*Short Name* - Ln IV Cult org #2)
- Code: 17945-7 (*Short Name* - Ln IV Cult org #5)
- Code: 616-3 (*Short Name* - Ln IV Cult)
- Code: 17944-0 (*Short Name* - Ln IV Cult org #4)
- Code: 17943-2 (*Short Name* - Ln IV Cult org #3)
- Code: 17946-5 (*Short Name* - Ln IV Cult org #6)

Cyanide measurement, blood

TEST DEFINITION

Measurement of cyanide level in blood or serum following intentional or inadvertent exposure

REFERENCE RANGE

- Smokers:
- Serum: 0.006 mg/L (0.23 micromol/L)
- Blood (fluoride/oxalate): 0.041 mg/L (1.57 micromol/L)
- Nonsmokers:
- Serum: 0.004 mg/L (0.15 micromol/L)
- Blood (fluoride/oxalate): 0.016 mg/L (0.61 micromol/L)
- Nitroprusside therapy:
- Serum: 0.01-0.06 mg/L (0.38-2.3 micromol/L)
- Blood (fluoride/oxalate): 0.05-0.5 mg/L (1.92-19.2 micromol/L)
  Please refer to your institution's reference ranges as lab normals may vary.

INDICATIONS

Suspected cyanide toxicity in smoke inhalation victims
      Strength of Recommendation: Class IIb
      Strength of Evidence: Category B
      Results Interpretation:
      Cyanide poisoning
      Cyanide levels of 1 mcg/mL (38.5 micromol/L) or greater are typically associated with significant symptoms. The length of exposure to carbon monoxide does not always correlate with a specific cyanide level.

Suspected cyanide exposure or poisoning
    Strength of Recommendation: Class IIb
    Strength of Evidence: Category C
Results Interpretation:
Cyanide poisoning
    Elevated blood cyanide levels may confirm the diagnosis of cyanide poisoning but are not clinically useful unless results are rapidly available. Treatment should be initiated based on clinical presentation and index of suspicion.
- Whole blood cyanide levels and associated symptoms:
  - 0.5-1 mcg/mL (20-38 micromol/L): Tachycardia, flushing
  - 1-2.5 mcg/mL (48-95 micromol/L): Depressed level of consciousness
  - 2.5-3 mcg/mL (95-114 micromol/L): Coma, respiratory depression
  - >3 mcg/mL (>114 micromol/L): Death

COLLECTION/STORAGE INFORMATION
- Prolonged time from specimen collection to analysis will result in falsely low readings.
- Store sample at 4°C to 8°C.

LOINC CODES
- Code: 5634-1 (*Short Name* - Cyanide Bld-mCnc)

Cyclosporine measurement

TEST DEFINITION
    The measurement of cyclosporine for therapeutic monitoring of transplant patients or autoimmune disease treatment

REFERENCE RANGE
- Therapeutic levels by transplant type:
- Renal: 100-200 nanograms/mL (83-166 nanomoles/L)
- Cardiac: 150-250 nanograms/mL (125-208 nanomoles/L)
- Hepatic: 100-400 nanograms/mL (83-333 nanomoles/L)
- Bone marrow: 100-300 nanograms/mL (83-250 nanomoles/L)
  Please refer to your institution's reference ranges as lab normals may vary.

INDICATIONS
Therapeutic monitoring of cyclosporine treatment
    Strength of Recommendation: Class I
    Strength of Evidence: Category A
Results Interpretation:
Therapeutic drug level - finding
    Therapeutic levels range from 100 to 400 nanograms/mL (83 to 166 nanomoles/L) and are affected by transplantation type and time of dosing.
    Toxicity may occur at levels greater than 400 nanograms/mL (333 nanomoles/L).
Timing of Monitoring
    Trough blood levels usually have been measured for therapeutic monitoring. Various time point sampling protocols are being investigated. Results also are affected by time after transplant.

CLINICAL NOTES
    Cyclosporine has a narrow therapeutic index. Monitoring blood levels on a regular basis is necessary to maintain a therapeutic dose while avoiding toxicity.

COLLECTION/STORAGE INFORMATION
- Specimen Collection and Handling:
  - Collect whole blood in tubes coated with EDTA
  - Store at 4° C if not analyzed immediately

LOINC Codes
- Code: 17807-9 (*Short Name* - Cyclosporin Fld-mCnc)

Cyst fluid cytology

Test Definition
Evaluation of cystic fluid to diagnose benign or malignant lesions or masses

Reference Range
- Adults and Children: Negative
  Please refer to your institution's reference ranges as lab normals may vary.

Indications
Cystic brain tumor
  Strength of Recommendation: Class IIb
  Strength of Evidence: Category C
  Results Interpretation:
  Positive cytology findings
  Cytologic evaluation of brain cyst fluid is unreliable, with limited diagnostic ability due to a high false negative rate (38%) and low sensitivity.

Neck mass
  Strength of Recommendation: Class IIa
  Strength of Evidence: Category C
  Results Interpretation:
  Positive cytology findings
  A positive needle biopsy of a neck mass is highly diagnostic for carcinomas, salivary gland tumors, and other lesions.

  False Results
  In highly suspicious cases, repeating the biopsy may be indicated because inadequate samples can produce high false-negative results.

Ovarian cyst
  Strength of Recommendation: Class IIa
  Strength of Evidence: Category B
  Results Interpretation:
  Positive cytology findings
  Overall, cytologic evaluation of the ovary does not appear to have sufficient sensitivity to predict malignancy but may be useful as a second-line diagnostic tool for ovarian cysts.

Thyroid cyst
  Strength of Recommendation: Class IIa
  Strength of Evidence: Category B
  Results Interpretation:
  Positive cytology findings
  Cyst fluid cytology from ultrasound-guided fine needle aspiration biopsy is beneficial for detection of benign or malignant cells from thyroid nodules.

Clinical Notes
Fine needle aspiration cytology is minimally invasive and can be both diagnostic and therapeutic in some cases.

Cystic fibrosis carrier detection

TEST DEFINITION
Molecular analysis to detect mutant alleles in the cystic fibrosis transmembrane regulator (CFTR) gene

SYNONYMS
- Cystic fibrosis DNA detection
- Cystic fibrosis mutation analysis

REFERENCE RANGE
- Negative

Please refer to your institution's reference ranges as lab normals may vary.

INDICATIONS
Cystic fibrosis screening
   Strength of Recommendation: Class IIa
   Strength of Evidence: Category B
   Results Interpretation:
   Positive laboratory findings
   Positive screening results identify infants at risk for cystic fibrosis (CF) but is not diagnostic. Detection of one mutation along with elevated levels of immunoreactive trypsinogen (IRT), or the presence of 2 mutations, indicate a high risk of CF. Positive results should be confirmed with a sweat test and clinical evaluation.
   Infants with a positive screening result and a negative sweat test are considered unaffected. Infants with two detectable mutations and a negative sweat test should be further evaluated, and those with one detectable mutation should be referred for family genetic counseling. Infants with 0 or 1 detectable mutation with a borderline sweat test should be evaluated with extensive CF mutation testing.
   Negative laboratory findings
   A negative screening result may indicate that the screening panel was not specific for a particular mutation. Further testing may be clinically indicated in certain cases (ie, an elevated immunoreactive trypsinogen (IRT) level, clinical suspicion).

CLINICAL NOTES
   The most commonly reported mutation is deltaF508, which is responsible for 70% of mutated alleles in Caucasians; however, more than 1,000 separate mutations in the CF transmembrane regulator protein (CFTR) have been identified for cystic fibrosis (CF). CF mutation analysis has become a complex and broad spectrum test, hence only the most common 25 mutations and 6 polymorphisms affecting particular location and ethnicity are included in population-based CF screening as recommended by the American College of Medical Genetics (ACMG)/ American College of Obstetrics and Gynecology (ACOG) guidelines.
   The most common mutations included in this test panel are deltaF508, R553X, R117H, G551D, G542X, N1303K and W1282. Detection rates can be improved by testing with a mutation panel that is associated with a specific ethnic or geographic group (eg, W1282X for Ashkenazi, 2143delT in Germany, Y122X in Reunion Island, T3381 in Sardinia and 2183AA>G and R1162X in northeast Italy).
   Laboratories classify CF DNA testing for better risk evaluation. These various classes include: diagnostic testing versus carrier testing, atypical CF versus classic CF, high risk testing versus population screening, and deltaF508 mutation testing versus a complete mutation panel.

COLLECTION/STORAGE INFORMATION
- Specimen Collection and Handling:
    - Collect whole blood in EDTA (lavender-top) or acid-citrate-dextrose (yellow-top) tube.
    - Collect buccal cells by vigorously twirling and brushing a cheekbrush for 30 seconds; place in appropriate container (eg, Cyto-pak®).
    - Prenatal Testing: Collect chorionic villus samples for DNA extraction.
    - Store whole blood at 4°C and tissue samples at -20°C if DNA extraction delayed.

LOINC CODES
- Code: 34718-7 (*Short Name* - CFTR Gene Mut Anal)
- Code: 21654-9 (*Short Name* - CFTR Gene Mut Anal)
- Code: 21656-4 (*Short Name* - CFTR Gene Mut Tested)

Cystic fibrosis sweat test

TEST DEFINITION
Measurement of chloride concentration in sweat for the diagnosis of cystic fibrosis

SYNONYMS
- Chloride measurement, sweat
- Sweat chloride
- Sweat chloride level

REFERENCE RANGE
- Adults and Children: <40 mmol/L
  Please refer to your institution's reference ranges as lab normals may vary.

INDICATIONS
Suspected cystic fibrosis
    Strength of Recommendation: Class I
    Strength of Evidence: Category C
    Results Interpretation:
    Increased level (laboratory finding)
        A sweat chloride concentration of 40 to 60 mmol/L is considered indeterminate or borderline, and a concentration greater than 60 mmol/L is diagnostic for cystic fibrosis (CF). A definitive diagnosis is established when elevations in the sweat chloride concentration by pilocarpine iontophoresis are demonstrated on 2 separate occasions.

        Sweat chloride concentrations increase with age and borderline concentrations (up to 60 mmol/L) are possible in normal adolescents and adults. Patients with clinical manifestations of CF and indeterminate chloride sweat concentration should undergo repeat testing. Although measurement of the sodium sweat concentration alone is not recommended, it may assist diagnosis in patients with borderline chloride values. About 1% to 2% of patients with clinical CF have normal sweat chloride levels. Test results should be interpreted in the clinical context.

        Low sweat chloride concentrations (less than 10 mmol/L) are the norm for healthy infants, although normal infants may have elevated sweat chloride levels in the first 48 hours and elevated levels may persist for 7 days. The likelihood of CF is high in infants (less than 3 months of age) with sweat chloride concentrations of 40 mmol/L or more; additional diagnostic testing is recommended for these individuals.

        In infants with CF, elevated sweat chloride concentrations occur between 3 and 5 weeks of age.

        Evaporation, leakage, or low sweat secretion rates may result in higher borderline sweat chloride concentration values.

        Patients diagnosed with CF in adulthood are characterized by indeterminate chloride sweat test concentrations, pulmonary sufficiency, and a myriad of genetic mutations typically not found in children diagnosed with CF. Thorough genetic mutation studies and repeat sweat chloride tests are necessary to confirm diagnosis in these patients.

CLINICAL NOTES
    In the absence of severe illness, infants weighing more than 3 kg and over 2 weeks of age can undergo chloride sweat testing.

    Do not perform the chloride sweat test on patients that are edematous, on steroids or on an open delivery oxygen system

    Sweat collected below the recommended sweat secretion rate should not be analyzed and inadequate sample weight/volume should not be pooled. The lab personnel and the individuals performing the sweat test should concur that a sufficient sweat weight/volume is collected and that those values are included in the results report.

    Quantitative pilocarpine iontophoresis chloride sweat testing can be technically demanding and requires experienced personnel. The sweat chloride test should be performed at a facility that does it frequently and follows the National Committee for Clinical Laboratory Standards guidelines.

    Sweat collection times greater than 30 minutes are not recommended because of minimal increases in yield and the risk of specimen evaporation.

COLLECTION/STORAGE INFORMATION
- Collect a minimum of 15 microliters of sweat within 30 minutes from a single site.

LOINC CODES
- Code: 2077-6 (*Short Name* - Chloride Swt-sCnc)

Cysticercosis antibody level

TEST DEFINITION
Detection of antibodies against *Taenia solium* in blood or cerebrospinal fluid for evaluation and management of neurocysticercosis

REFERENCE RANGE
- Negative
Please refer to your institution's reference ranges as lab normals may vary.

INDICATIONS
Suspected *Taenia solium* **infection causing neurocysticercosis**
>**Strength of Recommendation:** Class IIa
>**Strength of Evidence:** Category B
>**Results Interpretation:**
>**Antibody studies abnormal**
>>Diagnosis of cysticercosis is based on a combination of clinical presentation and neuroimaging with serology testing used to confirm rather than diagnose the infection.
>>A positive result may be of limited diagnostic value in areas where cysticercosis is endemic; conversely, a negative result does not exclude neurocysticercosis in patients with a single cyst or with brain calcifications.
>>Persistent seropositivity does not always indicate active infection; patients often remain seropositive for at least a year after successful antiparasitic therapy.

>**False Results**
>>In patients with a solitary parenchymal brain lesion or with inactive disease, false negatives are possible with both enzyme-linked immunotransfer blot assays and enzyme linked immunosorbent assays. False positives may occur in the presence of other helminthic infections.

CLINICAL NOTES
The electroimmunotransfer blot (EITB) is usually performed at special parasitology laboratories or at the Centers for Disease Control and may not be available routinely in clinical laboratories.

COLLECTION/STORAGE INFORMATION
- Collect serum in a red marble-top separation tube and freeze if not assayed immediately

Cystine measurement, Plasma

TEST DEFINITION
Measurement of cystine in plasma for detection of acquired and hereditary amino acid disorders.

REFERENCE RANGE
- Premature neonate, 1 day: 0.78 ± 0.12 mg/dL (65 ± 10 micromol/L)
- Neonate, 1 day: 0.43-1.01 mg/dL (36-84 micromol/L)
- Infants 1 to 3 months: 0.65 ± 0.25 mg/dL (54 ± 21 micromol/L)
- Infants 2 to 6 months: 0.64-0.97 mg/dL (53-81 micromol/L)
- Infants 3 to 10 years: 0.54-0.92 mg/dL (45-77 micromol/L)
- Children 6 to 18 years: 0.43-0.7 mg/dL (36-58 micromol/L)
- Adults: 0.4-1.4 mg/dL (33-117 micromol/L)
Please refer to your institution's reference ranges as lab normals may vary.

INDICATIONS
Suspected inborn error of metabolism
  Strength of Recommendation: Class IIa
  Strength of Evidence: Category C
  Results Interpretation:
  Increased amino acid
    Inherited amino acid disorders are directly related to the absence of an enzyme involved in the metabolism of one or more amino acids; therefore, an elevated plasma level of a particular amino acid is highly suggestive of an inherited metabolic defect. In the majority of cases amino acid and organic acid analysis together permit diagnostic confirmation in infants. Immediate treatment should be initiated when an inborn error of metabolism is suspected, even if a definitive diagnosis has not yet been determined.

COLLECTION/STORAGE INFORMATION
- Specimen Collection and Handling:
  - Immediately place sample in ice water.
  - Isolate plasma sample and freeze it within 1 hour; sample stable for 1 week at -20°C.
  - Sample should be deproteinized and stored at -70°C for protracted periods of usage.

Cytomegalovirus antibody avidity assay

TEST DEFINITION
Measurement of IgG avidity in serum for the evaluation of cytomegalovirus infection

REFERENCE RANGE
- Adults: seronegative
  Please refer to your institution's reference ranges as lab normals may vary.

INDICATIONS
Suspected primary cytomegalovirus in pregnancy
  Strength of Recommendation: Class IIa
  Strength of Evidence: Category B
  Results Interpretation:
  Laboratory test finding
    IgG avidity reflects the functional bonding affinity of IgG, which is lower at infection onset and increases over time. In the presence of cytomegalovirus (CMV) IgM antibodies in pregnant women, low avidity suggests primary CMV infection of less than 3 months duration. High avidity, with or without the concurrent presence of IgM antibodies, suggests past infection in the majority of pregnant women, particularly if testing is performed during the first trimester, although primary infection cannot be definitively ruled out.

LOINC CODES
- Code: 34403-6 (*Short Name* - CMV AB Avidity Ser-aCnc)

Cytomegalovirus antibody measurement

TEST DEFINITION
Measurement of cytomegalovirus (CMV) antibodies in serum for the detection and management of CMV infections

SYNONYMS
- CMV antibody level

REFERENCE RANGE
- Adults and children: nonreactive
  Please refer to your institution's reference ranges as lab normals may vary.

INDICATIONS

Suspected congenital cytomegalovirus
Strength of Recommendation: Class IIa
Strength of Evidence: Category B
Results Interpretation:
Positive immunology findings
A positive IgG titer in a previously negative patient is indicative of active maternal infection and suggests potential transmission of disease to the neonate. IgM titers peak 1 to 3 months after the onset of infection before gradually declining. Because the presence of IgM antibodies can be due to either active infection or persistent antibody response to past infection, IgM seropositivity alone cannot accurately diagnose active infection, nor can it predict the risk of congenital infection. Additional IgG avidity testing may help to differentiate primary from nonprimary infection.
Negative immunology findings
A negative IgM or IgG titer suggests no current or latent infection.

Suspected cytomegalovirus mononucleosis
Strength of Recommendation: Class IIb
Strength of Evidence: Category C
Results Interpretation:
Positive laboratory findings
In the presence of fever and atypical lymphocytes greater than 10%, a positive serologic test for cytomegalovirus (CMV) suggests CMV mononucleosis. During acute infection CMV IgG antibodies usually increase fourfold or more and may take 4 to 7 weeks to peak. IgM antibodies are present in the majority of patients during the acute phase of illness and can remain detectable for up to a year or longer in 20% or more of patients. CMV seropositivity does not differentiate between reactivation of latent infection or reinfection with a new CMV strain.

False Results
In patients with acute Epstein-Barr infection (EBV), false positive CMV IgM serologic results have been observed and are likely due to antigenic cross-reactivity among the herpes viruses.

Suspected or known cytomegalovirus infection
Strength of Recommendation: Class IIa
Strength of Evidence: Category B
Results Interpretation:
Positive immunology findings
A positive IgG titer in a previously seronegative patient is indicative of new primary infection. A fourfold or greater rise in antibody titer in a patient who was previously seropositive is consistent with a serologic diagnosis of CMV infection. IgG antibodies are usually detectable within 3 to 6 weeks after initial infection and IgG antibodies remain detectable for life; levels may drop with advanced age or immunosuppression. In patients whose previous antibody status is unknown, IgG seropositivity can indicate new primary infection, reactivation of latent virus, or new infection by a different viral strain. Nearly all HIV positive patients have detectable CMV IgG antibodies, and coinfection with more than one strain is common. In immunocompromised patients, positive IgM titers may be caused by new primary infection or reactivation of latent virus. Immunosuppressed patients may be IgM reactive for CMV for up to 1 year after initial infection.

False Results
Transplant patients who receive blood products may produce false positive low level titers to CMV due to passively transfused antibodies.
Negative immunology findings
A negative IgG titer suggests no current or past CMV infection, although CMV infection cannot definitively be ruled out; immunosuppressed patients with CMV infection can serorevert from seropositive to seronegative status. IgM titers are often nonreactive in immunocompromised patients with CMV due to their inability to mount an IgM response.

False Results
Transplant patients who receive blood products may produce false positive low level titers to CMV due to passively transfused antibodies.

Timing of Monitoring
Patients undergoing transplant should have baseline CMV serology status determined preoperatively and prior to the administration of any blood products. Postoperative monitoring for seroconversion or infection is imperative, as preoperative seronegative transplant patients are at high risk for developing CMV disease postoperatively, most often between the 30th and 100th postoperative day.

CLINICAL NOTES
The use of nonstandardized cytomegalovirus IgM-specific viral antigen preparations, which combine as many as 100 different antigenic proteins, can cause substantial interassay variability.

COLLECTION/STORAGE INFORMATION
• Draw serum sample in red-top or serum separator tube

LOINC CODES
• Code: 5121-9 (*Short Name* - CMV Ab Titr Ser LA)
• Code: 15377-5 (*Short Name* - CMV Ab Ser QI LA)
• Code: 16713-0 (*Short Name* - CMV Ab CSF-aCnc)
• Code: 5122-7 (*Short Name* - CMV Ab Ser IF-aCnc)
• Code: 16714-8 (*Short Name* - CMV Ab Ser LA-aCnc)
• Code: 9513-3 (*Short Name* - CMV Ab Titr Ser CF)
• Code: 16712-2 (*Short Name* - CMV Ab Fld-aCnc)
• Code: 7851-9 (*Short Name* - CMV Ab Ser-aCnc)
• Code: 9514-1 (*Short Name* - CMV Ab Titr CSF CF)
• Code: 32170-3 (*Short Name* - CMV Ab Titr Ser IF)
• Code: 22239-8 (*Short Name* - CMV Ab Ser QI)

Cytomegalovirus antigen assay

TEST DEFINITION
Antigen testing for diagnosis of cytomegalovirus (CMV) infection

REFERENCE RANGE
• Negative (pp65 antigenemia assay, negative: 0 positive cells/50,000 leukocytes examined)
  Please refer to your institution's reference ranges as lab normals may vary.

INDICATIONS
Suspected cytomegalovirus (CMV) infection in transplant recipients
  Strength of Recommendation: Class IIa
  Strength of Evidence: Category B
  Results Interpretation:
  Positive laboratory findings
  In a study that included 11 BMT recipients who developed CMV disease, mortality was 40% for patients with CMV antigenemia and disease, 0% for antigenemia without disease, and 1.3% for disease without antigenemia. The 1-year survival rate was 57% for patients with CMV antigenemia and disease, 82% for antigenemia without disease, and 63% for disease without antigenemia.
  The development of the CMV pp65 antigenemia assay allows for the surveillance of viremia in transplant recipients, leading to earlier antiviral treatment with a decrease in the incidence of CMV disease.
  Serology testing for CMV should only be used as an adjunct to tests that directly detect CMV due to the possibility of factors (eg, blood product transfusions, immunosuppressed response to antigen) that may yield false results.

Suspected cytomegalovirus infection in human immunodeficiency virus (HIV) positive patients
  Strength of Recommendation: Class IIa
  Strength of Evidence: Category B

Results Interpretation:
Positive laboratory findings

Significant factors for developing CMV disease in HIV-positive patients are cytomegalovirus (CMV) pp65 antigenemia greater than or equal to 100 nuclei/200,000 cells, a positive plasma polymerase chain reaction (PCR) for CMV DNA, and a CD4 T cell count of less than 75 X 10^6 cells/L.

Of HIV-positive patients with CMV pp65 antigenemia assay equal to or more than 100 nuclei/200,000 cells, up to 63% may develop CMV disease, compared to 3% without antigenemia.

Of HIV-positive patients with a positive CMV PCR result, up to 38% may develop CMV disease, compared to 3% with a negative PCR result.

Preemptive treatment for CMV is affected by test sensitivity where the detection pp65 antigenemia testing or CMV culture as compared to plasma PCR respectively yields a 2-month interval versus a 4-month interval between CMV detection and the onset of CMV disease.

ABNORMAL RESULTS

- Results increased in:
  - False positives for IgG testing can result following blood product transfusions.
- Results decreased in:
  - False negatives for pp65 antigenemia assay may result from autolysis of blood leukocytes.

CLINICAL NOTES

Cytomegalovirus (CMV) antigen testing can be performed on blood, CSF, urine, saliva or tissue. CMV culture takes 3 to 4 weeks for incubation.

Testing for CMV pp65 antigenemia assay can be performed within 5 hours.

COLLECTION/STORAGE INFORMATION

- Collect blood in EDTA (lavender) tube.

LOINC CODES

- Code: 6380-0 (*Short Name* - CMV Ag XXX EMIA)
- Code: 10660-9 (*Short Name* - CMV Ag Tiss Ql ImStn)
- Code: 6375-0 (*Short Name* - CMV Ag Bld EMIA)
- Code: 6378-4 (*Short Name* - CMV Ag Ur EMIA)
- Code: 6376-8 (*Short Name* - CMV Ag Ser Ql EIA)
- Code: 6379-2 (*Short Name* - CMV Ag XXX Ql EIA)
- Code: 6381-8 (*Short Name* - CMV Ag XXX Ql IF)
- Code: 6377-6 (*Short Name* - CMV Ag Ser Ql IF)

Cytomegalovirus culture

TEST DEFINITION

Culture of body fluid for detection of cytomegalovirus

REFERENCE RANGE

- Adults and Children: Negative growth
  Please refer to your institution's reference ranges as lab normals may vary.

INDICATIONS

Suspected cytomegalovirus infection in pregnancy
   Strength of Recommendation: Class IIa
   Strength of Evidence: Category B
Results Interpretation:
Positive microbiology findings

Culture of human fibroblasts is the benchmark method to diagnose congenital CMV infection in a newborn; amniotic fluid culture is preferred for diagnosing CMV prenatally.
   Timing of Monitoring

Neonatal testing by virus isolation in human fibroblasts in the first 2 weeks of life is required to confirm a prenatal diagnosis or to diagnose vertical transmission. Early testing limits the possibility of exposure acquired from the birth canal, breast milk, or blood products.

Suspected cytomegalovirus infection
    Strength of Recommendation: Class IIa
    Strength of Evidence: Category B
  Results Interpretation:
  Positive microbiology findings
    An incubation time of at least 7 days is required to obtain results. The rapid culture cytomegalovirus test can shorten detection time to 1 to 2 days.

COLLECTION/STORAGE INFORMATION

Collect a mid-void urine specimen during the acute phase of illness. Collect 2 to 3 specimens over successive days to maximize recovery of cytomegalovirus.

Immediately transport specimens in viral transport medium. Store all samples except blood at 4°C for no more than 5 days before processing. Do not freeze blood and urine samples. Store blood samples at room temperature at all times.

LOINC CODES

- Code: 5838-8 (*Short Name* - CMV XXX Cult)
- Code: 5837-0 (*Short Name* - CMV Ur Cult)
- Code: 5835-4 (*Short Name* - CMV Bld Cult)
- Code: 5836-2 (*Short Name* - CMV Tiss Cult)

Cytomegalovirus cytology

TEST DEFINITION

Cytologic detection of cytomegalovirus (CMV) in urine and other body fluids or tissues for the evaluation and management of CMV infections

SYNONYMS

- Cytomegalovirus inclusion body detection

REFERENCE RANGE

Negative
Please refer to your institution's reference ranges as lab normals may vary.

INDICATIONS

Suspected cytomegalovirus (CMV) infection
    Strength of Recommendation: Class IIa
    Strength of Evidence: Category B
  Results Interpretation:
  Positive laboratory findings
    The most frequent findings of cytomegalovirus (CMV) by urine cytology are intracytoplasmic inclusions, although intranuclear CMV inclusions are seen occasionally.

    A positive urine cytology finding for CMV in renal transplant recipients can help distinguish between acute allograft rejection and CMV infection. The mean period following renal transplantation for cytologic evidence of CMV infection to manifest is 8 weeks; patients can continue to shed CMV for months following transplant.

CLINICAL NOTES

Urine cytology is the most common microscopic examination done to detect cytomegalovirus (CMV)-related inclusions, but CMV inclusions also may be identified in epithelial cells from various tissue types.

COLLECTION/STORAGE INFORMATION

- Specimen Collection and Handling:
  - Collect urine clean catch or catheterized specimen in a sterile container.
  - Transport specimen to laboratory immediately after collection.

Cytomegalovirus nucleic acid assay

TEST DEFINITION
Detection and measurement of cytomegalovirus (CMV) by nucleic acid assay for evaluation and management of CMV infection and disease

SYNONYMS
• Cytomegalovirus nucleic acid detection

REFERENCE RANGE
• Adults and Children: Negative
Please refer to your institution's reference ranges as lab normals may vary.

INDICATIONS
Suspected cytomegalovirus (CMV) infection in immunocompromised patients
    Strength of Recommendation: Class I
    Strength of Evidence: Category B
    Results Interpretation:
    Positive laboratory findings
        A positive polymerase chain reaction (PCR) result for cytomegalovirus (CMV) does not differentiate between latent, active or reactivation of infection (with or without CMV disease), nor does a negative PCR result exclude the possibility of CMV disease. Results should be interpreted together with clinical presentation and other CMV tests, (eg, culture, serology), plus patient history.
        Cytomegalovirus is a common infection, with 40% to 100% of general populations being seropositive for CMV (rates are higher in underdeveloped countries).
        Patients at risk for CMV disease include immunocompromised patients (eg, HIV/AIDS, transplant) and immunoimmature patients (eg, fetus, newborn infants).
        While not always detectable without serial testing, CMV viremia always precedes CMV disease. Quantitative PCR blood results are valuable in diagnosing CMV disease and defining the extent of the disease. A positive PCR viremia finding in AIDS patients indicates a significant risk of developing CMV retinitis or other CMV disease complications. Quantitative PCR blood results are valuable in guiding antiviral therapy and demonstrating the effectiveness of antiviral treatment.
        Positive findings for nucleic acid sequence-based amplification (NASBA) testing for pp67 mRNA in whole blood are highly predictive and specific for the onset of CMV disease in renal transplant patients, but not for HIV patients where this test has low sensitivity and predictive value.
        In AIDS patients, the CMV viral load may be significantly higher in those with CMV retinitis.
        A single DNA PCR on blood with a positive result is highly associated with developing CMV disease in HIV patients within 1 year, whereas a single positive result for NASBA for pp67 mRNA or DNA PCR on throat swab is not.
        Early identification of CMV DNA in peripheral blood leukocytes (PBL) in bone marrow transplant (BMT) recipients and other immunocompromised patients is useful to identify patients who will need preemptive antiviral therapy.
        Up to 75% of patients with CMV retinitis may also have CMV encephalitis. The amount of CMV DNA identified in cerebrospinal fluid (CSF) correlates to brain lesion pattern and number, with higher CMV DNA CSF findings associated with more widespread ventriculoencephalitis. Quantitative PCR testing of CSF for CMV may also be useful in diagnosing CMV polyradiculopathy.
        The challenge of identifying CMV disease in immunocompromised patents is to distinguish between those developing CMV disease or at risk of developing CMV disease and those not at risk. Positive results for CMV late messenger RNA (mRNA), present during viral genome transcription, indicates active CMV replication.
    Negative laboratory findings
        Patients without CMV neurological sequelae usually have negative CSF PCR results for CMV.
        Patients with positive CMV nucleic acid tests who are HIV infected may subsequently have negative tests prior to developing CMV disease. This phenomena varies by test type: with NASBA testing for IEA mRNA, 50%

of patients may have subsequent negative test results; with DNA PCR testing on blood, 52.4%; with NASBA testing for pp67 mRNA, 45%; with DNA PCR testing on urine, 66.7%; and with DNA PCR testing on throat swabs, 31.6%.

Suspected congenital cytomegalovirus (CMV) infection in neonates
    Strength of Recommendation: Class IIa
    Strength of Evidence: Category C
    Results Interpretation:
    Positive laboratory findings

Although not used routinely as a screening test, detection of cytomegalovirus (CMV) by nucleic acid methods within the first 2 weeks of life indicates congenital CMV infection.

Cytomegalovirus is the most common cause of congenital infection, but it may be asymptomatic in up to 90% of infants at birth. Congenital CMV infection should be suspected in small-for-gestational-age infants, infants with microcephaly, and in infants with other signs of congenital infection (eg, prematurity, jaundice, hepatosplenomegaly, petechiae, lethargy).

CLINICAL NOTES

Cytomegalovirus (CMV) nucleic acid assays can be performed on a variety of specimen types: blood, serum, plasma, urine, cerebrospinal fluid (CSF), saliva, bronchoalveolar lavage, throat swab, intraocular fluid, amniotic fluid, dried blood spots, or body tissues.

Quantitative PCR testing may determine CMV 'viral load.' It is used to identify patients at risk for CMV disease and to guide treatment decisions.

COLLECTION/STORAGE INFORMATION

- Specimen Collection and Handling:
  - Collect blood in a lavender EDTA tube or a yellow ACD tube.
  - Store all body fluids at 4°C, store body tissues at -20°C.

LOINC CODES

- Code: 4998-1 (*Short Name* - CMV DNA Tiss QI PCR)
- Code: 4997-3 (*Short Name* - CMV DNA Tiss QI Prb)
- Code: 34719-5 (*Short Name* - CMV DNA Amn QI PCR)
- Code: 30326-3 (*Short Name* - CMV DNA CSF QI PCR)
- Code: 30247-1 (*Short Name* - CMV Viral Load SerPl PCR)
- Code: 28008-1 (*Short Name* - CMV DNA Bld QI bDNA)
- Code: 24041-6 (*Short Name* - CMV DNA XXX bDNA-aCnc)
- Code: 4996-5 (*Short Name* - CMV DNA Bld QI PCR)
- Code: 33006-8 (*Short Name* - CMV Viral Load XXX PCR)
- Code: 29590-7 (*Short Name* - CMV DNA Bld Prb-mCnc)
- Code: 5000-5 (*Short Name* - CMV DNA XXX QI PCR)
- Code: 34720-3 (*Short Name* - CMV DNA XXX PCR-aCnc)
- Code: 4999-9 (*Short Name* - CMV DNA Ur QI PCR)
- Code: 30246-3 (*Short Name* - CMV DNA SerPl QI PCR)
- Code: 29604-6 (*Short Name* - CMV Viral Load Bld PCR)

Cytomegalovirus nucleic acid assay, Quantitative

TEST DEFINITION

Quantitative measurement of cytomegalovirus (CMV) viral load in whole blood, serum, plasma, peripheral blood leukocytes, or cerebrospinal fluid for the diagnosis, evaluation, and management of CMV infection

SYNONYMS

- Cytomegalovirus nucleic acid detection

REFERENCE RANGE
- Adults and children: No virus detected
  Please refer to your institution's reference ranges as lab normals may vary.

INDICATIONS
Suspected or known cytomegalovirus (CMV) infection in immunocompromised patients
> **Strength of Recommendation:** Class IIa
> **Strength of Evidence:** Category B
> **Results Interpretation:**
> **Positive laboratory findings**
>> In bone marrow, renal, and liver transplant recipients, an increase in viral load is the major risk factor for symptomatic cytomegalovirus (CMV) infection. Elevated viral load may suggest the onset of end-organ involvement in immunosuppressed patients. Substantially higher CMV viral load has been observed in symptomatic, immunocompromised individuals when compared to asymptomatic patients with active CMV disease.
>> In HIV patients, the presence of CMV DNA is associated with a substantially higher risk of disease progression, and increasing viral load portends a poorer prognosis and shorter survival time.
>> The amount of CMV DNA identified in cerebrospinal fluid (CSF) correlates with both brain lesion pattern and the number of lesions, with higher CMV DNA CSF findings associated with more widespread ventriculoencephalitis. A CMV DNA count of up to 10^7 copies/mL may be observed in patients with CMV encephalitis. A decrease in viral load has been observed in CMV encephalitis patients following antiviral therapy. CMV detection by quantitative PCR is very uncommon in patients without CMV-related neurological conditions.

Suspected congenital cytomegalovirus (CMV) infection
> **Strength of Recommendation:** Class IIb
> **Strength of Evidence:** Category B
> **Results Interpretation:**
> **Increased level (laboratory finding)**
>> Elevated quantitative cytomegalovirus (CMV) nucleic acid levels in a newborn may suggest symptomatic congenital CMV.

COLLECTION/STORAGE INFORMATION
> Collect whole blood for suspected disseminated CMV. Collect organ samples for suspected organ syndromes.

LOINC CODES
- Code: 4998-1 (*Short Name* - CMV DNA Tiss Ql PCR)
- Code: 4997-3 (*Short Name* - CMV DNA Tiss Ql Prb)
- Code: 34719-5 (*Short Name* - CMV DNA Amn Ql PCR)
- Code: 30326-3 (*Short Name* - CMV DNA CSF Ql PCR)
- Code: 30247-1 (*Short Name* - CMV Viral Load SerPl PCR)
- Code: 28008-1 (*Short Name* - CMV DNA Bld Ql bDNA)
- Code: 24041-6 (*Short Name* - CMV DNA XXX bDNA-aCnc)
- Code: 4996-5 (*Short Name* - CMV DNA Bld Ql PCR)
- Code: 33006-8 (*Short Name* - CMV Viral Load XXX PCR)
- Code: 29590-7 (*Short Name* - CMV DNA Bld Prb-mCnc)
- Code: 5000-5 (*Short Name* - CMV DNA XXX Ql PCR)
- Code: 34720-3 (*Short Name* - CMV DNA XXX PCR-aCnc)
- Code: 4999-9 (*Short Name* - CMV DNA Ur Ql PCR)
- Code: 30246-3 (*Short Name* - CMV DNA SerPl Ql PCR)
- Code: 29604-6 (*Short Name* - CMV Viral Load Bld PCR)

D-dimer assay

TEST DEFINITION
Measurement of plasma D-dimer, a product of fibrin degradation, for the evaluation of conditions that involve intravascular thrombosis

REFERENCE RANGE
- Adults:<0.5 mcg/mL (<0.5 mg/L)
  Please refer to your institution's reference ranges as lab normals may vary.

INDICATIONS
Suspected acute aortic dissection
> **Strength of Recommendation:** Class IIa
> **Strength of Evidence:** Category B
> **Results Interpretation:**
> **Normal laboratory findings**

   D-dimer is the only known lab marker for acute aortic dissection (AD) for which a rapid assay is available. D-dimer levels appear to be higher earlier in the course of disease. Several small studies have demonstrated that D-dimer has a high sensitivity and negative predictive value for acute AD, indicating that a normal D-dimer would be helpful in excluding disease. Larger prospective trials would be helpful in confirming this role.

> **Timing of Monitoring**

   In a study of 78 coronary care unit patients with suspected acute aortic dissection (AD), time from symptom onset to measurement of D-dimer had no significant correlation with the D-dimer level in the acute AD group. Two patients had a level drawn by 1 hour, and the D-dimer was elevated in both.

   There was a statistically significant negative correlation between the interval from symptom onset to blood draw and the D-dimer concentration in a study of 10 patients who were prospectively evaluated for acute AD and 14 patients who were retrospectively identified by chart review and were diagnosed with AD and had a D-dimer sent. The interval in this study ranged from 1 hour to 120 hours.

   There was also a significant negative correlation between the interval from symptom onset to blood draw and the D-dimer concentration in a study that measured D-dimer levels by a latex-enhanced turbidimetric test in 64 consecutive chest pain patients and 32 controls with chronic AD.

Suspected acute coronary syndrome (ACS)
> **Strength of Recommendation:** Class III
> **Strength of Evidence:** Category B
> **Results Interpretation:**
> **Elevated D-dimer level**

   The low positive and negative predictive values of a D-dimer level in the setting of acute coronary syndrome make it difficult to draw any conclusions from either an elevated or a normal measurement. There is some evidence to suggest that an elevated D-dimer in the setting of a normal ECG and normal cardiac enzymes should heighten concern for recurrent events.

Suspected acute deep venous thrombosis (DVT)
> **Strength of Recommendation:** Class IIa
> **Strength of Evidence:** Category B
> **Results Interpretation:**
> **Normal laboratory findings**

   In outpatients with a low pretest probability for lower-extremity DVT, the following tests can be used to exclude DVT: a negative quantitative D-dimer assay (turbidimetric or ELISA) for exclusion of proximal and distal lower-extremity DVT, a negative whole blood cell qualitative D-dimer assay in conjunction with a Wells' scoring system for exclusion of proximal and distal DVT, or a negative whole blood D-dimer assay for exclusion of proximal lower-extremity DVT. A negative D-dimer cannot exclude DVT in patients with a moderate or high pretest probability.

> **Elevated D-dimer level**

   A positive D-dimer is not helpful in making the diagnosis of DVT, given its low positive predictive values and likelihood ratios.

Suspected acute pulmonary embolism
> **Strength of Recommendation:** Class IIa
> **Strength of Evidence:** Category B
> **Results Interpretation:**
> **Normal laboratory findings**

   In emergency department patients with a low pretest probability of PE, a negative ELISA or turbidimetric D-dimer assay or a negative whole blood cell qualitative D-dimer assay in conjunction with a Wells score of 2 or less is sufficient to exclude PE. A negative whole blood D-dimer assay (when not used with the Wells criteria) or a negative immunofiltration D-dimer assay can also exclude PE in the setting of low pretest probability.

In emergency department patients with low to moderate pretest probability of PE and a nondiagnostic ventilation/perfusion lung scan, a negative turbidimetric or ELISA D-dimer assay or a negative whole blood cell qualitative D-dimer assay in conjunction with a Wells score of 4 or less can exclude clinically significant PE, as can a negative whole blood D-dimer assay (when not used with the Wells criteria) or a negative immunofiltration D-dimer assay.

Suspected disseminated intravascular coagulation (DIC)
  Strength of Recommendation: Class IIa
  Strength of Evidence: Category B
  Results Interpretation:
  Elevated D-dimer level
    An elevated D-dimer level is suggestive of, though not conclusive for, DIC.
  Normal laboratory findings
    A normal D-dimer level has a high negative predictive value for DIC.

Suspected preeclampsia
  Results Interpretation:
  Elevated D-dimer level
    D-dimer assay is an early screen for coagulation abnormalities in women with a preeclamptic coagulopathy.

COMMON PANELS
- Disseminated intravascular coagulation screen

ABNORMAL RESULTS
- Results increased in:
  - Trauma
  - Cancer
  - Infection
  - Pregnancy
  - Increased age
  - Decreased renal function
  - Liver disease
  - Burns
  - Stroke/cerebrovascular disease
  - Peripheral vascular disease

COLLECTION/STORAGE INFORMATION
- Obtain plasma in sodium citrate tube
- Store at room temperature for 8 hours or at -20° C for up to 6 months

Dark field microscopy

TEST DEFINITION
Microscopic detection of *Treponema pallidum* in lesions, lymph nodes or other specimens for the detection of primary, secondary, and early congenital syphilis

SYNONYMS
- Darkfield microscopy
- Dark ground microscopy

REFERENCE RANGE
- Adults and children: negative
Please refer to your institution's reference ranges as lab normals may vary.

INDICATIONS
Suspected syphilis
> **Strength of Recommendation:** Class IIa
> **Strength of Evidence:** Category B
> **Results Interpretation:**
> **Abnormal laboratory findings**
>> The presence of *Treponema pallidum* by darkfield microscopy examination of lesions or lymph nodes can confirm the diagnosis of primary or secondary syphilis. A definitive diagnosis of neonatal congenital syphilis requires the presence of *T pallidum* by direct microscopic examination of umbilical cord, placental, nasal discharge or skin lesion specimens.
> **Negative laboratory findings**
>> An absence of *T pallidum* by darkfield microscopic examination does not exclude the diagnosis of syphilis.

COLLECTION/STORAGE INFORMATION
- Collect at least 3 specimens from each lesion onto a glass slide, removing all scabs, crust, secondary exudate, erythrocytes, tissue debris, and other organisms.
- Encrusted or obviously contaminated specimens should be cleansed with tap water or physiologic saline using a minimum amount of water, in order to prevent organism dilution. Antiseptics or soaps should be avoided.
- Place cover glass on each specimen and remove all air bubbles.
- Examine specimens immediately after collection.
- Darkfield microscopy should not be used to examine oral lesions due to the difficulty in differentiating *Treponema pallidum* from saprophytic spirochetes.

LOINC CODES
- Code: 6607-6 (*Short Name* - Dark Field Tiss)
- Code: 20884-3 (*Short Name* - Dark Field Stl)
- Code: 20883-5 (*Short Name* - Dark Field Ur)
- Code: 660-1 (*Short Name* - Dark Field XXX)
- Code: 20885-0 (*Short Name* - Dark Field Gast)

Dehydroepiandrosterone sulfate measurement

TEST DEFINITION
Measurement of dehydroepiandrosterone sulfate (DHEA-S) in plasma or serum for the evaluation and management of adrenal endocrine disorders

SYNONYMS
- Dehydroepiandrosterone sulphate measurement
- DHEA-S measurement

REFERENCE RANGE
- Adult males: 10-619 mcg/dL (100-6,190 mcg/L)
- Adult females (premenopausal): 12-535 mcg/dL (120-5,350 mcg/L)
- Adult females (postmenopausal): 30-260 mcg/dL (300-2,600 mcg/L)
  Please refer to your institution's reference ranges as lab normals may vary.

INDICATIONS
Hirsutism
> **Strength of Recommendation:** Class IIa
> **Strength of Evidence:** Category C
> **Results Interpretation:**
> **Increased level (laboratory finding)**
>> Increased levels of dehydroepiandrosterone sulfate (DHEA-S) suggest that hirsutism is caused by adrenal cortical hyperfunction.

Thirty percent to 50% of women with polycystic ovary syndrome have elevated DHEA-S levels. DHEA-S levels greater than 700 ng/dL warrant computed tomography (CT) or magnetic resonance imaging (MRI) of the adrenal glands to exclude an androgen-secreting tumor.

Normal laboratory findings

In a hirsute woman with normal ovulatory function, normal levels of DHEA-S and total and free testosterone are essentially diagnostic for idiopathic hirsutism.

Suspected adrenal cortical insufficiency

    Strength of Recommendation: Class IIb

    Strength of Evidence: Category B

Results Interpretation:

Normal laboratory findings

In one study, a normal dehydroepiandrosterone sulfate (DHEA-S) level essentially excluded the diagnosis of adrenal cortical insufficiency or adrenal corticotropic hormone (ACTH) deficiency, especially if the low-dose-Cortrosyn (LDC)-stimulation test was normal.

Decreased level (laboratory finding)

Because many factors can lower DHEA-S levels, a low level may not necessarily indicate adrenal insufficiency.

DRUG/LAB INTERACTIONS

- Veralipride - an increase in dehydroepiandrosterone sulfate (DHEAS) serum levels

ABNORMAL RESULTS

- Results increased in:
  - Low calorie diet
  - Acute submaximal exercise
  - Cigarette smoking
  - Primary biliary cirrhosis
- Results decreased in:
  - Burn trauma
  - Critical illness
  - Systemic lupus erythematosus (SLE)
  - Rheumatoid arthritis
  - Chronic liver disease
  - Diabetes mellitus type 2

COLLECTION/STORAGE INFORMATION

- Specimen Collection and Handling:
  - Collect sample in red-top (serum) or lavender-top (EDTA) tube.
  - May store at 4°C for 2 days or at -20°C for 2 months

LOINC CODES

- Code: 14688-6 (*Short Name* - DHEA-S SerPl-sCnc)
- Code: 35205-4 (*Short Name* - DHEA-S SerPl-msCnc)
- Code: 2192-3 (*Short Name* - DHEA-S 24H Ur-mRate)
- Code: 16728-8 (*Short Name* - DHEA-S sp7 p chal SerPl-mCnc)
- Code: 2190-7 (*Short Name* - DHEA-S Amn-mCnc)
- Code: 16722-1 (*Short Name* - DHEA-S sp10 p chal SerPl-mCnc)
- Code: 34281-6 (*Short Name* - DHEA-S 24H Ur-sCnc)
- Code: 16721-3 (*Short Name* - DHEA-S Sal-mCnc)
- Code: 16729-6 (*Short Name* - DHEA-S sp8 p chal SerPl-mCnc)
- Code: 16723-9 (*Short Name* - DHEA-S sp2 p chal SerPl-mCnc)
- Code: 15053-2 (*Short Name* - DHEA-S 24H Ur-sRate)
- Code: 2191-5 (*Short Name* - DHEA-S SerPl-mCnc)
- Code: 34280-8 (*Short Name* - DHEA-S Ur-sCnc)

Desipramine measurement

TEST DEFINITION
Measurement of desipramine levels in serum or plasma to facilitate therapeutic monitoring or assessment of toxicity

REFERENCE RANGE
- Adults: 75-300 ng/mL (281-1125 nmol/L)
  Please refer to your institution's reference ranges as lab normals may vary.

INDICATIONS
Suspected desipramine toxicity
  Strength of Recommendation: Class IIb
  Strength of Evidence: Category B
Results Interpretation:
Blood drug level high
- Toxic level (adults): >400 ng/mL (>1500 nmol/L)
- A plasma tricyclic antidepressant concentration greater than 500 microgram/L is associated with an increase in anticholinergic effects and levels above 1,000 micrograms/L have been associated with lethal cardiotoxicity.
- Lethal tricyclic antidepressant levels reported from forensic studies have ranged from 1,100 to 21,800 ng/mL (4,000 to 80,000 nmol/L). Serious side effects associated with tricyclic antidepressant overdose include sinus tachycardia, coma, QRS prolongation, hypotension, seizures, arrhythmias, cardiorespiratory arrest, and death. In addition, 35% of patients admitted for tricyclic antidepressant overdose show signs of CNS disturbances, including myoclonic twitches, seizures, and pyramidal signs.
- The development of seizures is associated with tricyclic antidepressant plasma levels above 1,000 ng/mL. However, seizures and other serious side effects may occur at levels less than 1,000 ng/mL.
Timing of Monitoring
  Patients who present with suspected tricyclic antidepressant overdose should have blood levels reported within 1 hour due to the potentially serious consequences of toxic blood levels.

Therapeutic drug monitoring during desipramine therapy
  Strength of Recommendation: Class I
  Strength of Evidence: Category C
Results Interpretation:
Blood drug levels - finding
  Desipramine levels aid in the evaluation of patient compliance, potential for toxicity, effects of drug-drug interactions, and individualized therapeutic concentrations The typical therapeutic concentration for desipramine is 75-300 ng/mL.
  There is a wide variation among individuals in their ability to metabolize desipramine. Patients who have an inactive CYP2D6 allele may be particularly poor metabolizers of tricyclic antidepressants, leading to high serum levels. Additionally, patients with hepatic cirrhosis or impaired renal function may have increased tricyclic drug concentrations.
  Plasma desipramine concentrations may not be as high as the plasma concentrations of its metabolite, 2-hydroxydesipramine
Blood drug level high
  Very high concentrations of desipramine (greater then 1,000 micrograms/liter) are associated with serious side effects, including cardiotoxicity.
Timing of Monitoring
  Specimens should be collected after steady state is achieved, which is 3-5 days after initiation of therapy or changes in dose. A trough sample should be collected either 10 to 14 hours after a single daily dose or 4 to 6 hours after divided daily dose. Due to the potential seriousness of elevated tricyclic antidepressant levels, results should be available within 24 hours for the purposes of therapeutic drug monitoring.

COLLECTION/STORAGE INFORMATION
- Specimen Collection and Handling:
  - Draw serum or plasma in an EDTA tube.
  - Do not use gel tubes, heparin tubes, or stoppers containing 2-butoxyethoxylphosphoryloxylethoxyl-butane (TBEP).
  - Collect at steady state, at least 3 to 6 days after the dose has been initiated.

- Collect trough sample 10 to 14 hours after last dose for once daily dosing and 4 to 6 hours after the last dose for divided daily dosing.
- Store up to 24 hours at room temperature, up to 4 months at 4°C, and at -20°C for any length greater than one year.

LOINC CODES

- Code: 3533-7 (*Short Name* - Desipramine Ur QI)
- Code: 14692-8 (*Short Name* - Desipramine Ur-sCnc)
- Code: 3534-5 (*Short Name* - Desipramine Ur-mCnc)

Digoxin measurement

TEST DEFINITION

Measurement of digoxin in serum for the evaluation and management of patients receiving digoxin or who have ingested digoxin-like compounds (eg, cardiac glycosides)

REFERENCE RANGE

- Therapeutic concentration: 0.8-2 ng/mL (1-2.6 nmol/L)
  Please refer to your institution's reference ranges as lab normals may vary.

INDICATIONS

Digitalized patients with hypomagnesemia
Results Interpretation:
Laboratory findings present
A serum digoxin level is indicated for all patients receiving digoxin who present with hypomagnesemia. Magnesium deficiency increases the risk of digitalis toxicity and arrhythmias, which may be caused by intracellular potassium depletion.

Suspected and known atrial fibrillation in patients receiving digoxin
Results Interpretation:
Digoxin level high
Digoxin toxicity is often associated with paroxysmal atrial tachycardia with a variable degree of block, and/or atrial fibrillation with complete heart block and a slow, regular, wide QRS complex ventricular escape rhythm.
Digoxin level low
Patients on digoxin may lack rate control due to low digoxin levels.

Drug level monitoring during digoxin therapy
Strength of Recommendation: Class I
Strength of Evidence: Category C
Results Interpretation:
Blood drug levels - finding
Although the official upper limit of the therapeutic range is 2 ng/mL, there is some evidence to suggest that mortality in heart failure is improved at levels of 0.5 ng/mL to 0.8 ng/mL, although others suggest that 1 ng/mL to 2 ng/mL is an appropriate therapeutic range.
Because an indication for digoxin is cardiac dysrhythmias and digoxin toxicity may manifest as arrhythmias, monitor serum digoxin levels, especially given the narrow therapeutic index. Also, check digoxin levels in patients who have decreased renal function or who are taking medications known to interact with digoxin such as quinidine, amiodarone, verapamil, flecainide, and clarithromycin.
Patients receiving digoxin who present with hypokalemia should have a digoxin level drawn due to increased risk of toxicity.
Renal function directly affects digoxin level as decreased renal function will prolong the half life of digoxin and increase the time it takes the patient to reach a steady-state drug level. Premature steady-state monitoring may yield a falsely-low digoxin level. Digoxin is not removed by dialysis effectively, and the digoxin steady-state distribution volume may be reduced in chronic renal failure, leading to elevated digoxin levels.
Timing of Monitoring
The timing of this test is crucial, as specimens obtained too soon after dose administration do not reflect equilibration and may yield falsely high results. The specimen should be obtained 12 hours after a dose of digoxin or just before the next dose is due to be given.

Monitor digoxin levels when a patient initially starts this medication because the therapeutic index is small.

Suspected and known atrial tachycardia
Strength of Recommendation: Class IIa
Strength of Evidence: Category C
Results Interpretation:
Digoxin level high
Digitalis is the the drug most commonly associated with drug-induced focal atrial tachycardia (AT), which typically presents as AT with atrioventricular (AV) block. In these cases, consideration should be given to discontinuation of digitalis or the administration of digitalis-binding agents for persistent, advanced AV block. Multifocal atrial tachycardia, conversely, is most often observed in patients with underlying pulmonary disease, and is not usually due to digoxin toxicity.

Suspected digoxin toxicity
Strength of Recommendation: Class I
Strength of Evidence: Category C
Results Interpretation:
Digoxin level high
- Adults: Toxic level: >2.5 ng/mL (>3.2 nmol/L)
- Children: Toxic level: >3 ng/mL (>3.8 nmol/L)
- Cardiotoxicity has been reported with serum digoxin concentrations in the therapeutic range. Patients have survived with levels as high as 48 ng/mL, and deaths have been reported with levels as low as 3.5 ng/mL

DRUG/LAB INTERACTIONS
- Canrenoate - false increases or decreases in digoxin levels
- Capromab Pendetide - falsely high digoxin serum levels
- Chan Su - false increases in digoxin concentrations
- Cortisone - false increases in digoxin levels
- Dexamethasone - false increases in digoxin levels
- Digitoxin - false increases in digoxin levels
- Digoxin Immune Fab (Ovine) - false increases in digoxin levels
- Fludrocortisone - false increases in digoxin levels
- Fluorescein - invalid digoxin assay results
- Ginseng, American - false readings in digoxin concentrations
- Ginseng, Chinese - false readings in digoxin concentrations
- Ginseng, Siberian - false readings in digoxin concentrations
- Hydrocortisone - false increases in digoxin levels
- Kyushin - false increases in digoxin concentrations
- Methylprednisolone - false increases in digoxin levels
- Prednisolone - false increases in digoxin levels
- Prednisone - false increases in digoxin levels
- Progesterone - false increases in digoxin levels
- Spironolactone - false increases in digoxin levels
- Tan-Shen - false increases in digoxin concentrations

ABNORMAL RESULTS
- Results increased in:
    - Renal failure
    - Older patients
    - Hypothyroidism
- Results decreased in:
    - Pregnancy
    - Hyperparathyroidism
    - Physical activity prior to testing

COLLECTION/STORAGE INFORMATION
- In the outpatient setting, patients should not exercise for at least 1 hour prior to sample collection.
- Collect venous blood specimen in heparin or EDTA tube 8 to 12 hours after last dose or prior to next dose.
- Store sample at 2°C to 8°C for up to 24 hours or at -20°C for 1 to 2 weeks.

LOINC CODES
- Code: 29216-9 (*Short Name* - Digoxin Fld-mCnc)

Direct Coombs test

TEST DEFINITION
Detection of immunoglobulin and/or complement bound to red blood cells for the evaluation of antibody-induced hemolysis

SYNONYMS
- Anti-human globulin test, direct
- DAT - Direct antiglobulin test
- DCT - Direct Coombs test
- Direct antiglobulin test

REFERENCE RANGE
- Adults and Children: Negative
  Please refer to your institution's reference ranges as lab normals may vary.

INDICATIONS
Hemolytic uremic syndrome (HUS)
    Results Interpretation:
    Direct Coombs test negative
       Patients with typical hemolytic uremic syndrome (HUS) have Coombs' negative microangiopathic hemolytic anemia.
    Coombs positive hemolytic anemia
       Patients with pneumococcal-associated HUS may have a Coombs' positive hemolytic anemia.

Suspected autoimmune hemolytic anemia
    Strength of Recommendation: Class IIa
    Strength of Evidence: Category C
    Results Interpretation:
    Direct Coombs test positive
       A positive direct Coombs test is a characteristic finding in autoimmune hemolytic anemia. It demonstrates the presence of antibodies or complement on the red blood cell surface. The degree of the agglutination is proportional to the amount of antibody or complement on the RBCs, which correlates with the probability of hemolysis. To ascertain the hemolytic mechanism involved, further analysis of IgG or complement is indicated.
    Direct Coombs test negative
       A negative direct Coombs test occasionally occurs in patients with clinical evidence of autoimmune hemolysis due to rare incidences of IgA or IgM autoantibodies, low-affinity IgG autoantibodies, or low numbers of IgG antibodies below the sensitivity threshold for the routine manual test.

Suspected blood group antibody-antigen mismatch blood transfusion
    Strength of Recommendation: Class IIa
    Strength of Evidence: Category C
    Results Interpretation:
    Direct Coombs test positive
       A positive direct Coombs test is diagnostic of immune hemolytic anemias, the most severe type being acute intravascular hemolysis after ABO incompatible RBC transfusion. The positive direct Coombs test identifies the presence of antibodies to red blood cell surface antigens. Further identification of the specific antigen requires additional studies.

Suspected cold autoimmune hemolytic anemia
    Strength of Recommendation: Class IIa
    Strength of Evidence: Category C

Results Interpretation:
Direct Coombs test positive

In cold hemagglutinin disease, a positive direct Coombs test indicates the presence of IgM autoantibodies that temporarily bind to red blood cells, activate complement, and lead to the deposition of complement factor C3 on the cell surface. The IgM antibodies are usually monoclonal and secondary to lymphoprolifer-ative disorders. These antibodies react with RBCs at temperatures below 37°C, causing hemolysis.

The direct Coombs test is always positive with anti-C3 and should be negative with anti-IgG in cold auto-immune hemolytic anemia.

Suspected hemolytic disease of the newborn due to ABO immunization
Strength of Recommendation: Class IIa
Strength of Evidence: Category B
Results Interpretation:
Direct Coombs test positive

A positive direct Coombs test is seen in hemolytic disease of the newborn due to ABO incompatibility, when the mother is group O and baby is group A or B. A positive direct Coombs test, in combination with an increased reticulocyte count and a sibling with neonatal jaundice, is a good predictor of severe hemolytic disease of the newborn in ABO incompatibility. A positive direct Coombs test may occur in newborns with ABO incompatibility but no hemolysis.
Direct Coombs test negative

A negative direct Coombs test can occur in newborns with significant hemolysis due to causes other than ABO incompatibility.

Suspected paroxysmal cold hemoglobinuria
Strength of Recommendation: Class IIa
Strength of Evidence: Category C
Results Interpretation:
Direct Coombs test positive

A positive direct Coombs test is found in paroxysmal cold hemoglobinuria, indicating complement coating of anti-P antibodies (ie, Donath-Landsteiner antibodies) on the red blood cell surface when anti-C3d reagents are used.
Direct Coombs test negative

Direct Coombs test using anti-IgG alone may be negative in paroxysmal cold hemoglobinuria.

DRUG/LAB INTERACTIONS

- Clavulanic Acid - a false positive Coombs' test
- Ticarcillin - a false positive Coombs' test

ABNORMAL RESULTS

- Results increased in:
    - Hypergammaglobulinemia

CLINICAL NOTES

A direct Coombs test is important in establishing immune hemolysis, but for differential diagnosis an extended work-up is required which includes: elution, autoabsorptions, serum studies to detect alloantibodies, and the uti-lization of drugs and/or drug-treated reagent cells to test serum/eluate.

COLLECTION/STORAGE INFORMATION

- Specimen Collection and Handling:
    - Collect specimen in an EDTA, lavender top tube and separate red cells to prevent uptake of complement components.
    - Avoid clotted blood if possible. If clotted blood is used, store specimen at 37°C until cells separate.
    - May store specimen at 4°C for 1 week.

Direct burn culture

TEST DEFINITION

Detection and isolation of microorganism(s) from a burn site to monitor for bacterial colonization and infection

REFERENCE RANGE
- Adults and Children: Negative
  Please refer to your institution's reference ranges as lab normals may vary.

INDICATIONS
Suspected bacterial infection of skin in burn patients
  Strength of Recommendation: Class IIa
  Strength of Evidence: Category B
  Results Interpretation:
  Positive microbiology findings
  A positive wound surface culture provides both quantitative and qualitative information regarding bacterial colonization; however wound biopsy is more useful in diagnosing infection. Any clinical evidence of a wound infection should be confirmed with a burn wound biopsy and examined histologically to rule out invasion of bacteria into the underlying tissue.
  The most common bacteria cultured are Staphylococcus, Streptococcus, and Pseudomonas. Bacteroides fragilis, other gram-negative enteric rods, and group D streptococcus are frequently cultured from burns around the anus.
  Timing of Monitoring
  While skin cultures have often been obtained in the first 24 hours of treatment following burns, early specimen testing has not been shown to affect therapy significantly, and adds to the cost.

ABNORMAL RESULTS
- Results increased in:
  - Sampling taken from pooled secretions or exudate or sloughing eschar (overgrowth)
  - Prolonged incubation of swab in transport media prior to analysis
- Results decreased in:
  - Sampling taken from a nonrepresentative desiccated area or area with residual topical agent (undergrowth)
  - Delay in transport to lab

CLINICAL NOTES
  Monitoring for bacterial colonization using surface culture techniques is useful, but infected areas should be biopsied, evaluated histologically, and cultured quantitiatively. Subeschar microorganism proliferation which can result in invasion of viable tissue is not accessible to surface culture; therefore, wound biopsy should also be performed to determine and diagnose the presence of a wound infection.
  The most commonly isolated pathogens from burn sites are S aureus including methicillin-sensitive and methicillin-resistant strains, Candida spp. Enterococcus spp, Pseudomonas aeruginosa, various gram-negative rods of the family Enterobacteriaceae, Streptococcus agalactiae and Streptococcus dysgalactiae.

COLLECTION/STORAGE INFORMATION
- Specimen Collection and Handling:
  - Swab burn site.
  - Collect as much fluid as possible in sterile tube or syringe.
  - Transport specimen to lab as soon as possible.

LOINC CODES
- Code: 17938-2 (*Short Name* - Burn Cult org #3)
- Code: 17941-6 (*Short Name* - Burn Cult org #6)
- Code: 17940-8 (*Short Name* - Burn Cult org #5)
- Code: 17937-4 (*Short Name* - Burn Cult org #2)
- Code: 17939-0 (*Short Name* - Burn Cult org #4)
- Code: 603-1 (*Short Name* - Burn Cult)

Direct fluorescent antibody test for syphilis

TEST DEFINITION
  Direct microscopic detection of *Treponema pallidum* in tissues, body fluids or lesions for the diagnosis of primary and congenital syphilis

SYNONYMS
- DFA-TP test

REFERENCE RANGE
- Adults and children: negative
  Please refer to your institution's reference ranges as lab normals may vary.

INDICATIONS
Suspected syphilis
   Strength of Recommendation: Class IIa
   Strength of Evidence: Category B
   Results Interpretation:
   Positive microbiology findings
      Detection of *T. pallidum* by direct fluorescent antibody microscopy is considered diagnostic for early and congenital syphilis.
   Negative microbiology findings
      A negative direct fluorescent antibody (DFA) test does not exclude the diagnosis of syphilis, since results may be affected by sample quality, storage and transport conditions, and laboratory technique.

CLINICAL NOTES
   Unlike darkfield examination, organism motility is not a requirement for adequate identification of *Treponema pallidum* by direct fluorescent antibody (DFA) examination.

COLLECTION/STORAGE INFORMATION
   Encrusted or obviously contaminated specimens should be cleansed with tap water or physiologic saline using a minimum amount of water, in order to prevent organism dilution. Antiseptics or soaps should be avoided.

LOINC CODES
- Code: 9826-9 (*Short Name* - T pallidum Ab CSF Ql IF)
- Code: 17727-9 (*Short Name* - T pallidum IgG Ser IF-aCnc)
- Code: 17729-5 (*Short Name* - T pallidum IgM Ser Ql IF)
- Code: 5393-4 (*Short Name* - T pallidum Ab Ser Ql IF)
- Code: 17728-7 (*Short Name* - T pallidum IgM Ser IF-aCnc)
- Code: 17726-1 (*Short Name* - T pallidum IgG Ser Ql IF)
- Code: 34382-2 (*Short Name* - T pallidum Ab Titr Ser IF)
- Code: 17724-6 (*Short Name* - T pallidum Ab Ser IF-aCnc)
- Code: 29310-0 (*Short Name* - T pallidum XXX Ql IF)
- Code: 13288-6 (*Short Name* - T pallidum Ab Bld IF-aCnc)

Disopyramide measurement

TEST DEFINITION
   Measurement of disopyramide levels in serum for the monitoring of antiarrhythmic therapy

REFERENCE RANGE
   Therapeutic range for atrial arrhythmia: 2.8-3.2 mcg/mL (8.2-9.4 micromol/L)
   Therapeutic range for ventricular arrhythmia: 3.3-7.5 mcg/mL (9.7-22.1 micromol/L)
   Please refer to your institution's reference ranges as lab normals may vary.

INDICATIONS
Monitoring of disopyramide treatment
   Results Interpretation:
   Blood drug levels - finding
      Disopyramide levels of 2.8 to 3.2 mcg/mL for atrial arrhythmias and 3.3 to 7.5 mcg/mL for ventricular arrhythmias are considered therapeutic.
      Therapeutic blood levels of disopyramide are crucial to the success of antiarrhythmic therapy, and can be used as an indicator of patient compliance.

Serum levels of disopyramide below the lower analytical range of the assay should be investigated further for the possibility of inappropriate collection technique or mixed samples.

Timing of Monitoring

Specimen should be collected at trough concentration. Peak levels occur within 1 to 1.5 hours of ingestion of rapid-release medication, and 4.7 to 5.6 hours of sustained-release.

Suspected disopyramide toxicity
  Results Interpretation:
  Blood drug levels - finding

Serum levels of disopyramide greater than 7 mcg/mL may be toxic.

Protein binding of disopyramide is non-linear and concentration-dependent. This indicates that a given dosage increase would not yield a proportional increase in free fraction and, therefore, may not be predictive of toxicity.

COLLECTION/STORAGE INFORMATION

- Specimen Collection and Handling:
  - Collect specimen in an EDTA (lavender) or heparin (green) tube.
  - Collect at trough concentration.

LOINC CODES

- Code: 16780-9 (*Short Name* - Disopyramide Ur-mCnc)
- Code: 14702-5 (*Short Name* - Disopyramide SerPl-sCnc)
- Code: 29401-7 (*Short Name* - Disopyramide Gast-mCnc)
- Code: 12366-1 (*Short Name* - Disopyramide Ur Ql)
- Code: 29217-7 (*Short Name* - Disopyramide Fld-mCnc)
- Code: 3576-6 (*Short Name* - Disopyramide SerPl-mCnc)
- Code: 13558-2 (*Short Name* - Disopyramide SerPl Ql)

Disseminated intravascular coagulation screen

TEST DEFINITION

Measurement of selected blood coagulation tests for the evaluation of disseminated intravascular coagulation (DIC)

SYNONYMS

- Blood coagulation panel, DIC
- Consumptive coagulopathy screen
- DIC - Disseminated intravascular coagulation screen
- DIC screen
- Disseminated intravascular coagulation screening
- Disseminated intravascular coagulation screening panel

INDICATIONS

Ovarian hyperstimulation syndrome
  Results Interpretation:
  Increased prothrombin time

Ovarian hyperstimulation syndrome is associated with abnormal coagulation studies, including a prolonged prothrombin time.

  Increased partial thromboplastin time

Ovarian hyperstimulation syndrome is associated with abnormal coagulation studies, including a prolonged partial thromboplastin time.

Suspected and known disseminated intravascular coagulation (DIC)
    Strength of Recommendation: Class IIa
    Strength of Evidence: Category B

Results Interpretation:
Abnormal hematology findings

The diagnosis of DIC should be based on clinical and global coagulation tests in addition to a screening assay, when available, to assess intravascular soluble fibrin formation or fibrin degradation products (FDP). Global coagulation tests, however, may lack sufficient sensitivity to diagnose early DIC, and are less reliable diagnostic markers in patients with chronic or recurrent inflammatory conditions, liver impairment, ischemia-reperfusion disorders, and impaired nutritional states.

- The International Society on Thrombosis and Haemostasis recommends a 5-point algorithm system for diagnosing overt DIC. A score of greater than or equal to 5 is compatible with overt DIC, while a score of less than 5 is suggestive of, but not diagnostic for, non-overt (early) DIC. Daily testing is recommended for a score of 5 or above, and repeat testing in 1 to 2 days is recommended for a score of less than 5:
  - Platelet count: greater than 100,000/microL = 0 points; less than 100,000/microL = 1 point; less than 50,000/microL = 2 points
  - Elevated fibrin-related marker (eg, soluble fibrin monomers, FDP): no increase = 0 points; moderate increase = 2 points; strong increase = 3 points
  - Prolonged prothrombin time (PT): less than 3 seconds = 0 points; greater than 3 seconds but less than 6 seconds = 1 point; greater than 6 seconds = 2 points
  - Fibrinogen: greater than 1 g/L = 0 points; less than 1 g/L = 1 point
- A proposed 8-point scoring system for diagnosing DIC gives 1 point each for the following events: a disease associated with fulminant DIC; thrombohemorrhagic events; elevated PT, PTT, or thrombin time; thrombocytopenia less than 130,000/microL; fibrinogen less than 150 mg/dL; FDP greater than 10 mcg/mL; D-dimer greater than 0.25 mcg/mL; and decreased antithrombin (AT) less than 75%. A score of 5 points or above suggests a diagnosis of DIC.
- Another proposed system for determining a laboratory diagnosis of DIC requires documentation of at least one abnormal finding from group I, group II, and group III and at least 2 abnormal findings from group IV:
  - Group I (indicates procoagulant activation):
    - Elevated prothrombin fragment 1+2
    - Elevated fibrinopeptide A
    - Elevated fibrinopeptide B
    - Elevated thrombin-antithrombin (TAT) complex
    - Elevated D-dimer
  - Group II (indicates fibrinolytic action):
    - Elevated D-dimer
    - Elevated FDP
    - Elevated plasmin
    - Elevated plasmin-antiplasmin complex
  - Group III (indicates inhibitor consumption):
    - Decreased antithrombin-III
    - Decreased alpha-2-antiplasmin
    - Decreased heparin cofactor II
    - Decreased protein C or S
    - Elevated TAT complex
    - Elevated plasmin-antiplasmin complex
  - Group IV (indicates end-organ damage or failure):
    - Elevated LDH
    - Elevated creatinine
    - Decreased pH
    - Decreased PaO2

Suspected and known toxic shock syndrome
Results Interpretation:
Blood coagulation disorder

DIC may develop in streptococcal toxic shock syndrome (TSS). Isolated aPTT prolongation has also been reported, suggesting that kallikrein-kinin system activation leading to bradykinin release may occur and contribute to several key features of this syndrome.

In staphylococcal TSS, evidence of DIC has been rarely reported with the associated findings of prolonged prothrombin and partial thromboplastin times, decreased fibrinogen, and increased fibrin split products.

COMMON PANELS
- Disseminated intravascular coagulation screen

Drugs of abuse urine screening test

TEST DEFINITION
Screening of urine for detection of drugs of abuse

REFERENCE RANGE
- Adults and children: Negative
  Please refer to your institution's reference ranges as lab normals may vary.

INDICATIONS
Known or suspected substance abuse
>**Strength of Recommendation:** Class IIa
>**Strength of Evidence:** Category B
>**Results Interpretation:**
>**Urine drug levels - finding**
>   A positive urine drug screen is generally qualitative, intended only to verify exposure to the assayed substances. Drug screening provides no information regarding degree of functional impairment or the timing, chronicity, route or quantity of exposure. In cases where the integrity of the results is in doubt, confirmatory testing is indicated. Results must be evaluated in conjunction with clinical assessment and patient history. A negative test does not eliminate the possibility of substance abuse. If drug abuse is suspected a referral for counseling and treatment may be appropriate even in the presence of a negative urine screen.
>   The threshold concentration or cutoff value for each substance measured varies by laboratory, method, and specific test; the threshold concentration does not specify the sensitivity or detection limit of the assay. Evaluation of results is aided by an understanding of the drugs screened and the cutoff thresholds used for each substance.

COMMON PANELS
- Drugs of abuse testing, urine

COLLECTION/STORAGE INFORMATION
- Ensure proper chain of custody as appropriate.

Duchenne/Becker muscular dystrophy DNA detection

TEST DEFINITION
Evaluation of gene mutations and dystrophin abnormalities in whole blood and tissue for the identification of Duchenne/Becker variant muscular dystrophies.

SYNONYMS
- Duchenne muscular dystrophy carrier detection
- Genetic detection of Duchenne/Becker muscular dystrophy

REFERENCE RANGE
- Negative for gene mutation or dystrophin abnormality
  Please refer to your institution's reference ranges as lab normals may vary.

INDICATIONS
Patients with, and carriers of, suspected Duchenne or Becker muscular dystrophy
>**Strength of Recommendation:** Class IIa
>**Strength of Evidence:** Category B

Results Interpretation:
X-linked muscular dystrophy with abnormal dystrophin
   Southern blot and PCR analysis are diagnostic in the 65% of Duchenne and Becker muscular dystrophy patients who have detectable mutations. Because the absence of a detectable abnormality does not rule out the diagnosis, further testing is warranted in the remaining 35% of patients with no detectable mutations.
   Patients with Duchenne muscular dystrophy have no detectable dystrophin; those with Becker muscular dystrophy have abnormal quantities of, or abnormally sized, dystrophin.

COLLECTION/STORAGE INFORMATION
- Collect whole blood in yellow top (ACD) or lavender top (EDTA) tube.
- Preserve blood sample at 4°C if not processed immediately.
- Immediately freeze muscle tissue at -70°C (skeletal, smooth or cardiac muscle).

LOINC CODES
- Code: 21247-2 (*Short Name* - DMD Gene Mut Anal)
- Code: 22075-6 (*Short Name* - DMD Gene Mut Tested)

Eastern equine encephalitis virus antibody assay

TEST DEFINITION
   Measurement of eastern equine encephalitis virus serology in serum for the evaluation of viral infection

SYNONYMS
- Serologic test for Eastern equine encephalitis virus

REFERENCE RANGE
- Negative
   Please refer to your institution's reference ranges as lab normals may vary.

INDICATIONS
Suspected Eastern equine encephalitis
      Strength of Recommendation: Class IIb
      Strength of Evidence: Category C
   Results Interpretation:
   Serology positive
      A single positive Eastern equine encephalitis (EEE)-specific IgM antibody level with IgM antibody-capture enzyme-linked immunosorbent assay (MAC-ELISA) found in cerebrospinal fluid (CSF) is sufficient to confirm an EEE central nervous system infection.
      The presence of EEE-specific IgM identified by enzyme-linked immunoassay (EIA)/MAC-ELISA testing plus a EEE-positive IgG antibody in the same or a later specimen by another serologic assay (eg, neutralization or hemagglutination) is diagnostic for EEE disease.
      A 4-fold or greater change in a PRNT antibody titer in paired sera specimens is diagnostic for EEE disease.
      Complement fixation titers greater than or equal to 1:8 and hemagglutination inhibition titers greater than or equal to 1:10 are suggestive of EEE. A 4-fold increase in antibody levels between sera of acute and convalescent stage is confirmatory.
      A specimen (collected within 45 days of symptom onset) that is positive for IgG but negative for IgM, may indicate a past infection.
      Some laboratory methods demonstrate cross-reactivity between the various arboviruses. Therefore, IgM testing may yield more specific results than IgG.
   Timing of Monitoring
      Serum specimens should be collected at disease onset and 2 to 4 weeks later for acute and convalescent specimen analysis.
      IgG antibodies to arboviruses are increased by the 12th day following symptom onset and can persist for years after the acute infection.

CLINICAL NOTES

Laboratory workers involved in the isolation of eastern equine encephalitis virus are at risk for a serious infection.

COLLECTION/STORAGE INFORMATION

- Obtain the serum sample at the onset of disease and after a time period of 2 to 4 weeks.
- Freeze the sample if testing is delayed.

LOINC CODES

- Code: 10899-3 (*Short Name* - EEEV IgM Titr CSF IF)
- Code: 10898-5 (*Short Name* - EEEV IgM Titr Ser IF)
- Code: 29811-7 (*Short Name* - EEEV IgG Ser QI IF)
- Code: 7860-0 (*Short Name* - EEEV IgG Ser-aCnc)
- Code: 22257-0 (*Short Name* - EEEV Ab Titr Ser)
- Code: 13229-0 (*Short Name* - EEEV IgM CSF-aCnc)
- Code: 22258-8 (*Short Name* - EEEV IgG Titr CSF)
- Code: 10896-9 (*Short Name* - EEEV IgG Titr Ser IF)
- Code: 29785-3 (*Short Name* - EEEV IgG XXX QI IF)
- Code: 24287-5 (*Short Name* - EEEV Ab sp1 Titr Ser)
- Code: 22255-4 (*Short Name* - EEEV Ab CSF QI)
- Code: 22259-6 (*Short Name* - EEEV IgG Titr Ser)
- Code: 23044-1 (*Short Name* - EEEV Ab Ser QI Nt)
- Code: 20793-6 (*Short Name* - EEEV Ab Ser QI CF)
- Code: 22256-2 (*Short Name* - EEEV Ab Ser QI)
- Code: 24288-3 (*Short Name* - EEEV Ab #2 Titr Ser)
- Code: 7861-8 (*Short Name* - EEEV IgM Ser-aCnc)
- Code: 13918-8 (*Short Name* - EEEV Ab Titr Ser IF)
- Code: 20792-8 (*Short Name* - EEEV Ab CSF QI IF)
- Code: 23042-5 (*Short Name* - EEEV Ab Titr Ser HAI)
- Code: 20794-4 (*Short Name* - EEEV Ab CSF QI CF)
- Code: 10897-7 (*Short Name* - EEEV IgG Titr CSF IF)
- Code: 5134-2 (*Short Name* - EEEV Ab Ser-aCnc)
- Code: 23043-3 (*Short Name* - EEEV Ab Ser QI Aggl)
- Code: 20795-1 (*Short Name* - EEEV Ab Titr Ser Nt)
- Code: 23046-6 (*Short Name* - EEEV IgM Ser QI)
- Code: 29824-0 (*Short Name* - EEEV IgG XXX QI)
- Code: 13228-2 (*Short Name* - EEEV IgG CSF-aCnc)
- Code: 29848-9 (*Short Name* - EEEV IgG Ser QI)
- Code: 23045-8 (*Short Name* - EEEV IgM Ser QI EIA)
- Code: 29836-4 (*Short Name* - EEEV IgG CSF QI)
- Code: 22260-4 (*Short Name* - EEEV IgM Titr CSF)
- Code: 22261-2 (*Short Name* - EEEV IgM Titr Ser)
- Code: 24006-9 (*Short Name* - EEEV Ab Ser-Imp)

Endometrial cytology

TEST DEFINITION

Cytologic evaluation of an endometrial specimen to identify endometrial abnormalities

REFERENCE RANGE

- Negative cytologic examination
  Please refer to your institution's reference ranges as lab normals may vary.

INDICATIONS

Suspected endometrial carcinoma
Strength of Recommendation: Class IIa
Strength of Evidence: Category B

Results Interpretation:
Abnormal cytology specimen findings from female genital organs
Smears showing tumor diathesis, containing histiocyte aggregates with nuclear debris, leukocytes and degenerated tumor cells in the background indicate malignancy. In addition, the architecture of the endometrial tissue fragments is abnormal in endometrial carcinoma.

Suspected endometrial hyperplasia
    Strength of Recommendation: Class IIa
    Strength of Evidence: Category B
Results Interpretation:
Abnormal cytology specimen findings from female genital organs
Cytologic features of endometrial hyperplasia without atypia may be similar to disordered proliferative endometrium. Hyperplasia has more bulbous, 3-dimensional papillary clusters and lesser straight tubules compared with disordered proliferative endometrium.

Atypical hyperplasia shows nuclear atypia, which includes nuclear hyperchromatism, pleomorphism, prominent nucleoli, and a large nuclear/cytoplasmic ratio. Several bulbous and 3-dimensional papillary clusters may be seen on the smears.

COLLECTION/STORAGE INFORMATION
- Specimen Collection and Handling
  - Endometrial Brush Biopsy:
    - Place brush into fixative solution (eg, CytoRich Red® solution, PreservCyt® solution); cut brush if necessary. Alternatively, place brush in fixative solution and vigorously rotate several times and remove brush.
    - Tissue fragments can be removed by fine forceps and placed in the fixative to be used as a cell block or mini-biopsy.
    - Deliver to histology laboratory for further processing.
  - Endometrial Suction Catheter:
    - Fix sample in formalin.
    - Deliver to histology laboratory for further processing.

Endomysial antibody measurement

TEST DEFINITION
Detection of antiendomysial antibodies in serum for the evaluation and management of celiac disease and dermatitis herpetiformis

SYNONYMS
- Endomysium antibody level

REFERENCE RANGE
- Negative
Please refer to your institution's reference ranges as lab normals may vary.

INDICATIONS
Suspected and known celiac disease
    Strength of Recommendation: Class IIa
    Strength of Evidence: Category B
Results Interpretation:
Serology positive
There is a positive correlation between IgA-EMA titers and the severity of intestinal villous atrophy. High rates of positivity generally reflect more severe villous atrophy, whereas patients with milder villous atrophy are less likely to have a positive IgA-EMA test.

EMA titers respond to a gluten-free diet and levels are typically not detectable in serum after 6 to 12 months on such a diet; however, if initial titers were high, it may take up to 31 months until levels become undetectable.

False Results

In celiac disease, false negative EMA results may occur in patients with mild enteropathy, IgA deficiency, and in children less than 2 years of age.

Suspected dermatitis herpetiformis (DH)
    Strength of Recommendation: Class IIa
    Strength of Evidence: Category B
Results Interpretation:
Serology positive

Endomysial antibody (EMA) assays are both sensitive and specific for dermatitis herpetiformis (DH). In addition to being minimally invasive studies, serological tests for EMA are useful in DH diagnosis when performed in conjunction with direct immunofluorescence of skin biopsy specimens.

There is a positive correlation between the presence of EMA and the severity of villous atrophy in DH patients. In addition, IgA-EMA titers respond to gluten dietary intake, and thus serum levels are useful for monitoring clinical response to dietary treatment as opposed to repeat jejunal biopsy.

In one study, the prevalence of EMA in the DH subjects was approximately 65%. This data suggests that EMA serology has limited utility as a screening test for DH and jejunal biopsy may be necessary for accurate diagnosis. There is generally less jejunal involvement associated with DH than in celiac disease and this may account for the lower incidence of EMA in DH patients.

COLLECTION/STORAGE INFORMATION

- Collect serum and store specimen at -20°C

Entamoeba histolytica antibody assay

TEST DEFINITION

Detection of serum antibodies to *Entamoeba histolytica* for the diagnosis of amebiasis

SYNONYMS

- Entameba histolytica antibody assay

REFERENCE RANGE

- <1:64 titer
  Please refer to your institution's reference ranges as lab normals may vary.

INDICATIONS

Suspected amebic liver abscess
    Strength of Recommendation: Class IIa
    Strength of Evidence: Category B
Results Interpretation:
Positive immunology findings

Serology is helpful in making the diagnosis of amebic liver abscess; antibodies are present in 70% to 80% of patients at the time of initial presentation.

Serology has a high specificity for amebic liver abscess.

IgM may be better at diagnosing acute infection, whereas IgG may be a better indicator of prior exposure.

Suspected intestinal amebiasis
    Strength of Recommendation: Class IIb
    Strength of Evidence: Category C
Results Interpretation:
Positive immunology findings

While some experts recommend that serology not be used for the routine diagnosis of intestinal amebiasis, others state that the diagnosis should be made by positive serology and the presence of *Entamoeba histolytica* DNA or antigen in the stool.

Many serologic tests have detectable titers up to 2 years after treatment, making it difficult to distinguish acute from prior infection; consequently, diagnosis by serology is particularly problematic in endemic areas.

The sensitivity of serology for the diagnosis of amebic colitis is higher during the convalescent phase of illness.

CLINICAL NOTES
False-positive results are minimized when *Entamoeba histolytica* antibody titers exceed 1:256.

COLLECTION/STORAGE INFORMATION
- Collect acute and convalescent serum specimens in marble-top tubes, approximately 2 to 3 weeks apart.
- May store at $-20°C$

LOINC CODES
- Code: 16820-3 (*Short Name* - E histolyt Ab Ser CF-aCnc)
- Code: 22287-7 (*Short Name* - E histolyt IgA Ser-aCnc)
- Code: 27090-0 (*Short Name* - E histolyt IgA Sal QI)
- Code: 9523-2 (*Short Name* - E histolyt IgM Ser EIA-aCnc)
- Code: 16817-9 (*Short Name* - E histolyt Ab Ser QI ID)
- Code: 16819-5 (*Short Name* - E histolyt Ab Ser IF-aCnc)
- Code: 22289-3 (*Short Name* - E histolyt IgM Ser-aCnc)
- Code: 21259-7 (*Short Name* - E histolyt Ab Titr Ser HA)
- Code: 25400-3 (*Short Name* - E histolyt Ab Titr Ser IF)
- Code: 16818-7 (*Short Name* - E histolyt Ab CSF-aCnc)
- Code: 22285-1 (*Short Name* - E histolyt Ab Ser QI)
- Code: 9420-1 (*Short Name* - E histolyt Ab Titr Ser CF)
- Code: 9521-6 (*Short Name* - E histolyt IgA Ser EIA-aCnc)
- Code: 5151-6 (*Short Name* - E histolyt Ab Ser HA-aCnc)
- Code: 9421-9 (*Short Name* - E histolyt Ab Ser ID-aCnc)
- Code: 9522-4 (*Short Name* - E histolyt IgG Ser EIA-aCnc)
- Code: 22286-9 (*Short Name* - E histolyt Ab Titr Ser)
- Code: 22288-5 (*Short Name* - E histolyt IgG Ser-aCnc)

Entamoeba histolytica antigen assay

TEST DEFINITION
Detection of *Entamoeba histolytica* antigen in stool and serum for the diagnosis and management of amoebiasis

SYNONYMS
- Entameba histolytica antigen assay

REFERENCE RANGE
- Adults and children: negative assay
  Please refer to your institution's reference ranges as lab normals may vary.

INDICATIONS
Suspected amoebic dysentery
> **Strength of Recommendation:** Class IIa
> **Strength of Evidence:** Category B
> **Results Interpretation:**
> **Raised microbiology findings**
> Positive findings of *Entamoeba histolytica* antigen in serum and stool, when associated with acute and chronic diarrhea, abdominal pain, and tenesmus, are often diagnostic for *E histolytica* dysentery.
> If *Entamoeba dispar* is the only organism identified, treatment is unnecessary, and in persons with gastrointestinal symptoms, other causes should be investigated. In asymptomatic individuals, treatment is not appropriate unless *E histolytica* has been specifically identified or is highly suspected. Optimally *E histolytica* should be specifically identified and treated, if present.
> *E histolytica* antigens are present in serum during invasive amoebiasis and clear within 1 week after treatment.

Suspected amoebic liver abscess
> **Strength of Recommendation:** Class IIa
> **Strength of Evidence:** Category B

Results Interpretation:
Positive immunology findings
The presence of *Entamoeba histolytica* antigen in serum is indicative of active infection; this finding, when associated with a clinically enlarged and tender liver, toxemia, and a palpable abscess yielding 'anchovy sauce' pus on aspiration, is often diagnostic for *E histolytica* liver abscess.
E histolytica antigens are present in serum during invasive amoebiasis and clear within 1 week after treatment.

CLINICAL NOTES
The ability to distinguish between intestinal infection with *Entamoeba histolytica* and the non-pathogenic *Entamoeba dispar* will be determined by the antisera of the testing kit used.
Antigen tests are limited to fresh or frozen stool specimens.

LOINC CODES
- Code: 6399-0 (*Short Name* - E histolyt Ag XXX EIA-aCnc)
- Code: 31812-1 (*Short Name* - E histolyt Ag XXX-aCnc)
- Code: 29905-7 (*Short Name* - E histolyt Ag Stl Ql EIA)
- Code: 6398-2 (*Short Name* - E histolyt Ag Stl EIA-aCnc)

Enterovirus culture

TEST DEFINITION
Detection of enterovirus in cerebrospinal fluid (CSF) and other body fluids for the evaluation of enterovirus infection

REFERENCE RANGE
- Adults and children: no growth
  Please refer to your institution's reference ranges as lab normals may vary.

INDICATIONS
Suspected enterovirus meningitis
   Strength of Recommendation: Class IIa
   Strength of Evidence: Category B
   Results Interpretation:
   Positive microbiology findings
   The presence of an enteroviral cytopathic effect (CPE) on cell culture of cerebrospinal fluid, or isolation of enterovirus from the stool or throat in conjunction with a positive serology to the same serotype, supports the diagnosis of enterovirus meningitis.

CLINICAL NOTES
Enteroviral cytopathic effects in cell culture may be evident within the first 24 to 48 hours after inoculation, while most cytopathic responses will be occur within one week.

COLLECTION/STORAGE INFORMATION
- Specimen Collection and Handling:
  - Obtain specimen during acute phase of illness.
  - Transport and process immediately.
  - May be refrigerated for a short time.
  - A minimum volume of 0.5 mL of cerebrospinal fluid is typically required, while 1 mL is preferred.

LOINC CODES
- Code: 5843-8 (*Short Name* - EV XXX Cult)
- Code: 5842-0 (*Short Name* - EV Stl Cult)
- Code: 5839-6 (*Short Name* - EV CSF Cult)

Enterovirus polymerase chain reaction

TEST DEFINITION

Rapid detection of enterovirus RNA in cerebrospinal fluid (CSF) (most commonly), blood, urine, lymph nodes and myocardium

SYNONYMS

- Enterovirus ribonucleic acid detection
- Enterovirus RNA assay
- PCR test for enterovirus

REFERENCE RANGE

- Adults and children: No enterovirus genome detected
  Please refer to your institution's reference ranges as lab normals may vary.

INDICATIONS

Suspected enteroviral meningitis
  Strength of Recommendation: Class IIa
  Strength of Evidence: Category B
  Results Interpretation:
  Polymerase chain reaction observation
  A positive polymerase chain reaction assay confirms the diagnosis of enteroviral meningitis.

Suspected hand, foot, and mouth disease due to enterovirus 71 (EV71) infection
  Strength of Recommendation: Class IIb
  Strength of Evidence: Category B
  Results Interpretation:
  Polymerase chain reaction observation
  In one outbreak, polymerase chain reaction assay genotypically identified enterovirus 71 directly from a broad range of clinical specimens 71% of the time, which was statistically superior to viral cell culture.

CLINICAL NOTES

Although polymerase chain reaction testing is expensive, it appears to be cost-effective, with savings related to shorter hospital stays.

COLLECTION/STORAGE INFORMATION

- Specimen Collection and Handling:
  - Collect cerebrospinal fluid samples in a glass or plastic tube
  - Use an EDTA tube for blood samples
  - Store samples at −80°C

LOINC CODES

- Code: 27952-1 (*Short Name* - EV RNA CSF QI Prb)
- Code: 29591-5 (*Short Name* - EV RNA XXX QI PCR)
- Code: 29558-4 (*Short Name* - EV RNA CSF QI PCR)

Eosinophil count

TEST DEFINITION

Measurement of eosinophils in whole blood for the evaluation and management of allergic, hematologic, and infectious diseases, as well as parasitic infestations

SYNONYMS

- Eosinophil count - observation

REFERENCE RANGE

- Adults:
- Relative: 0%-8%
- Absolute: 0-0.45 cells X 10^9 /L
- Neonates, birth to 28 days :
- Absolute: 0-0.9 X 10^3 cells/microL
- Infants, 1 week to 6 months :
- Absolute: 0.2-0.3 X 10^3 cells/microL
- Infants, 1 year:
- Relative: 2.6%
- Absolute: 0.3 X 10^3 cells/microL
- Infants, 2 years :
- Absolute: 0-0.7 X 10^3 cells/microL
- Children, 4 to 10 years:
- Relative: 2.4%-2.8%
- Absolute: 0-0.6 X 10^3 cells/microL
  Please refer to your institution's reference ranges as lab normals may vary.

INDICATIONS

Evaluation of asthma severity
   Strength of Recommendation: Class IIa
   Strength of Evidence: Category B
   Results Interpretation:
   Eosinophil count - finding
      The eosinophil count is normally only 2% to 3%, but in asthmatics, the count may be elevated to 5% or more, and the absolute total eosinophil count may increase to more than 350/mm^3.
      Elevated eosinophil count in asthma is a marker of severity and risk of death. Eosinophilia persisting after bronchodilator therapy is a strong marker for increased risk of subsequent death.
      Acute asthma exacerbations may be associated with decreased eosinophil counts, which correlate with decreases in arterial oxygen tension (PaO2).
      Eosinophilia is associated with the development of Churg-Strauss syndrome (systemic vasculitis) in asthmatics.

HIV/AIDS
   Strength of Recommendation: Class IIb
   Strength of Evidence: Category B
   Results Interpretation:
   Eosinophil count raised
      Eosinophilia in HIV infection is associated with a high incidence of cutaneous disease (eg, atopic dermatitis, eosinophilic pustular folliculitis) but not with other conditions commonly associated with eosinophilia (eg, parasitic infections, malignancy, allergic reactions). Therefore, extensive work-up for asymptomatic eosinophilia in HIV-infected persons with cutaneous disease is probably unwarranted.
      In HIV infection, eosinophil counts increase as CD4 cell counts decrease; therefore, eosinophilia may be prompted by HIV infection itself as other cell components decline.

Suspected anisakiasis
   Results Interpretation:
   Eosinophil count raised
      Modest eosinophilia from 30% to 40% is a common finding in patients with gastric anisakiasis. Eosinophil counts are normal with intestinal involvement.

Suspected atopic dermatitis
   Strength of Recommendation: Class IIb
   Strength of Evidence: Category B
   Results Interpretation:
   Eosinophil count raised
      Eosinophilia is associated with atopic dermatitis, particularly in conjunction with respiratory allergic disease.
      Elevated eosinophil counts during infancy is predictive of allergic disease during the first six years of life.

Suspected hypereosinophilic syndrome
    Strength of Recommendation: Class I
    Strength of Evidence: Category C
Results Interpretation:
Eosinophil count raised
    In the absence of other known causes, absolute eosinophil counts at or above 1500 cells/microL sustained for at least 6 months, in conjunction with organ damage, may be classified as hypereosinophilic syndrome.

Suspected schistosomiasis
    Strength of Recommendation: Class IIb
    Strength of Evidence: Category C
Results Interpretation:
Eosinophil count raised
    During the acute phase of schistosomal infection, eosinophilia may be as high as 70%.
    In nonimmune travelers, eosinophilia is often present during the early stages of schistosomiasis, along with cough, dyspnea or fever, possibly in response to an immunologic process.

Suspected *Strongyloides* infection
    Strength of Recommendation: Class IIa
    Strength of Evidence: Category C
Results Interpretation:
Eosinophil count raised
    Tissue-invasive parasitosis, including strongyloidiasis, is a common cause of secondary eosinophilia, with values often exceeding 400 cells/microL.

Suspected *Trichinella spiralis* infection (trichinosis)
    Strength of Recommendation: Class IIb
    Strength of Evidence: Category C
Results Interpretation:
Eosinophil count raised
    Eosinophilia occurs in more than 50% of cases of trichinosis. Typically levels rise within days, peak during the third or fourth week, then gradually decline over a period of months. An eosinophil count that does not increase with *Trichinella spiralis* infection may be a poor prognostic sign.
    Trichinosis is associated with a relative eosinophilia of at least 20%, commonly exceeds 50%, and may reach a maximum of 90%. An absolute eosinophil count of 350 to 3,000/microL is associated with 75% of trichinosis cases. Twenty percent of patients have eosinophil counts of 3,000 to 8,000/microL, while few cases may have normal or near-normal values. Absolute eosinophil counts as high as high as 15×10^9/L have been noted.

COMMON PANELS
- Complete blood count with automated differential

ABNORMAL RESULTS
- Results increased in:
  - Smoking
- Results decreased in:
  - Labor

COLLECTION/STORAGE INFORMATION
- Collect whole blood in purple top EDTA tube or use capillary blood.

LOINC CODES
- Code: 32173-7 (*Short Name* - Eosinophil Bld Ql Wright Stn)
- Code: 712-0 (*Short Name* - Eosinophil # Bld Manual)
- Code: 5785-1 (*Short Name* - Eosinophil UrnS Qn HPF)
- Code: 29993-3 (*Short Name* - Eosinophil Spt Ql Wright Stn)
- Code: 711-2 (*Short Name* - Eosinophil # Bld Auto)
- Code: 20472-7 (*Short Name* - Eosinophil XXX Ql Wright Stn)
- Code: 26449-9 (*Short Name* - Eosinophil # Bld)

Epstein-Barr virus serology

TEST DEFINITION
Serologic diagnosis of Epstein-Barr virus (EBV) infection

REFERENCE RANGE
• Negative
Please refer to your institution's reference ranges as lab normals may vary.

INDICATIONS
Suspected infectious mononucleosis, with atypical clinical findings or severe prolonged illness and heterophile-negative test results.
     Strength of Recommendation: Class IIa
     Strength of Evidence: Category C
  Results Interpretation:
  Serology positive
• Serologic antibody titer profiles of EBV-induced infectious mononucleosis:
  • VCA-IgG: Positive in current, recent, past, reactivated, and indeterminate infections
  • VCA-IgM: Positive in current and recent infections
  • anti-EA: Positive in current, recent, reactivated, and indeterminate infections
  • anti-EBNA: Positive in past, reactivated, and indeterminate infections

CLINICAL NOTES
The ELISA and IF assays are the preferred tests in patients with either atypical or severe illness and heterophile-negative test results.

COLLECTION/STORAGE INFORMATION
• Specimen Collection and Handling:
  • Collect serum samples in red top tube
  • Freeze specimens if immediate testing not anticipated

Erythrocyte mean corpuscular volume determination

TEST DEFINITION
Measurement of the average volume of RBCs calculated from the hematocrit and the RBC count for the evaluation and management of hematologic disorders

SYNONYMS
• MCV - Mean cell volume

REFERENCE RANGE
• Adults: 80-100 mcm^3 (80-100 fL)
• Fetal blood:
• 18 to 20 weeks' gestation: 133.9 +/- 8.8 fL
• 21 to 22 weeks' gestation: 130.1 +/- 6.2 fL
• 23 to 25 weeks' gestation: 126.2 +/- 6.2 fL
• 26 to 30 weeks' gestation: 118.2 +/- 5.8 fL
• Neonates, cord blood: 98-118 fL (2 SD) (whole blood)
• Neonates, 2 weeks: 88-140 fL (whole blood)
• Neonates, 1 month: 91-112 fL (whole blood)
• Infants, 2 months: 84-106 fL (whole blood)
• Infants, 4 months: 76-97 fL (whole blood)
• Infants, 6 months: 68-85 fL (whole blood)
• Infants, 9 months: 70-85 fL (whole blood)

- Infants, 12 months: 71-84 fL (whole blood)
- Infants, 2 weeks to 2 years: 70-84 fL (95% range) (whole blood)
- Children, 2 to 5 years: 73-85 fL (whole blood)
- Children, 5-9 years: 75-87 fL (whole blood)
- Children, 9-12 years: 76-90 fL (whole blood)
- Adolescent males, 12 to 14 years: 77-94 fL (whole blood):
- Adolescent females, 12 to 14 years: 73-95 fL (whole blood):
- Adolescent males, 15 to 17 years: 79-95 fL (whole blood):
- Adolescent females, 15 to 17 years: 78-98 fL (whole blood):
- Neonates, 1 day: 119 +/- 9.4 (SD) (capillary blood)
- Neonates, 4 days: 114 +/- 7.5 fL (capillary blood)
- Neonates, 7 days: 118 +/-11.2 fL (capillary blood)
- Neonates, 1 to 2 weeks: 112 +/- 19.0 fL (capillary blood)
- Neonates, 3 to 4 weeks: 105 +/- 7.5 fL (capillary blood)
- Infants, 5 to 6 weeks: 102 +/- 10.2 fL (capillary blood)
- Infants, 7 to 8 weeks: 100 +/- 13.0 fL (capillary blood)
- Infants, 9 to 10 weeks: 91 +/- 9.3 fL (capillary blood)
- Infants, 11 to 12 weeks: 88 +/- 7.9 fL (capillary blood)
  Please refer to your institution's reference ranges as lab normals may vary.

INDICATIONS
Screening for suspected alcohol abuse
    Strength of Recommendation: Class IIb
    Strength of Evidence: Category C
    Results Interpretation:
    Raised hematology findings
    Mean corpuscular volume (MCV) increases with excessive alcohol consumption. Sustained and regular drinking appears necessary to elevate MCV levels.

Suspected iron deficiency anemia
    Strength of Recommendation: Class IIa
    Strength of Evidence: Category C
    Results Interpretation:
    Lowered hematology findings
    A low mean corpuscular volume (MCV) (less than 80 femtoliters), together with a low RBC count and high red cell distribution width, favors the diagnosis of iron deficiency. Severe microcytic anemia (MCV less than 70 fL) is caused mainly by iron deficiency or thalassemia.

Suspected thalassemia
    Strength of Recommendation: Class IIa
    Strength of Evidence: Category C
    Results Interpretation:
    Lowered hematology findings
    Clinically symptomatic thalassemias are characterized by microcytosis and a low (less than 75 fL) mean corpuscular volume (MCV). In patients who are heterozygous for beta-thalassemia, the MCV is less than 75 fL, but the Hct is usually greater than 33% and the RBC count is normal or slightly elevated.
    Patients with beta-thalassemia trait typically have marked hypochromia and microcytosis, some degree of anisocytosis, and a large portion of target cells. Although these latter findings also may be present in patients with severe iron deficiency anemia, patients with beta-thalassemia trait usually have more prominent target cell formation and proportionally a lower MCV for the equivalent packed cell volume valuel

COMMON PANELS
- Complete blood count
- Red blood cell indices

COLLECTION/STORAGE INFORMATION
- Specimen Collection and Handling:
    - Collect whole blood sample in EDTA (lavender-top) tube or capillary blood sample in heparin (green-top) tube.
    - Collect fetal blood by percutaneous umbilical blood sampling (PUBS).
    - Store sample up to 6 hours at 25°C or for 24 hours at 4°C.

LOINC CODES
- Code: 30428-7 (*Short Name* - MCV RBC Qn)
- Code: 11272-2 (*Short Name* - MCV BldCo Fet Qn Auto)
- Code: 787-2 (*Short Name* - MCV RBC Qn Auto)

Estrone measurement

TEST DEFINITION
Measurement of estrone in serum for evaluation and management of sex steroid hormone disorders in men and women

SYNONYMS
- Oestrone measurement

REFERENCE RANGE
- Prepubertal children 1 to 10 years: <1.5 ng/dL (<56 pmol/L)
- Male Tanner Stages:
- Tanner stage 1: 0.5-1.7 ng/dL (18-63 pmol/L)
- Tanner stage 2: 1-2.5 ng/dL (37-92 pmol/L)
- Tanner stage 3: 1.5-2.5 ng/dL (55-92 pmol/L)
- Tanner stage 4: 1.5-4.5 ng/dL (56-166 pmol/L)
- Tanner stage 5: 2-4.5 ng/dL (74-166 pmol/L)
- Female Tanner Stages:
- Tanner stage 1: 0.4-2.9 ng/dL (15-107 pmol/L)
- Tanner stage 2: 1-3.3 ng/dL (37-122 pmol/L)
- Tanner stage 3: 1.5-4.3 ng/dL (55-159 pmol/L)
- Tanner stage 4: 1.6-7.7 ng/dL (59-285 pmol/L)
- Tanner stage 5: 2.9-10.5 ng/dL (107-388 pmol/L)
- Adult males: 1.5-6.5 pg/mL (55-240 pmol/L)
- Adult females (menstrual phase):
- Early follicular phase: 1.5-15 pg/mL (55-555 pmol/L)
- Luteal phase: 1.5-20 pg/mL (55-740 pmol/L)
- Pregnant women: Estrone increases 10-fold from 24th to 41st week
- Postmenopausal women: 1.5-5.5 pg/mL (55-204 pmol/L)
  Please refer to your institution's reference ranges as lab normals may vary.

INDICATIONS
Prepubertal gynecomastia evaluation in males
    Strength of Recommendation: Class IIa
    Strength of Evidence: Category C
Results Interpretation:
Increased estrone level
Elevated serum estrone levels in the presence of normal 17 beta-estradiol levels may be the only indicative serum parameter of prepubertal gynecomastia.

Suspected breast cancer in postmenopausal women
    Strength of Recommendation: Class IIb
    Strength of Evidence: Category B
Results Interpretation:
Increased estrone level
Elevated estrone levels may be associated with an increased risk of breast cancer in postmenopausal women.

High serum estrone levels (greater than 8 pg/mL) in postmenopausal women may significantly increase the risk for estrogen receptor-positive breast cancer.

Postmenopausal women with a history of cigarette smoking and elevated estrone levels may be at increased risk for developing breast cancer, with ex-smokers within the last 5 years having the greatest risk.

Postmenopausal women who consume more than 25 grams of alcohol per day may potentially increase estrone levels, thereby increasing their risk for breast cancer.

COLLECTION/STORAGE INFORMATION
- Patient Preparation:
  - Have patient fast for 8 hours prior to sampling
- Specimen Collection and Handling:
  - Separate serum from sample immediately by centrifugation
  - Store samples at -20° C until use

LOINC CODES
- Code: 2258-2 (*Short Name* - Estrone SerPl-mCnc)
- Code: 6776-9 (*Short Name* - Estrone 24H Ur-mRate)
- Code: 27998-4 (*Short Name* - Estrone Sal-mCnc)
- Code: 2260-8 (*Short Name* - u Estrone Amn-mCnc)
- Code: 2257-4 (*Short Name* - Estrone Smn-mCnc)
- Code: 31177-9 (*Short Name* - Estrone Amn-mCnc)
- Code: 2261-6 (*Short Name* - u Estrone SerPl-mCnc)
- Code: 14971-6 (*Short Name* - Estrone Bioavail % SerPl)
- Code: 22663-9 (*Short Name* - Estrone SerPl-sCnc)
- Code: 2262-4 (*Short Name* - u Estrone 24H Ur-mRate)
- Code: 2259-0 (*Short Name* - Estrone Ur-mCnc)
- Code: 14160-6 (*Short Name* - u Estrone % SerPl)
- Code: 25403-7 (*Short Name* - Estrone Ur-sCnc)
- Code: 14970-8 (*Short Name* - Estrone Bioavail SerPl-mCnc)

Ethosuximide measurement

TEST DEFINITION
Measurement of ethosuximide levels in blood for evaluation and management of antiepileptic therapy

REFERENCE RANGE
- Adults: 40-100 mcg/mL (283-708 micromol/L)
  Please refer to your institution's reference ranges as lab normals may vary.

INDICATIONS
Therapeutic drug monitoring for ethosuximide
      Strength of Recommendation: Class IIa
      Strength of Evidence: Category C
      Results Interpretation:
      Drug therapy finding
      Routine monitoring of ethosuximide blood levels may maximize effectiveness, minimize adverse effects, and determine patient compliance. However, toxic effects do not necessarily correlate with blood levels.

      Ethosuximide blood levels are generally considered therapeutic between 40 mcg/mL and 100 mcg/mL, becoming toxic over 150 mcg/mL, and associated with possible adverse effects when levels exceed 100 mcg/mL (eg, gastric distress, loss of appetite, sedation). Levels below 40 mcg/mL are rarely effective.

      Ethosuximide doses of 20 mg/kg typically equate to blood levels between 20 to 60 mcg/mL, doses of 40 mg/kg typically equate to blood levels between 60 to 160 mcg/mL, and doses of 750 mg/day should equate to blood levels between 30 to 100 mcg/mL. It takes approximately one week of drug therapy for blood levels to stabilize. Levels may increase more rapidly, relative to dose, in females than in males, and may be decreased in children.

CLINICAL NOTES
Micellar electrokinetic chromatography (MEKC) allows the simultaneous analysis of ethosuximide, primidone, phenytoin, and carbamazepine in a short amount of time, without complex preparation.

COLLECTION/STORAGE INFORMATION
- Specimen Collection and Handling:
  - Collect venous blood sample in a purple top tube (heparin, EDTA)
  - Collect trough level
  - May keep sample at room temperature for several hours; for longer storage (up to one year), freeze at -20°C

• Code: 29218-5 (*Short Name* - Ethosuximide Fld-mCnc)

Ethylene glycol measurement

TEST DEFINITION
Measurement of ethylene glycol in serum or plasma for the evaluation of poisoning

SYNONYMS
• Antifreeze measurement

REFERENCE RANGE
Negative
Please refer to your institution's reference ranges as lab normals may vary.

INDICATIONS
Suspected ethylene glycol poisoning
   Strength of Recommendation: Class IIa
   Strength of Evidence: Category C
   Results Interpretation:
   Positive laboratory findings
• Toxic Concentration:
   • The toxic serum ethylene glycol concentration is approximately 3 mmol/L (20 mg/dL).
   • One swallow of ethylene glycol (120 mg/kg body weight or 0.1 mL/kg body weight) can result in a toxic concentration.
• Lethal Concentration:
   • An approximate lethal ethylene glycol dose in adults is approximately 100 cc; however, individuals reportedly have survived much higher doses.
   • An estimated lethal oral ethylene glycol dose is 1.4 mL/kg or 1.56 g/kg.
   • Death has been reported with ingestion of as little as 30 to 60 mL; however, survival has been reported with ingestion of more than 3,000 mL.
   Ethylene glycol level may be undetectable due to conversion of the parent compound to toxic metabolites (glycoaldehyde, glycolate, glyoxalate, oxalate).

CLINICAL NOTES
Ethylene glycol is used as a solvent, in antifreeze, industrial humectant, and hydraulic brake fluids, and as a glycerin substitute in commercial products such as paints, lacquers, detergents, and cosmetics.

COLLECTION/STORAGE INFORMATION
Collect plasma in EDTA (ethylene diamine tetraacetic acid) tube, or draw serum blood sample.

LOINC CODES
• Code: 22734-8 (*Short Name* - Ethylene Glycol XXX-sCnc)
• Code: 14721-5 (*Short Name* - Ethylene Glycol SerPl-sCnc)
• Code: 31082-1 (*Short Name* - Ethylene Glycol Gast-mCnc)
• Code: 29279-7 (*Short Name* - Ethylene Glycol Ur Ql)
• Code: 5647-3 (*Short Name* - Ethylene Glycol Ur-mCnc)
• Code: 5646-5 (*Short Name* - Ethylene Glycol SerPl-mCnc)

Factor V Leiden test

TEST DEFINITION
Molecular genetic analysis to detect the factor V Leiden mutation (an inherited condition and predisposing factor for thrombosis)

REFERENCE RANGE

Negative
Please refer to your institution's reference ranges as lab normals may vary.

INDICATIONS

Suspected factor V Leiden mutation predisposing to spontaneous abortion
> **Strength of Recommendation:** Class IIb
> **Strength of Evidence:** Category C
> **Results Interpretation:**
> **Positive laboratory findings**

The factor V Leiden mutation has been identified as a cause of second-trimester pregnancy loss, which may be secondary to placental thrombosis. In a study of 50 patients with second-trimester pregnancy loss, there was a 20% prevalence of resistance to activated protein C, significantly higher than in women with a history of first-trimester miscarriage only (5.7%) or in controls (4.3%). In a large cohort of women, those with factor V Leiden had an elevated risk of fetal loss after 28 weeks' gestation (OR=2). In another study, the risk of fetal loss after 20 weeks' gestation was tripled in carriers of factor V Leiden. Carriers of factor V Leiden also have an increased risk of fetal loss at less than 25 weeks' gestation.

Factor V Leiden has also been identified as a cause of recurrent pregnancy loss, documented in 9% of women experiencing three or more pregnancy losses. The risk is increased in homozygous carriers as compared to heterozygous carriers.

Fetal expression of factor V Leiden mutation prenatally may result in spontaneous abortion during the first half of pregnancy or in placental infarction in the second half of pregnancy. A cohort study of 396 high-risk pregnancies found a significant increase in the frequency of factor V Leiden mutation in those with greater than 10% placental infarction.

Suspected factor V Leiden mutation predisposing to thromboembolic stroke
> **Results Interpretation:**
> **Positive laboratory findings**

Factor V Leiden mutation is one of the most prevalent inherited coagulation defects associated with cerebral venous thrombosis, occurring in 10% to 20% of patients.

Factor V Leiden mutation was found to be a particularly important contributing factor in childhood strokes. A retrospective case-control analysis found that the presence of factor V Leiden mutation increased stroke risk by a factor of 5.

In one group of young women, factor V Leiden was not found to be an important risk factor for stroke; however, in some cases, the factor V Leiden mutation in combination with additional prothrombotic states (eg, homocystinemia), or non-factor V Leiden-related activated protein C resistance in certain ethnic populations (eg, Hispanics), may be an important contributor to arterial strokes.

Some data suggest that postmenopausal hormone replacement may be a risk factor for ischemic stroke in women with the factor V Leiden mutation.

Some studies have found that the factor V Leiden mutation is not a risk factor for cerebrovascular disease caused by arterial thromoboembolism.

Suspected factor V Leiden mutation predisposing to venous thromboembolism
> **Strength of Recommendation:** Class IIa
> **Strength of Evidence:** Category C
> **Results Interpretation:**
> **Positive laboratory findings**

In heterozygous carriers of factor V Leiden, the risk of deep venous thrombosis (DVT) is increased by a factor of 5 to 10. Despite this increased risk, most carriers will never have a thromboembolic event; the risk for thrombosis by mid-adulthood in a heterozygote is about 20%. In homozygotes, the risk of DVT is increased by about 80-fold. The increased risk of venous thromboembolism conferred by the factor V Leiden mutation does not necessarily warrant lifelong anticoagulation after an isolated episode of DVT.

CLINICAL NOTES

Genotyping is a confirmatory test for factor V Leiden and can distinguish between homozygous and heterozygous states.

COLLECTION/STORAGE INFORMATION

- Specimen Collection and Handling:
  - May collect crude cell lysate, serum, or whole blood
  - Avoid contaminating sample with extraneous DNA or RNA

- Avoid anticoagulants except citrate and EDTA.
- Store nucleic acids frozen at -20°C.

Factor VIII assay

TEST DEFINITION
Measurement of coagulation factor VIII in plasma for the evaluation and management of hemophilia A

REFERENCE RANGE
- 50%-200% (0.5-2) of normal plasma activity
  Please refer to your institution's reference ranges as lab normals may vary.

INDICATIONS
Suspected and known hemophilia A
> **Strength of Recommendation:** Class I
> **Strength of Evidence:** Category C
> **Results Interpretation:**
> **Coag./bleeding tests normal**
>> A normal factor VIIIC concentration does not exclude carrier status. In this case, carrier status should be identified by mutation detection.
>> Both hemophilia A and B will have normal factor VIII related antigen levels.

> **Coag./bleeding tests abnormal**
- Severity of disease based on concentration of factor VIIIC:
  - Mild disease is indicated by a factor VIIIC level of 5% to 40% (less than 0.05 to 0.4 International Units/mL); bleeding occurs after accidents or surgery.
  - Moderate disease is indicated by a factor VIIIC level of 1% to 5% (0.01 to 0.05 International Units/mL); marked bleeding after dental procedures or surgery and bleeding into joints and muscles after minor injuries.
  - Severe disease is indicated by a factor VIIIC level of less than 1% of normal (less than 0.01 International Units/mL); marked bleeding occurs after accidents, injuries, dental procedures, and surgery and spontaneous bleeding occurs into joints and muscles.

  A deficiency of factor VIII is diagnostic for hemophilia A.

  Factor VIII coagulant activity is decreased in hemophilia A.

> **Frequency of Monitoring**
>> Because the concentration of factor VIIIC can increase under stress, factor VIIIC concentrations should be measured more than once.

COMMON PANELS
- Coagulation factor assay

ABNORMAL RESULTS
- Results increased in:
  - Third trimester of pregnancy
  - Renal insufficiency
  - Post-exercise
  - Stress

COLLECTION/STORAGE INFORMATION
- Specimen Collection and Handling:
  - Collect 4.5 mL plasma in blue top tube (citrate).
  - May store on ice for up to 2 hours; freeze if longer (factor VIII levels decrease at room temperature)

LOINC CODES
- Code: 21001-3 (*Short Name* - FVIII XXX-Imp)
- Code: 3209-4 (*Short Name* - FVIII Act/Nor PPP Qn)
- Code: 3210-2 (*Short Name* - FVIII PPP Chro-aCnc)
- Code: 3208-6 (*Short Name* - FVIIIa PPP Coag-aCnc)
- Code: 3211-0 (*Short Name* - FVIII Act/Nor PPP Qn 2Stg Coag)

Fecal elastase 1 level

TEST DEFINITION
Measurement of proteolytic pancreas-specific enzyme elastase 1 in stool for diagnosis of exocrine pancreatic insufficiency

SYNONYMS
- Faecal elastase 1 level

REFERENCE RANGE
- Adults and children: >200 mcg pancreatic elastase/g stool
  Please refer to your institution's reference ranges as lab normals may vary.

INDICATIONS
Suspected exocrine pancreatic insufficiency in chronic pancreatitis
   Strength of Recommendation: Class IIb
   Strength of Evidence: Category B
   Results Interpretation:
   Decreased level (laboratory finding)
   - 100 to 200 microg pancreatic elastase/g stool = mild to moderate exocrine pancreatic insufficiency
   - Less than 100 microg pancreatic elastase/g stool = severe exocrine pancreatic insufficiency

Suspected exocrine pancreatic insufficiency in cystic fibrosis
   Strength of Recommendation: Class I
   Strength of Evidence: Category A
   Results Interpretation:
   Decreased level (laboratory finding)
   - 100 to 200 mcg pancreatic elastase/g stool = Mild to moderate exocrine pancreatic insufficiency
   - Less than 100 mcg pancreatic elastase/g stool = Severe exocrine pancreatic insufficiency

Suspected exocrine pancreatic insufficiency in diabetes mellitus
   Strength of Recommendation: Class IIa
   Strength of Evidence: Category B
   Results Interpretation:
   Decreased level (laboratory finding)
   - 100 to 200 mcg pancreatic elastase/g stool = Mild to moderate exocrine pancreatic insufficiency
   - Less than 100 mcg pancreatic elastase/g stool = Severe exocrine pancreatic insufficiency

ABNORMAL RESULTS
- Results decreased in nonpancreatic diarrhea due to alterations in stool composition or water content.

COLLECTION/STORAGE INFORMATION
- Specimen collection and handling:
   - Collect a random sample of 20 g of formed stool
   - Store sample at room temperature
   - Ship the specimen within 5 days of collection in an approved lab pack

LOINC CODES
- Code: 25907-7 (*Short Name* - Elastase Panc Stl-mCnt)

Fecal occult blood test

TEST DEFINITION
Detection of occult blood in feces for the evaluation and management of gastrointestinal disorders and colorectal cancers.

SYNONYMS
- Faecal occult blood test
- FOBT - Faecal occult blood test
- FOBT - Fecal occult blood test

REFERENCE RANGE
- Adults and children: negative
  Please refer to your institution's reference ranges as lab normals may vary.

INDICATIONS
Abdominal pain
   Results Interpretation:
   Fecal occult blood: positive
      Blood in the stool suggests underlying peptic ulcer disease, polyps, inflammatory bowel disease, vascular ischemia, or intussusception.

Screening for colorectal cancer
      Strength of Recommendation: Class I
      Strength of Evidence: Category A
   Results Interpretation:
   Fecal occult blood: positive
      Colonoscopy is recommended whenever a patient presents with a positive fecal occult blood test on any specimen. There is no justification for repeating the test if the initial result is positive.
   Frequency of Monitoring
      The American Cancer Society recommends 5 colorectal cancer screening options for all men and women at average risk beginning at age 50: (1) Fecal occult blood test (FOBT) annually; (2) flexible sigmoidoscopy every 5 years; (3) annual FOBT plus flexible sigmoidoscopy every 5 years; (4) double-contrast barium enema every 5 years; or (5) colonoscopy every 10 years. The American Gastroenterological Association recommends annual guaiac-based FOBT testing. Higher surveillance screening, including colonoscopy, is recommended for patients at increased risk of developing colorectal cancer. The appropriate age for discontinuation of colorectal screening is not known; consideration should be given to the patient's age and life expectancy. Significant decreases in cancer mortality are first measurable within 5 years after the initiation of screening.

Suspected gastrointestinal bleeding
      Strength of Recommendation: Class IIa
      Strength of Evidence: Category B
   Results Interpretation:
   Fecal occult blood: positive
      A guaiac test for occult blood in stool will detect 0.5 to 1 mg of Hgb per mL of aqueous solution, while the Hematest® technique is capable of detecting as little as 0.1 mg of blood in aqueous solution.
      The combination of a highly sensitive guaiac test with an immunochemical test may differentiate upper from lower gastrointestinal bleeding.

      False Results
         Betadine® or ingestion of preparations containing the expectorant guaifenesin will result in a positive guaiac test.
   Fecal occult blood: trace
      The Hematest® will at times paradoxically give only a trace or 1+ reaction with tarry stools.

      False Results
         Betadine® or ingestion of preparations containing the expectorant guaifenesin will result in a positive guaiac test.

Suspected infectious diarrhea
   Results Interpretation:
   Fecal occult blood: positive
      Blood may be found in any diarrheal stool; however, it is more common in infections caused by pathogens that produce injury to the mucosa, particularly *Shigella*, *Yersinia*, enterohemorrhagic *E coli*, *Campylobacter*, and *Salmonella*.

Suspected irritable bowel syndrome (IBS)
   Results Interpretation:
   Fecal occult blood: negative
      Negative occult blood test results are expected in IBS.
   Fecal occult blood: positive
      Positive results from a stool specimen may indicate organic or structural disease such as colon cancer requiring diagnostic colonoscopy.

Suspected or known Henoch-Schonlein purpura
   Strength of Recommendation: Class IIb
   Strength of Evidence: Category C
   Results Interpretation:
   Positive laboratory findings
      Fecal occult blood tests may be positive in Henoch-Schonlein purpura patients.

LOINC CODES

- Code: 27926-5 (*Short Name* - Hemocult #8 Stl Ql)
- Code: 12504-7 (*Short Name* - Hemocult #5 Stl Ql)
- Code: 29771-3 (*Short Name* - Hemocult Stl Ql Imm)
- Code: 2335-8 (*Short Name* - Hemocult Stl Ql)
- Code: 27401-9 (*Short Name* - Hemocult sp6 Stl Ql)
- Code: 27925-7 (*Short Name* - Hemocult sp7 Stl Ql)
- Code: 27396-1 (*Short Name* - Hemocult Stl-mCnt)
- Code: 14565-6 (*Short Name* - Hemocult #3 Stl Ql)
- Code: 14564-9 (*Short Name* - Hemocult sp2 Stl Ql)
- Code: 14563-1 (*Short Name* - Hemocult sp1 Stl Ql)
- Code: 12503-9 (*Short Name* - Hemocult sp4 Stl Ql)

Fetal fibronectin measurement

TEST DEFINITION
   Measurement of fetal fibronectin in cervicovaginal secretions to assess risk of preterm delivery.

REFERENCE RANGE
- Pregnancy (cervicovaginal fluid): <50 ng/mL
   Please refer to your institution's reference ranges as lab normals may vary.

INDICATIONS
Prediction of preterm delivery in preterm labor
   Strength of Recommendation: Class I
   Strength of Evidence: Category A
   Results Interpretation:
   Positive biochemistry findings
      Presence of greater than or equal to 50 ng/mL fetal fibronectin (FFN) in a cervicovaginal sample defines a positive FFN test. The ability of a positive test to predict preterm birth is best before 34 weeks gestation in asymptomatic women, but is most predictive of delivery within 7 to 10 days in symptomatic women with cervical dilation less than 3 cm; approximately 20% will deliver in this interval.
   Negative biochemistry findings
      Negative fetal fibronectin testing is the most predictive result when obtained between 24 and 34 weeks gestation. When negative, less than 1% of women will deliver within the next 1 to 2 weeks.
   Frequency of Monitoring
      Fetal fibronectin may be repeated in 7 to 14 days if labor symptoms persist and the first test was negative.
   Timing of Monitoring
      Fetal fibronectin testing is performed in women between 24 and 36 weeks gestation experiencing labor symptoms.

Prediction of successful induction of labor in pregnancy
   Strength of Recommendation: Class IIb
   Strength of Evidence: Category B

Results Interpretation:
Positive biochemistry findings
   Presence of greater than or equal to 50 ng/mL vaginal fetal fibronectin has been shown to be be a predictor of successful induction of labor.

ABNORMAL RESULTS

- Results increased in: '
  - Recent sexual intercourse
  - Pre-eclampsia
- Results decreased in:
  - Severe infection
  - Protein loss (as seen in trauma, vascular collapse, and coagulopathies)

COLLECTION/STORAGE INFORMATION

- Patient Preparation:
  - Patient should abstain from sexual intercourse for 24 hours prior to test
- Specimen Collection and Handling:
  - Collect cervicovaginal secretions from the posterior fornix using a Dacron swab
  - Place specimen in a buffered collection tube (ie, albumin with protease inhibitors) for transport
  - May store specimen at 4°C for up to 72 hours and at -20°C for up to 6 months

LOINC CODES

- Code: 20404-0 (*Short Name* - Fibronectin Fetal GenV QI)
- Code: 20403-2 (*Short Name* - Fibronectin Fetal GenV-mCnc)

Fibrinogen measurement

TEST DEFINITION

   Measurement of plasma fibrinogen for the evaluation of coagulopathies

SYNONYMS

- Fibrinogen level

REFERENCE RANGE

- Adults: 150-400 mg/dL (1.5-4 g/L)
- Neonates: 125-300 mg/dL (1.25-3 g/L)
  Please refer to your institution's reference ranges as lab normals may vary.

INDICATIONS

Suspected and known preeclampsia
   Results Interpretation:
   Laboratory test finding
      Fibrinogen levels less than 250 mg/dL are abnormal and levels less than 200 mg/dL are associated with a higher risk of significant hemorrhage.
   Timing of Monitoring
      Fibrinogen measurements (as well as other coagulation studies) are only necessary when there is evidence of coagulopathy such as bleeding, a platelet count less than 150,000/microL, or an LDH level above the upper nonpregnant limit.

Suspected DIC
   Strength of Recommendation: Class IIb
   Strength of Evidence: Category C
   Results Interpretation:
   Decreased fibrinogen
      While a panel of tests including fibrinogen is usually ordered in patients suspected to have DIC, the clinical picture is paramount, as no single laboratory test can confirm or exclude the diagnosis of DIC.
      Low levels of fibrinogen may be seen only in the most severe cases of DIC, as plasma fibrinogen is an acute-phase reactant with increased levels in response to conditions such as inflammation, infection, or trauma.

Decreased levels of fibrinogen have been found in less than 50% of patients with DIC.

A low level of fibrinogen will not differentiate between DIC and liver disease because low levels may result from decreased synthesis (fibrinogen is produced in the liver) as well as from increased consumption.

Suspected meningococcemia
Results Interpretation:
Decreased fibrinogen

A serum fibrinogen concentration less than 150 mg/dL (4.4 micromol/L) may predict poor outcome in children with purpuric sepsis syndrome.

Suspected or known hemolytic uremic syndrome (HUS)
Results Interpretation:
Increased fibrinogen

In postdiarrheal hemolytic uremic syndrome (HUS), the fibrinogen concentrations are either normal or high.

Suspected sepsis
Strength of Recommendation: Class IIb
Strength of Evidence: Category C
Results Interpretation:
Abnormal laboratory findings

Baseline fibrinogen levels should be obtained in patients with sepsis.

COMMON PANELS

- Disseminated intravascular coagulation screen
- Disseminated intravascular coagulopathy panel

ABNORMAL RESULTS

- Results increased in:
  - Pregnancy

COLLECTION/STORAGE INFORMATION

- Collect venous specimen in blue top tube containing sodium citrate.
- Specimen may be stored for several months at -20°C.

LOINC CODES

- Code: 21002-1 (*Short Name* - Fibrinogen PPP-Imp)

Filaria antibody assay

TEST DEFINITION

Qualitative screening for parasitic organisms associated with the filarial group

REFERENCE RANGE

- Adults and Children: Negative
  Please refer to your institution's reference ranges as lab normals may vary.

INDICATIONS

Suspected filarial infection
Results Interpretation:
Serology positive

A positive serology test is a useful adjunct to direct microfilariae detection in the diagnosis of filariasis.

CLINICAL NOTES

Antibody detection that is based on whole parasite extracts can result in cross-reactivity in individuals with other filarial infections. Serology tests for parasitic diseases are infrequently requested; specimens are usually sent to the Center for Disease Control and Prevention (CDC) or reference laboratories with the interpretative criteria established by reagent manufacturers.

Serology testing is unable to distinguish between active and past infection, which may be significant when testing is performed in endemic areas.

COLLECTION/STORAGE INFORMATION

- Specimen Collection and Handling:
    - Collect serum in separation tube.
    - Freeze specimen if analysis delayed.

LOINC CODES

- Code: 25410-2 (*Short Name* - Filaria IgG Ser EIA-aCnc)
- Code: 30044-2 (*Short Name* - D immitis Ab Titr Ser)
- Code: 25409-4 (*Short Name* - Filaria Ab Titr Ser IF)
- Code: 25344-3 (*Short Name* - Filaria Ab Titr Ser)
- Code: 5165-6 (*Short Name* - Filaria Ab Ser HA-aCnc)
- Code: 13244-9 (*Short Name* - Filaria IgG Ser-aCnc)
- Code: 13245-6 (*Short Name* - Filaria IgM Ser-aCnc)
- Code: 7887-3 (*Short Name* - Filaria Ab Ser-aCnc)

Fluorescent antibody measurement, Influenzavirus, type A, avian

TEST DEFINITION

Detection of influenza A virus in respiratory specimens or cell culture for the diagnosis of avian influenza A.

REFERENCE RANGE

- Adults and children: negative titer
  Please refer to your institution's reference ranges as lab normals may vary.

INDICATIONS

Suspected avian influenza A
    Strength of Recommendation: Class IIa
    Strength of Evidence: Category C
Results Interpretation:
Positive laboratory findings
    One or more intact cells showing intracellular fluorescence is considered a positive result. Nuclear and/or cytoplasmic fluorescence may be seen. Staining should produce an intense intracellular apple-green fluorescence. Due to cross-reactivity between commercially available influenza A subtype antibodies, positive results require confirmatory testing using the World Health Organization (WHO) approved monoclonal antibody kit.
Timing of Monitoring
    Specimens should be obtained as soon as possible after symptoms first appear.

COLLECTION/STORAGE INFORMATION

Infected respiratory epithelial cells are fragile; specimens should be kept on ice during processing to minimize damage. Cell cultures are the preferred specimen in order to make viral amplification possible.

Serial specimen collection over several days is optimal; specimens collected within the first 3 days of illness onset are more likely to detect the virus.

Oropharyngeal swab specimens and lower respiratory tract specimens, such as bronchoalveolar lavage and tracheal aspirates, are preferred because they appear to contain more virus; nasal and nasopharyngeal swab specimens are less optimal because they may contain a lower viral count.

Clinicians should contact their local or state health departments in all cases of suspected infection with any novel influenza A virus; state and local health departments should in turn contact the Centers for Disease Control (CDC) Emergency Response Hotline.

To obtain a nasopharyngeal aspirate/wash, instill 1 ml to 1.5 ml nonbacteriostatic saline (pH) into one nostril. Flush a plastic catheter or tubing with 2 ml to 3 ml of saline. Insert tubing into nostril parallel to the palate and aspirate nasopharyngeal secretions. Repeat procedure with second nostril.

To obtain a nasopharyngeal or oropharyngeal swab, insert a swab into the nostril parallel to the palate. Leave the swab in place for a few seconds to absorb secretions. Repeat with second nostril. All swabs used for specimen collection should have an aluminum or plastic shaft and a Dacron tip. Calcium alginate swabs, cotton-tipped swabs, or swabs with wooden shafts should not be used for specimen collection. Place specimen at 4°C immediately after collection.

To collect sputum, have patient rinse mouth with water then expectorate deep cough sputum directly into a sterile screw-cap sputum collection cup or sterile dry container. Use cold packs to keep sample at 4°C for domestic shipping. For international shipping pack in dry ice.

During bronchoalveolar lavage or tracheal aspirate, use a double-tube system to maximize shielding from oropharyngeal secretions; bronchoalveolar lavage is a high-risk, aerosol generating procedure. Centrifuge half of the specimen and fix the cell pellet in formalin. Place the remaining unspun fluid in sterile vials with external caps and internal O-rings. If no O-rings are available, seal tightly with available cap and secure with Parafilm®. Label each specimen with patient's ID and collection date. For domestic shipping use cold packs to keep sample at 4°C. For international shipping, ship fixed cells at room temperature and unfixed cells frozen.

Fluorescent treponemal antibody absorption test

TEST DEFINITION
Detection of antibodies in serum for the confirmatory diagnosis of syphilis

SYNONYMS
- FTA(Abs) - Fluorescent treponemal antibody test
- FTA-ABS test

REFERENCE RANGE
- Adults and children: nonreactive
  Please refer to your institution's reference ranges as lab normals may vary.

INDICATIONS
Suspected congenital syphilis
>**Strength of Recommendation:** Class IIa
>**Strength of Evidence:** Category B
>**Results Interpretation:**
>**Positive laboratory findings**
>>For infants born to syphilitic mothers, a positive fluorescent treponemal antibody absorption (FTA-ABS) test confirming a reactive nontreponemal test is suggestive of congenital syphilis, particularly if the treponemal test remains positive over a 3-month period.
>>
>>A reactive treponemal and nontreponemal test in an asymptomatic mother may indicate recent or previous infection. A positive FTA-ABS result following a negative nontreponemal test may suggest late syphilis infection, successful past treatment of syphilis in the mother, or another medical condition such as Lyme disease. A negative treponemal test and a reactive nontreponemal test is consistent with a false positive nontreponemal test result.
>
>**Negative laboratory findings**
>>When a treponemal test such as a fluorescent treponemal antibody absorption (FTA-ABS) assay fails to confirm a positive nontreponemal test for syphilis in a pregnant woman, the result is suggestive of a negative syphilis diagnosis.
>
>**Frequency of Monitoring**
>>Maternal and fetal testing for syphilis should be conducted at 28 weeks gestation and again at delivery. If a negative fluorescent treponemal antibody absorption (FTA-ABS) result fails to confirm a positive nontreponemal test, then both assays should be repeated within 4 weeks.

Suspected syphilis
    Strength of Recommendation: Class IIa
    Strength of Evidence: Category B
    Results Interpretation:
    Positive laboratory findings
        A positive nontreponemal test followed by a positive FTA-ABS is suggestive of syphilis. Up to 85% of patients who undergo treatment for syphilis will remain seropositive indefinitely regardless of disease state or treatment rendered, while the remaining 15% to 25% of patients will return to seronegative status in 2 to 3 years.
        Results are reported as reactive, reactive minimal, nonreactive or atypical fluorescence observed. Specimens which produce reactive minimal findings require retesting. If retesting produces the same result, the results should be reported as equivocal and repeat serologic testing should be performed 1 to 2 weeks after the initial specimen was obtained. A finding of atypical fluorescence can occur in serum from patients with active lupus or other autoimmune disorders.

ABNORMAL RESULTS

False results are rare but have been reported in patients with viral infection, autoimmune disease, mixed connective tissue disease and in pregnancy.

CLINICAL NOTES

Positive tests results require mandatory health department reporting.

LOINC CODES

- Code: 29310-0 (*Short Name* - T pallidum XXX QI IF)
- Code: 34382-2 (*Short Name* - T pallidum Ab Titr Ser IF)
- Code: 13288-6 (*Short Name* - T pallidum Ab Bld IF-aCnc)
- Code: 17729-5 (*Short Name* - T pallidum IgM Ser QI IF)
- Code: 17726-1 (*Short Name* - T pallidum IgG Ser QI IF)
- Code: 9826-9 (*Short Name* - T pallidum Ab CSF QI IF)
- Code: 5393-4 (*Short Name* - T pallidum Ab Ser QI IF)
- Code: 17728-7 (*Short Name* - T pallidum IgM Ser IF-aCnc)
- Code: 17724-6 (*Short Name* - T pallidum Ab Ser IF-aCnc)
- Code: 17727-9 (*Short Name* - T pallidum IgG Ser IF-aCnc)

Fluorescent treponemal antibody absorption test, Cerebrospinal fluid

TEST DEFINITION

Detection of antibodies in cerebrospinal fluid for the evaluation of suspected neurosyphilis

SYNONYMS

- FTA(Abs) - Fluorescent treponemal antibody test
- FTA-ABS test

REFERENCE RANGE

- Adults and children: nonreactive
  Please refer to your institution's reference ranges as lab normals may vary.

INDICATIONS

Suspected neurosyphilis
    Strength of Recommendation: Class IIb
    Strength of Evidence: Category B

Results Interpretation:
Positive laboratory findings

A positive fluorescent treponemal antibody absorption (FTA-ABS) may be indicative of current neurosyphilis infection, or of previously treated early or latent syphilis. Antibodies may remain in the cerebrospinal fluid (CSF) long after successful treatment.

Negative laboratory findings

A negative fluorescent treponemal antibody absorption (FTA-ABS) test may rule out a diagnosis of neurosyphilis.

ABNORMAL RESULTS

- Contamination with sera during specimen collection may produce false positive results.

LOINC CODES

- Code: 29310-0 (*Short Name* - T pallidum XXX QI IF)
- Code: 34382-2 (*Short Name* - T pallidum Ab Titr Ser IF)
- Code: 13288-6 (*Short Name* - T pallidum Ab Bld IF-aCnc)
- Code: 17729-5 (*Short Name* - T pallidum IgM Ser QI IF)
- Code: 17726-1 (*Short Name* - T pallidum IgG Ser QI IF)
- Code: 9826-9 (*Short Name* - T pallidum Ab CSF QI IF)
- Code: 5393-4 (*Short Name* - T pallidum Ab Ser QI IF)
- Code: 17728-7 (*Short Name* - T pallidum IgM Ser IF-aCnc)
- Code: 17724-6 (*Short Name* - T pallidum Ab Ser IF-aCnc)
- Code: 17727-9 (*Short Name* - T pallidum IgG Ser IF-aCnc)

Fluphenazine measurement

TEST DEFINITION

Measurement of fluphenazine levels in serum or plasma to facilitate therapeutic or toxicity monitoring

REFERENCE RANGE

- Therapeutic range: 0.2-4 ng/mL (0.4-8.4 nmol/L)
  Please refer to your institution's reference ranges as lab normals may vary.

INDICATIONS

Therapeutic drug monitoring for fluphenazine therapy
  Strength of Recommendation: Class IIb
  Strength of Evidence: Category B
  Results Interpretation:
  Therapeutic drug level - finding

Patients with fluphenazine concentrations less than 0.5 ng/mL may run a higher risk of psychotic exacerbations than patients with fluphenazine concentrations greater than 1 ng/mL.

Monitoring plasma concentrations of fluphenazine may be useful for clinical management and the prediction of psychotic exacerbations.

Higher plasma fluphenazine levels may suggest an excessive drug dosage, as the levels appear to correlate with extrapyramidal side effects, while lower fluphenazine concentrations may be adequate to prevent most psychotic relapses.

A so-called therapeutic level does not necessarily predict a clinical response; there are a subset of patients who show no symptomatic improvement regardless of their fluphenazine levels.

ABNORMAL RESULTS

Radioimmunoassay techniques used for fluphenazine monitoring may be affected by interfering compounds, including prochlorperazine, trifluoperazine, perphenazine, and fluphenazine metabolites.

COLLECTION/STORAGE INFORMATION

- Specimen Collection and Handling:
  - Draw plasma in heparinized tube.
  - Store up to 3 weeks at -20°C.

LOINC CODES
- Code: 3651-7 (*Short Name* - Fluphenazine Ur-mCnc)
- Code: 3650-9 (*Short Name* - Fluphenazine SerPl-mCnc)

Folic acid measurement, RBC

TEST DEFINITION
Measurement of folic acid (folate) levels in red blood cells for the evaluation and management of certain anemias or neurologic dysfunction

SYNONYMS
- RBC folate measurement
- Red cell folic acid level

REFERENCE RANGE
- Adults: 150-450 ng/mL/cells (340-1020 nmol/L/cells)
- Children, 2 to 16 years (competitive protein binding radioassay): >160 ng/mL (>362 nmol/L)
- Adolescents, older than 16 years (competitive protein binding radioassay): 140-628 ng/mL (317-1422 nmol/L)
  Please refer to your institution's reference ranges as lab normals may vary.

INDICATIONS
Screening for pregnancy risk of fetal neural tube defect
   Results Interpretation:
   Decreased folic acid
   A decreased level of RBC folic acid may indicate an increased risk of a woman having a child with a neural tube defect, though some data suggests there is no correlation.

Suspected folic acid (folate) deficiency
   Strength of Recommendation: Class IIb
   Strength of Evidence: Category B
   Results Interpretation:
   Decreased folic acid
   RBC folate has testing limitations because of sensitivity and specificity issues. Only about 70% of pregnant women and alcoholics with megaloblastic erythropoiesis thought to be due to folate deficiency have low RBC folate levels, while approximately 20% to 30% of pregnant women and alcoholics had low RBC folate levels in the absence of megaloblastic erythropoiesis.
   RBC folate values may be superior to serum folate values for the assessment of folate tissue stores; however, there is controversy over whether RBC folate is a better test than or comparable to serum folate for the diagnosis of folate deficiency.

CLINICAL NOTES
RBC folate levels, unlike serum folate levels, are not affected by recent dietary intake or drugs.

COLLECTION/STORAGE INFORMATION
- Specimen Collection and Handling:
  - Collect whole blood in EDTA (competitive protein binding radioassay or automated chemiluminescence) or heparinized tube (automated chemiluminescence).
  - Specimen stable for 4 hours at 8°C and 8 weeks at -20°C

LOINC CODES
- Code: 14731-4 (*Short Name* - Folate RBC-sCnc)

Free erythrocyte protoporphyrin measurement

TEST DEFINITION
Assessments of possible iron deficiency or lead toxicity by measurement of non-complexed, non-heme protoporphyrin concentration

REFERENCE RANGE
- Adults: 16-36 mcg/dL red cells (0.28-0.64 micromol/L red cells)
  Please refer to your institution's reference ranges as lab normals may vary.

INDICATIONS
Suspected erythropoietic protoporphyria
> **Strength of Recommendation:** Class I
> **Strength of Evidence:** Category C
> **Results Interpretation:**
> **Increased protoporphyrin**
> > In differentiating between the cutaneous porphyrias (ie, variegate porphyria, hereditary coproporphyria, and porphyria cutanea tarda), an elevated free erythrocyte protoporphyrin (FEP) indicates erythropoietic protoporphyria.

Suspected iron deficiency
> **Strength of Recommendation:** Class IIb
> **Strength of Evidence:** Category B
> **Results Interpretation:**
> **Increased protoporphyrin**
> > An elevated erythrocyte protoporphyrin (EP) level suggests iron deficiency, especially in preschool children.
> > Because the prevalence of severe lead toxicity has declined, an elevated EP level is more likely to be a positive screen for iron deficiency.
> > There has been some confusion between zinc protoporphyrin (ZnPP or ZPP) and erythrocyte protoporphyrin (EP), also known as free erythrocyte protoporphyrin (FEP); and in some studies these may have been inaccurately considered equivalent.

Suspected severe lead poisoning in children
> **Strength of Recommendation:** Class IIb
> **Strength of Evidence:** Category B
> **Results Interpretation:**
> **Increased protoporphyrin**
> > Erythrocyte protoporphyrin (EP) levels greater than or equal to 35 mcg/dL suggest elevated blood lead (BPb) levels in children. The EP level increases exponentially with increasing BPb levels and is less accurate in identifying BPb levels less than 25 mcg/dL than levels 25 mcg/dL or greater.
> > Changes in free erythrocyte protoporphyrin (FEP) occur slowly over a period of days to weeks and may remain for the entire lifespan of the red blood cell.
> > There has been some confusion between zinc protoporphyrin (ZnPP or ZPP) and erythrocyte protoporphyrin (EP), also known as free erythrocyte protoporphyrin (FEP); and in some studies these may have been inaccurately considered equivalent.

ABNORMAL RESULTS
- Results increased in:
  - Markedly increased erythropoiesis:
    - Sickle cell disease
    - Severe hemolytic anemias
    - Thalassemia major

CLINICAL NOTES
Advantages of the erythrocyte protoporphyrin test are that it is inexpensive and easy to perform.

* Specimen Collection and Handling:
  * Collect whole blood in a tube containing either heparin or EDTA.
  * Avoid exposure to light.
  * Blood sample is stable at 4°C for up to 5 days.

LOINC CODES
* Code: 2892-8 (*Short Name* - FEP Bld-mCnc)
* Code: 15093-8 (*Short Name* - FEP Bld-sCnc)

Free prostate specific antigen level

TEST DEFINITION
Measurement of free prostate specific antigen (fPSA) in serum or plasma for the evaluation of prostatic disorders

SYNONYMS
* Free PSA level

REFERENCE RANGE
* Men ages 40-49: 0.5 ng/mL
* Men ages 50-59: 0.7 ng/mL
* Men ages 60-69: 1 ng/mL
* Men ages 70-79: 1.2 ng/mL
  Please refer to your institution's reference ranges as lab normals may vary.

INDICATIONS
Suspected prostate cancer
> **Strength of Recommendation:** Class IIb
> **Strength of Evidence:** Category B
> **Results Interpretation:**
> **Abnormal biochemistry findings**
> The clinical utility or interpretation of a single free prostate specific antigen (fPSA) value for prostate cancer has not been established. In clinical practice, fPSA is most often evaluated in combination with total PSA as percent free PSA.

COLLECTION/STORAGE INFORMATION
Plasma samples may be stored up to 20 years at -20°C.
If long term storage of samples is planned, plasma samples are recommended, since long term storage of serum samples results in random variability of fPSA measurements and produces significantly lower values than those obtained from plasma samples. Short term storage of plasma and serum samples produce equivalent results.
* Collect plasma samples in EDTA tube.

LOINC CODES
* Code: 10886-0 (*Short Name* - Free PSA SerPl-mCnc)
* Code: 19201-3 (*Short Name* - Free PSA SerPl-aCnc)
* Code: 19206-2 (*Short Name* - Free PSA Smn-sCnc)

Fungal blood culture

TEST DEFINITION
Detection of fungi in blood in the setting of suspected invasive or disseminated fungal disease

REFERENCE RANGE
Adults and Children: Negative or No Growth
Please refer to your institution's reference ranges as lab normals may vary.

INDICATIONS
Suspected systemic mycosis
    Strength of Recommendation: Class IIa
    Strength of Evidence: Category B
    Results Interpretation:
    Positive microbiology findings
        Blood cultures are the primary test used in the diagnosis of systemic mycosis. Positive fungal cultures should be correlated with clinical evidence and histopathology when available. *Candida spp.* are commonly found in blood cultures and are the fourth most common cause of nosocomial blood stream infection.

        Since many fungal organisms also occur as normal flora (ie, *Candida spp*) or are widespread in the environment (ie, *Aspergillus spp*) it may be difficult to determine the clinical significance of a positive laboratory culture in the absence of clinical findings.

        Negative cultures can occur in patients with disseminated fungal illness.

        Over 150 species of fungi can produce human disease. *Candida albicans* is the most common fungal pathogen that produces illness; however non-*C. albicans* is increasingly isolated from cultures. *Aspergillus spp.* are the most common mold organisms producing illness. The two organisms are responsible for greater than 80% of fungal infections reported in solid organ and bone marrow transplant patients.

        Other pathogens that are likely to cause fungemia are: *H capsulatum* and *C neoformans* ; pathogens that have been occasionally isolated include: *Trichosporon spp., Malassezia spp., Acremonium spp.,* and *Fusarium spp.*.

CLINICAL NOTES
    Fungal infections may occur in both community- and hospital-acquired infections, due to an increase in broad spectrum antibiotics, use of central venous catheters, and immunosuppression. Fungemias have become more prevalent than anaerobic bacteremias during the past two decades.

    Standard bacteriological media (ie, routine aerobic culture bottles) can be used in the growth of most fungi, however, media specifically formulated for the isolation and detection of fungi have been developed. These culture techniques (ie, lysis centrifugation technique {Wampole Isolator}) can improve sensitivity for fungal growth.

    Candida spp. is the most common isolate recovered from blood cultures. Other commonly reported fungal pathogens include: *Histoplasma capsulatum, Coccidioides immitis, Candida albicans, Cryptococcus neoformans, Aspergillus spp.,* and *Blastomyces dermatitidis.*

    In one study, the growth of *Candida* improved with larger inocula in an automatic blood culture system (Bactec 9240). Although not statistically significant, increasing inoculum size (ie, 1000 CFU/bottle) was associated with better growth detection.

    Lysis centrifugation has become the 'gold standard' for recovery of pathogenic yeast and thermally dimorphic fungi from blood, although the method can be more labor intensive and has been associated with a higher rate of contamination

    In areas that are endemic for *Histoplasma capsulatum* and *Coccidioides immitis* or in severely immunocompromised patients (ie, HIV infection), the lysis centrifugation method may improve recovery rates in suspected fungal infection.

    Typical fungal cultures may take up to 4 weeks to rule out the presence of fungi. A single negative culture does not rule out the diagnosis of fungemia.

COLLECTION/STORAGE INFORMATION
- Specimen Collection and Handling:
  - Collect 5 mL blood per 50 mL blood culture bottle; ratio of blood to culture should be 1:10 to 1:20
    - Collect 20 mL to 30 mL of blood in adults for the lysis centrifugation technique
  - Use vented vacuum blood culture bottles
  - Process specimens immediately; may refrigerate samples up to 15 hours

LOINC CODES
- Code: 601-5 (*Short Name* - Fungus Bld Cult)

Fungal culture, body fluid, Cerebrospinal fluid

TEST DEFINITION
Fungal culture of cerebrospinal fluid to aid in the diagnosis of central nervous system fungal infection

REFERENCE RANGE
Adults and children: no growth
Please refer to your institution's reference ranges as lab normals may vary.

INDICATIONS
Suspected and known cryptococcal meningitis
> **Strength of Recommendation:** Class IIa
> **Strength of Evidence:** Category C
> **Results Interpretation:**
> **Positive microbiology findings**

Cryptococcus neoformans is the most common worldwide pathogen associated with fungal meningitis; *Candida* species have also been reported in newborns and children. Diagnosis requires evaluation of cultures, direct smears, antigen and antibody testing.

Although fungal meningitis has been diagnosed in immunocompetent patients, it occurs more frequently in patients who are immunocompromised (eg, AIDS, organ transplant, immunosuppressive chemotherapy, and chronic corticosteroid therapy); up to 10% of AIDS patients will develop cryptococcal meningitis.

If fungal meningitis is suspected subsequent cerebrospinal fluid samples should be obtained, even if the initial specimen is negative. A single negative fungal culture does not rule out infection, and false positive results are possible due an opportunistic pathogen or environmental contamination. Four weeks or more may be required to detect the presence of fungi.

> **Timing of Monitoring**

An additional cerebrospinal fluid culture 2 weeks after the initiation of treatment is recommended to assess patient response; a positive culture may necessitate a longer course of induction therapy.

Suspected fungal infection of central nervous system
> **Strength of Recommendation:** Class IIb
> **Strength of Evidence:** Category C
> **Results Interpretation:**
> **Positive microbiology findings**

Cerebrospinal fluid (CSF) examination results can be nonspecific, with elevated protein level and cell count. In only rare cases are CSF cultures positive. Fungal brain abscess occurs most commonly in immunocompromised patients (eg, diabetics, those receiving corticosteroid therapy, AIDS patients).

In endemic areas, *Candida, Aspergillosis,* and *Coccidioides* species have been cultured from the CSF of patients with fungal central nervous system infections.

In addition to CSF culture, direct smears and antigen and antibody testing are required to make a diagnosis of fungal CNS infection. Generally, viral meningitis and encephalitis are the hardest CNS infections to diagnose.

COLLECTION/STORAGE INFORMATION
A minimum of 1 mL of CSF is required per culture request, although 3 mL has been recommended. The diagnosis of some fungi requires volumes of 10 mL to 20 mL of ventricular or cisternal CSF. Specimen should obtained in a sterile tube and kept at room temperature during transport and storage. Anaerobic culture requires specimen collection in an oxygen-free container. Specimen should not be refrigerated or placed on ice.

LOINC CODES
- Code: 576-9 (*Short Name* - Fungus Snv Cult)
- Code: 570-2 (*Short Name* - Fungus Fld Cult)
- Code: 569-4 (*Short Name* - Fungus CSF Cult)
- Code: 574-4 (*Short Name* - Fungus Prt Cult)

Fungal culture, body fluid, Synovial fluid

TEST DEFINITION

Detection of fungus by culture of synovial fluid for evaluation and management of potential fungal infections (eg, *Candida*, *Aspergillus*, *Cryptococcus*, and *Histoplasma* species).

REFERENCE RANGE

Adults and Children: No growth or negative
Please refer to your institution's reference ranges as lab normals may vary.

INDICATIONS

Suspected fungal arthritis
   Strength of Recommendation: Class IIa
   Strength of Evidence: Category C
Results Interpretation:
Positive microbiology findings
   Diagnosis is made by the presence of fungal organisms in synovial fluid.
   Clinical presentation of fungal infection can appear similar to other septic or noninfectious arthritides. Infection may be either localized or systemic. A high index of suspicion in a high risk patient population (eg, decreased immunity; history of a parenteral catheter in neonates, surgery or trauma to the knee or intraarticular injection) should prompt synovial fluid analysis.
   Fungal organisms most frequently isolated from synovial fluid are *Coccidioides immitis*, *Histoplasma capsulatum*, *Blastomyces dermatitidis*, and rarely *Sporothrix schenkii*. Fungal organisms do not frequently affect joints, but the risk of opportunistic fungal infection can occur in immunocompromised patients (eg, AIDS). *Candida*, *Aspergillus*, *Cryptococcus*, and *Histoplasma* have been associated with fungal infections in immunocompromised patients.
   Fusarium and *Trichosporon spp.* have been reported as emerging opportunistic fungal infections that can cause articular infection.

CLINICAL NOTES

It usually takes up to 4 weeks to completely rule out fungal growth; *Histoplasma capsulatum* may take up to 8 weeks. A single negative culture does not rule out infection.

COLLECTION/STORAGE INFORMATION

• Specimen Collection and Handling:
   • Collect as much fluid as possible in a sterile tube or syringe; swabs are unsuitable for specimen collection.
   • Transport to lab immediately; may refrigerate specimen for up to 12 to 15 hours if unable to process immediately.
   • Avoid contamination with normal body fluids.

LOINC CODES

• Code: 576-9 (*Short Name* - Fungus Snv Cult)
• Code: 570-2 (*Short Name* - Fungus Fld Cult)
• Code: 569-4 (*Short Name* - Fungus CSF Cult)
• Code: 574-4 (*Short Name* - Fungus Prt Cult)

Fungal culture, sputum

TEST DEFINITION

Culture of sputum to aid in the diagnosis of lower respiratory tract fungal infection or systemic mycoses

SYNONYMS

• Sputum fungus culture

REFERENCE RANGE
- Adults and Children: Negative or no growth
  Please refer to your institution's reference ranges as lab normals may vary.

INDICATIONS
Suspected pulmonary fungal infection
>**Strength of Recommendation:** Class IIa
>**Strength of Evidence:** Category C

Results Interpretation:
Positive microbiology findings
The presence of fungal organisms in sputum, along with clinical and radiologic evidence supports the diagnosis of a respiratory fungal infection. There are a limited number of fungal organisms that can produce a respiratory fungal infection, as a result of either opportunistic infection (eg, aspergillosis, mucormycosis, or candidiasis) or endemic mycoses (ie, histoplasmosis blastomycosis, coccidioidomycosis and paracoccidioidomycosis).

OPPORTUNISTIC INFECTIONS
Pulmonary aspergillosis is primarily caused by a few species (*Aspergillus fumigatus, A. flavus, A. niger*) that are pathogenic to humans. Sputum cultures are negative in up to 50% of patients diagnosed with aspergilloma. Invasive pulmonary aspergillosis is difficult to diagnose and the presence of *Aspergillus spp* in the sputum may be due to colonization, however, in immunocompromised patients sputum cultures can be useful in the diagnosis. The diagnosis of aspergilloma and chronic necrotizing aspergillosis are usually strongly suggested by a positive sputum culture and and positive radiologic evidence. Additionally, sputum cultures are not essential in the diagnosis of allergic bronchopulmonary aspergillosis.

Candida is easy to culture from sputum, but is not useful in the diagnosis of pulmonary infection in the absence of clinical evidence.

Mucormycosis is usually difficult to diagnose and positive cultures should be interpreted with caution because the organism is so commonly found in the environment. Diagnosis is often made at autopsy.

ENDEMIC MYCOSES
In general, acute pneumonias caused by endemic mycoses are difficult to diagnose and timely data is rare during the course of acute illness.

Histoplasmosis is endemic in the Ohio and Mississippi River valleys and acute illness is difficult to diagnose by sputum culture, which may require up to 30 days for culture identification. Sputum cultures are positive in less than 10% of cases of primary pulmonary histoplasmosis.

Culture remains the 'gold standard' for the diagnosis of blastomycosis, although the method is time consuming. If the inoculum size is large enough, preliminary results may be available within 5 days, and a tentative diagnosis can be made based on clinical suspicion. Most cases of both acute and chronic pulmonary blastomycosis are readily diagnosed by sputum culture or direct sputum smears. Final confirmation may take up to 4 to 5 weeks.

Coccidioidomycosis occurs in semiarid desert locations and is caused by the organism *Coccidioides immitis* which can be easily cultured. However, the fragile arthroconidia can break off easily and aerosolize the fungus. Extra caution is usually required to culture this organism.

Other potential pulmonary fungal infections can include paracoccidiodomycosis and cryptococcosis. Paracoccidiodomycosis has a distinct morphology that can be observed in cultures from sputum, while a positive sputum culture is predictive of cryptococcal pneumonia in immunosuppressed patients.

CLINICAL NOTES
Prior to culture, the quality of the specimen should be evaluated by screening with Gram stain examination.
Specimens can easily be contaminated with saliva (greater than 25 squamous epithelial cells per low power field); these samples are rejected for culture in some laboratories. To avoid cultures becoming contaminated with rapidly growing molds (fungi growing as mycelia) the specimen should be refrigerated immediately.

COLLECTION/STORAGE INFORMATION
- Collect expectorated or induced sputum sample.
- Instruct patient to rinse mouth and gargle with water and to cough deeply and expectorate sputum (preferably 5 to 10 mL) into sterile container. For patients with a non-productive cough, have patient breathe aerosolized droplets of a solution of 15% sodium chloride and 10% glycerin for about 10 minutes to induce cough reflex.
- Collect lower respiratory secretions via a tracheal aspirate into a Luken's trap in patients with a tracheostomy.
- Collect early morning sample to improve sample quality..
- Transport specimen to lab immediately (less than one hour) or refrigerate.
- All specimens collected for fungal culture should be handled in a biological safety cabinet.

LOINC CODES

- Code: 6409-7 (*Short Name* - Fungus SptT Cult)
- Code: 577-7 (*Short Name* - Fungus Spt Cult)

Fungal culture, urine

TEST DEFINITION

Detection of fungi in urine for the diagnosis and management of fungal urinary tract infections

SYNONYMS

- Fungal urine culture
- Urine fungus culture

REFERENCE RANGE

Adults and Children: Negative, or rare growth (described as 10^2 to 10^3 colony forming units/mL urine)
Please refer to your institution's reference ranges as lab normals may vary.

INDICATIONS

Suspected candiduria
Strength of Recommendation: Class IIa
Strength of Evidence: Category B
Results Interpretation:
Positive microbiology findings

Positive cultures may be a transient sign that represent colonization or contamination rather than infection. Cultures should be evaluated in the context of clinical evidence of disease. Pyuria also does not differentiate between colonization and infection. Two consecutive positive cultures are recommended prior to the start of antifungal therapy.

- Positive urine culture is delineated as follows:
  - Abundant: Greater than 10^5 colony forming units (CFU)/mL for yeast
  - Moderate: 10^4 to 10^5 CFU/mL
  - Few: 10^3 to 10^4 CFU/mL

Urinary count of greater than 10,000 to 15,000 CFU/mL urine in a noncatherized patient likely represents infection by *Candida*.

Candiduria and fungal urinary tract infections have become more prevalent due in part to the extensive use of broad-spectrum antimicrobial agents, corticosteroids, immunosuppressive and cytotoxic therapy, advanced age, and chronic diseases (eg, diabetes, AIDS).

Most frequent organism isolated from urine and associated with fungal urinary tract infections (UTIs) is *Candida albicans* (up to 50% of isolates) followed by *C (Torulopsis) glabrata* (25% to 35%), and other *Candida spp* (8% to 28%), which have included *C tropicalis*, and *C krusei*.

The presence of Candida in the urine must be evaluated to determine if colonization or low-grade infection is present. Candiduria often resolves with the cessation of antibiotic therapy or catheter removal. Persistent fungi in the urine can lead to disseminated infection.

Candiduria may be predictive of fungemia in infants.

Suspected fungal infection of the genitourinary tract, by organisms other than *Candida spp.*
Strength of Recommendation: Class IIa
Strength of Evidence: Category C
Results Interpretation:
Positive microbiology findings

- Positive urine culture is described as follows:
  - Abundant: Greater than 10^5 colony forming units (CFU)/mL for yeast
  - Moderate: 10^4 to 10^5 CFU/mL
  - Few: 10^3 to 10^4 CFU/mL

Aspergillus, Cryptococcosis, and *Mucormycosis* are infrequently associated with descending urinary tract infections (UTI). Diabetics, patients with AIDS, and aged or immunocompromised patients tend to be at greatest risk for developing these opportunistic infections.

Renal transplant recipients receiving immunosuppression are at risk for invasive fungal infections (ie, *Candida , Aspergillus,* or *Cryptococcus* species.

Aspergillosis is rarely associated with urinary tract-only infection; disseminated disease is usually present.

Cryptococcus neoformans is an opportunistic fungus found throughout the environment. Infection most often occurs by inhalation, and the presence of genitourinary cryptococcosis infection usually implies disseminated illness.

Histoplasma capsulatum is endemic to the central United States and found in soil with high nitrogen content provided by birds. Illness is acquired by inhalation, and genitourinary infection is suggestive of disseminated illness that can be diagnosed by urine culture.

Blastomycosis, a soil fungus found frequently in the Ohio, Mississippi and Missouri River valleys, and the western shores of Lake Michigan, is acquired by respiratory inhalation. Dissemination can affect multiple body systems, and genitourinary involvement can range from 15% to 56%.

Coccidioides immitis is a soil saprophyte and the only etiologic agent of coccidioidomycosis, which is endemic in southwestern United States. Infection results from inhalation, and genitourinary tract involvement may be difficult to identify.

ABNORMAL RESULTS
- Other:
  - Risk factors for funguria:
    - Antibiotic use (broad-spectrum)
    - Chronic renal failure and hemodialysis patients
    - Diabetes
    - Female gender
    - Hematologic malignancies
    - Indwelling catheters for urinary drainage
    - Intravenous catheters used for total parenteral nutrition

CLINICAL NOTES

Candida albicans is the most common species isolated (estimated to be 40% to 65% of all fungal isolates) from urine along with *C glabrata* which accounts for 25% to 35% of infections while other *Candida spp.* {*C tropicalis, C krusei*} make up 8% to 28% of infections.

Fungi associated with genitourinary fungal infections are usually characterized in two separate groups: *Candida, Aspergillus,* and *Cryptococcus* which are opportunistic organisms of low virulence. The second group are pathogens endemic to localized areas: *Histoplasma, Blastomyces,* and *Coccidioides*.

COLLECTION/STORAGE INFORMATION
- Specimen Collection and Handling
  - Collect midvoid urine sample in a sterile container; percutaneous needle aspiration is an optimal specimen
  - Refrigerate specimens if they cannot be processed immediately; limit refrigeration to 12 to 15 hours

Galactose screening test for galactosemia

TEST DEFINITION
Screening test for an inherited disorder of galactose metabolism in neonates

SYNONYMS
- Beutler test
- Galactose screening test for galactosaemia
- Paigen test

REFERENCE RANGE
- Neonates:
- Inhibition assay: Bacterial growth
- Paigen test: No bacterial growth
- Qualitative fluorometric assay: Bright fluorescence at 1 and 2 hours
- Quantitative fluorometric assay: 18-30[149] micromol/hour/g Hgb (19-32 kilounits/mol Hgb)
  Please refer to your institution's reference ranges as lab normals may vary.

INDICATIONS

Screening for suspected galactosemia in neonates
>**Strength of Recommendation:** Class I
>**Strength of Evidence:** Category C
>**Results Interpretation:**
>**Screened - abnormality**
>>An enzyme deficiency in red cells or an accumulation of galactose and/or galactose-1-phosphate in red cells in infants ingesting milk is diagnostic of galactosemia.
>>An abnormal screening test for galactosemia should prompt confirmatory testing using quantitative assays or DNA analysis that measure the enzymes of galactose metabolism.

>>**False Results**
>>>As screening tests are designed to prevent false negatives, a large number of false positives can occur.
>>>Utilization of the Beutler test in hot summer months can lead to false-positive results. Blood transfusions may cause false negative Beutler test results for up to 3 months.
>>**Timing of Monitoring**
>>>This test should be performed no later than 3 to 4 days of life and before hospital discharge or transfer from the nursery.
>>>Early screening is important as a galactose-free diet and knowledgeable supportive care are essential in the successful management of this disease.

CLINICAL NOTES

>Screening tests vary by state, and not all states test for galactosemia.
>Tests that assess galactose levels, eg, the Paigen test, are dependent on milk ingestion.
>Fluorescent assay will detect reduced galactose-1-phosphate uridyl transferase (GALT) activity in circumstances under which the enzyme may deteriorate, such as in hot, humid conditions or when the specimens are batched, leading to many false positives.
>Partial enzyme deficiencies, such as occur in heterozygotes, may be missed.

COLLECTION/STORAGE INFORMATION

- Collect whole blood on filter paper, or cord or capillary blood (heparin) from newborn

Galactose-1-phosphate uridyltransferase measurement

TEST DEFINITION

>Measurement of galactose-1-phosphate uridyltransferase in whole blood or erythrocytes for the evaluation and management of galactosemia

REFERENCE RANGE

- The normal range depends on type of test:
- Radiometric after diethylaminoethyl (DEAE) separation (for erythrocytes):
- Normal patients: 5.9-9.5 micromols/h/mL (98 units/L-158 units/L)
- Galactosemia heterozygotes: 2-4.8 micromols/h/mL (33 units/L-80 units/L)
- Galactosemia homozygotes: 0 micromols/h/mL (0 units/L)
- Uridine diphosphoglucose (UDPG) consumption assay (for erythrocytes)
- Normal patients:
- 18.5-28.5 units/g hemoglobin (1.19-1.84 megaunits/mol hemoglobin)
- 537-827 units/10^{12} erythrocytes (0.54-0.83 nanounits/erythrocytes)
- 6.29-9.69 units/mL erythrocytes (6.29-9.69 kilounits/L erythrocytes)
- Heterozygotes (Duarte variant):
- 13.5-18.5 units/g hemoglobin (0.87-1.19 megaunits/mol hemoglobin)
- Galactosemia heterozygotes and homozygotes for the Duarte variant:
- 8.5-13.5 units/g hemoglobin (0.55-0.87 megaunits/mol hemoglobin)
- Double heterozygotes for galactosemia and the Duarte variant:
- 3.5-8.5 units/g hemoglobin (0.23-0.55 megaunits/mol hemoglobin)
- Galactose-1-phosphate uridyltransferase assay:

- Qualitative fluorometry (no other enzyme deficiency): Bright fluorescence at 1 and 2 hours
- Quantitative fluorometry:
- Normal: 18-30 micromols/h/g hemoglobin (19-32 kilounits/mol hemoglobin)
- Galactosemia homozygotes: <3 micromol/h/g hemoglobin (3.2 kilounits/mol hemoglobin)
- Galactosemia heterozygotes: Intermediate values
  Please refer to your institution's reference ranges as lab normals may vary.

INDICATIONS
Suspected classic galactosemia
      Strength of Recommendation: Class IIa
      Strength of Evidence: Category C
      Results Interpretation:
Decreased level (laboratory finding)
      An absence or deficiency in galactose-1-phosphate uridyl transferase (GALT) confirms a diagnosis of galactosemia.
      Heat and humidity can cause reduced GALT activity and may lead to false positive test results.
      High levels of galactose-1-phosphate may indicate acute neonatal toxicity due to GALT enzyme deficiency. Levels may remain higher in galactosemia patients than normal patients, even after dietary galactose restriction.
Timing of Monitoring
      Newborn screening conducted at 3 days of age improves the clinical course of newborns with galactosemia, particularly when combining tests measuring galactose and GALT enzyme activity.

COLLECTION/STORAGE INFORMATION
- Specimen Collection and Handling:
  - Erythrocyte Samples:
    - Draw whole blood in EDTA or heparinized tube.
    - Store up to 14 days at room temperature and up to 4 weeks at 4°C.
    - Do not freeze.
  - Whole Blood Samples:
    - Draw whole blood, cord, or capillary sample in heparinized tube.

LOINC CODES
- Code: 24082-0 (*Short Name* - Gal1PUT RBC-cCnt)
- Code: 2314-3 (*Short Name* - Gal1PUT RBC-cCnc)

Genital microscopy, culture and sensitivities

TEST DEFINITION
      Detection by culture of routine bacterial organisms (eg, *Neisseria gonorrhoeae,Chlamydia trachomatis,* and *Gardnerella vaginalis*) from genital exudate or discharge

REFERENCE RANGE
- Adults and Children: Negative
  Please refer to your institution's reference ranges as lab normals may vary.

INDICATIONS
Suspected genital infection
      Strength of Recommendation: Class IIa
      Strength of Evidence: Category B
      Results Interpretation:
Positive microbiology findings
      Genital cultures detect genital infections with a high degree of accuracy for *N gonorrhoeae* but are less useful for detection of *Chlamydial* infections or bacterial vaginosis..
      Positive results indicate the presence of a given microorganism(s) and further studies may be indicated (eg, gram-stain, gas chromatography, antibiotic susceptibility)

Evidence of *N gonorrhoeae* on Gram stain and oxidase testing from a genital culture can provide a presumptive diagnosis, but additional tests are required to confirm the findings; however, antimicrobial therapy may be initiated.

A minimum of 24 to 72 hours are required to report a presumptive culture for *N gonorrhoeae*.

Suspected preterm labor
Results Interpretation:
Vaginal swab culture positive

Even without maternal fever, culture of the high vaginal area and endocervical canal may reveal the presence of pathogens associated with preterm labor.

- Organisms associated with preterm labor
  - Group B beta-hemolytic *Streptococcus*
  - *Chlamydia trachomatis*
  - *Ureaplasma urealyticum*
  - *Gardnerella vaginalis*
  - *Bacteroides spp*
  - *Neisseria gonorrhoeae*
  - *Mycoplasma hominis*
  - Herpes simplex
  - *Listeria monocytogenes*

COLLECTION/STORAGE INFORMATION

- Specimen Collection and Handling:
- Routine:
  - Swab urethral exudate (males) or swab cervical scrapings or skin lesion for routine culture
  - Place specimen in sterile tube or transport system.
  - Transport to lab immediately; do not refrigerate.
- *Neisseria gonorrhoeae* :
  - Collect fluid from genital discharge or exudate (if no fluid present, place an unmoistened alginate swab into the distal urethra and gently rotate).
  - Collect endocervical specimens by direct visualization using a speculum.
  - Transport to lab immediately; do not refrigerate.
  - Use a buffered holding medium (ie, Stuart's or Ames's) to maintain viability of gonococci if transport is 12 hours or less. For delayed transport (>12 hours) use a transport system (ie, JEMBEC by Miles Laboratories, Gono-Pak System or Bio Bag)
- *Haemophilus ducreyi* :
  - Cleanse ulcer area with gauze saturated with non-bacteriostatic saline
  - Irrigate ulcer with nonbacteriostatic saline and aspirate with Pasteur pipet; mix and use as inoculum or use a cotton swab moistened with saline to obtain specimen and streak onto appropriate media.

Giardia lamblia antigen assay

TEST DEFINITION

Detection of *Giardia lamblia* antigen in stool for the diagnosis of giardiasis

REFERENCE RANGE

- Adults and children: Negative
  Please refer to your institution's reference ranges as lab normals may vary.

INDICATIONS
Suspected giardiasis
   Strength of Recommendation: Class IIa
   Strength of Evidence: Category B
   Results Interpretation:
   Positive immunology findings

A positive *Giardia lamblia* antigen test is diagnostic of *G lamblia* infection, and appears to be highly sensitive and specific for disease detection.

Antigen assays for *Giardia lamblia* have been positive for up to 3 days after effective treatment for the active infection; therefore, a positive follow-up assay in patients treated for the infection must be interpreted accordingly.

LOINC CODES

- Code: 31831-1 (*Short Name* - G lamblia Ag sp2 Stl Ql)
- Code: 27265-8 (*Short Name* - Giardia Ag Stl Ql)
- Code: 16899-7 (*Short Name* - G lamblia Ag XXX Ql)
- Code: 6412-1 (*Short Name* - G lamblia Ag Stl Ql EIA)
- Code: 21302-5 (*Short Name* - G lamblia Ag #2 Stl Ql EIA)
- Code: 14210-9 (*Short Name* - G lamblia Ag Stl Ql IF)
- Code: 23744-6 (*Short Name* - G lamblia Ag XXX Ql IF)
- Code: 6413-9 (*Short Name* - G lamblia Ag XXX Ql EIA)
- Code: 31830-3 (*Short Name* - G lamblia Ag Stl Ql)

Gliadin antibody measurement

TEST DEFINITION

Detection of antigliadin antibodies in serum for the evaluation and management of celiac disease and dermatitis herpetiformis

REFERENCE RANGE

- Negative

Please refer to your institution's reference ranges as lab normals may vary.

INDICATIONS

Suspected and known celiac disease

    Strength of Recommendation: Class IIb

    Strength of Evidence: Category B

Results Interpretation:

Serology positive

Antigliadin antibody (AGA) levels are elevated in 60% to 100% of untreated celiac disease patients.

Patients with partial villous atrophy usually have antibodies against gliadin.

Although IgG-AGA is less specific than IgG-AGA for celiac disease, concurrent testing with both assays generally provides a high level of detection.

After a patient has initiated a gluten-free diet, IgA-AGA levels usually fall and become undetectable within 3 to 6 months. AGA levels often remain undetectable (along with endomysial antibodies) as long the patient is compliant with the gluten diet restriction.

Testing patients with suspected celiac disease with AGA assays in conjunction with endomysial antibody assays, may offer both 100% diagnostic sensitivity and elimination of false results.

In IgA deficient patients, the IgG-AGA assay may better reflect disease activity that the IgG tissue transglutaminase test.

Results of this assay should be used in conjunction with other serologic tests and with clinical findings because it is not a reliable diagnostic test on its own.

    False Results

    False positive results for antigliadin antibody (AGA) test may occur in patients without celiac disease, and patients with other gastrointestinal disorders.

Suspected dermatitis herpetiformis

    Strength of Recommendation: Class IIb

    Strength of Evidence: Category C

Results Interpretation:

Serology positive

The antigliadin antibody (AGA) test may be a useful diagnostic aide for confirmation of dermatitis herpetiformis (DH) in patients with severe celiac disease, and for identifying patients in which jejunal biopsy may not be necessary.

AGA measurements may not accurately reflect the severity of villous atrophy in patients with DH.

AGA titers are affected by gluten consumption, and research suggests that this antibody is useful for assessing response and compliance to a gluten free diet in DH patients.

COLLECTION/STORAGE INFORMATION
- Collect 1-2 mL of serum and store specimen at -70°C.

LOINC CODES
- Code: 7893-1 (*Short Name* - Gliadin Ab Ser-aCnc)
- Code: 16900-3 (*Short Name* - Gliadin Ab Sal-aCnc)

Glucose measurement, CSF

TEST DEFINITION
Measurement of glucose in cerebrospinal fluid for evaluation and management of bacterial meningitis.

REFERENCE RANGE
- Adults: 40-70 mg/dL (2.22-3.89 mmol/L)
- Infants and children: 60-80 mg/dL (3.3-4.4 mmol/L)
  Please refer to your institution's reference ranges as lab normals may vary.

INDICATIONS
Suspected and known bacterial meningitis
    Strength of Recommendation: Class IIa
    Strength of Evidence: Category B
    Results Interpretation:
    Lowered biochemistry findings
    Cerebrospinal fluid (CSF) glucose concentrations of less than or equal to 20 mg/dL are highly correlated with bacterial meningitis; glucose levels of 20 mg/dL to 40 mg/dL are suggestive of bacterial meningitis. CSF glucose concentrations will normally remain low for 2 to 3 days after initiation of antibiotic therapy. Reduced CSF glucose concentrations are characteristically associated with bacterial, fungal, and tuberculous meningitis, while normal CSF glucose levels are associated with viral meningitis. CSF glucose concentrations are normal in 9% of patients with bacterial meningitis. Low CSF glucose in the presence of a negative gram stain is considered presumptive evidence of bacterial meningitis.

    Restoration of normal CSF glucose levels during recovery from meningitis typically occurs more rapidly than normalization of CSF cell counts and protein levels, suggesting CSF glucose measurement may be an effective parameter for monitoring response to antimicrobial therapy.

    Ventricular fluid glucose levels are typically 6 to 18 mg/dL higher than lumbar fluid glucose levels.

    CSF glucose concentrations depend directly upon blood glucose concentrations, with a normal CSF:blood glucose ratio of 0.6 in adults, and 0.74 to 0.96 in premature and term infants, respectively. Because equilibration between blood and CSF glucose levels generally requires 2 to 4 hours, blood samples should be obtained prior to CSF samples for more accurate ratio results. Hyperglycemia and hypoglycemia will result in elevated and lowered CSF glucose levels, respectively, even in the presence of bacterial meningitis. Central nervous system sarcoidosis and subarachnoid hemorrhage can also cause low CSF glucose.

Suspected or known status epilepticus
    Results Interpretation:
    CSF: glucose level - finding
    Cerebrospinal fluid glucose level is normal in patients with status epilepticus if no underlying cause exists that would alter the results; however, one study found a positive correlation between duration of seizure and the cerebrospinal fluid glucose level in children with seizures.

COLLECTION/STORAGE INFORMATION
- Process specimen immediately to avoid a lower result due to glycolysis.
- Store specimen at −20°C.

LOINC CODES
- Code: 2342-4 (*Short Name* - Glucose CSF-mCnc)

Glucose tolerance test, Plasma, Serum

TEST DEFINITION

Measurement of plasma or serum glucose following oral glucose administration for the evaluation of suspected diabetes

SYNONYMS

- Glucose challenge test
- GTT - Glucose tolerance test
- OGTT - Oral glucose tolerance test

REFERENCE RANGE

- Adult, nonpregnant, 2-hour 75 gm oral glucose tolerance test (OGTT):
- < 200 mg/dL (11.1 mmol/L)
  Please refer to your institution's reference ranges as lab normals may vary.

INDICATIONS

Suspected diabetes mellitus in nonpregnant adults
    Strength of Recommendation: Class IIb
    Strength of Evidence: Category C
    Results Interpretation:
    Abnormal glucose tolerance test
    A 2-hour plasma glucose of 200 mg/dL (11.1 mmol/L) or greater during an oral glucose tolerance test (OGTT) meets the diagnostic criteria for diabetes mellitus.
    The OGTT is not recommended for routine clinical use, but may be required in the evaluation of patients with impaired fasting glucose or when diabetes is still suspected despite a normal fasting plasma glucose.

Evaluation of gestational diabetes mellitus in at-risk pregnant women
    Strength of Recommendation: Class IIa
    Strength of Evidence: Category C
    Results Interpretation:
    Pregnancy with abnormal glucose tolerance test
    Diagnose gestational diabetes mellitus (GDM) in a woman who exceeds 2 or more of the following plasma glucose levels with a 100 g glucose load:

100g glucose load	mg/dL	mmol/L
Fasting	≥95	≥5.3
1-hour	≥180	≥10.0
2-hour	≥155	≥8.6
3-hour	≥140	≥7.8

    Diagnose gestational diabetes mellitus (GDM) in a woman who exceeds 2 or more of the following plasma glucose levels with a 75 g glucose load:

75g glucose load	mg/dL	mmol/L
Fasting	≥95	≥5.3
1-hour	≥180	≥10.0
2-hour	≥155	≥8.6

Timing of Monitoring

High-risk women should be tested as soon as possible.

Average-risk women and women who do not have GDM at the initial screening should be tested between 24 and 28 weeks gestation using either the one-step or two-step oral glucose tolerance test.

Women who meet criteria for low risk do not require testing.

Women with gestational diabetes mellitus (GDM) should be screened 6 weeks postpartum, and should be followed up with subsequent screening for the development of diabetes or prediabetes. Low-risk status requires no glucose testing.

COLLECTION/STORAGE INFORMATION
- Have the patient remain seated and abstain from smoking throughout the test.

Glucose-6-phosphate dehydrogenase test

TEST DEFINITION
Measurement of glucose-6-phosphate dehydrogenase (G6PD) in red blood cells for the evaluation and management of enzyme deficiency

REFERENCE RANGE
- Adults: 5-14 units/g Hgb (0.1-0.28 microkat/L)
  Please refer to your institution's reference ranges as lab normals may vary.

INDICATIONS
Suspected glucose-6-phosphate dehydrogenase (G6PD) deficiency
    Strength of Recommendation: Class IIa
    Strength of Evidence: Category C
    Results Interpretation:
    Decreased level (laboratory finding)
    A decreased glucose-6-phosphate dehydrogenase (G6PD) level indicates a hereditary enzyme deficiency that can predispose affected persons to hemolytic anemia.
    The absence of G6PD leaves the erythrocyte vulnerable to oxidative damage, with the most frequent clinical manifestation being anemia.

Suspected glucose-6-phosphate dehydrogenase deficiency as cause of neonatal hyperbilirubinemia
    Strength of Recommendation: Class IIa
    Strength of Evidence: Category B
    Results Interpretation:
    Decreased level (laboratory finding)
    Neonates (especially males) with glucose-6-phosphate dehydrogenase (G6PD) deficiency are at increased risk of developing hyperbilirubinemia.

Suspected sepsis
    Strength of Recommendation: Class IIb
    Strength of Evidence: Category B
    Results Interpretation:
    Decreased level (laboratory finding)
    A decreased of glucose-6-phosphate dehydrogenase level predisposes to septic complications and anemia in trauma patients.

COLLECTION/STORAGE INFORMATION
- Specimen Collection and Handling:
  - Perform a glucose-6-phosphate dehydrogenase screen prior to test.
  - Collect 5 mL of whole blood in a lavender or green top tube.

LOINC CODES
- Code: 2360-6 (*Short Name* - G6PD WBC-cCnc)
- Code: 33287-4 (*Short Name* - G6PD Bld.Dot Ql)
- Code: 2358-0 (*Short Name* - G6PD Ser Ql)
- Code: 2357-2 (*Short Name* - G6PD RBC-cCnc)
- Code: 2359-8 (*Short Name* - G6PD Ser-cCnc)
- Code: 18228-7 (*Short Name* - G6PD Tiss Ql)
- Code: 2356-4 (*Short Name* - G6PD RBC Ql)
- Code: 32546-4 (*Short Name* - G6PD RBC-cCnt)

Glycine measurement, cerebrospinal fluid

TEST DEFINITION
Measurement of glycine levels in cerebrospinal fluid for the evaluation of nonketotic hyperglycinemia

REFERENCE RANGE
- Adults: 0.044 ± 0.002 mg/dL (5.8 ± 0.3 micromol/L)
- Neonates: 0.083 ± 0.032 mg/dL (11 ± 4.2 micromol/L)
- Infants, 3 months to 2 years: 0.036 ± 0.015 mg/dL (4.8-2 micromol/L)
- Children, 2 to 10 years: 0.034 ± 0.011 mg/dL (4.6 ± 1.5 micromol/L)
  Please refer to your institution's reference ranges as lab normals may vary.

INDICATIONS
Suspected non-ketotic hyperglycinemia
    Strength of Recommendation: Class IIa
    Strength of Evidence: Category C
Results Interpretation:
Raised biochemistry findings
    A marked elevation of glycine concentration in cerebrospinal fluid (CSF) may indicate an accumulation of glycine in the brain due to a defect of the glycine cleavage system, resulting in glycine encephalopathy.
    CSF glycine levels can be elevated more than 30 times the upper limit of normal in neonatal non-ketotic hyperglycinemia (NKH).
    Elevated glycine levels in CSF may be found in genetic disorders and clinical conditions other than NKH, and can be affected by therapeutic agents and iatrogenic and technical factors.
    In atypical cases of NKH, glycine levels may be minimally elevated or normal.
Timing of Monitoring
    As plasma glycine levels correlate well with the cerebrospinal fluid (CSF) glycine levels, these 2 tests should be done concurrently to improve the diagnostic accuracy in patients with non-ketotic hyperglycinemia.

COLLECTION/STORAGE INFORMATION
- Specimen Collection and Handling:
  - Collect cerebrospinal fluid in sterile tubes.
  - Store frozen; stable at −20°C for 1 week, or at −70°C for 2 months.
  - Avoid blood in cerebrospinal fluid.
  - Plasma and cerebrospinal samples should be collected simultaneously, if possible.

LOINC CODES
- Code: 22650-6 (*Short Name* - Glycine CSF-sCnc)
- Code: 2389-5 (*Short Name* - Glycine CSF-mCnc)

Glycine measurement, urine

TEST DEFINITION
Quantification of urine glycine for diagnostic screening of suspected metabolic disorders

REFERENCE RANGE
- Infants, 10 days to 7 weeks: 14.6-59.2 mg/day (194-787 micromol/day)
- Children, 3 to 12 years: 12.4-106.8 mg/day (165-1420 micromol/day)
- Adults: 59-294.6 mg/day (785-3918 micromol/day)
  Please refer to your institution's reference ranges as lab normals may vary.

INDICATIONS
Measurement of glycine in urine to evaluate suspected inborn errors of metabolism
    Strength of Recommendation: Class IIb
    Strength of Evidence: Category C

Results Interpretation:
Increased level (laboratory finding)
   The measurement of organic acids and glycine conjugates in urine may be of value in the diagnosis and management of multiple inborn errors of metabolism (IEM). Interpretation of results is complicated by difficulty in identifying the sources of some urinary organic acids and glycine conjugates, the variability of the compounds excreted, and the lack of agreement as to the significance of a given compound or excretion pattern consistent with IEM.

CLINICAL NOTES
   Glycinuria without glycinemia may occur in urinary tract infections and contaminated urine specimens as a result of bacterial hydrolysis of glycine conjugates excreted in urine.

COLLECTION/STORAGE INFORMATION
- Obtain 24-hour urine collection. A random first morning voided specimen may be an acceptable alternative.
- Add 20 ml of toluene at start of collection.
- Refrigerate specimen during collection.
- Store at -18°C or below without preservative.
- Sample collection during fasting or metabolic decompensation is recommended, if possible, as key compounds are excreted selectively or in higher amounts under these conditions.

LOINC CODES
- Code: 30066-5 (*Short Name* - Glycine/creat Ur-Rto)
- Code: 13750-5 (*Short Name* - Glycine/creat Ur-mRto)
- Code: 27325-0 (*Short Name* - Glycine Ur-sCnc)
- Code: 25921-8 (*Short Name* - Glycine 24H Ur-sCnc)
- Code: 16919-3 (*Short Name* - Glycine Ur QI)
- Code: 25431-8 (*Short Name* - Glycine 24H Ur-sRate)
- Code: 22709-0 (*Short Name* - Glycine/creat Ur-sRto)
- Code: 2392-9 (*Short Name* - Glycine Ur-mCnc)
- Code: 2393-7 (*Short Name* - Glycine 24H Ur-mRate)
- Code: 26807-8 (*Short Name* - Glycine 24H Ur QI)

Gram stain, sputum

TEST DEFINITION
   Detection of bacterial microorganisms or inflammatory cells in sputum for presumptive evidence of infection.

SYNONYMS
- Identification of organism on gram stain of sputum
- Sputum: organism on gram stain

REFERENCE RANGE
- Adults and Children: No organisms
   Please refer to your institution's reference ranges as lab normals may vary.

INDICATIONS
Community-acquired pneumonia
      Strength of Recommendation: Class IIa
      Strength of Evidence: Category B
   Results Interpretation:
   Positive microbiology findings
      Abundant organisms are typically present in samples of patients with *Haemophilus* pneumonia. A finding of lancet-shaped gram-positive diplococci suggests *S. pneumoniae*.
      A finding of multiple polymorphonuclear leukocytes with abundant bacteria consistent with a likely pulmonary pathogen may be adequate for guiding initial therapy, assuming the absence of previous antibiotic use, cytological confirmation of lower airway secretions and appropriate specimen handling. Culture results should be correlated with Gram stain results.

Negative microbiology findings
　　A negative Gram stain may suggest an increased likelihood of the presence of an atypical pathogen. The finding of abundant white blood cells and no bacteria in a patient who has not received antibiotics is consistent with an absence of infection caused by most common bacterial pathogens.
Timing of Monitoring
　　Sputum specimens for Gram stain should be obtained before antibiotic treatment is initiated.

Suspected and known aspiration pneumonia
Results Interpretation:
Positive microbiology findings
　　Gram-positive cocci, gram-negative rods, and (rarely) anaerobes may be found on the Gram stain.
　　The most common organisms in community-acquired aspiration pneumonia are *S pneumoniae, S aureus, H influenzae*, and *Enterobacteriaceae*. Gram-negative organisms, including *P aeruginosa*, predominate in hospital-acquired cases.

Suspected and known aspiration pneumonitis
Results Interpretation:
Positive microbiology findings
　　Bacterial infections do not play an important role in the early stages of aspiration pneumonitis because gastric contents are sterile.

Suspected plague
Results Interpretation:
Positive microbiology findings
　　Yersinia pestis is a Gram-negative, bipolar staining pleomorphic coccobacilli. When stained with Wayson's or Giemsa's stain, it shows a bipolar 'safety pin' structure.

Suspected respiratory infection
Strength of Recommendation: Class IIa
Strength of Evidence: Category B
Results Interpretation:
Positive microbiology findings
　　Positive Gram stain results can provide a presumptive diagnosis and can be used to guide initial empiric antimicrobial therapy.
　　The presence of staphylococci on Gram stain is considered virtually diagnostic.
Negative microbiology findings
　　A negative tracheal aspirate strongly suggests the absence of ventilator-associated pneumonia.

LOINC CODES
· Code: 648-6 (*Short Name* - Gram Stn Spt)

Group B Streptococcus screen, rapid

TEST DEFINITION
Rapid detection of the presence of group B streptococcus

SYNONYMS
· Streptococcus agalactiae latex screen
· Streptococcus Group B latex screen

INDICATIONS
Suspected group B streptococcus carrier status in women
Strength of Recommendation: Class IIb
Strength of Evidence: Category B
Results Interpretation:
Positive laboratory findings
　　Rapid screens for group B streptococcus (GBS) appear to have a consistently high specificity, implying that if the test is positive, there is a fair certainty that the disease is present; however, the sensitivity may be lower for some screens.

According to the CDC, currently available rapid tests that detect GBS antigen from swab specimens are insufficiently sensitive to detect light colonization, and therefore are not adequate to replace culture-based prenatal screening or to use in place of the risk-based approach when culture results are unknown at the time of labor. Drawbacks of rapid tests include delays in administration of intrapartum antibiotic prophylaxis while test results are pending and lack of an isolate for susceptibility testing, which is of particular concern for penicillin-allergic women.

CLINICAL NOTES

Fluorogenic polymerase chain reaction (PCR) yields results within 30 to 45 minutes, compared with 100 minutes for conventional PCR, while rapid antigen tests (eg, enzyme-linked immunosorbent assay [ELISA]) yield results within 2 hours or less.

COLLECTION/STORAGE INFORMATION

- Specimen Collection and Handling :
  - Polymerase chain reaction (PCR):
    - For anal specimens, insert swab approximately 2.5 cm beyond the anal sphincter and gently rotate, touching anal crypts.
    - For vaginal specimens, wipe away excessive secretions or discharge and swab secretions from mucosa of lower third of vaginal vault.
    - For combined vaginal and anal specimens, swab vaginal area before obtaining anal specimen.
    - Soak swab with transport medium immediately after obtaining sample.
    - Transport sample to laboratory at room temperature.
  - Enzyme-linked immunosorbent assay (ELISA):
    - Rotate cotton-tipped swab in posterior fornix and place in dry swab holder.

HIV genotyping

TEST DEFINITION

Detection of drug resistant HIV mutations in plasma for the management of HIV retroviral therapy.

SYNONYMS

- HIV resistance testing, genotype

REFERENCE RANGE

- Absence of drug resistance mutations
  Please refer to your institution's reference ranges as lab normals may vary.

INDICATIONS

Suspected antiretroviral drug resistance in HIV patients
> **Strength of Recommendation:** Class IIa
> **Strength of Evidence:** Category B
> **Results Interpretation:**
> **Increased drug resistance**
> Detection of drug resistant HIV mutations aid in the identification of viral strains and in the determination of treatment strategies.
> Results from genotyping are interpreted manually or by computerized rules-based complex algorithms that specify the level of resistance associated with the determined strain of HIV; substantial differences exist among available algorithms. The lack of standardization and failure to update mutation databases may affect the reliability of genotype results, particularly in the cases of newly developed drugs or drugs used together in novel combinations. For these reasons it is recommended that clinicians consult with an HIV drug resistance specialist who can interpret the complex results generated by each genetic variation.
> Phenotyping results are reported as either IC_{50} or IC_{90} relative to wild-type strains. Values greater than 10-fold the wild-type are classified as highly resistant while values between 2.5-fold and 10-fold are reported as intermediate or low-level resistant.
> Drug-resistant strains comprising less than 10% to 20% of the circulating virus population are not likely to be detected by available assays, but can lead to re-emergence of virus 4 to 6 weeks after discontinuation of drug therapy.

Timing of Monitoring

Drug testing is optimally conducted after virological failure has been determined but before, or within 4 weeks after, antiretroviral drugs are discontinued. Baseline resistance testing is recommended when initiating therapy in patients with active HIV infection. In cases when newly infected patients are genotyped for drug resistance, patients should be started on an antiretroviral regimen before the genotype results are received, since waiting may negate the immunologic benefits of early antiretroviral therapy treatment.

HIV genotyping may be useful during the initiation of antiretroviral therapy in chronically infected patients, particularly in patients suspected of having been infected by a drug resistant virus, or in previously untreated patients who may have had the infection for to 2 years or longer.

LOINC Codes

- Code: 34700-5 (*Short Name* - HIV RT+Prot Gene Mut Tested)
- Code: 33630-5 (*Short Name* - HIV Prot Gene Mut)
- Code: 30554-0 (*Short Name* - HIV RT Gene Mut)

HIV p24 antigen test

Test Definition

Measurement of p24 antigen levels in serum or plasma for the evaluation and management of human immunodeficiency virus

Synonyms

- HIV p24 antigen level

Reference Range

- Negative
  Please refer to your institution's reference ranges as lab normals may vary.

Indications

Screening of donated blood for human immunodeficiency virus infection
   Strength of Recommendation: Class IIa
   Strength of Evidence: Category B
   Results Interpretation:
   Human immunodeficiency virus p24 antigen positive

A positive result on an enzyme immunosorbant assay for p24 antigen should be followed by a repeat testing. After the test and the repeat test return positive, a neutralization test should be conducted before confirming diagnosis.
   Negative laboratory findings

Negative results of p24 antigen may not rule out human immunodeficiency virus because levels sink significantly after the acute phase of infection. However, levels of p24 antigen may reappear during the late and symptomatic stages of infection.

Suspected acquired immune deficiency syndrome (AIDS)
   Strength of Recommendation: Class IIa
   Strength of Evidence: Category B
   Results Interpretation:
   Human immunodeficiency virus p24 antigen positive

In patients receiving treatment for HIV-infection, failure to sustain a decrease of p24 antigen levels may indicate loss of therapeutic effect or advanced stage of disease, such as progression to acquired immunodeficiency syndrome (AIDS).
   Negative laboratory findings

Negative p24 antigen results may not rule out human immunodeficiency virus, because detectable levels sink significantly after the acute phase of infection. However, levels of p24 antigen may reappear during the late and symptomatic stages of infection.

Suspected HIV infection
   Strength of Recommendation: Class IIa
   Strength of Evidence: Category B

Results Interpretation:
HIV infection
 A positive result on an enzyme immunosorbant assay for p24 antigen should be followed by repeat testing. After the test and the repeat test return positive, a neutralization test should be conducted before confirming the HIV diagnosis. In patients receiving treatment for HIV-infection, failure to sustain a decrease of p24 antigen levels may indicate loss of therapeutic effect.
Negative laboratory findings
 Negative results of p24 antigen may not rule out HIV because levels sink significantly after the acute phase of infection. However, levels of p24 antigen may reappear during the late and symptomatic stages of infection.

COLLECTION/STORAGE INFORMATION
* Specimen Collection and Handling
  * Draw serum or plasma in a marbled, green, or yellow-topped tube
  * Store sample for less than 7 days at 4°C and more than 7 days at -20°C

HIV viral load

TEST DEFINITION
 Quantification of HIV-1 viral load in serum, whole blood, or plasma for monitoring clinical status and therapeutic response

REFERENCE RANGE
* Adults and children: no detectable virus
  Please refer to your institution's reference ranges as lab normals may vary.

INDICATIONS
Monitoring HIV infection and evaluating treatment for HIV
  Strength of Recommendation: Class IIa
  Strength of Evidence: Category B
Results Interpretation:
Increased HIV viral load level
 An increase in plasma viral load indicates progression of HIV infection and may indicate failure of antiretroviral therapy. Initial antiretroviral therapy suppression followed by rebound RNA levels may indicate suboptimal patient compliance, emergence of drug-resistant HIV variants, decreased absorption of antiretroviral drugs, altered drug metabolism, drug interactions, vaccinations, or concurrent infections, and should be confirmed with a second test before making any treatment changes. In clinically stable HIV positive patients, HIV RNA levels can vary by threefold ($0.5 \log_{10}$) in either direction with repeated measurements. While changes greater than $0.5 \log_{10}$ are usually clinical significant, variations greater than $0.5 \log_{10}$ at low plasma HIV RNA levels may be caused by inherent biological or assay variability at the test's lower limits of sensitivity.
 Baseline viral load greater than 30,000 copies/mL, regardless of CD4+ count, is suggestive of HIV disease progression and antiretroviral therapy is recommended. Antiretroviral therapy is recommended for patients with a baseline viral load of between 5,000 and 30,000 copies/mL when the CD4+ cell count is 500×10^6 /L or less, and when viral load is less than 5,000 copies/mL and the CD4+ count is less than 350×10^6 /L. Therapy should be considered with a viral load of 5,000 to 30,000 copies/mL when the CD4+ count is greater than 500×10^6 /L, and with a viral load of less than 5,000 copies/mL when the CD4+ count is 350 to 500×10^6 /L. Therapy should be deferred when the viral load is less than 5,000 copies/mL and the CD4+ count is greater than 500^6 /L. The initial change in viral load after initiation of antiretroviral therapy is predictive of the patient's long-term response to the treatment regimen.
 After initially low levels during the first few weeks of life, the viral load of vertically-infected infants typically peaks at 4 to 8 weeks and then slowly declines over the first 2 years. Infants generally have higher HIV-1 RNA levels than asymptomatic adults.
Decreased level (laboratory finding)
 HIV RNA levels less than 50 copies/mL are associated with a longer period of viral suppression as compared to viral loads of 50 to 500 copies/mL. If viral load remains detectable after 16 to 24 weeks of therapy, a confirmatory repeat test should be performed and a change in therapy considered. A rapid decrease of at least 1.5- to 2-log should be observed within 4 weeks after antiretroviral therapy is initiated; a rapid decline by 4 or 8 weeks is predictive of subsequent HIV suppression. Patients with greater than 100,000 copies/mL may take longer to achieve maximum suppression.

Frequency of Monitoring

Quantitative viral load testing is indicated at the time of diagnosis, every 3 to 4 months for untreated patients to assess changes in the viral load, immediately prior to, and 2 to 8 weeks after initiation of antiretroviral therapy to obtain an initial assessment of drug efficacy, monthly until levels below detection are reached, and every 2 to 4 months after initiation of antiretroviral therapy to evaluate therapy response.

Timing of Monitoring

Plasma HIV RNA levels should not be obtained within 4 weeks of immunization, or during or within, 4 weeks after the successful treatment of any infection or symptomatic illness. Before initiating or changing antiretroviral therapy, HIV RNA and CD4+ levels should be obtained twice to improve the accuracy of results, preferably from the same laboratory on 2 different days. However, patients with advanced HIV disease should have therapy initiated after just one level is obtained, in order to prevent unnecessary treatment delay.

ABNORMAL RESULTS

- Results increased in:
  - Concurrent acute infectious illness
  - Status post vaccination (usually resolving 4-6 weeks after vaccination)

CLINICAL NOTES

The reporting laboratory should report test results according to the reportable range stated in the manufacturer's package insert. Values outside the reportable range should be reported as less than or greater than the lower or upper limit of quantification, respectively (eg <400 copies/mL); the specific value should not be reported in these instances. Results must be reported as a value in copies/mL as well as the log_{10} transformation. Test kit name, manufacturer and version should also be provided.

Due to the increasing number of nonB infections being identified worldwide, along with the inability of most viral test kits to identify non HIV-1 B viruses, the development of an international standard to ensure accurate quantification of divergent, nonclade B viruses is essential.

COLLECTION/STORAGE INFORMATION

- General testing information:
  - If possible, use the same type of collection tube, laboratory, and assay for individual patient monitoring
  - EDTA-treated plasma samples may have higher values than EDTA-treated serum samples.
  - The number of HIV-1 RNA molecules detected is impacted by the type of anticoagulant agent used and the time interval between sample collection and freezing. Generally, samples should be separated and frozen within 6 hours of collection to limit the extent of DNA degradation.
- Reverse transcriptase-polymerase chain reaction (RT-PCR):
  - Collect sample in acid citrate dextrose (ACD) or EDTA tube. Do not use heparin.
- Branched chain DNA (bDNA):
  - Collect sample in EDTA tube. Do not use heparin.
- Nucleic acid sequence-based amplification (NASBA):
  - Collect sample in acid citrate dextrose (ACD) or EDTA tube. Do not use heparin.

LOINC CODES

- Code: 29539-4 (*Short Name* - HIV Log Viral Load Plas Bdna)
- Code: 25836-8 (*Short Name* - HIV1 Viral Load XXX)
- Code: 29541-0 (*Short Name* - HIV Log Viral Load Plas PCR)
- Code: 20447-9 (*Short Name* - HIV Viral Load SerPl PCR)

HIV-1 Western blot assay

TEST DEFINITION

Measurement of antibodies in serum or plasma for the confirmatory diagnosis of HIV infection

REFERENCE RANGE

- Adults and children: negative

Please refer to your institution's reference ranges as lab normals may vary.

INDICATIONS
Confirmatory HIV testing for patients with positive enzyme immunoassay results
  Strength of Recommendation: Class IIa
  Strength of Evidence: Category C
  Results Interpretation:
  Positive laboratory findings
      Results are reported as positive, indeterminate, or negative. The Centers for Disease Control criteria require any 2 of the following bands to be present in order for a sample to be reported as positive: p24, gp41, and gp120/160.
  Negative laboratory findings
      A negative Western blot (WB) result has no bands present.
  Borderline laboratory findings
      An indeterminate Western blot (WB) is reported when the band patterns do not satisfy the criteria for a positive test. Most indeterminate patterns involve p18, p24, p55, or any combination of these 3 proteins.
      Indeterminate WB tests that follow repeatedly positive enzyme immunoassays could be due to incomplete antibody responses in HIV infected persons, nonspecific reactions in uninfected persons, or insufficient specimen quantity. Patients without recent exposure to HIV who remain WB indeterminate after 1 month are unlikely to be infected with HIV. Persons with no known risk factors, no clinical symptoms or other findings, and indeterminate results for at least 6 months, are considered negative for antibodies to HIV-1. Persons with indeterminate results who have a history of exposure, or who are exhibiting clinical symptoms, require clinical monitoring to include serial WB testing. FDA guidelines prohibit the donation of blood or plasma from any individual with an indeterminate WB result.
  Frequency of Monitoring
      A patient who has indeterminate results on the Western blot (WB) assay for HIV should be retested 1 month or later, since most patients with indeterminate WB results who are infected with HIV will develop detectable antibodies within 1 month.

COLLECTION/STORAGE INFORMATION
• Draw serum or plasma in a red-top or serum separator tube
• Store sample for 2 weeks or less at 2 to 8°C, or longer at -20°C

LOINC CODES
• Code: 34592-6 (*Short Name* - HIV1 Ab Fld QI IB)
• Code: 5221-7 (*Short Name* - HIV 1 Ab Ser QI IB)
• Code: 32571-2 (*Short Name* - HIV 1 Ab Ur QI IB)
• Code: 21009-6 (*Short Name* - HIV 1 Ser IB-Imp)

HTLV 1 AND 2 antibody assay

TEST DEFINITION
    Detection and measurement of retroviral antibodies in serum for the identification and management of human T-lymphotropic virus (HTLV) types 1 and 2

REFERENCE RANGE
    Negative
    Please refer to your institution's reference ranges as lab normals may vary.

INDICATIONS
Screening of donated blood for human T-lymphotropic virus (HTLV) types I and II
  Strength of Recommendation: Class IIa
  Strength of Evidence: Category B
  Results Interpretation:
  Positive immunology findings
      A positive enzyme immunoassay result for HTLV types I and II should be retested to ensure accuracy. Once seropositivity is confirmed, immunoreactivity to gag gene product p24 and to an env gene product must be demonstrated before diagnosis can be made.
      Higher human T-lymphotropic (HTLV) type I or type II viral loads may be associated with higher seroconversion rates in patients receiving infected blood products.

In general, individuals with HTLV-I have a higher viral load than patients with HTLV-II (0.2 copies per 100 peripheral blood mononuclear cell (PBMC) vs 0.04 per 100 PBMC, respectively). Patients who have higher HTLV proviral load may have a higher incidence of disease, such as myelopathy, tropical spastic paraparesis, cutaneous lymphoma, and peripheral neuropathy, particularly in patients co-infected with HIV. Patients with lower proviral loads have milder disease-related signs and symptoms.

COLLECTION/STORAGE INFORMATION
- Draw serum sample in red-top or serum separator tube.

LOINC CODES
- Code: 22363-6 (*Short Name* - HTLV1+2 Ab Ser-aCnc)
- Code: 13247-2 (*Short Name* - HTLV1+2 Ab CSF-aCnc)
- Code: 21345-4 (*Short Name* - HTLV 1+2 Ab CSF QI IB)
- Code: 22361-0 (*Short Name* - HTLV 1+2 Ab CSF QI)
- Code: 29901-6 (*Short Name* - HTLV 1+2 Ab Ser QI EIA)
- Code: 16982-1 (*Short Name* - HTLV 1+2 Ab Ser QI IB)
- Code: 22362-8 (*Short Name* - HTLV 1+2 Ab Ser QI)
- Code: 5226-6 (*Short Name* - HTLV 1+2 Ab Ser EIA-aCnc)

Haloperidol measurement

TEST DEFINITION
Measurement of haloperidol levels in serum or plasma to facilitate therapeutic monitoring

SYNONYMS
- Haldol measurement

REFERENCE RANGE
- Therapeutic concentration: 6 to 245 ng/mL (tentative) [x 2.66 = 16 to 652 nmol/l]
  Please refer to your institution's reference ranges as lab normals may vary.

INDICATIONS
Drug level monitoring during haloperidol therapy
   Strength of Recommendation: Class IIa
   Strength of Evidence: Category B
   Results Interpretation:
   Blood drug levels - finding
      There is wide interindividual variability among patients in determining the most effective therapeutic dose, but serum concentrations of haloperidol appear to be reasonable predictors of clinical response in patients with schizophrenia. Haloperidol plasma concentrations between 12 and 59 ng/mL (maximum therapeutic efficacy was reached at concentrations of approximately 35.7 ng/mL) were found to be the limits of the therapeutic window for schizophrenic patients. A second study found the average effective range to be 4 to 22 ng/mL. Higher serum concentrations were not associated with clinical improvement, but rather increased the risk for adverse effects.
      Serum concentrations over 6 to 9 ng/mL have been associated with an increased in side effects in psychotic patients. Sedation has been observed at lower levels in patients with Gilles de la Tourette Syndrome. In schizophrenic patients, haloperidol concentrations of 20 to 26 ng/mL were more frequently associated with extrapyramidal reactions. Adverse effects (ie, intense sedation, fatigue, muscular weakness, psychomotor agitation, aggressive episodes, and increased hallucinations) have been reported at haloperidol concentrations of 50 to 200 ng/mL.
      In children, daily doses of haloperidol from 15 to 285 mcg/kg resulted in varied steady-state plasma concentrations from 0.7 to 19 ng/mL without an apparent relationship to dose. However, a correlation between an increase in side effects and haloperidol plasma levels over 6 ng/mL was observed. Plasma concentrations of 15 to 20 micrograms/mL were associated with deep coma following accidental high doses of haloperidol in children. Although a correlation apparently exists between adverse events and plasma concentration in children, this correlation remains controversial.

COLLECTION/STORAGE INFORMATION
- Collect serum in purple (EDTA) or green top (heparin) tube.

LOINC CODES
- Code: 14774-4 (*Short Name* - Haloperidol SerPl-sCnc)
- Code: 3669-9 (*Short Name* - Haloperidol SerPl-mCnc)
- Code: 3671-5 (*Short Name* - Haloperidol Ur-mCnc)
- Code: 19478-7 (*Short Name* - Haloperidol Ur Ql Scn)
- Code: 3670-7 (*Short Name* - Haloperidol Ur Ql)
- Code: 19479-5 (*Short Name* - Haloperidol Ur Ql Cnfrn)
- Code: 26847-4 (*Short Name* - Haloperidol SerPl Ql)
- Code: 20530-2 (*Short Name* - Haloperidol Ur Cnfrn-mCnc)
- Code: 19480-3 (*Short Name* - Haloperidol CtO Ur Scn-mCnc)
- Code: 19481-1 (*Short Name* - Haloperidol CtO Ur Cfm-mCnc)

Ham test

TEST DEFINITION
Measurement of red cell lysis in an acidic environment for the detection of certain red cell disorders (Ham's test)

SYNONYMS
- Acid haemolysin assay
- Acid hemolysin assay
- Acidified serum lysis test, RBC
- Acidified serum test, RBC

REFERENCE RANGE
- Negative
  Please refer to your institution's reference ranges as lab normals may vary.

INDICATIONS
Suspected congenital dyserythropoietic anemia type II (CDA II)/hereditary erythroblastic multinuclearity associated with a positive acidified-serum test (HEMPAS)
  Strength of Recommendation: Class IIa
  Strength of Evidence: Category C
  Results Interpretation:
  Acidified serum test positive
   A positive result on the acidified serum lysis test, when paired with a negative sucrose hemolysis test, strongly suggests the diagnosis of CDA II.

Suspected paroxysmal nocturnal hemoglobinuria (PNH)
  Strength of Recommendation: Class IIb
  Strength of Evidence: Category B
  Results Interpretation:
  Acidified serum test positive
   A positive Ham's test result is determined when greater than 5% of red blood cells are lysed. A positive result on Ham test confirms the diagnosis of either PNH or CDA II, the latter of which can be ruled out by a bone marrow biopsy and a negative sucrose hemolysis test.

  False Results
   A false negative Ham's test may occur in complement depletion

COLLECTION/STORAGE INFORMATION
- Draw blood in EDTA (lavender), heparin (green), oxalate, or citrate (blue) tubes

LOINC CODES
- Code: 18297-2 (*Short Name* - Ac Lysis RBC-mCnc)

Helicobacter pylori antibody assay

TEST DEFINITION
Detection of *helicobacter pylori* in serum for the evaluation and management of gastrointestinal disorders

SYNONYMS
- Serologic test for Helicobacter pylori

REFERENCE RANGE
- Negative
  Please refer to your institution's reference ranges as lab normals may vary.

INDICATIONS
Suspected *Helicobacter pylori* **associated gastric cancer**
> **Strength of Recommendation:** Class IIa
> **Strength of Evidence:** Category B
> **Results Interpretation:**
> **Helicobacter serology positive**
> *Helicobacter pylori* antibody titers are associated with the development of gastric cancer.

Suspected *Helicobacter pylori* **gastritis**
> **Strength of Recommendation:** Class IIa
> **Strength of Evidence:** Category B
> **Results Interpretation:**
> **Helicobacter serology positive**
> A drop in antibody levels of 20% to 50% from baseline is suggestive of cure. However, because levels drop slowly and inconsistently, *Helicobacter pylori* -specific antibody tests are not useful for monitoring response to treatment or for measuring reinfection rates. Levels should be limited to establishing an initial diagnosis.

> **False Results**
> False negative serology results for *Helicobacter pylori* have been correlated with chronic atrophic gastritis in the elderly.
> Because serologic assay cutoff values may be different in children, cut-off values may require a downward adjustment in pediatric patients to avoid false negatives. In one study, 50% of children with *Helicobacter pylori* gastritis would have presented as seronegative using the adult cut-off value.
> **Timing of Monitoring**
> Antibody titers gradually decrease after successful treatment, but the rate of decline is variable. A drop in titer from baseline may occur as early as 6 weeks after successful eradication, but seronegativity may take up to 1 year. Studies have reported wide variability in both 6 month seronegativity (85%) and 1 year seronegativity conversion (36%, 50% and 95%).

Suspected *Helicobacter pylori* **peptic ulcer disease**
> **Strength of Recommendation:** Class IIa
> **Strength of Evidence:** Category C
> **Results Interpretation:**
> **Helicobacter serology positive**
> *Helicobacter pylori* eradication leads to a substantial reduction in type B gastritis and a lower duodenal ulcer relapse rate.

CLINICAL NOTES
The enzyme-linked immunosorbent assay (ELISA) must be locally validated because of regional variability in antibody levels.

COLLECTION/STORAGE INFORMATION
- Enzyme-linked immunosorbent assay (ELISA):
  - Collect specimen in marble-top tube.
- Rapid antibody serology test:
  - Draw fingerstick specimen into glass or plastic capillary tube.

LOINC CODES

- Code: 7900-4 (*Short Name* - H pylori Ab Ser-aCnc)
- Code: 16533-2 (*Short Name* - H pylori Ab Titr Ser)
- Code: 7901-2 (*Short Name* - H pylori IgA Ser-aCnc)
- Code: 6419-6 (*Short Name* - H pylori Ab Ser Ql IF)
- Code: 6420-4 (*Short Name* - H pylori IgA Ser EIA-aCnc)
- Code: 5174-8 (*Short Name* - H pylori Ab Ser EIA-aCnc)
- Code: 16127-3 (*Short Name* - H pylori IgM Ser Ql)
- Code: 16929-2 (*Short Name* - H pylori Ab Ser IF-aCnc)
- Code: 7903-8 (*Short Name* - H pylori IgM Ser-aCnc)
- Code: 5177-1 (*Short Name* - H pylori IgM Ser EIA-aCnc)
- Code: 5175-5 (*Short Name* - H pylori Ab Titr Ser LA)

Helicobacter pylori breath test

TEST DEFINITION

Detection of *Helicobacter pylori* urease activity by measurement of exhaled CO_2 following ingestion of radiolabeled urea for the diagnosis and management of *H pylori* infection

REFERENCE RANGE

Adults and Children: Below cut-off value for radiolabeled CO_2
- Adults: Below cut-off value for radiolabeled CO_2
Please refer to your institution's reference ranges as lab normals may vary.

INDICATIONS

Suspected *Helicobacter pylori* **gastritis**
    Strength of Recommendation: Class IIa
    Strength of Evidence: Category B
    Results Interpretation:
    Positive biochemistry findings
    A positive urea breath test may be considered diagnostic of *Helicobacter pylori* -associated gastritis and may be useful in monitoring response to therapy.
    Frequency of Monitoring
    When monitoring response to anti-*H pylori* treatment, re-testing should be postponed for at least one month after completing antibiotic, bismuth, or proton pump inhibitor therapy to prevent false-negative test results.
    Timing of Monitoring
    To avoid false-negative results, testing should be delayed for at least 2 weeks after discontinuing proton pump inhibitors or high-dose H2 receptor antagonists and 4 weeks after antibiotic or bismuth therapy.

DRUG/LAB INTERACTIONS

- Lansoprazole - false-negative 13C-urea breath test results
- Omeprazole - false-negative 13C-urea breath test results
- Ranitidine - false-negative 13C-urea breath test results

CLINICAL NOTES

The timing of the breath collection, the substance choice, the form in which the urea is delivered (liquid versus tablet), the adequacy of the collection technique, and the gastric emptying time will all influence the accuracy of the test.

Contraindications

Avoid the use of ^{14}C-labeled urea in children and pregnant women.

Helicobacter pylori culture

TEST DEFINITION
Detection of *Helicobacter pylori* by culture of gastric antrum and corpus biopsy specimens

REFERENCE RANGE
• Negative
Please refer to your institution's reference ranges as lab normals may vary.

INDICATIONS
Treatment-resistant peptic ulcer
    Strength of Recommendation: Class IIa
    Strength of Evidence: Category C
    Results Interpretation:
    Positive microbiology findings
    Helicobacter pylori usually can be detected in culture of gastric biopsy specimens after 3 to 5 days of incubation, although it may take up to 10 days.
    Reduced sensitivity in detecting *H pylori* in bleeding peptic ulcers may be a result of actual decreased bacterial load due to a suppression effect of intraluminal blood on *H pylori*, removal by gastric lavage before endoscopy, or use of antisecretory drugs.
    Overall prevalence of antibiotic-resistant *H pylori* is highest with use of metronidazole and clarithromycin; resistance to amoxicillin and tetracycline is rare.

    False Results
    Possibility of false-negative results increases in patients with recent use of antibiotics, bismuth compounds, or proton pump inhibitors.

CLINICAL NOTES
Recent antibiotic use, ingestion of topical anesthetic or simethicone during endoscopy, and contamination of biopsy forceps with glutaraldehyde can affect culture results.

COLLECTION/STORAGE INFORMATION
• Specimen Collection and Handling:
    • Process specimen within 2 to 3 hours of collection.
    • For transport under 6 hours, use sterile saline.
    • For delayed processing and transport greater than 6 hours, use an enriched medium such as Brucella or cysteine Albemi broth with 20% glycerol, isotonic sterile saline with 4% glucose, or Stuart's.
    • May store tissue specimen at 4°C for up to 5 hours. For long-term storage, freeze specimen immediately at -70°C or in medium with glycerol.

LOINC CODES
• Code: 587-6 (*Short Name* - H pylori XXX QI Cult)

Hematocrit determination

TEST DEFINITION
Ratio of the volume of red blood cells (RBC) to volume of whole blood expressed as a percentage (conventional) or as a decimal fraction (SI units)

SYNONYMS
• Haematocrit
• Haematocrit determination
• Haematocrit - PCV
• Hct - Haematocrit
• Hct - Hematocrit
• Hematocrit

- Hematocrit - PCV

REFERENCE RANGE
- Adult females, whole blood: 36%-46% (0.36-0.46):
- Adult males, whole blood: 41%-53% (0.41-0.53):
- Fetal and cord blood:
- 18 to 20 weeks' gestation: 35.86% +/- 3.29 (0.36 +/- 0.03)
- 21 to 22 weeks' gestation: 38.53% +/- 3.21 (0.39 +/- 0.03)
- 23 to 25 weeks' gestation: 38.59% +/- 2.41 (0.39 +/- 0.02)
- 26 to 30 weeks' gestation: 41.54% +/- 3.31 (0.42 +/- 0.03)
- Cord Blood: 42%-60% (0.42-0.6)
- Neonates, 1 day (capillary whole blood): 61% +/- 7.41 (0.61 +/- 0.07)
- Neonates, 4 days (capillary whole blood): 57% +/- 8.1 (0.57 +/- 0.08)
- Neonates, 7 days (capillary whole blood): 56% +/- 9.4 (0.56 +/- 0.09)
- Neonates, 1-2 weeks (capillary whole blood): 54% +/- 8.3 (0.54 +/- 0.08)
- Neonates, 3-4 weeks (capillary whole blood): 43% +/- 5.7 (0.43 +/- 0.06)
- Infants, 5-6 weeks (capillary whole blood): 36% +/- 6.2 (0.36 +/- 0.06)
- Infants, 7-8 weeks (capillary whole blood): 33% +/- 3.7 (0.33 +/- 0.04)
- Infants, 9-10 weeks (capillary whole blood): 32% +/- 2.7 (0.32 +/- 0.03)
- Infants, 11-12 weeks (capillary whole blood): 33% +/- 3.3 (0.33 +/- 0.03)
- Infants, 2 weeks (whole blood): 41%-65% (0.41-0.65)
- Infants, 1 month (whole blood): 33%-55% (0.33-0.55)
- Infants, 2 months (whole blood): 28%-42% (0.28-0.42)
- Infants, 4 months (whole blood): 32%-44% (0.32-0.44)
- Infants, 6 months (whole blood): 31%-41% (0.31-0.41)
- Infants, 9 months (whole blood): 32%-40% (0.32-0.40)
- Infants, 12 months (whole blood): 33%-41% (0.33-0.41)
- Infants, 1-2 years (whole blood): 32%-40% (0.32-0.40)
- Children, 3-5 years (whole blood): 32%-42% (0.32-0.42)
- Children, 6-8 years (whole blood): 33%-41% (0.33-0.41)
- Children, 9-11 years (whole blood): 34%-43% (0.34-0.43)
- Females, 12-14 years (whole blood): 34%-44% (0.34-0.44)
- Males, 12-14 years (whole blood): 35%-45% (0.35-0.45)
- Females, 15-17 years (whole blood): 34%-44% (0.34-0.44)
- Males, 15-17 years (whole blood): 37%-48% (0.37-0.48)
Please refer to your institution's reference ranges as lab normals may vary.

INDICATIONS
Pre-eclampsia
   Results Interpretation:
   Decreased hematocrit level
      Evidence of microangiopathic hemolytic anemia (with increased LDH concentration), alone or with thrombocytopenia, increases the certainty of a preeclampsia diagnosis. A decreased hematocrit is a marker of severe disease.
   Hematocrit - PCV - high
      Hemoconcentration supports a diagnosis of preeclampsia (with or without proteinuria) and is an indicator of disease severity.

Assessment of anemia in patients with a suspected or known femoral shaft fracture
   Results Interpretation:
   Decreased hematocrit level
      The typical adult femoral shaft fracture causes 1,500 to 2,500 mL of blood loss with a resultant drop in hematocrit.

Abnormal uterine bleeding
   Results Interpretation:
   Decreased hematocrit level
      A decreased hematocrit indicates significant chronic or acute blood loss.
      Blood loss of more than 80 mL can occur without anemia. Failure to demonstrate anemia may be due to excessive production of red blood cells that allows the body to compensate for excessive blood loss. The presence of hypochromic microcytic anemia may provide supportive evidence for excessive blood loss.

Iron balance in a normal woman is only marginally adequate. Excessive menstrual bleeding usually depletes iron stores, which results in iron deficiency anemia in almost 70% of women, unless they are taking extra sources of iron in their diet. Low serum ferritin levels may be more sensitive, indicating depletion of iron stores before anemia develops.

End-stage renal disease
Strength of Recommendation: Class I
Strength of Evidence: Category A
Results Interpretation:
Decreased hematocrit level
Anemia is present in most patients with chronic renal failure and glomerular filtration rate of less than 30 mL/min secondary to decreased quantities of endogenous erythropoietin.
Based on guidelines by the National Kidney Foundation, a target hematocrit (Hct) level of 33% to 36% is desirable to improve overall morbidity and mortality in end-stage renal disease patients.

Hemolytic uremic syndrome (HUS)
Results Interpretation:
Decreased hematocrit level
Patients with typical hemolytic uremic syndrome (HUS) usually have a normochromic and microcytic anemia with a hematocrit less than 25%. Hemolysis may be brisk, with a corresponding hematocrit drop of 10% or more in 24 hours.
The mean corpuscular volume (MCV) is low secondary to mechanical counting of RBC fragments.

HIV infection
Results Interpretation:
Decreased hematocrit level
Mild to moderate anemia (hematocrit 31% to 39%) is usually present in patients with HIV infection, but more severe anemia may occur. The degree of anemia does not correlate with any clinical manifestations of AIDS. Inadequate increments in serum erythropoietin may be involved in HIV-associated anemia.
Autoimmune hemolytic anemia may occur, often without reticulocytosis, despite bone marrow erythroid hyperplasia. The disorder should be suspected in all anemic HIV-infected patients who have positive direct antiglobulin tests.
Persistent parvovirus B19 infection may be a major contributing factor to anemia in patients with AIDS. This should be considered whenever cytopenia occurs, particularly in the setting of severe anemia.

Infectious mononucleosis
Results Interpretation:
Anemia is rare in infectious mononucleosis. It may be secondary to hemolysis and can be severe and life-threatening.
Aplastic anemia has also been described.

Initial laboratory evaluation of patients with blunt head trauma.
Results Interpretation:
Decreased hematocrit level
Hematocrit value may be decreased if there is significant blood loss from scalp or associated extracranial injuries, or in children with cephalhematoma.

Malaria
Results Interpretation:
Decreased hematocrit level
Decreased hematocrit is the most common lab abnormality in patients with malaria, and the cause is multifactorial. The pathogenesis varies with the Plasmodium species, stage of disease, and host factors. Dehydration may mask the presence or degree of anemia.
Hemolysis results primarily from rupture of infected RBCs during schizogony, although the magnitude of hemolysis tends to be greater than can be accounted for by this process alone.
Other mechanisms of hemolysis include splenic clearance of infected RBCs in association with the development of splenomegaly, autoimmune destruction of infected and noninfected coated RBCs, increased fragility of RBCs caused by dysfunction of the sodium-potassium pump, decreased incorporation of iron into heme, and impaired erythropoiesis.
Severity is positively correlated with the number of infected RBCs and the host response to infection. The most severe anemia occurs with falciparum infections because erythrocytes of all ages are invaded, and parasite counts ultimately may exceed 50%.

In vivax and ovale malaria, parasites invade only reticulocytes, and therefore, the parasite count rarely exceeds 2% to 5%. In *P malariae* infection, only older erythrocytes are invaded, and the parasite count is usually less than 2%. The majority of patients with 1 of these nonfalciparum infections compensate sufficiently that anemia does not occur.

Pancreatitis
Results Interpretation:
Hematocrit - finding
- Normal hematocrit:
  - A normal hematocrit (ie, the absence of hemoconcentration) in otherwise stable patients is helpful in ruling out pancreatic necrosis
- Increased hematocrit:
  - An elevated hematocrit value may occur secondary to volume depletion
- Decreased hematocrit:
  - A decreased hematocrit value may occur secondary to hemorrhage
  - A >10% decrease in hematocrit within 48 hours of admission is one of Ranson's criteria suggesting severe pancreatitis

Screening for iron-deficiency anemia
Strength of Recommendation: Class IIa
Strength of Evidence: Category C
Results Interpretation:
Decreased hematocrit level
A screening cutoff value below the accepted threshold requires a confirmatory test in all patients. In patients who are not ill a presumptive diagnosis of iron-deficiency anemia can be made, and treatment initiated, if the second test result also falls below the acceptable threshold for the patient's age. If HCT rises to 3% or more after 4 weeks of iron supplementation therapy the diagnosis of iron-deficiency anemia can be confirmed. Patients who do not respond favorably after 4 weeks of iron supplementation therapy and who are not acutely ill should have further testing done, to include mean cell volume, red blood cell distribution width and serum ferritin concentration.

In iron deficiency anemia, Hgb levels fall first, followed by HCT levels.

Blacks have lower HCT values than whites. Because the cause of this disparity is not yet understood, recommended race-specific cutoff values have not been determined by the Centers for Disease Control. Other tests such as serum ferritin and transferrin saturation may be appropriate alternative tests in this population.

Thalassemia minor or sickle cell trait should be considered in women of African, Mediterranean or Southeast Asian ancestry with mild anemia refractory to therapy.

Pregnant women with an HCT below 27% should be referred to a physician with expertise in treating anemia during pregnancy.

False Results
Vigorous squeezing of the finger during capillary specimen collection can cause false low results due to contamination of the sample by excessive tissue fluid. Low results obtained by the capillary collection method should be confirmed with a repeat capillary sample or by venipuncture.

Hematocrit - PCV - high
High Hgb and HCT levels in pregnancy are associated with poor pregnancy outcomes. HCT levels greater than 43% at 26 to 30 weeks gestation have been associated with an increased risk of preterm delivery and fetal growth retardation. HCT levels above 45%, especially in the second trimester, require further evaluation for potential pregnancy complications due to inadequate blood volume expansion. High levels of either HCT or Hgb in the second or third trimester are not reflective of desirable iron status.

False Results
Vigorous squeezing of the finger during capillary specimen collection can cause false low results due to contamination of the sample by excessive tissue fluid. Low results obtained by the capillary collection method should be confirmed with a repeat capillary sample or by venipuncture.

Hematocrit - finding
- Cutoff HCT values (<%) for anemia by age, sex, and pregnancy are as follows. The values for children ages 1 to <2 can be used for infants ages 6 to 12 months:
  - Children (age in years):
    - 1 - <2: 32.9
    - 2 - <5: 33
    - 5 - <8: 34.5
    - 8 - <12: 35.4

- Men (age in years):
  - 12 - <15: 37.3
  - 15 - <18: 39.7
  - ≥18: 39.9
- Nonpregnant women and lactating women (age in years):
  - 12 - <15: 35.7
  - 15 - <18: 35.9
  - ≥18: 35.7
- Pregnant women by weeks gestation:
  - 12 wks: 33
  - 16 wks: 32
  - 20 wks: 32
  - 24 wks: 32
  - 28 wks: 32
  - 32 wks: 33
  - 36 wks: 34
  - 40 wks: 36
- Pregnant women by trimester:
  - First trimester: 33
  - Second trimester: 32
  - Third trimester: 33
- People that live at elevations of 3,000 feet or higher for long periods of time will have slightly higher Hgb and HCT levels, as will smokers. HCT values (%) should therefore be adjusted upward as follows:
  - Altitude (feet)
    - 3,000 - 3,999: +0.5
    - 4,000 - 4,999: +1
    - 5,000 - 5,999: +1.5
    - 6,000 - 6,999: +2
    - 7,000 - 7,999: +3
    - 8,000 - 8,999: +4
    - 9,000 - 9,999: +5
    - 10,000 - 11,000: +6
  - Cigarette smoking (packs per day)
    - 0.5 - <1: +1
    - 1 - <2: +1.5
    - ≥2: +2%
    - All smokers: +1

HCT values cannot identify the cause of anemia. However, iron-deficiency anemia can be diagnosed if either Hgb or HCT values rise following iron supplementation therapy. Other red blood cell indices such as mean cell volume, red blood cell distribution width and serum ferritin, can also be used to differentiate iron-deficiency anemia from other causes of anemia.

False Results

Vigorous squeezing of the finger during capillary specimen collection can cause false low results due to contamination of the sample by excessive tissue fluid. Low results obtained by the capillary collection method should be confirmed with a repeat capillary sample or by venipuncture.

Frequency of Monitoring

In infants, children, and adolescents, a repeat Hgb or HCT test should be performed 1 month after iron supplementation therapy is initiated. If HCT results still indicate anemia continue iron supplementation and repeat an HCT test in 2 more months. An HCT test should also be obtained 6 months after completion of successful treatment.

Timing of Monitoring

The Centers for Disease Control recommends screening all high-risk infants and children between 9 and 12 months, 6 months later, and annually in children ages 2 to 5. Preterm and low birthweight infants who are not fed iron-fortified formula should be screened before 6 months of age. Children between the ages of 2 and 5 should be assessed annually and screened if risk factors are present (low-iron diet, limited access to food, or special health-care needs). At age 9 to 12 months and again at age 15 to 18 months, screen children who have one or more of the following risk factors: (1) preterm or low birthweight infants; (2) infants fed a non iron-fortified infant formula for more than 2 months; (3) infants fed cow's milk before 1 year of age; (4) breast-fed infants who are consuming an inadequate amount of iron from supplementary foods; (4) children who drink more than 24 oz of cow's milk daily; (5) children with special health-care needs, eg children with chronic infection or inflammatory conditions, children who have experienced significant blood loss through injury or surgery, children on restricted diets, or children who take medication that interferes with iron absorption. School age children and adolescent boys require screening only if they have a history of iron-deficiency anemia, have special health-care needs, or have a history of low iron intake.

The American Academy of Pediatrics recommends routine universal HCT or Hgb screening at 9 to 12 months of age and annual screening in menstruating adolescents. Additional screening is recommended in early childhood (15 months of age through 5 years of age) for children at risk. Screening prior to 9 months should be considered for high risk infants.

Adolescent nonpregnant girls should be screening every 5 to 10 years throughout their childbearing years as part of routine health examinations. Annual screening in this population is suggested if risk factors are present such as excessive menstrual blood loss, low iron intake or a history of iron-deficiency anemia.

Routine screening of all asymptomatic pregnant women is recommended. Pregnant women should be tested at their first prenatal visit and again 4 to 6 weeks postpartum if risk factors are present, ie anemia throughout the third trimester, extensive blood loss during delivery, and multiple birth.

Severe heart failure
Strength of Recommendation: Class I
Strength of Evidence: Category B
Results Interpretation:
Decreased hematocrit level
A moderate anemia (hematocrit 25% to 35%) may aggravate underlying heart failure, and a severe anemia (hematocrit less than 25%) may precipitate heart failure even in a patient without underlying structural heart disease.

According to data from the Prospective Randomized Amlodipine Survival Evaluation (PRAISE), anemia (hematocrit less than 37.5%) is a significant predictor of mortality in patients with severe heart failure, particularly death due to progressive pump failure.

Suspected acute hemorrhage
Strength of Recommendation: Class I
Strength of Evidence: Category B
Results Interpretation:
Decreased hematocrit level
A low HCT level on initial presentation suggests significant ongoing hemorrhage and a high risk of death.
Hematocrit - finding
A normal HCT level in hemorrhagic shock may be due to endogenous intravascular volume expansion by transcapillary refill.

Endogenous hemodilution by movement of fluid from interstitial to intravascular space equilibration according to Starling's forces requires several hours, so initial HCTs may be normal.

Suspected alcoholic ketoacidosis
Results Interpretation:
Hematocrit - borderline high
With significant dehydration seen in alcoholic ketoacidosis, the hematocrit can be mildly elevated.
Decreased hematocrit level
Following rehydration for alcoholic ketoacidosis, the hematocrit usually falls to anemic values consistent with chronic alcoholism.

Suspected and known bowel obstruction
Results Interpretation:
Patients with large bowel obstruction may show evidence of anemia, particularly when presenting with neoplasms or inflammatory bowel disease.
Raised hematology findings
Dehydration secondary to fluid sequestration and vomiting may cause an increase in hematocrit.

Suspected and known ovarian hyperstimulation syndrome
Results Interpretation:
Raised hematology findings
An increased hematocrit is a frequent finding associated with fluid shifts into the peritoneal and thoracic cavities. Values may be directly related to the plasma concentrations of vasoactive substances (plasma renin activity, aldosterone, norepinephrine, and antidiuretic hormone).

A hematocrit greater than 48% indicates possible grade 5 ovarian hyperstimulation syndrome and is an indication for hospital admission.

Decreased hematocrit level
Some investigators have reported a decreased hematocrit in patients with ovarian hyperstimulation syndrome, possibly as a consequence of intravenous fluid therapy.

Suspected and known rheumatoid arthritis
Results Interpretation:
Decreased hematocrit level
Moderate normocytic normochromic anemia is the most common extraarticular manifestation of rheumatoid disease, but microcytic or macrocytic anemia also may occur. The anemia is closely correlated to the extent of the disease activity. Some drug therapies used for rheumatoid arthritis may be associated with anemia such as in nonsteroidal antiinflammatory drug-induced iron deficiency.

Suspected anemia
Results Interpretation:
Decreased hematocrit level
Very mild anemias are associated with few or no clinical signs or symptoms; therefore, a mild anemia usually is first detected from a screening measurement of Hgb or HCT.
A markedly decreased HCT level should prompt additional laboratory investigation, including a CBC, a reticulocyte count, and measurements of iron supply, including the serum iron, total iron-binding capacity (TIBC), and serum ferritin.
In children and adolescents, a HCT level less than 20% with a Hgb level less than 7 g/dL may be associated with increased mortality.

Suspected decompression sickness
Results Interpretation:
Raised hematology findings
An increased hematocrit value secondary to plasma loss and hemoconcentration may be seen.

Suspected ectopic pregnancy
Results Interpretation:
Decreased hematocrit level
Continued or worsening anemia in a woman with abdominal pain should alert the physician to the possibility of ruptured ectopic pregnancy.
Hematocrit - finding
A hematocrit value in the normal range is expected unless the patient has had repeated blood loss.

Suspected ehrlichiosis
Strength of Recommendation: Class IIa
Strength of Evidence: Category C
Results Interpretation:
Decreased hematocrit level
Mild anemia (usually normocytic normochromic) is a common finding in ehrlichiosis, noted in about 50% of cases. Mild anemia develops after first week of illness and is usually transient, but may indicate more serious illness, particularly in elderly patients.

Suspected hantavirus pulmonary syndrome
Results Interpretation:
Raised hematology findings
Hemoconcentration is a characteristic laboratory finding in hantavirus pulmonary syndrome and indicates capillary leak. It has been noted on admission in 75% of patients. A median peak hematocrit reported is 56.3% (range, 49.9% to 67.8%) in men and 48.5% (range, 36.5% to 60.3%) in women.
The combination of maximal increases in hematocrit and either serum LDH or partial thromboplastin time during hospitalization is predictive of death.

Suspected hemorrhagic shock
Results Interpretation:
Hematocrit - finding
A normal hematocrit is due to endogenous intravascular volume expansion by transcapillary refill.

Suspected infective endocarditis
Results Interpretation:
Decreased hematocrit level
Anemia is present in 50% to 80% of patients and is usually normocytic and normochromic, without reticulocytosis. May develop rapidly secondary to intravascular hemorrhage.
Hemolytic anemia may occur secondary to splenic sequestration.

Suspected Kawasaki disease
Results Interpretation:
Decreased level (laboratory finding)
Mild-to-moderate normocytic anemia that is not associated with reticulocytosis may develop with normal red blood cell indices during a more prolonged phase of active inflammation.
A hematocrit level of less than 35% is one of several criteria used in the Harada scoring system for predicting coronary artery aneurysms.
Severe hemolytic anemia may rarely occur and may be related to immunoglobulin therapy.

Suspected necrotizing soft tissue infection
Results Interpretation:
Hematocrit - finding
An increase in the hematocrit occurs during the late stages of necrotizing fasciitis and clostridial myonecrosis, secondary to large third-space plasma losses into the necrotic tissue. This occasionally results in shock.
Marked hemolysis and a loss of blood into the necrotic tissue sometimes results in a decrease in the hematocrit and hemoglobin in necrotizing fasciitis and clostridial myonecrosis. Hematocrit is less than 30 mg/dL in 40% of patients with synergistic necrotizing cellulitis and in 70% of patients with necrotizing fasciitis due to hemolysis. A decreased hematocrit is also reported in Fournier's gangrene.

Suspected or known cardiogenic shock
Results Interpretation:
Raised hematology findings
Increased HCT occurs during the first few days following infarction as a consequence of hemoconcentration.
Decreased hematocrit level
Anemia rarely occurs within the first 12 hours of the onset of shock.

Suspected or known gastrointestinal bleeding
Results Interpretation:
Hematocrit - PCV abnormal
- An initial HCT level less than 28% and a Hgb level less than 11 g/dL represent significant hemorrhage or an acute bleeding episode superimposed on chronic bleeding.
- Even with massive bleeding, the HCT and Hgb levels may remain normal for several hours. However, the plasma refill rate is proportional to the degree of hemorrhagic shock.
  - A 10% to 20% loss results in a 40 to 90 mL/hour movement of fluid from the interstitial space into the intravascular space. Thirty to 40 hours are needed for completion of this process.
  - Patients with blood loss greater than 40% have intravascular fluid space refill rates as high as 1,500 mL in the first 90 minutes following injury.
  - Therefore, even without exogenous crystalloid transfusion, a significant dilution in RBC mass with a decrease in the HCT level can occur relatively quickly.
  - Repeated HCT level measurements may reflect the rate of replenishment of the intravascular fluid space.
- In children and adolescents, a HCT level less than 20% with a Hgb level less than 7 g/dL may be associated with increased mortality.
- Microcytic anemia is most commonly associated with occult upper gastrointestinal bleeding.
- Macrocytic anemia may occur with an achlorhydric stomach in gastric carcinoma, in hamartomas, or following acute hemorrhage with increased reticulocytosis.

Suspected or known Meckel diverticulum
Results Interpretation:
Anemia may be present in patients with a Meckel diverticulum who are experiencing either acute or chronic bleeding. Anemia may be especially severe in children less than 2 years of age, necessitating blood transfusions in some cases.
If bleeding has been chronic, a Meckel diverticulum may be associated with iron-deficiency anemia, which may be the presenting feature.

Fluid loss from vomiting or fluid sequestration in obstruction, diverticulitis, or perforation may cause a falsely elevated hematocrit.

Suspected polycythemia
Strength of Recommendation: Class IIa
Strength of Evidence: Category C
Results Interpretation:
Increased level (laboratory finding)

An increased hemoglobin or hematocrit is often the first sign of erythrocytosis. Serial blood counts are valuable for documenting the onset of elevated levels.

Patients with persistently elevated packed red cell volume (greater than 51% in males; greater than 48% in females) should be referred to a hematologist for further evaluation.

A hematocrit of more than 60% (hemoglobin 20%) in males and more than 55% (hemoglobin 18%) in females is usually diagnostic for absolute erythrocytosis. Red cell mass and plasma volume, however, should be evaluated to exclude a contracted plasma volume state.

In mountainous areas, baseline hematocrit levels will be higher. A hematocrit level of more than 48% in women and 54% or higher in men generally indicates the presence of erythrocytosis, but a change in hematocrit level is a more important indicator.

In infants, a venous hematocrit of 65% or higher is usually diagnostic of neonatal polycythemia. The diagnosis needs to be confirmed with a venous sample, because a peripheral capillary sample will overestimate the venous hematocrit in many infants.

False Results
In infants, peripheral capillary sampling can overestimate hematocrit levels; venous sampling is required to confirm neonatal polycythemia.
Timing of Monitoring
In well infants, hematocrit testing should be performed after the peak hematocrit at 6 to 8 hours of age; symptomatic infants should be evaluated as clinically indicated.

Suspected porphyria
Results Interpretation:
Decreased level (laboratory finding)
Hematocrit may be decreased with erythrocytic porphyria.

Suspected post-streptococcal glomerulonephritis
Strength of Recommendation: Class I
Strength of Evidence: Category C
Results Interpretation:
Decreased level (laboratory finding)
Anemia may occur in patients with active post-streptococcal glomerulonephritis and may persist until diuresis occurs. The anemia is due to hemodilution rather than to blood loss.

Suspected preterm labor
Results Interpretation:
Decreased hematocrit level
The hematocrit is generally slightly depressed in most third trimester patients. This may be a reflection of the total increase in maternal blood volume throughout pregnancy. The total amount of hemoglobin is increased.

Suspected ruptured abdominal aortic aneurysm
Results Interpretation:
Decreased hematocrit level
An initial HCT of less than 28% and Hgb of less than 11 g/dL represents significant hemorrhage or an acute bleeding episode superimposed on chronic bleeding in patients with AAA.

Suspected tetanus
Results Interpretation:
Decreased hematocrit level
Decreased hematocrit in patients with tetanus may be due to the activity of hemolysin exotoxin.

Suspected toxic shock syndrome
> **Results Interpretation:**
> **Decreased hematocrit level**
>> The presence of normochromic normocytic anemia which normalizes within 4 to 6 weeks, is common in staphylococcal toxic shock syndrome (TSS).
>> Hemolytic anemia secondary to splenic sequestration may occur in streptococcal TSS.

Thermal burn
> **Results Interpretation:**
> **Decreased hematocrit level**
>> Blood volume decreases as a result of red blood cell destruction and loss of plasma from the vascular compartment immediately following a burn injury. This is directly related to the extent of the burn injury.
>> Hematocrit begins to decrease within 48 to 72 hours of burn injury due to intravascular fluid resorption, red blood cell lysis from thermal injury, and a characteristic anemia that develops in burn patients. Some extravasation of red blood cells occurs following burn injury, though the need for transfusion is rare.
> **Timing of Monitoring**
>> A baseline hematocrit measurement should be obtained immediately upon arrival in the emergency department. Hematocrit levels are obtained frequently in all burn victims requiring admission for fluid status monitoring, including blood status.

Traumatic amputation
> **Results Interpretation:**
> **Decreased hematocrit level**
>> The hematocrit is decreased in patients with traumatic amputation.

COMMON PANELS

- Anemia panel
- Complete blood count
- Complete blood count with automated differential
- Disseminated intravascular coagulopathy panel
- Enteral/Parenteral nutritional management panel
- General health panel
- Hemolysis panel
- Human immunodeficiency virus panel
- Prenatal screening panel
- Renal panel
- Transfusion reaction workup
- Transplant panel

ABNORMAL RESULTS

- Results increased in:
  - Prolonged venous status during venipuncture
  - Strenuous exercise
  - High altitude
- Results decreased in:
  - Hematocrit is slightly lower between 5 pm and 7 am
  - Hematocrit is up to 5.7% lower in recumbent patients
  - Men aged 65 to 74 years

COLLECTION/STORAGE INFORMATION

- Specimen Collection and Handling:
  - Collect whole blood sample in EDTA (lavender-top) tube or capillary blood sample in heparin (green-top) tube.
  - Obtain fetal blood by percutaneous umbilical blood sampling.
  - Sample stable for 48 hours at 4°C or 6 hours at 23°C.

LOINC CODES

- Code: 32354-3 (*Short Name* - Hct % BldA)
- Code: 31100-1 (*Short Name* - Hct % Bld Imped)
- Code: 17809-5 (*Short Name* - Hct % Ur)
- Code: 11153-4 (*Short Name* - Hct % Fld)

- Code: 11271-4 (*Short Name* - Hct % BldCo Fetus Auto)
- Code: 11151-8 (*Short Name* - Hct % BldCo Fet)
- Code: 4544-3 (*Short Name* - Hct % Bld Auto)
- Code: 20570-8 (*Short Name* - Hct % Bld)
- Code: 30398-2 (*Short Name* - Hct % CSF)

Hemochromatosis gene screening test

TEST DEFINITION
Detection of C282Y gene mutations in serum for the evaluation of hereditary hemochromatosis

SYNONYMS
- Haemochromatosis gene screening test

REFERENCE RANGE
- Negative
  Please refer to your institution's reference ranges as lab normals may vary.

INDICATIONS
Suspected hereditary hemochromatosis
 Strength of Recommendation: Class I
 Strength of Evidence: Category B
Results Interpretation:
Positive laboratory findings
 The hereditary hemochromatosis (HH) C282Y detection test can be used to confirm HH in symptomatic patients. In addition, the test may be used to identify homozygotes with presymptomatic iron overload for whom phlebotomy therapy may be warranted to prevent future chronic disease. With a test sensitivity of 90%, failure to detect C282Y homozygosity does not rule out HH; consequently, a liver biopsy may be warranted.

COLLECTION/STORAGE INFORMATION
- Collect serum in a lavender-topped tube.
- Store sample at -20°C.

LOINC CODES
- Code: 21695-2 (*Short Name* - HFE Gene p.C282y Ql)
- Code: 34519-9 (*Short Name* - HFE Gene Mut Anal)
- Code: 21694-5 (*Short Name* - HFE Gene Mut Anal)
- Code: 21697-8 (*Short Name* - HFE Gene Mut Tested)

Hemoglobin A1c measurement

TEST DEFINITION
Measurement of hemoglobin A1C in whole blood for the management of diabetes mellitus

SYNONYMS
- Haemoglobin A1c measurement
- HbA1c - Haemoglobin A1c level
- HbA1c - Hemoglobin A1c level

REFERENCE RANGE
- Adults: 3.8%-6.4% (0.038-0.064 hemoglobin fraction)
  Please refer to your institution's reference ranges as lab normals may vary.

INDICATIONS

Diabetes mellitus

> **Strength of Recommendation:** Class I
> **Strength of Evidence:** Category B

Results Interpretation:

Hemoglobin A1C - diabetic control finding

Hemoglobin A1C (HbA1C) should be used to monitor glycemic control but not to diagnose diabetes. The goal of diabetes management for patients in general is an HbA1C level of less than 7%. The goal for an individual patient is an A1C level as close to normal (less than 6%) as possible without significant hypoglycemia. These goals may not be appropriate for patients with a history of severe hypoglycemia, patients with limited life expectancies, very young children or older adults, and patients with comorbidities.

Point-of-care testing: Therapy is frequently intensified and glycemic control is improved when A1C results are available at the time the patient is seen.

A reduction of microvascular and neuropathic complications has been associated with lowering A1C levels. HbA1C reflects the development and progression of complications of diabetes mellitus, as well as a patient's overall glycemic control.

- In general, A1C levels correlate to mean plasma glucose (MPG) levels over the preceding 2 to 3 months as follows:
  - An A1C level of 4% reflects an MPG of 65 mg/dL (3.5 mmol/L)
  - An A1C level of 5% reflects an MPG of 100 mg/dL (5.5 mmol/L)
  - An A1C level of 6% reflects an MPG of 135 mg/dL (7.5 mmol/L)
  - An A1C level of 7% reflects an MPG of 170 mg/dL (9.5 mmol/L)
  - An A1C level of 8% reflects an MPG of 205 mg/dL (11.5 mmol/L)
  - An A1C level of 9% reflects an MPG of 240 mg/dL (13.5 mmol/L)
  - An A1C level of 10% reflects an MPG of 275 mg/dL (15.5 mmol/L)
  - An A1C level of 11% reflects an MPG of 310 mg/dL (17.5 mmol/L)
  - An A1C level of 12% reflects an MPG of 345 mg/dL (19.5 mmol/L)

There is little individual variation in A1C levels; however, wide interindividual variation has been reported regardless of glycemic status.

Frequency of Monitoring

Hemoglobin A1C levels should be obtained at every diabetic patient's initial assessment to ascertain the degree of glycemic control, and then at least every 3 months to assess ongoing metabolic control. A1C levels should be obtained twice a year for patients who are meeting treatment goals and exhibit stable glycemic control, and quarterly in patients whose therapy has changed or who are not meeting glycemic goals.

ABNORMAL RESULTS

- Results affected in:
  - Conditions that affect erythrocyte turnover (hemolysis, blood loss)
  - Hemoglobin variants

COLLECTION/STORAGE INFORMATION

- Draw whole blood in heparin, EDTA or oxalate tube.
- Store up to 7 days at 4°C ; store up to 30 days at 70°C.

LOINC CODES

- Code: 17855-8 (*Short Name* - Hgb A1c % Bld Calc)
- Code: 4548-4 (*Short Name* - Hgb A1c % Bld)
- Code: 17856-6 (*Short Name* - Hgb A1c % Bld HPLC)
- Code: 4549-2 (*Short Name* - Hgb A1c % Bld Elph)

Hemoglobin A2 measurement

TEST DEFINITION

The measurement of hemoglobin A^2 in whole blood for the evaluation of inherited hemoglobinopathies

SYNONYMS

- Haemoglobin A2 level
- Haemoglobin A2 measurement

- Hemoglobin A2 level

REFERENCE RANGE
- Adults: 1.5% - 3.5% (0.015 - 0.035 SI units)
  Please refer to your institution's reference ranges as lab normals may vary.

INDICATIONS
Antepartum and neonatal screening for hemoglobinopathies
> **Strength of Recommendation:** Class IIb
> **Strength of Evidence:** Category C
> **Results Interpretation:**
> **Abnormal hematology findings**
>> Beta-thalassemia is associated with a hemoglobin A_2 level above 3.5%. The partner of any individual who has elevated hemoglobin A_2, or other hemoglobin abnormalities, should be offered testing to evaluate reproductive risk.

Suspected hemoglobinopathy
> **Strength of Recommendation:** Class IIa
> **Strength of Evidence:** Category C
> **Results Interpretation:**
> **Abnormal hematology findings**
>> A diagnosis of heterozygous beta-thalassemia (beta thalassemia trait) can be made when the mean corpuscular hemoglobin (MCH) is below 27 pg and the hemoglobin A_2 (Hb A_2) is above 3.5%. Most beta-thalassemia carriers will have an MCH between 19 and 23 pg, and an Hb A_2 in the 4% to 6% range. An Hb A_2 between 3.5% and 4% is typically seen in mild beta$^+$-thalassemia carriers. Mild beta-thalassemia may also present as a combination of MCH less than 27 pg, Hb A_2 below 3.5%, and normal Hb F level; this presentation is also associated with iron deficiency and (epsilon-, gamma-, delta-, beta-)^0-thalassemia traits. Heterozygote carriers, most often seen in Asian, Indian, or Mediterranean populations, may present with low MCV and MCH values, and Hb A_2 levels between 3.4% and 3.8%. A highly unusual silent beta-thalassemia phenotype is associated with an Hb A_2 level less than 3.5% in the presence of mild beta-globin deficiency.
>> Patients with co-inherited alpha-thalassemia and beta-thalassemia can present with elevated Hb A_2 levels and nearly normal MCH levels. In geographic areas where combined alpha- and beta-thalassemia deficiencies are more common, such as the Middle East, Far East, and some Mediterranean countries, beta thalassemia carriers should also be screened for alpha^0-thalassemia mutations.
>> Hb A_2 is not increased in homozygous beta-thalassemia.

Suspected sickle cell disease
> **Strength of Recommendation:** Class IIb
> **Strength of Evidence:** Category C
> **Results Interpretation:**
> **Abnormal hematology findings**
>> Hemoglobin A_2 levels of 0.2% to 1% higher than the reference values have been reported in patients with sickle cell trait or sickle cell anemia, although this difference has not always been statistically significant.
>> Sickle cell disease typically presents with a normal or elevated mean corpuscular volume (MCV), hemoglobin A_2 less than 3.6%, and hemoglobin F (Hb F) less than 25%.

ABNORMAL RESULTS

CLINICAL NOTES
Although electrophoresis is more commonly utilized in American laboratories, the precision and accuracy of the electrophoretic gels for Hb A_2 is inferior as compared to high performance liquid chromatography (HPLC) techniques. HPLC may be preferred for initial screening of Hb variants, and for quantification of Hb A_2 concentrations. Any clinically relevant hemoglobinopathy finding by HPLC should be confirmed by an alternative method.

LOINC CODES
- Code: 4550-0 (*Short Name* - Hgb A2 Bld Column Chrom-sCnc)
- Code: 4552-6 (*Short Name* - Hgb A2 % Bld Elph)
- Code: 4551-8 (*Short Name* - Hgb A2 % Bld)
- Code: 4553-4 (*Short Name* - Hgb A2' % Bld Elph Acid)
- Code: 4554-2 (*Short Name* - Hgb A2 % Bld Elph Alk)

- Code: 27345-8 (*Short Name* - Hgb A2 Bld Ql Elph)
- Code: 28559-3 (*Short Name* - Hgb A2 Bld Ql)

Hemoglobin determination

TEST DEFINITION
Measurement of hemoglobin in whole blood for the evaluation of the oxygen carrying capacity and management of red blood cell disorders

SYNONYMS
- Haemoglobin determination

REFERENCE RANGE
- Adult males: 13.5-17.5 g/dL (8.4-10.9 mmol/L)
- Adult females: 12-16 g/dL (7.4-9.9 mmol/L)
- Pregnant females: 15% below the nonpregnant value
  Please refer to your institution's reference ranges as lab normals may vary.

INDICATIONS
Screening for iron deficiency anemia
> **Strength of Recommendation:** Class IIa
> **Strength of Evidence:** Category C

Results Interpretation:
Decreased hemoglobin
A screening cutoff value below the accepted threshold requires a confirmatory test in all patients. In patients who are not ill a presumptive diagnosis of iron-deficiency anemia can be made, and treatment initiated, if the second test result also falls below the acceptable threshold for the patient's age. If Hgb rises to 1 g/dL or greater after 4 weeks of iron supplementation therapy the diagnosis of iron-deficiency anemia can be confirmed. Patients who do not respond favorably after 4 weeks of iron supplementation therapy and who are not acutely ill should have further testing done, to include mean cell volume, red blood cell distribution width and serum ferritin concentration.

In iron deficiency anemia, Hgb levels fall first, followed by HCT levels.

Thalassemia minor or sickle cell trait should be considered in women of African, Mediterranean or Southeast Asian ancestry with mild anemia refractory to therapy.

Pregnant women with an Hgb less than 9 g/dL should be referred to a physician with expertise in treating anemia during pregnancy.

False Results
Vigorous squeezing of the finger during capillary specimen collection can cause false low results due to contamination of the sample by excessive tissue fluid. Low results obtained by the capillary collection method should be confirmed with a repeat capillary sample or by venipuncture.

Increased hemoglobin
High Hgb and HCT levels in pregnancy are associated with poor pregnancy outcomes. Hgb levels above 15 g/dL, especially in the second trimester, require further evaluation for potential pregnancy complications due to inadequate blood volume expansion. High levels of either HCT or Hgb in the second or third trimester are not reflective of desirable iron status.

False Results
Vigorous squeezing of the finger during capillary specimen collection can cause false low results due to contamination of the sample by excessive tissue fluid. Low results obtained by the capillary collection method should be confirmed with a repeat capillary sample or by venipuncture.

Hemoglobin finding
- Cutoff Hgb values (<g/dL) for anemia by age, sex, and pregnancy are as follows. The values for children ages 1 to <2 can be used for infants ages 6 to 12 months:
  - Children (age in years):
    - 1 - <2: 11
    - 2 - <5: 11.1
    - 5 - <8: 11.5
    - 8 - <12: 11.9

- Men (age in years):
  - 12 - <15: 12.5
  - 15 - <18: 13.3
  - ≥18: 13.5
- Nonpregnant women and lactating women (age in years):
  - 12 - <15: 11.8
  - 15 - <18: 12
  - ≥18: 12
- Pregnant women by weeks gestation:
  - 12 wks: 11
  - 16 wks: 10.6
  - 20 wks: 10.5
  - 24 wks: 10.5
  - 28 wks: 10.7
  - 32 wks: 11
  - 36 wks: 11.4
  - 40 wks: 11.9
- Pregnant women by trimester:
  - First trimester: 11
  - Second trimester: 10.5
  - Third trimester: 11
- People that live at elevations of 3,000 feet or higher for long periods of time will have slightly higher hgb and HCT levels, as will smokers. Hgb values (g/dL) should therefore be adjusted upward as follows:
  - Altitude (feet)
    - 3,000 - 3,999: +0.2
    - 4,000 - 4,999: +0.3
    - 5,000 - 5,999: +0.5
    - 6,000 - 6,999: +0.7
    - 7,000 - 7,999: +1.0
    - 8,000 - 8,999: +1.3
    - 9,000 - 9,999: +1.6
    - 10,000 - 11,000: +2.0
  - Cigarette smoking (packs per day)
    - 0.5 - <1: +0.3
    - 1 - <2: +0.5
    - ≥2: +0.7
    - All smokers: +0.3

Hgb values cannot identify the cause of anemia. However, iron-deficiency anemia can be diagnosed if either Hgb or HCT values rise following iron supplementation therapy. Other red blood cell indices such as mean cell volume, red blood cell distribution width and serum ferritin, can also be used to differentiate iron-deficiency anemia from other causes of anemia.

False Results

Vigorous squeezing of the finger during capillary specimen collection can cause false low results due to contamination of the sample by excessive tissue fluid. Low results obtained by the capillary collection method should be confirmed with a repeat capillary sample or by venipuncture.

Frequency of Monitoring

In infants, children, and adolescents, a repeat Hgb or HCT test should be performed 1 month after iron supplementation therapy is initiated. If HCT results still indicate anemia continue iron supplementation and repeat a HCT test in 2 more months. An HCT test should also be obtained 6 months after completion of successful treatment.

Timing of Monitoring

The Centers for Disease Control recommends screening all high-risk infants and children between 9 and 12 months, 6 months later, and annually in children ages 2 to 5. Preterm and low birthweight infants who are not fed iron-fortified formula should be screened before 6 months of age. Children between the ages of 2 and 5 should be assessed annually and screened if risk factors are present (low-iron diet, limited access to food, or special health-care needs). At age 9 to 12 months and again at age 15 to 18 months, screen children who have one or more of the following risk factors: (1) preterm or low birthweight infants; (2) infants fed a non iron-fortified infant formula for more than 2 months; (3) infants fed cow's milk before 1 year of age; (4) breast-fed infants who are consuming an inadequate amount of iron from supplementary foods; (4) children who drink more than 24 oz of cow's milk daily; (5) children with special health-care needs, eg children with chronic infection or inflammatory conditions, children who have experienced significant blood loss through injury or surgery, children on restricted diets, or children who take medication that interferes with iron absorption. School age children and adolescent boys require screening only if they have a history of iron-deficiency anemia, have special health-care needs, or have a history of low iron intake.

The American Academy of Pediatrics recommends routine universal HCT or hgb screening at 9 to 12 months of age and annual screening in menstruating adolescents. Additional screening is recommended in early childhood (15 months of age through 5 years of age) for children at risk. Screening prior to 9 months should be considered for high risk infants.

Adolescent nonpregnant girls should be screening every 5 to 10 years throughout their childbearing years as part of routine health examinations. Annual screening in this population is suggested if risk factors are present such as excessive menstrual blood loss, low iron intake or a history of iron-deficiency anemia.

Routine screening of all asymptomatic pregnant women is recommended. Pregnant women should be tested at their first prenatal visit and again 4 to 6 weeks postpartum if risk factors are present, ie anemia throughout the third trimester, extensive blood loss during delivery, and multiple birth.

Suspected fat embolism
Results Interpretation:
Decreased hemoglobin
Unexplained anemia is present in 67% to 95% of patients with fat emboli, with hemoglobin levels decreased by 3 to 5 g/dL.

Suspected lactic acidosis
Results Interpretation:
Decreased hemoglobin
Acute hypoxia due to hemorrhagic shock or an acute decrease in hemoglobin or hemoglobin oxygen-carrying capacity results in increased lactate production.

A hemoglobin concentration less than 6 g/dL may be associated with a modest increase in blood lactate (ie, less than 2 mmol/L). Therefore, severe anemia is not an important cause of lactic acidemia.

Suspected sickle cell disease
Results Interpretation:
Decreased hemoglobin
The average steady-state hemoglobin level in patients with sickle cell disease is 7.5 g/dL.

Hemoglobin levels drop acutely during splenic sequestration and hyperhemolytic crises. Decreases are more gradual, but may be just as profound during aplastic crises.

Abnormal hemoglobin levels can signify an abnormality of solubility and stability or capacity to transport oxygen in patients with sickle cell disease.
Increased hemoglobin
High hemoglobin levels (greater than 8.5 g/dL) appear to be an important risk factor for painful crises in homozygous sickle cell disease. In one study, the frequency of painful crises correlated positively with hemoglobin levels and reticulocyte counts in both sexes and negatively with mean corpuscular volume in females.

Suspected West Nile viral encephalitis
Results Interpretation:
Decreased hemoglobin
Decreased hemoglobin is reported in 40% of patients with West Nile virus infection. In one study, presence of anemia was an independent predictor of mortality.

COMMON PANELS
- Complete blood count
- Hemolysis panel

ABNORMAL RESULTS
- Results increased in:
    - Vigorous exercise or excitement
    - Hemoconcentration (dehydration, burns, severe vomiting, intestinal obstruction)
    - Long-term residence at high altitude
    - Smoking
- Results decreased in:
    - Recumbency

COLLECTION/STORAGE INFORMATION

- Collect sample in a lavender top tube.
- Store specimen at 23°C for 24 hours or at 4°C for 48 hours.

LOINC CODES

- Code: 722-9 (*Short Name* - Hgb Plr-mCnc)
- Code: 724-5 (*Short Name* - Hgb Snv-mCnc)
- Code: 30350-3 (*Short Name* - Hgb BldV-mCnc)
- Code: 14775-1 (*Short Name* - Hgb BldA Oximetry-mCnc)
- Code: 20509-6 (*Short Name* - Hgb Bld Calc-mCnc)
- Code: 30313-1 (*Short Name* - Hgb BldA-mCnc)
- Code: 14134-1 (*Short Name* - Hgb Ser-mCnc)
- Code: 723-7 (*Short Name* - Hgb Prt-mCnc)
- Code: 30353-7 (*Short Name* - Hgb BldCoV-mCnc)
- Code: 719-5 (*Short Name* - Hgb CSF-mCnc)
- Code: 30354-5 (*Short Name* - Hgb BldCoA-mCnc)
- Code: 30352-9 (*Short Name* - Hgb BldC-mCnc)
- Code: 718-7 (*Short Name* - Hgb Bld-mCnc)
- Code: 30351-1 (*Short Name* - Hgb BldMV-mCnc)

Hemoglobin electrophoresis

TEST DEFINITION

Detection and differentiation of hemoglobin (Hb) variants for evaluation and management of inherited disorders of hemoglobin

SYNONYMS

- Haemoglobin electrophoresis

REFERENCE RANGE

- Adults:
- Hemoglobin A: 95%-98% (0.95-0.98 mass fraction)
- Hemoglobin F: 0%-2%: (0-0.02 mass fraction)
- Hemoglobin A_2 : 1.5%-3.5% (0.01-0.03 mass fraction)
- Neonates aged 1 day: 77% ± 7.3% (0.77 ± 0.073 mass fraction)
- Neonates aged 5 days: 76.8% ± 5.8% (0.768 ± 0.058 mass fraction)
- Neonates aged 3 weeks: 70% ± 7.3% (0.7 ± 0.073 mass fraction)
- Infants aged 6 to 9 weeks: 52.9% ± 11% (0.529 ± 0.11 mass fraction)
- Infants aged 3 to 4 months: 23.2% ± 16% (0.232 ± 0.16 mass fraction)
- Infants aged 6 months: 4.7% ± 2.2% (0.047 ± 0.022 mass fraction)
- Infants aged 8 to 11 months: 1.6% ± 1% (0.16 ± 0.01 mass fraction)
  Please refer to your institution's reference ranges as lab normals may vary.

INDICATIONS

Infants with suspected sickle cell disease
   Results Interpretation:
   The finding of only hemoglobin S (HbS) and fetal hemoglobin (HbF) indicates sickle cell disease.

Screening for hemoglobinopathies
      Strength of Recommendation: Class IIa
      Strength of Evidence: Category C
   Results Interpretation:
   Hemoglobin abnormal
   Hemoglobin electrophoresis (EP) detects hemoglobin (Hb) variants. The presence of significant levels of abnormal hemoglobin may indicate sickle cell anemia, Hb S disease, or a rare hemoglobinopathy. In normal adults, only Hb A and Hb A_2 are present at significant levels.
   Common variants -- Hb S (populations of African origin, associated with sickle cell anemia), Hb E (populations from Southeast Asia), Hb C (associated with hemolytic anemia), and Hb D-Pungab -- comprise 90% of

abnormal hemoglobins observed. Other less common variants cause anemias of varying degrees of severity, and many cannot be definitively identified. Most infants are heterozygotes with no clinical or laboratory evidence of disease. Neonates with clinical or laboratory evidence of hemolysis or abnormal oxygen affinity, and those without hemoglobin A, require definitive hemoglobin identification either by protein sequencing, DNA analysis or high performance liquid chromatography combined with electrospray mass spectrometry.

Although the definitive diagnosis of thalassemia syndromes requires direct DNA-based techniques, hemoglobin EP is a useful ancillary test to differentiate thalassemias from the sickle hemoglobinopathies and to help differentiate among the thalassemias. In the beta-thalassemias, the deficient synthesis of beta-globulin results in the partial compensatory increase in delta and gamma chains, which in turn lead to elevated levels of Hb A_2 (alpha-2 delta-2) or fetal hemoglobin (Hb F), and alpha-2 (gamma-2). Thus, in the beta-thalassemias, Hb A_2 and/or Hb F are typically elevated. In contrast, in the alpha-thalassemias, there is no compensatory increase in delta or gamma chains, so neither the Hb A_2 nor the Hb F level is usually increased. Hb F may vary in sickle cell disease ranging from 2% to 20%. Other electrophoretic techniques may be necessary to identify some of the other double heterozygous sickle cell syndromes.

Timing of Monitoring

It is recommended that all newborns be screened and that screening be undertaken prior to any blood transfusion, regardless of age. Infants with positive screening tests should have confirmatory testing repeated at 2 months of age by a complementary method. In addition, all high risk infants not screened at birth should have hemoglobinopathy screening by 2 months of age. There is no consensus on the appropriate follow-up of infants with unidentified hemoglobin variants.

COMMON PANELS
- Hemolysis panel

ABNORMAL RESULTS
- Results decreased in:
  - Blood transfusion

COLLECTION/STORAGE INFORMATION
- Specimen Collection and Handling:
  - Collect whole blood in EDTA, citrate, or heparin tube
  - Use fresh or refrigerate at 4°C

LOINC CODES
- Code: 13514-5 (*Short Name* - Hgb Fractions Bld Elph-Imp)
- Code: 13515-2 (*Short Name* - Hgb Fractions Bld Elph Citrate-Imp)
- Code: 24469-9 (*Short Name* - Hgb XXX % Bld Elph)
- Code: 32017-6 (*Short Name* - Hgb Other % Bld Elph)
- Code: 12710-0 (*Short Name* - Hgb Fract Bld-Imp)

Heparin induced thrombocytopenia screening test

TEST DEFINITION
Several available techniques, functional or observational, intended to evaluate possible heparin induced thrombocytopenia (HIT)

REFERENCE RANGE
Negative: Defined by the specific test methodology being utilized
Please refer to your institution's reference ranges as lab normals may vary.

INDICATIONS
Evaluation of suspected heparin induced thrombocytopenia (HIT)
  Strength of Recommendation: Class IIa
  Strength of Evidence: Category C

Results Interpretation:
Abnormal laboratory findings

The diagnosis of type II heparin-induced thrombocytopenia (HIT) is dependent upon clinical and laboratory evidence. Diagnostic criteria include evidence of relative or absolute thrombocytopenia (>50% drop in platelet count relative to preheparin levels or a count below 100,000/mm^3), the exclusion of other causes of thrombocytopenia (besides heparin administration), and the resolution of thrombocytopenia with discontinuation of heparin therapy. Diagnostic test interpretation should reflect both the clinical context and the relative abnormality of HIT antibody testing results.

Of key importance is interpretation of the study based on clinical context. Both types of assays (functional and observational) have high sensitivity and high negative predictive values; however, the specificity varies. First, not all patients with antibodies have type II HIT; in fact, most patients do not have HIT. Second, particularly in the observational assay but to some extent in the functional assay, there can be cross-reaction with other antibodies, thus making the test nonspecific. As a result, a positive test needs to be confirmed by the correct clinical setting, including the degree of platelet decline, timing after heparin onset, presence of thrombosis, and presence of other causes of platelet fall.

Because antibody assays can be nonspecific, particularly in the postoperative period, interpretation of a positive HIT antibody test should be done in context with the clinical setting.

Accuracy

Clinical Notes

A diagnosis of heparin induced thrombocytopenia (HIT) necessitates a clinicopathologic approach. Diagnostic interpretation should reflect both the clinical context and the relative abnormality of HIT antibody testing results.

Hepatitis A antibody level

Test Definition

Measurement of serum for IgM or total (IgM and IgG) hepatitis A virus (HAV) antibody levels for the evaluation of HAV infection or immunity

Reference Range

• Adults and Children: Negative
  Please refer to your institution's reference ranges as lab normals may vary.

Indications

Detection of hepatitis A viral (HAV) antibodies in serum to identify active HAV infection, prior HAV infection, or to determine immunity to HAV
       Strength of Recommendation: Class I
       Strength of Evidence: Category B
       Results Interpretation:
       Positive laboratory findings

Hepatitis A virus (HAV) antibodies include IgM, which appear early in HAV infection, and IgG, which appear during recovery from HAV infection and persist indefinitely.

Following vaccination against HAV, 94% to 100% of adults developed protective levels of IgG by 1 month after the first dose; after the second dose, all had acquired protective antibody levels.

• IgM HAV antibody (anti-HAV IgM)
  • The presence of anti-HAV IgM may indicate an active HAV infection with or without symptoms, a previous HAV infection with prolonged presence of anti-HAV IgM, or a false-positive result.
  • Positive test results for IgM anti-HAV IgM confirm an active HAV infection. Anti-HAV IgM becomes detectable 5 to 10 days prior to symptom onset and may remain elevated for 3 to 6 months following infection.
  • Confirmed case criteria for public health purposes include patients with symptomatic HAV infection plus positive serology results for anti-HAV IgM antibodies.
  • Up to 20% of symptomatic patients have a biphasic or relapsing form of HAV, in which a second or third incidence of acute HAV infection occurs following the resolution of the initial HAV symptoms and development of positive IgM serology.
  • Positive anti-HAV IgM serology test results in asymptomatic older patients may indicate a previous HAV infection from months or years earlier, or may be a false-positive result.

- Screening patients without active HAV symptoms may lead to false-positive anti-HAV IgM antibody results and consequently may lack clinical importance.
- Total (IgM and IgG) HAV antibodies
  - A positive test result for total HAV antibodies (IgM and IgG) may indicate an active HAV infection, a previous HAV infection, or immunity related to vaccination against HAV.
  - A patient with acute HAV infection symptoms and a positive total anti-HAV serology result should be immediately retested for anti-HAV IgM antibody.
  - The presence of anti-HAV IgG antibody confirms prior HAV infection or vaccination against HAV and is the indicator for immunity against HAV.

Negative laboratory findings

A negative test result for anti-HAV IgM antibodies indicates no active HAV infection. A negative total HAV antibody (IgM and IgG) test result indicates no current or previous HAV infection, and no immunity to HAV.

Following vaccination, persons who are anti-HAV negative by standard assays may still have protective levels of antibody.

COMMON PANELS

- Acute hepatitis panel

CLINICAL NOTES

Because active hepatitis A virus (HAV) infection is a communicable disease capable of causing community-wide outbreaks and typically affecting children, adolescents, and young adults in the US, positive IgM HAV antibody (anti-HAV) results are reportable to state and national public health agencies, such as the Centers for Disease Control and Prevention.

COLLECTION/STORAGE INFORMATION

- Collect blood in a marbled serum separator tube (SST).
- Serum is stable for up to 7 days at room temperature and indefinitely at 4°C or -20°C.

LOINC CODES

- Code: 5184-7 (*Short Name* - Hep A Ab Ser RIA-aCnc)
- Code: 5183-9 (*Short Name* - Hep A Ab Ser EIA-aCnc)
- Code: 20575-7 (*Short Name* - Hep A Ab Ser Ql)

Hepatitis A virus RNA assay

TEST DEFINITION

The detection of hepatitis A virus (HAV) ribonucleic acid (RNA) in serum for the evaluation and management of HAV

REFERENCE RANGE

- Adults and Children: Negative

Please refer to your institution's reference ranges as lab normals may vary.

INDICATIONS

Suspected viral hepatitis, type A

    Strength of Recommendation: Class IIb

    Strength of Evidence: Category C

Results Interpretation:

Positive laboratory findings

A positive nucleic acid test for the presence of hepatitis A virus (HAV) is diagnostic of HAV.

CLINICAL NOTES

Nucleic acid assays are not routinely performed for the diagnosis or management of hepatitis A virus (HAV).

COLLECTION/STORAGE INFORMATION

- Store body fluids at 4°C and tissue at -20°C or lower.

Hepatitis B core antibody measurement

TEST DEFINITION
Detection of hepatitis B core antibodies as a serologic marker for evaluation of current or past exposure to hepatitis B virus

SYNONYMS
• HBcAB measurement

REFERENCE RANGE
• Adults and Children: Negative
Please refer to your institution's reference ranges as lab normals may vary.

INDICATIONS
Suspected acute hepatitis B viral infection
> **Strength of Recommendation:** Class I
> **Strength of Evidence:** Category C
> **Results Interpretation:**
> **Hepatitis B antibody present**
> A positive total hepatitis B core antibody (anti-HBc) test includes both IgM and IgG class antibody to the core protein and indicates a current or prior hepatitis B exposure.
> IgM and IgG fractions are useful in differentiating between acute and past infections. Anti-HBc IgM begins to rise during acute hepatitis, persists for generally 4-6 months, then declines. Anti-HBc IgG rises with the anti-HBc IgM, but to a much higher level and persists for a long time.
> The presence of anti-HBc IgM, with or without hepatitis B surface antigen, indicates the presence of acute (HBV) infection. Low-titer anti-HBc IgG is usually the most persistent marker of past hepatitis B infection.
> A positive anti-HBc test indicates the presence of anti-HBc antibodies that confirm immunity following HBV infection.
> **Timing of Monitoring**
> Hepatitis B core antibody (anti-HBc) is readily detectable 1-2 weeks after the appearance of hepatitis B surface antigen and may precede the detection of hepatitis B surface antibody (anti-HBs) by weeks to months, but may also remain detectable longer than anti-HBs. Levels may be undetectable 6-18 months after infection.

COMMON PANELS
• Acute hepatitis panel

COLLECTION/STORAGE INFORMATION
• Specimen Collection and Handling:
  • Collect the serum sample in a marbled red top tube.
  • The sample is stable for a period of 7 days at room temperature and indefinitely at 4°C or -20°C.

LOINC CODES

Hepatitis B surface antibody measurement

TEST DEFINITION
Detection of hepatitis B surface antibody (anti-HBs) in serum for the evaluation of infection or immunity

SYNONYMS
• HBsAb measurement

REFERENCE RANGE
• Adults and children: Negative (limits of detection 2-10 International Units/L)
  Please refer to your institution's reference ranges as lab normals may vary.

INDICATIONS
Confirmation of immunity following hepatitis B vaccination
    Strength of Recommendation: Class IIb
    Strength of Evidence: Category B
Results Interpretation:
Hepatitis B antibody present
    Hepatitis B surface antibody (anti-HBs) is the only hepatitis B (HBV) antibody marker present following HBV vaccination. Titers fall, often rapidly, following the completion of the HBV vaccination series. The highest anti-HBs titers generally occur 1 month after a booster vaccination, with a sharp decline over the next 12 months and a slow decline thereafter. The generally accepted titer level associated with the minimal level of protection against HBV is 10 International Units/L, although this is debatable. A titer level between 10 and 100 International Units/L may be an indication for revaccination of immunocompromised patients. The anti-HBs level may be elevated within 4 days of administration of the booster immunization.

    A positive anti-HBs titer combined with a negative hepatitis B surface antigen (HBsAg) titer at 12 to 15 months of age indicates effective treatment for infants born to HBsAg-positive mothers and treated with hepatitis B immunoglobulin (HBIG) and HBV vaccination.

Suspected hepatitis B exposure from sexual assault
    Strength of Recommendation: Class IIb
    Strength of Evidence: Category B
Results Interpretation:
Blood - infectious titer negative
    Some experts recommend that sexual assault victims who have previously been immunized but have a negative hepatitis B surface antibody (anti-HBs) titer should be revaccinated for hepatitis B (HBV); however, the CDC does not consider revaccination necessary in patients who have completed the full HBV vaccination series.
Timing of Monitoring
    Hepatitis B virus (HBV) testing should be performed at the time of the initial sexual assault examination to determine the need for HBV immunization. HBV tests should be repeated in 6 weeks.

Suspected hepatitis B infection
    Strength of Recommendation: Class IIb
    Strength of Evidence: Category C
Results Interpretation:
Hepatitis B antibody present
    Hepatitis B surface antibody (anti-HBs) is generated during the resolution phase of acute hepatitis B and is usually a marker for recovery and immunity.

    A positive hepatitis B surface antibody may also indicate a chronic HBV infection. The appearance of anti-HBs generally follows the disappearance of detectable levels of hepatitis B surface antigen (HBsAg). In chronic HBV, the anti-HBs level can remain positive for decades, and some patients may have detectable levels of both HBsAg and anti-HBs.

    In one study, concurrence of HBsAg and anti-HBs was found in 32% of 228 HBsAg-positive patients. This was significantly more common in patients with chronic active hepatitis than in those with acute hepatitis, chronic persistent hepatitis, or the asymptomatic carrier state. Concurrence was associated with evidence of viral replication and active hepatic inflammation.
Blood - infectious titer negative
    Of patients who are chronic HBV carriers, 60% to 80% have no detectable level of anti-HBs.

COLLECTION/STORAGE INFORMATION
- Collect venous specimen in a marbled serum separator tube (SST).

LOINC CODES
- Code: 16935-9 (*Short Name* - Hep Bs Ab Ser-aCnc)
- Code: 21006-2 (*Short Name* - Hep B Surf Ab Ser Donr EIA-aCnc)
- Code: 5193-8 (*Short Name* - Hep B Surf Ab Ser EIA-aCnc)
- Code: 5194-6 (*Short Name* - Hep Bs Ab Ser RIA-aCnc)
- Code: 10900-9 (*Short Name* - Hep Bs Ab Ser QI EIA)
- Code: 22323-0 (*Short Name* - Hep B Surf Ab Ser Donr-aCnc)
- Code: 32019-2 (*Short Name* - Hep Bs Ab Titr Ser)
- Code: 22322-2 (*Short Name* - Hep Bs Ab Ser QI)

Hepatitis B surface antigen measurement

TEST DEFINITION
Detection of serologic marker on surface of hepatitis B virus (HBsAg) for evaluation of current hepatitis B infection

SYNONYMS
- HBsAg measurement

REFERENCE RANGE
Negative (limits of detection 0.02-10 ng/mL)
Please refer to your institution's reference ranges as lab normals may vary.

INDICATIONS
Suspected acute or chronic type B viral hepatitis
>   **Strength of Recommendation:** Class I
>   **Strength of Evidence:** Category C
>   **Results Interpretation:**
>   **Hepatitis B surface antigen positive**
>   The finding of hepatitis B surface antigen (HBsAg) without other serologic markers indicates (1) acute hepatitis B, (2) superimposed hepatitis A in a chronic HBV carrier, or (3) reactivation of chronic hepatitis B.
>   HBsAg can be identified in serum 30-60 days after exposure to hepatitis B virus (HBV) and persists for variable periods. It rises rapidly during the first 1-3 weeks of the presymptomatic stage and persists during the icteric and symptomatic phase of acute illness, peaking at or shortly after the increase in liver function tests.
>   Duration of HBsAg positivity depends on levels of HBsAg titers. HBsAg typically becomes undetectable in early convalescence (1-3 months after onset of jaundice), but it may persist for up to 6 months if high titers occur early. After HBsAg disappears, antibody to HBsAg (anti-HBs) appears, indicating recovery and immunity to reinfection.
>   The presence of HBsAg for 6 months or more is diagnostic for chronic HBV. Patients with chronic HBV usually have continuing levels of HBsAg, often for life, plus detectable levels of HBV DNA, indicating viremia and conferring chronic carrier status.
>   **Hepatitis B surface antigen negative**
>   Some chronic low-level HBV carriers may lack detectable HBsAg in their serum, despite presence of HBV in liver and peripheral blood. One reason for the lack of HBsAg may be genetic alterations in the HBV S gene leading to an escape from recognition by routinely used assays. Therefore, when HBsAg is negative and suspicion for acute viral hepatitis is high, an assay for IgM antibody to hepatitis B core antigen (IgM anti-HBc) may be indicated.
>   In cases of fulminant HBV infection, HBsAg may clear rapidly and not be detectable in the serum at the time of initial symptoms.

COMMON PANELS
- Acute hepatitis panel
- Hepatitis chronic carrier panel
- Prenatal screening panel

- Transplant panel

CLINICAL NOTES
Commercial diagnostic assays vary in their ability to detect expressed hepatitis B surface antigen (HBsAg) variants.

COLLECTION/STORAGE INFORMATION
- Specimen Collection and Handling:
    - Collect serum sample in red top tube.
    - May keep serum at room temperature for up to 7 days; for longer storage, freeze at 4°C or -20°C.

LOINC CODES
- Code: 10674-0 (*Short Name* - Hep B Surf Ag Tiss Ql ImStn)
- Code: 5197-9 (*Short Name* - Hep B Surf Ag Ser Ql RIA)
- Code: 7905-3 (*Short Name* - Hep B Surf Ag Ser Ql Nt)
- Code: 5195-3 (*Short Name* - Hep Bs Ag Ser Ql)
- Code: 5196-1 (*Short Name* - Hep B Surf Ag Ser Ql EIA)
- Code: 10675-7 (*Short Name* - Hep B Surf Ag Tiss Orcein Stn)

Hepatitis B virus polymerase DNA assay

TEST DEFINITION
Detection of hepatitis B virus DNA in serum, liver tissue and polymorphonuclear neutrophils for the evaluation and management of hepatitis B virus infection

REFERENCE RANGE
- Adults and Children: Negative
  Please refer to your institution's reference ranges as lab normals may vary.

INDICATIONS
Suspected acute or chronic type B viral hepatitis
    Strength of Recommendation: Class IIa
    Strength of Evidence: Category C
Results Interpretation:
Polymerase chain reaction observation
    Hepatitis B virus (HBV) DNA appears to be the first detectable serologic marker of HBV infection and it may persist in serum for months, even in self-limiting infections. HBV-DNA positivity is seen during the peak of HBV replication, at 1 to 2 1/2 months postexposure. Increasing levels of HBV replication appear to be closely correlated with liver injury, presumably through immunologically-mediated mechanisms. When HBV replication diminishes spontaneously or as a result of treatment with interferon or lamivudine, HBV DNA and hepatitis Be antigen (HBeAg) may diminish or become undetectable in serum, and elevated levels of serum aminotransferase return to the normal range. Low levels of HBV DNA may persist, nonetheless, in hepatocytes.
    Persistence of HBsAg for more than 6 months, accompanied by positive tests for HBV DNA or HBeAg, indicates chronic HBV infection and ongoing HBV replication. Hepatitis B surface antigen (HBsAg)-positive patients should be tested for the presence of HBeAg and HBV DNA to assess the level of HBV replication. Only those who are replicating HBV and have elevated serum aminotransferase levels are likely to respond to treatment with antiviral or immunomodulatory drugs. HBsAg-positive patients with progressive disease who are HBeAg-negative but HBV DNA-positive are likely to have the precore mutant.
    Patients with multiple normal alanine transaminase (ALT) levels in conjunction with high viral DNA levels are not likely to have advanced liver disease, and biopsy is not always required in these patients.

CLINICAL NOTES
Hepatitis B virus (HBV)-DNA polymerase chain reaction assay is utilized currently for the confirmation of HBV infection in immunosuppressed patients with inconsistent serological markers, and in the assessment of treatment for HBV.

COLLECTION/STORAGE INFORMATION
- Specimen Collection and Handling:
  - Freeze specimen if test cannot be performed immediately.
  - Specimen is stable for at least 7 days at $-20°C$.
  - Collect sample in an EDTA tube (lavender top).

LOINC CODES
- Code: 16934-2 (*Short Name* - Hep B DNAp Bld QI PCR)

Hepatitis Be antibody measurement

TEST DEFINITION
Measurement of antibodies to hepatitis Be antigen in hepatitis B infection

SYNONYMS
- HBeAB measurement

REFERENCE RANGE
- Negative
Please refer to your institution's reference ranges as lab normals may vary.

INDICATIONS
Hepatitis B viral infection
> **Strength of Recommendation:** Class IIb
> **Strength of Evidence:** Category B
> **Results Interpretation:**
> **Serology positive**
> Hepatitis Be antibody (anti-HBe) usually appears after the disappearance of hepatitis Be antigen (HBeAg), however, both may exist together for a short time. Anti-HBe may persist for years after an acute infection.
> Conversion from HBeAg to anti-HBe indicates remission of active disease and reduced infectivity.
> In chronic hepatitis B infection, HBeAg disappears in about half the patients over time and anti-HBe appears. Reactivation of chronic hepatitis B may occur even in the presence of anti-HBe. Usually, there is a return of HBeAg, which may be transient or sustained but recurrent episodes of reactivation may lead to severe progressive liver disease.
> Anti-HBe and HBeAg should be ordered together in patients with chronic positive hepatitis B surface antigen (HBsAg). The anti-HBe is suggestive of low infectivity risk despite the presence of HBsAg. However, a study of 45 HBsAg carriers with anti-HBe detected Dane particle-HBeAg- a marker of a highly infectious carrier state- in 18% of the patients, suggesting that some carriers with anti-HBe may be infective.

COMMON PANELS
- Hepatitis chronic carrier panel

COLLECTION/STORAGE INFORMATION
- Specimen Collection and Handling:
  - Collect serum sample.
  - Store sample indefinitely at 4°C or -20°C.

LOINC CODES
- Code: 5190-4 (*Short Name* - Hep Be Ab Ser RIA-aCnc)
- Code: 22321-4 (*Short Name* - Hep Be Ab Ser-aCnc)
- Code: 5189-6 (*Short Name* - Hep Be Ab Ser EIA-aCnc)
- Code: 22320-6 (*Short Name* - Hep Be Ab Ser QI)

Hepatitis Be antigen measurement

TEST DEFINITION

Measurement of hepatitis B e antigen in serum for evaluation of infectivity and management of hepatitis B virus infection

SYNONYMS

- HBeAg measurement
- Hepatitis B e antigen level

REFERENCE RANGE

- Negative
  Please refer to your institution's reference ranges as lab normals may vary.

INDICATIONS

Hepatitis B viral infection
  Strength of Recommendation: Class IIa
  Strength of Evidence: Category B
  Results Interpretation:
  Hepatitis e antigen present
    High levels of serum hepatitis B virus (HBV) are associated with hepatitis Be antigen (HBeAg) and indicate high infectivity, either early in an acute infection or in chronic disease. Hepatitis B surface antigen (HBsAg)-postive patients with progressive disease who are HBeAg-negative, but HBV DNA-positive are likely to have the precore mutant.
    The level of HBeAg begins to decline with the onset of clinical illness and usually disappears after the conversion to anti-HBe, which indicates remission and reduced infectivity.
    If HBeAg persists in the serum for 10 weeks, there is an increased risk for progression to chronic disease. In chronic hepatitis B infection, HBeAg disappears in about half the patients over time and anti-HBe appears. Disappearance of HBeAg with conversion to a positive anti-HBe suggests resolution of virus replication and resolution of disease. Reactivation of chronic hepatitis B may occur even in the presence of anti-HBe. Usually, there is a return of HBeAg, which may be transient or sustained, but recurrent episodes of reactivation may lead to severe, progressive liver disease.
    Anti-HBe and HBeAg should be ordered together in patients with chronic positive HBsAg.
    The presence of HBeAg in HBsAg carriers suggests infectivity.
    In patients with HBV-related hepatocellular carcinoma, the presence of HBeAg may be an indicator of exacerbation of liver damage during or after chemotherapy.
    The presence of HBeAg in patients with chronic progressive hepatitis may be suggest a poorer prognosis.

COMMON PANELS

- Hepatitis chronic carrier panel

CLINICAL NOTES

Patients infected with hepatitis B virus (HBV) precore mutant have undetectable levels of Hepatitis B e-antigen (HBeAg) because the mutant virus is unable to synthesize precore or core protein from which HBeAg is derived.
Mutant strains of HBV that do not produce HBeAg are common in the Middle East and Asia. Testing for HBeAg is not very useful in areas where these mutant strains are common.

COLLECTION/STORAGE INFORMATION

- Collect serum sample in a marble-top tube.
- Specimen is stable at room temperature for 7 days and indefinitely at 40°C or -20°C.

LOINC CODES

- Code: 31845-1 (*Short Name* - Hep Be Ag Ser-aCnc)
- Code: 5192-0 (*Short Name* - Hep Be Ag Ser Ql RIA)
- Code: 32178-6 (*Short Name* - Hep Be Ag Titr Ser)
- Code: 31844-4 (*Short Name* - Hep Be Ag Ser Ql)

Hepatitis C nucleic acid assay, Qualitative

TEST DEFINITION

Qualitative nucleic acid assay measured in blood to detect the presence or absence of active hepatitis C virus (HCV) infection, as a confirmatory test for anti-HCV antibody detection in screening tests, and useful for monitoring successful antiviral therapy (ie, absence of viremia)

SYNONYMS

• Hepatitis C nucleic acid detection

REFERENCE RANGE

• Adults and Children: Negative
Please refer to your institution's reference ranges as lab normals may vary.

INDICATIONS

Suspected viral hepatitis C
    Strength of Recommendation: Class IIa
    Strength of Evidence: Category C
    Results Interpretation:
    Serology positive
    A single positive qualitative assay for HCV RNA confirms active HCV replication, which is valuable in detecting the absence or presence of infection. Positive findings can occur 1 to 3 weeks following exposure. In general, qualitative HCV RNA assays have a detection of 50 international units/mL (100 viral genes/mL) or less, and are used to confirm hepatitis C virus infection following a positive enzyme immunoassay screening test. A transcription mediated amplification (TMA) based assay has a lower detection limit of 10 international units/mL for all of the major HCV genotypes.

    Qualitative assays for HCV RNA have become the gold standard in determining the effectiveness of antiviral therapy (ie, the absence of viremia), while quantitative (ie, assessment of viral load) and HCV genotype are used to guide response and tentative duration of therapy.

    Absence of HCV RNA at 12 weeks post-treatment for hepatitis C has been associated with resolution of liver injury, a reduction in liver fibrosis, and a low likelihood of relapse from HCV.

    Of note, it is possible that active infection may still exist if the level of viremia transiently drops below the assay's limit of detection. However, negative HCV RNA for all genotypes 24 weeks after the completion of therapy indicates a sustained virological response, and an overall good indicator of recovery.

    Frequency of Monitoring
    Qualitative HCV RNA can be useful in determining individuals with prior infection who no longer have detectable virus from those with persistent HCV infection. In some individuals, repeat testing may be necessary to identify those patients with chronic HCV that are only intermittently viremic. Sustained virologic response is defined as continued absence of HCV RNA for at least 6 months following the completion of therapy.

    Timing of Monitoring
    Hepatitic C virus ribonucleic acid can be found in the blood of acutely infected patients within 7 to 21 days of exposure, and when symptoms become apparent. HCV RNA will be detected in the blood of those with chronic infection for 6 months.

    When hepatitic C is suspected and the first HCV RNA is negative, a follow-up test is suggested. Untreated patients may be given the test to ascertain if acute infection has resolved. In post antiviral treatment, HCV RNA testing is required periodically to determine whether sustained virological response (SVR) is being maintained. Testing should be obtained after a needlestick injury from an HCV positive patient at the time of exposure and 2 to 8 weeks following exposure. Infants born to hepatitis C virus positive mothers, should also be tested between the ages of 2 to 6 months.

    HIV positive patients with a negative anti-HCV test and suspicion of chronic hepatitis C infection should have the HCV RNA assay performed initially, and repeated intermittently during therapy.

CLINICAL NOTES

Amplcor HCV test (version 2.0) obtained FDA approval, and has a lower limit of detection of 50 international units/mL.

Transcription mediated amplification (TMA) has been approved by the FDA for the screening of blood donations to identify HCV-positive donors who are antibody negative. A PCR-assay is also expected to attain approval.

COLLECTION/STORAGE INFORMATION
- Collect serum or plasma in an ACD (yellow-top) or EDTA (lavendar-top) tube.
- Separate serum or plasma from whole blood within 4 hours of collection to minimize RNA degradation by ribonucleases, and freeze at less than -20°C.
- Rapidly store specimens at less than -70°C, avoid thawing and refreezing.
- Specimen analysis should be done within 2 weeks of collection.

Hepatitis C nucleic acid assay, Quantitative

TEST DEFINITION
Quantitative nucleic acid assay measured in blood for the detection of hepatitis C virus to determine viral load, monitor patient response to therapy, and assess prognosis

SYNONYMS
- Hepatitis C nucleic acid detection

REFERENCE RANGE
- Adults and Children: the lower detection cut-off of various assays ranges from less than 30 international units/mL to 615 international units/mL, and the upper end of the range is less than 500,000 international units/mL to 7,700,000 international units/mL
  Please refer to your institution's reference ranges as lab normals may vary.

INDICATIONS
Assess prognosis, determine therapeutic options, and monitor response to therapy in patients with viral hepatitis C (HCV)
> **Strength of Recommendation:** Class IIa
> **Strength of Evidence:** Category C
Results Interpretation:
Serology positive
> Quantitative testing can be useful to provide information on the likelihood of response to antiviral therapy and monitor therapeutic response. Results may be variable and depend on the individual assay. Serial measurements using the same assay is recommended.

> Assays have been standardized and are expressed in international units per mL serum. A viral load over 800,000 international units/mL is considered elevated regardless of the assay used.

> The upper end of linear ranges for various assays can be less than 500,000 international units/mL to 7,700,000 international units/mL. A sample with a viral level at the upper end of the range for that assay must be diluted and retested to report accurate results.

> Untreated patients with hepatitis C may have circulating HCV RNA levels of 50,000 international units/mL to 5,000,000 international units/mL. It is thought that patients with a high viral load have a lower likelihood of response to antiviral therapy.

> Following antiviral therapy, quantitative retesting may show low or undetectable viral levels, indicating a positive response. However, the level yields no information about disease progression or severity.

False Results
> Regardless of the assay chosen, RNA is inherently unstable in biological specimens; therefore, the RNA extraction process requires strict quality control. Improperly handled specimens can produce false-negative results.

Frequency of Monitoring
> The frequency of quantitative HCV RNA measurement during therapy is based in part on HCV genotype. Baseline HCV RNA quantification is useful in patients with genotype 1 and those with genotype 4, 5, and 6, but not necessary with genotype 2 or 3. A minimum 2-log decrease or undetectable HCV RNA at week 12, is described as early virologic response (EVR) and has a low positive predictive value, but a good negative predictive value to sustained virological response. The absence of EVR correlates poorly with sustained virological response, which can be useful in determining whether therapy should be continued or stopped after 12 weeks.

Timing of Monitoring

Hepatitis C virus ribonucleic acid can be detected in the blood of acutely infected patients within 7 to 21 days of exposure, and when symptoms become apparent. Persistence of chronic hepatitis C infection can be detected in the blood by HCV RNA for at least 6 months.

HIV positive patients with a negative anti-HCV test and suspicion of chronic hepatitis C infection should have HCV RNA levels checked initially and during treatment.

CLINICAL NOTES

Quantitative assays are used to monitor viral load in patients with confirmed hepatitis C virus (HCV) infection. Diagnosis of active HCV infection should be confirmed with qualitative HCV RNA, because quantitative assays are not reliable in detecting low-level viremia. Complete viral clearance cannot also be reliably determined by quantitative HCV RNA during treatment or in the posttreatment phase, due to the extremely low levels of virus that may still be present. Of note, previous or current infection, or patients whose infection has disappeared cannot be determined by this method.

The World Health Organization designated international units as the international standard for measurement of HCV RNA quantity in blood. This standard should be used in lieu of 'copy' or 'genome equivalent' levels. One international unit is equivalent to approximately 2.5 copies of HCV RNA, and approximately 6.3 genomes.

Serial measurements using the same assay is recommended to increase the clinical reliability of HCV viral load analysis.

Baseline values of HCV RNA are also valuable for the management of patients with HCV genotypes 1, 4, 5, and 6, but not genotypes 2 and 3.

COLLECTION/STORAGE INFORMATION

- Collect plasma or serum in an ACD (yellow-top) or EDTA (purple-top) tube.
- Separate serum or plasma from whole blood within 4 hours of collection to minimize RNA degradation by ribonucleases, and freeze at less than -20°C.
- If storage required, rapidly freeze specimen at -70°C; avoid thawing and refreezing.
- Specimen analysis should be done within 2 weeks of collection.

Hepatitis D virus measurement

TEST DEFINITION

Detection of delta antigen or antibody in serum for evaluation of hepatitis D virus (HDV) infection

SYNONYMS

- HDV measurement
- Hepatitis delta agent measurement

REFERENCE RANGE

Negative
Please refer to your institution's reference ranges as lab normals may vary.

INDICATIONS

Suspected hepatitis D (delta) infection
>   **Strength of Recommendation:** Class IIa
>   **Strength of Evidence:** Category C
>   **Results Interpretation:**
>   **Serology positive**
>   - A positive hepatitis D (HDV) serology test indicates infection with the delta agent. Serologic markers for HDV may indicate acute or chronic infection as noted in the following table

Marker/Technique	Acute HDV (2-3 weeks after symptom onset)	Chronic HDV
Serum IgM anti-HD/RIA, EIA	Positive	Positive
Serum IgG anti-HD/RIA, EIA	Positive	Positive
HDAg (Antigen)/RIA, EIA	Positive or Negative	Negative
HDAg/Immunoblot	Positive	Positive

- HDV serologic markers may be associated with HBV markers, indicating coinfection, superinfection, or chronic infection, as noted in the following table.

Marker	HBV/HDV Coinfection	HBV/HDV Superinfection	Chronic HBV/HDV
Total anti-HBsAg	Negative	Negative	Negative
IgM anti-HBcAg	Positive	Negative	Negative
Serum HBsAb (Antibody)	Positive	Negative	Negative
Total anti-HDV	Positive (late/transient)	Positive	Positive (late, persistent)
IgM anti-HDAg	Positive (late/transient)	Positive	Positive (late, persistent)
Serum HDAg	Positive (early/transient)	Positive	Positive (early, persistent)

Distinguishing coinfection and superinfection is important due to their prognoses.

Presence of both anti-HDV and HBsAg indicates acute hepatitis D infection.

In patients with chronic HDV infection, delta antibodies persist.

In HBsAg-positive patients with known chronic hepatitis, if an exacerbation is recognized or if HDV infection is suspected, the presence of anti-HDV suggests that chronic HDV infection is present and may be contributing to progression of the disease.

HDV antigen appears transiently early in the course of delta hepatitis. In acute coinfection with hepatitis B, anti-delta IgM antibody may be present for about two weeks, followed by appearance of IgG antibody by the sixth week of illness.

The results of one long-term study suggest that the evolution to cirrhosis is significantly more common in patients with chronic HBV who have serologic evidence of HDV infection.

The presence of IgM antibody to delta virus distinguishes HBsAg carriers who have underlying inflammatory HDV liver disease from those with past HDV infection, and provides prognostic information on the course of chronic HDV hepatitis. Some evidence suggests that IgM persistence is associated with progressive, unremitting liver disease.

In immunocompetent patients with HDV/HBV coinfection, and in whom HBsAg and IgM anti-HBc are identified, anti-HDV is present in a minority at the time of clinical presentation. However, repeat testing 1 month after onset reveals anti-HDV in nearly all. IgM anti-HDV with or without the subsequent appearance of IgG anti-HDV may be identified.

Active infection is not always indicated by HDV antibodies.

COLLECTION/STORAGE INFORMATION
- Specimen Collection and Handling:
    - Collect serum sample in red top or marble top tube.
    - Allow blood to clot at room temperature for no more than 1 hour.
    - Process immediately, or store sample at 4°C or in wet ice for 2 to 4 hours.
    - Transport sample on dry ice.

Hepatitis E antibody measurement

TEST DEFINITION
Detection of hepatitis E antibodies in serum for the evaluation of hepatitis E virus infection

REFERENCE RANGE
Negative
Please refer to your institution's reference ranges as lab normals may vary.

INDICATIONS
Suspected hepatitis E viral infection
   Strength of Recommendation: Class IIa
   Strength of Evidence: Category C
Results Interpretation:
Hepatitis e antigen present
The detection of anti-hepatitis E (anti-HEV) antibodies indicates infection. The presence of IgM anti-HEV suggests acute infection. The presence of IgG anti-HEV suggests prior infection and can be detected for long periods.

The IgG response occurs after the IgM response, with an increasing titer during the acute phase into the convalescent phase, and remaining high 1 to 4.5 years after the acute illness.

The duration of detection of anti-HEV antibodies is unknown; however, anti-HEV antibodies have been detected in persons 14 years after acute infection.

Early detection of HEV in pregnancy is essential due to high mortality (15% to 25%), particularly in the third trimester.

Timing of Monitoring

By the time antibodies appear, individuals may have recovered from the acute phase of hepatitis E virus (HEV) infection. Reverse transcription polymerase chain reaction (RT-PCR) should then be performed. If RT-PCR is unavailable, antibody testing should be repeated in 2 weeks after an initial negative test. RT-PCR should be completed as soon as possible following exposure in pregnancy due to the high mortality of HEV in pregnancy.

CLINICAL NOTES

Hepatitis E virus was previously known as enterically-transmitted non-A, non-B hepatitis.

COLLECTION/STORAGE INFORMATION

- Specimen Collection and Handling:
  - Collect serum sample in red top or marble top tube.
  - Allow blood to clot at room temperature for no more than 1 hour.
  - If unable to immediately process, store at 4°C or in wet ice for 2 to 4 hours.
  - Transport samples on dry ice.

LOINC CODES

- Code: 13294-4 (*Short Name* - Hep E Ab Ser Ql)

Herpes simplex virus 1 AND 2 antibody assay

TEST DEFINITION

Detection of herpes simplex 1 and 2 serum antibody. Serologic tests have only a minor role in initial diagnosis of HSV infection, but can be used to diagnose primary infection. Often used to identify patients with asymptomatic HSV infection (eg, pregnant women).

REFERENCE RANGE

- Adults and Children: Negative (less than a 4-fold rise in antibody titer)
  Please refer to your institution's reference ranges as lab normals may vary.

INDICATIONS

Suspected genital infection with herpes simplex virus
> **Strength of Recommendation:** Class IIa
> **Strength of Evidence:** Category B

Results Interpretation:
Positive immunology findings

Detection of a 4-fold increase in glycoprotein-type specific antibodies to herpes simplex serotypes 1 and 2 between acute and convalescent sera is thought to confirm the presence of herpes simplex virus (HSV) infection.

Suspected herpes simplex encephalitis
> **Strength of Recommendation:** Class IIb
> **Strength of Evidence:** Category B

Results Interpretation:
Positive immunology findings

A 4-fold increase in herpes simplex 1 and 2 antibody titer between acute and convalescent sera is thought to confirm the presence of infection. However, negative serologic findings in isolation do not exclude CNS HSV infection, and the mounting of an intrathecal (CSF) immune response to infection may be delayed by early institution of antiviral therapy.

COMMON PANELS
- Prenatal screening panel
- Transplant panel

CLINICAL NOTES
Although serological tests are not considered useful for initial diagnosis of herpesvirus (HSV) infection, they have proven useful for the confirmation of a diagnosis based upon clinical signs and positive viral culture, as well as for confirming a diagnosis of infection in asymptomatic patients, patients with symptomatic yet culture-negative lesions, and patients with atypical presentations of disease.

Antibody titers for HSV serotypes 1 and 2 generally rise to peak levels within 4 to 6 weeks after the onset of infection. While titers will decline with time, they are known to persist at low levels in the absence of active disease.

Distinguishing between HSV serotypes 1 and 2 may be difficult due to the antibody cross-reactivity between serotype 1 and 2 antigens.

COLLECTION/STORAGE INFORMATION
- Specimen Collection and Handling:
  - Collect serum at onset of disease and 2 to 4 weeks later for both acute and convalescent titers.
  - Freeze specimens if not processed immediately.

LOINC CODES
- Code: 27948-9 (*Short Name* - HSV 1+2 IgG Ser EIA-aCnc)
- Code: 13249-8 (*Short Name* - HSV1+2 IgG CSF-aCnc)
- Code: 31411-2 (*Short Name* - HSV 1+2 IgG Ser-aCnc)

Herpes simplex virus DNA assay

TEST DEFINITION
Detection of herpes simplex virus using polymerase chain reaction assay

REFERENCE RANGE
Adults and Children: No herpes simplex virus detected
Please refer to your institution's reference ranges as lab normals may vary.

INDICATIONS
Suspected congenital herpes simplex
>**Results Interpretation:**
>**Polymerase chain reaction observation**
>>A positive polymerase chain reaction test for herpes simplex virus (HSV) is diagnostic of congenital HSV infection.
>
>>**False Results**
>>>A negative polymerase chain reaction test does not rule out a diagnosis of herpes simplex virus infection. Sensitivities are not high enough to exclude the diagnosis with a negative assay.

Suspected genital herpes simplex
>**Strength of Recommendation:** Class IIa
>**Strength of Evidence:** Category C
>**Results Interpretation:**
>**Polymerase chain reaction observation**
>>A positive polymerase chain reaction test for herpes simplex virus is diagnostic of genital herpes.

Suspected herpes simplex encephalitis
>**Strength of Recommendation:** Class IIa
>**Strength of Evidence:** Category B
>**Results Interpretation:**
>**Polymerase chain reaction observation**
>>A positive PCR test for HSV in CSF is generally diagnostic of HSV encephalitis.

Higher numbers (>100 copies/mm^3) of HSV DNA copies are associated with increased morbidity and mortality.

False Results
Initial negative PCR results have been reported in a small, but notable, number of patients with confirmed HSV encephalitis. This generally occurs during the first 48 hours of symptoms.

Timing of Monitoring
HSV is generally detectable by PCR in CSF for at least 1 week following symptom onset in cases of central nervous system HSV infection.

Suspected herpes simplex meningitis
Results Interpretation:
Polymerase chain reaction observation
A positive polymerase chain reaction (PCR) for herpes simplex virus (HSV) in cerebrospinal fluid is diagnostic of herpes meningitis.

CLINICAL NOTES

The LightCycler method uses a closed system, minimizing possible carry over contamination and provides results in 30 to 40 minutes.

Polymerase chain reaction (PCR) is inhibited by the presence of heparin or heme.

COLLECTION/STORAGE INFORMATION

- Specimen Collection and Handling :
  - Collect serum, cerebrospinal fluid, biopsies of skin lesions, ocular specimens or other tissue samples.
  - Store nucleic acid samples at ≤-20°C.
  - Avoid cross-contamination with extraneous DNA or RNA (polymerase chain reaction by its extreme sensitivity is susceptible to DNA contaminants).

LOINC CODES

- Code: 32364-2 (*Short Name* - HHV 8 DNA Ser QI PCR)

Herpes simplex virus antigen assay

TEST DEFINITION

Measurement of herpes simplex antigen in serum for the evaluation of herpes simplex viral infections

REFERENCE RANGE

- Negative
  Please refer to your institution's reference ranges as lab normals may vary.

INDICATIONS

Suspected herpes simplex keratitis
  Strength of Recommendation: Class IIa
  Strength of Evidence: Category B
  Results Interpretation:
  Presence of viral antigen - finding
  A positive immunofluorescence assay and/or polymerase chain reaction strongly suggests herpes simplex virus (HSV) keratitis. Giemsa stain showing multinucleated giant cells, lymphocytes or intranuclear inclusions is positive for HSV keratitis and is a good general screen for patients with microbial keratitis.

Suspected herpes simplex viral infection
  Strength of Recommendation: Class IIa
  Strength of Evidence: Category B
  Results Interpretation:
  Presence of viral antigen - finding
  Both the direct fluorescent-antibody assay and shell vial direct immunoperoxidase staining give faster results than the viral culture but are less accurate in diagnosing herpes simplex viral infections.

False Results

Direct fluorescent-antibody assay has at least a 20% to 30% false-negative rate when compared with culture.

False-negative results may occur with the enzyme-linked immunosorbent assay for the detection of herpes simplex virus (HSV), especially in the early stages of infection. False positive results may also occur, especially in patients with a low likelihood of HSV infection.

CLINICAL NOTES

Direct microscopic examination can be done; however, the presence of multinucleated giant cells is not specific to herpes simplex virus. Immunostaining of direct smears labeled with fluorescein or immunoperoxidase is better because it can identify viral antigen that does not yet have nuclear inclusions or syncytium formation.

Direct immunofluorescence assay (DFA) is most sensitive on vesicles and less for pustules. Because of technical difficulties, Tzanck smear is better for crusts than immunofluorescence.

COLLECTION/STORAGE INFORMATION

Using a cotton-tipped applicator, swab base of ulcerated lesion or unroofed vesicle, or scrape base of lesion with a scalpel or curette.

To transfer specimen from swab to glass microscope slide, gently roll applicator tip along slide, or transport swab in a container containing appropriate viral transport medium.

LOINC CODES

- Code: 31854-3 (*Short Name* - HSV Ag Skn Ql)
- Code: 31853-5 (*Short Name* - HSV Ag Ser Ql)
- Code: 5855-2 (*Short Name* - HSV Ag XXX Ql IF)
- Code: 16945-8 (*Short Name* - HSV Ag XXX Ql)
- Code: 5853-7 (*Short Name* - HSV Ag Skn Ql IF)
- Code: 5851-1 (*Short Name* - HSV Ag Gen Ql IF)
- Code: 31852-7 (*Short Name* - HSV Ag Gen Ql)
- Code: 29957-8 (*Short Name* - HSV Ag Ser Ql IB)

Herpes simplex virus culture

TEST DEFINITION

Detection of herpes simplex by culture from mucocutaneous lesions, blood, urine, or cerebrospinal fluid

REFERENCE RANGE

- No growth
  Please refer to your institution's reference ranges as lab normals may vary.

INDICATIONS

Suspected genital herpes simplex viral infection
　　Strength of Recommendation: Class IIa
　　Strength of Evidence: Category B
　Results Interpretation:
　Positive microbiology findings
　　Genital herpes infection can be confirmed by the isolation of herpes simplex virus (HSV) in cell culture. Cytopathic effects generally develop within 24 to 48 hours after inoculation and 90% to 95% of cultures are positive within 5 days.

　False Results
　　Viral shedding decreases over time, and therefore, false negative results may occur if the specimen is obtained later in the course of the infection or if the specimen was not transported appropriately.
　Timing of Monitoring
　　For the best results, lesions should be cultured early (within 3 days) in the course of illness.

Suspected herpes simplex infection
Results Interpretation:
Herpesvirus infection

Herpes simplex virus (HSV) isolated from cervix, urethra, anogenital region, skin lesions, cerebrospinal fluid, and other body fluids by culture methods is diagnostic of a herpes simplex infection. A cytopathic effect is evident in 1 to 3 days, and 90% to 95% of cultures are positive in 5 days. Low titer specimens may require 7 to 10 days to become positive.

Suspected herpes virus infection of the central nervous system
Strength of Recommendation: Class III
Strength of Evidence: Category C
Results Interpretation:
Abnormal microbiological findings in CSF

Herpes simplex virus (HSV) cultures of cerebrospinal fluid (CSF) are of limited value in the diagnosis of herpes simplex encephalitis (HSE) in children greater than 6 months and adults.

CSF cultures may be positive for HSV-2 in up to 75% of patients presenting with meningitis and initial episode of primary HSV infection, but is not helpful in recurrent infections.

Suspected neonatal herpes simplex infection
Strength of Recommendation: Class IIa
Strength of Evidence: Category B
Results Interpretation:
Positive microbiology findings

A positive herpes simplex virus (HSV) culture of the neonate confirms the diagnosis of neonatal HSV infection. Positive HSV cultures of skin lesions are diagnostic of neonatal herpes; however, many infants do not have lesions.

Cytopathic effects may be seen in 80% of the cultures within 2 days and in 90% of cultures by 4 days.

CLINICAL NOTES

The best specimen is fluid from the vesicle obtained within 3 days of its appearance, if possible, because the virus rapidly decreases after 4 days following symptom onset.

COLLECTION/STORAGE INFORMATION

- When obtaining a specimen from a vesicle or pustule, break it with a sterile needle and then swab with a dacron- or cotton-tipped swab.
- Transport specimen in a viral transport media.
- Process specimen as quickly as possible.
- Store blood samples at room temperature at all times. Store other viral specimens at 4°C. For longer delays, freeze at -70°C then thaw slowly at about 25°C per minute.
- Swab specimens in viral transport media with antibiotics may remain at room temperature for 12 to 24 hours. It is best to inoculate to cell culture the same day but overnight refrigeration is acceptable.

LOINC CODES

- Code: 5856-0 (*Short Name* - HSV Gen Cult)
- Code: 32689-2 (*Short Name* - HSV Eye Cult)
- Code: 5858-6 (*Short Name* - HSV Skn Cult)
- Code: 5859-4 (*Short Name* - HSV XXX Cult)

Heterophile antibody measurement

TEST DEFINITION

Serologic test for Epstein-Barr virus-induced infectious mononucleosis by detecting heterophile antibodies

REFERENCE RANGE

- Negative
Please refer to your institution's reference ranges as lab normals may vary.

INDICATIONS
Suspected infectious mononucleosis
      Strength of Recommendation: Class IIa
      Strength of Evidence: Category B
    Results Interpretation:
    Heterophile agglutin test abnormal
      A positive heterophile antibody test strongly support the diagnosis of infectious mononucleosis (IM).
      A positive slide test correlates with a heterophile titer of 1:128 or greater.
      In 60% of patients with IM, heterophile antibodies appear within the first or second week and in 80% to 90% by the first month. Titers usually decline in 3 to 6 months but the tests may remain positive for 6 to 12 months after IM.

      False Results
      False negative results occur, particularly in young children who develop fewer heterophile antibodies. The Paul-Bunnell test may not detect infectious mononucleosis (IM) heterophile antibodies in more than 50% of children under 4 years of age and in 10% to 20% of adults. The rate of heterophile antibody responses increases progressively with advancing age from infancy up to 4 years.
      In an analysis of different methodologies, including latex agglutination, false positive reactions were seen from samples of patients with cytomegalovirus, hepatitis A virus, parvovirus, and leptospira infection. Samples containing rheumatoid factor also produced a false positive reaction.
      The false-positive rate for the Paul-Bunnell absorption test is about 3%, and the false-negative rate is 10% to 15%. The slide test has a less than or equal to 2% false negative and a 3% to 6% false positive rate.
    Negative laboratory findings
      A negative heterophile antibody test may indicate the absence of IM; however, it may also represent a false-negative result, or the presence of an IM-like illness, such as toxoplasmosis or cytomegalovirus infection.

      False Results
      False negative results occur, particularly in young children who develop fewer heterophile antibodies. The Paul-Bunnell test may not detect infectious mononucleosis (IM) heterophile antibodies in more than 50% of children under 4 years of age and in 10% to 20% of adults. The rate of heterophile antibody responses increases progressively with advancing age from infancy up to 4 years.
      In an analysis of different methodologies, including latex agglutination, false positive reactions were seen from samples of patients with cytomegalovirus, hepatitis A virus, parvovirus, and leptospira infection. Samples containing rheumatoid factor also produced a false positive reaction.
      The false-positive rate for the Paul-Bunnell absorption test is about 3%, and the false-negative rate is 10% to 15%. The slide test has a less than or equal to 2% false negative and a 3% to 6% false positive rate.
    Frequency of Monitoring
      If a heterophile antibody test is negative and infectious mononucleosis is suspected, repeat the test in 1 to 2 weeks.

COLLECTION/STORAGE INFORMATION
- Specimen Collection and Handling:
  - May need acute and convalescent (2 to 4 weeks later) serum samples
  - Freeze specimens, if not tested immediately

LOINC CODES
- Code: 12221-8 (*Short Name* - Heteroph Ab Ser Ql Shp Aggl)
- Code: 11610-3 (*Short Name* - Heteroph Ab Ser-aCnc)
- Code: 6425-3 (*Short Name* - Heteroph Ab Ser Ql EIA)

Hexosaminidase A and total hexosaminidase measurement, serum and leukocytes

TEST DEFINITION
    Measurement of beta-hexosaminidase A and total hexosaminidase activity in serum and leukocytes for the detection of Tay-Sachs and Sandhoff disease

SYNONYMS
- Hexosaminidase A and total hexosaminidase measurement, serum and leucocytes

REFERENCE RANGE
The normal range is method specific.
Please refer to your institution's reference ranges as lab normals may vary.

INDICATIONS
Screen for at-risk carriers of Sandhoff disease
> **Strength of Recommendation:** Class IIa
> **Strength of Evidence:** Category C
> **Results Interpretation:**
> **Abnormal laboratory findings**
> A deficiency or absence of hexosaminidase A and B indicates Sandhoff disease; present but lowered levels may indicate a heterozygote carrier state.

Screen for at-risk carriers of Tay-Sachs disease
> **Strength of Recommendation:** Class IIa
> **Strength of Evidence:** Category C
> **Results Interpretation:**
> **Abnormal laboratory findings**
> A deficiency or absence of beta-hexosaminidase A indicates Tay-Sachs disease; a present but lowered level may indicate a heterozygote carrier state.
>
> If the serum hexosaminidase level is inconclusive, as it may be with pregnancy, use of oral contraceptives and certain illnesses, measurement of enzyme activity in white blood cells is more accurate in defining carrier status.

COLLECTION/STORAGE INFORMATION
- Specimen Collection and Handling:
  - Draw serum specimen in red top tube.
  - Allow specimen to clot at 3°C, then centrifuge at 3°C.
  - Store specimen at −20°C.

High density lipoprotein measurement

TEST DEFINITION
Measurement of high-density lipoprotein (HDL) cholesterol in serum or plasma for the prevention of coronary heart disease

SYNONYMS
- HDL measurement

REFERENCE RANGE
- Adults, men and women, low level: <40 mg/dL (<1.03 mmol/L)
- Adults, men and women, high level: ≥60 mg/dL (≥1.55 mmol/L)
- Starting in puberty, high density lipoprotein levels average 10 mg/dL lower in men than women.
Please refer to your institution's reference ranges as lab normals may vary.

INDICATIONS
Screening and primary prevention of coronary heart disease
> **Strength of Recommendation:** Class I
> **Strength of Evidence:** Category A
> **Results Interpretation:**
> **Decreased HDL level**
> Low levels of high density lipoprotein (HDL) cholesterol are strongly and inversely correlated with a risk of coronary heart disease (CHD) and CHD-associated morbidity and mortality. While no threshold has been

identified, a level below 40 mg/dL is predictive for CHD in both men and women. Raising HDL reduces the risk of CHD, although an independent association between elevated HDL and lowered CHD has not been determined.

Variations in HDL levels between individuals are due to genetic and acquired factors in about equal proportions. Acquired factors include elevated serum triglycerides, obesity, physical inactivity, cigarette smoking, very high carbohydrate intake, type 2 diabetes, and drugs such as beta-blockers, anabolic steroids and progestational agents. A more substantial HDL-lowering effect is seen in individuals with a genetic predisposition to low HDL who are also overweight or obese.

A targeted HDL goal level has not been identified; low-density lipoprotein (LDL) is the primary target of cholesterol-lowering therapy. Drug and nondrug interventions that raise HDL should be encouraged as part of the overall management of all lipid and nonlipid risk factors. Reversal of the primary causes of low HDL levels (ie, obesity and overweight, physical inactivity, and smoking) will further reduce CHD risk.

Frequency of Monitoring

High density lipoprotein (HDL) testing should be performed as part of a fasting lipid profile every 5 years in low-risk adults starting at age 20. No further testing is necessary in otherwise low-risk persons if HDL is greater than or equal to 40 mg/dL and total cholesterol is less than 200 mg/dL. More frequent testing is necessary for those with multiple risk factors, or for those with 0 or 1 risk factors if the LDL (low-density lipoprotein) level is slightly below the target level.

COMMON PANELS

- Diabetic management panel
- General health panel
- Lipid profile

ABNORMAL RESULTS

Abnormal results can occur in the presence of acute illness, pregnancy, or recent changes in diet. All lipid measurements should be obtained when individuals are in a baseline stable condition.

CLINICAL NOTES

Results from plasma samples are approximately 3% lower than serum samples.

COLLECTION/STORAGE INFORMATION

- Instruct the patient to fast for 9 to 12 hours before the test.
- Have the individual sit for at least 5 minutes prior to phlebotomy to avoid hemoconcentration.
- Collect sample in tube without anticoagulant for serum, or with EDTA for plasma. Due to potential enzyme inhibition, do not use oxalate, citrate, or fluoride tubes.
- Store up to 4 days at 4°C; frozen samples should be stored -70°C and thawed rapidly to 37°C immediately before use.
- To prevent RBC hemolysis, do not agitate tube.
- For fingerstick collection, accurate sample collection is critical to avoid fluid dilution, and to obtain accurate results.

LOINC CODES

- Code: 26822-7 (*Short Name* - A-Lipoprotein Fld QI)
- Code: 2573-4 (*Short Name* - A-LP SerPl-mCnc)
- Code: 19250-0 (*Short Name* - A-LP Plr-mCnc)
- Code: 17845-9 (*Short Name* - A-Lipoprotein SerPl QI)

Histidine measurement

TEST DEFINITION

Measurement of histidine in plasma or serum for detection of acquired and hereditary amino acid disorders

REFERENCE RANGE

- Premature neonate, 1 day: 0.78 ± 0.31 mg/dL (50 ± 20 micromol/L)
- Neonate, 1 day: 0.76-1.77 mg/dL (49-114 micromol/L)
- Infants 1 to 3 months: 0.98 ± 0.16 mg/dL (63 ± 10 micromol/L)
- Infants 2 to 6 months: 1.49-2.12 mg/dL (96-137 micromol/L)

- Infants 9 to 24 months: 0.37-1.74 mg/dL (24-112 micromol/L)
- Children 3 to 10 years: 0.37-1.32 mg/dL (24-85 micromol/L)
- Children 6 to 18 years: 0.99-1.64 mg/dL (64-106 micromol/L)
- Adults: 0.50-1.66 mg/dL (32-107 micromol/L)
  Please refer to your institution's reference ranges as lab normals may vary.

INDICATIONS

Suspected inborn error of metabolism
> **Strength of Recommendation:** Class IIa
> **Strength of Evidence:** Category C
> **Results Interpretation:**
> **Increased amino acid**
> Inherited amino acid disorders are directly related to the absence of an enzyme involved in the metabolism of one or more amino acids; therefore, an elevated plasma level of a particular amino acid is highly suggestive of an inherited metabolic defect. In the majority of cases amino acid and organic acid analysis together permit diagnostic confirmation in infants. Immediate treatment should be initiated when an inborn error of metabolism is suspected, even if a definitive diagnosis has not yet been determined.
> Histidinemia is associated with elevated blood levels of both histidine and alanine.

COLLECTION/STORAGE INFORMATION

- Specimen Collection and Handling:
  - Immediately place sample in ice water.
  - Isolate plasma sample and freeze it within 1 hour; sample stable for 1 week at -20°C.
  - Sample should be deproteinized and stored at -70°C for protracted periods of usage.

LOINC CODES

- Code: 2418-2 (*Short Name* - Histidine Bld Ql)
- Code: 2422-4 (*Short Name* - Histidine Ur Ql)
- Code: 25440-9 (*Short Name* - Histidine 24H Ur-sRate)
- Code: 26808-6 (*Short Name* - Histidine 24H Ur Ql)
- Code: 32247-9 (*Short Name* - Histidine Vitf-sCnc)
- Code: 13398-3 (*Short Name* - Histidine Amn-mCnc)
- Code: 30047-5 (*Short Name* - Histidine/creat Ur-Rto)
- Code: 27111-4 (*Short Name* - Histidine Amn-sCnc)
- Code: 9453-2 (*Short Name* - Histidine CSF-sCnc)
- Code: 2423-2 (*Short Name* - Histidine Ur-mCnc)
- Code: 25926-7 (*Short Name* - Histidine 24H Ur-sCnc)
- Code: 25927-5 (*Short Name* - Histidine/creat 24H Ur-sRto)
- Code: 13757-0 (*Short Name* - Histidine/creat Ur-mRto)
- Code: 22717-3 (*Short Name* - Histidine XXX-sCnc)
- Code: 2419-0 (*Short Name* - Histidine Bld-mCnc)
- Code: 2424-0 (*Short Name* - Histidine 24H Ur-mRate)
- Code: 22703-3 (*Short Name* - Histidine/creat Ur-sRto)
- Code: 27904-2 (*Short Name* - Histidine Ur-sCnc)
- Code: 32246-1 (*Short Name* - Histidine Fld-sCnc)

Histoplasma antibody assay

TEST DEFINITION

Measurement of histoplasma antibodies in blood for the evaluation and management of acute, disseminated or chronic infection

SYNONYMS

- Serologic test for Histoplasma

REFERENCE RANGE

- Adults and Children: Negative
  Please refer to your institution's reference ranges as lab normals may vary.

INDICATIONS

Suspected histoplasmosis
>**Strength of Recommendation:** Class IIa
>**Strength of Evidence:** Category B
>**Results Interpretation:**
>**Serology positive**
>
>In patients with mild histoplasmosis, a positive serology test can be diagnostic. Anti-*Histoplasma* antibodies can be detected in 90% of patients with histoplasmosis; however a two to six week delay following exposure is necessary for antibodies to be present.
>
>The complement fixation (CF) test is standardized and readily available in most state health departments. CF titers of 1:32 or greater are highly suggestive of active histoplasmosis. Weakly positive titers of 1:8 or 1:16 are less helpful in differentiating active infection from past infection, but in about one-third of cases, titers in this range are due to active histoplasmosis.
>
>The presence of M or H precipitin bands using commercial immunodiffusion kits can also provide strong evidence for active histoplasmosis.

ABNORMAL RESULTS

- Results increased in:
  - Past histoplasmosis infection can result in persistent antibody levels.
  - Infections that cross-react with *Histoplasma capsulatum* or other fungal infections
  - Endemic areas can have background levels ranging from 0.5% (immunodiffusion) to 4% (by complement fixation).
- Results decreased in:
  - Immunosuppressed patients

CLINICAL NOTES

Serologic testing for Histoplasma antibodies may have limited value in the assessment of acute illness, because a two to six week delay following exposure is required for antibodies to be produced.

Complement fixation is useful as a screening tool, and results are usually more sensitive and available sooner than immunodiffusion.

Testing with immunodiffusion can be positive for several years and exposure to other fungal diseases can produce a false-positive result. Findings can indicate active or past infection.

COLLECTION/STORAGE INFORMATION

- Specimen Collection and Handling:
  - Collect serum for acute and convalescent measurement; obtain levels approximately 2 to 3 weeks apart

LOINC CODES

- Code: 27266-6 (*Short Name* - Histoplasma Ab Titr Ser ID)
- Code: 31429-4 (*Short Name* - Histoplasma Ab Ser-aCnc)
- Code: 23748-7 (*Short Name* - Histoplasma Ab Ser QI ID)
- Code: 26641-1 (*Short Name* - Histoplasma Ab Ser QI)

Histoplasma capsulatum antigen assay, serum

TEST DEFINITION

Detection of *Histoplasma capsulatum* antigen in serum for the evaluation and management of histoplasmosis

REFERENCE RANGE

- <1 unit
  Please refer to your institution's reference ranges as lab normals may vary.

INDICATIONS

Suspected histoplasmosis.
>**Strength of Recommendation:** Class IIb
>**Strength of Evidence:** Category B

Results Interpretation:
Histoplasmosis test positive
- Positive results:
  - 1 to 2 units: Probable histoplasmosis
  - 2.1 to >10 units: Indicates histoplasmosis
- Increase in post-treatment levels:
  - <1.9 units: Stable
  - 2 to 4 units: Possible therapy failure
  - >4 units: Probable therapy failure

Antigen levels should decrease with treatment and increase with relapse. With treatment, antigen levels decrease more quickly in blood than in urine.

Antigen detection is highest using samples taken from patients exposed within the preceding 30 days or who have disseminated histoplasmosis.

Serum antigen testing is less sensitive than urine antigen testing in the diagnosis of *Histoplasma capsulatum*, but the use of both tests increases diagnostic accuracy. If a positive serum antigen but a negative urine antigen are obtained from the same patient, a diagnosis of histoplasmosis is unlikely.

Serum antigen tests may yield results in 24 to 48 hours, whereas cultures may take up to 4 weeks to become positive.

Serum antigen tests are best used for the diagnosis of disseminated or acute histoplasmosis, rather than chronic pulmonary, self-limited, or asymptomatic disease, which are often associated with low fungal burdens.

Histoplasmosis test negative
Negative antigen test results can occur in up to 20% of disseminated histoplasmosis and 25% to 30% of diffuse pulmonary cases.

ABNORMAL RESULTS
- Results increased in:
  - Collagen diseases
  - Cirrhosis
  - Plasma-cell dyscrasias
  - Malignancy

COLLECTION/STORAGE INFORMATION
- Collect 5 mL of serum in a marble-topped tube.

LOINC CODES
- Code: 19108-0 (*Short Name* - H capsul Ag Ser QI)
- Code: 31855-0 (*Short Name* - H capsul Ag Ser-aCnc)
- Code: 19107-2 (*Short Name* - H capsul Ag Ser RIA-aCnc)
- Code: 6428-7 (*Short Name* - H capsul Ag Ser EIA-aCnc)

Histoplasma capsulatum antigen assay, urine

TEST DEFINITION
Detection of *Histoplasma capsulatum* antigen in urine for the evaluation and management of histoplasmosis

REFERENCE RANGE
- <1 unit
  Please refer to your institution's reference ranges as lab normals may vary.

INDICATIONS
Suspected histoplasmosis
  Strength of Recommendation: Class IIa
  Strength of Evidence: Category B
  Results Interpretation:
  Histoplasmosis test positive
  - Positive results:
    - 1 to 2 units: Probable histoplasmosis

- 2.1 to >10 units: Indicates histoplasmosis
- Increase in post-treatment levels:
  - <1.9 units: Stable
  - 2 to 4 units: Possible therapy failure
  - >4 units: Probable therapy failure
  Antigen levels should decrease with treatment and increase with relapse. With treatment, antigen levels decrease more slowly in urine than in blood.
  Antigen detection is highest using samples taken from patients exposed within the preceding 30 days or who have disseminated histoplasmosis.
  Urine antigen testing is more sensitive than serum antigen testing in the diagnosis of *Histoplasma capsulatum*, but the use of both tests increases diagnostic accuracy.
  Results from antigen tests take 24 to 48 hours to obtain, whereas cultures may take up to 4 weeks to become positive.
  Urine antigen tests are best used for the diagnosis of disseminated or acute histoplasmosis, rather than chronic pulmonary, self-limited, or asymptomatic disease, which are often associated with low fungal burdens.
  Histoplasmosis test negative
  Negative antigen test results can occur in up to 20% of disseminated histoplasmosis and 25% to 30% of diffuse pulmonary cases.
  If a negative urine antigen but a positive serum antigen are obtained from the same patient, a diagnosis of histoplasmosis is unlikely.

ABNORMAL RESULTS
- Results increased in:
  - Collagen diseases
  - Cirrhosis
  - Plasma-cell dyscrasias
  - Malignancy

COLLECTION/STORAGE INFORMATION
- Collect at least 5 mL of urine in a clean plastic or glass container.

LOINC CODES
- Code: 31856-8 (*Short Name* - H capsul Ag Ur-aCnc)
- Code: 13971-7 (*Short Name* - H capsul Ag Ur EIA-aCnc)

Human herpesvirus 6 culture

TEST DEFINITION
Detection of human herpesvirus 6 (HHV-6) in body fluid or tissue for the evaluation of suspected HHV-6 infection

SYNONYMS
- HHV-6 culture

REFERENCE RANGE
- Adults and children: no growth
  Please refer to your institution's reference ranges as lab normals may vary.

INDICATIONS
Suspected roseola infantum in infants
  Strength of Recommendation: Class IIa
  Strength of Evidence: Category B
  Results Interpretation:
  Positive microbiology findings
  A positive human herpesvirus 6 (HHV-6) blood culture is consistent with a retrospective diagnosis of HHV-6 roseola infantum. The rate of virus isolation is highest during the first 3 days of the disease course. HHV-6 has been observed in the cerebrospinal fluid of children with roseola infantum.

CLINICAL NOTES

Viral culture for human herpesvirus 6 (HHV-6) is considered the gold standard for detecting the virus in peripheral blood mononuclear lymphocytes. A more rapid shell vial culture technique can detect HHV-6 within 72 hours, as opposed to the traditional cell culture isolation technique which requires 5 to 21 days for detection. Immunohistochemical staining of tissue and PCR assay are alternative methods for detecting HHV-6.

COLLECTION/STORAGE INFORMATION

- Specimen Collection and Handling:
  - Obtain specimen during acute phase of illness.
  - Transport blood specimen immediately at room temperature, in viral transport medium.
  - Ideally, viral cultures should be inoculated within 36 hours of specimen collection.
  - Hold blood sample at room temperature; do not freeze specimen.

Human immunodeficiency virus antibody titer measurement

TEST DEFINITION

Detection of HIV antibodies in serum or plasma for the diagnosis of HIV

SYNONYMS

- HIV - Human immunodeficiency virus antibody titer
- HIV - Human immunodeficiency virus antibody titre
- Human immunodeficiency virus antibody level
- Human immunodeficiency virus antibody titer
- Human immunodeficiency virus antibody titre
- Human immunodeficiency virus antibody titre measurement

REFERENCE RANGE

- Adults and children: nonreactive
  Please refer to your institution's reference ranges as lab normals may vary.

INDICATIONS

HIV exposure
> **Strength of Recommendation:** Class IIa
> **Strength of Evidence:** Category C

Results Interpretation:

HIV positive
> A repeatedly reactive enzyme immunoassay (EIA) result is highly suggestive of HIV infection. Although results should be confirmed by Western blot or immunofluorescent antibody before informing the source person, these confirmatory results are not necessary to make initial decisions about postexposure management in the exposed person. Most infected persons will develop antibodies within 3 months of exposure.

HIV negative
> Enzyme immunoassay seronegative results indicate the absence of HIV infection. If the source person is HIV seronegative and no clinical evidence of AIDS or HIV infection exists, no further testing or follow-up of the source person is necessary.

Frequency of Monitoring
> Because time to seroconversion can be up to 3 months, testing of the victim should be repeated at 6, 12, and 24 weeks after a sexual assault, if the initial test results are negative and infection is likely to be present in the assailant. For health care providers (HCP) with occupational exposure to HIV, follow-up antibody testing should continue for at least 6 months postexposure (eg, at 6 weeks, 12 weeks, and 6 months). Testing beyond 6 months is not routinely recommended, as delayed seroconversion is rare, but may be appropriate in given situations based on clinical judgment.

Timing of Monitoring
> An HIV antibody test should be completed within 24 to 48 hours of exposure -- ideally within a few hours -- in order to establish infection status at the time of exposure.

Suspected HIV exposure
    Strength of Recommendation: Class IIa
    Strength of Evidence: Category C
Results Interpretation:
Finding of HIV status

- The World Health Organization suggests 3 different testing strategies depending on the testing objective and the HIV prevalence in the geographic area. Strategy I is recommended for diagnosing HIV in symptomatic patients when the disease prevalence in the geographic area is greater than 30%. Strategy II is suggested for diagnosing HIV in symptomatic patients when the disease prevalence is 30% or less, and for diagnosing HIV in asymptomatic patients when the disease prevalence is greater than 10%. Strategy III is recommended for diagnosing asymptomatic patients when the disease prevalence is 10% or less:
  - Strategy I: Test each serum or plasma sample once using an enzyme-linked immunosorbent assay (ELISA) or a rapid test. A single reactive test is considered HIV antibody positive while a nonreactive test is considered HIV antibody negative.
  - Strategy II: Test all plasma with one ELISA or rapid test. Retest any single reactive test with another ELISA or rapid test that utilizes a different antigen preparation and/or test methodology. Serum that is reactive on both assays is considered HIV antibody positive. Serum that is nonreactive on the first test is considered HIV antibody negative. Any test that is positive on the first assay and negative on the second assay should be retested with the same 2 assays. Discordant results are interpreted as indeterminate.
  - Strategy III: Test each serum or plasma sample with one ELISA or rapid test. All reactive tests should be retested using a different assay. If a test is initially reactive and then non-reactive when tested again using a second assay, both tests should be repeated. If the first assay is repeatedly positive, or both the first and second assays are positive, a third test should be performed. The test strategies for all 3 steps should utilize different antigen preparations and/or different test methodologies. Discordant results are considered indeterminate. Serum that is seropositive on the first assay and nonreactive on the second and third assays is considered indeterminate for those who may have been exposed within the previous 3 months, and negative for those with no exposure or HIV risk. Serum reactive on all 3 tests is considered HIV antibody positive. Serum that is nonreactive on the first test is considered HIV antibody negative.

False Results
    Individuals who have been vaccinated against HIV or influenzamay have false positive test results.
HIV positive
    Patients newly diagnosed as seropositive on the basis of their first sample should have an additional sample drawn and tested, to decrease the potential for a false positive result due to technical or clerical error.
    A positive result in an infant born to an HIV-infected mother may not be indicative of HIV status until the age of 18 months due to passively acquired maternal antibodies.

False Results
    Individuals who have been vaccinated against HIV or influenzamay have false positive test results.
HIV negative
    All non-reactive tests are generally considered HIV antibody negative. Patients may test negative after recent exposure prior to the development of detectable antibodies, although this window period has been reduced substantially by the improved analytical sensitivity of the assays. Enzyme immunoassay may fail to detect HIV infection in patients with variant strains of HIV (including HIV-2 or HIV-1 subtype O).

False Results
    Individuals who have been vaccinated against HIV or influenzamay have false positive test results.
Equivocal laboratory findings
    Patients who continue to have indeterminate results after one year are considered HIV negative. Patients in later stages of HIV disease may produce indeterminate results because of a decrease in antibodies and retesting is not necessary in these cases. In order to diagnose HIV in asymptomatic patients with indeterminate results, a second sample should be tested at least 2 weeks after the first sample is drawn, and a confirmatory test should be performed if this second sample also proves indeterminate; extended follow up testing may be necessary if the confirmatory test results are also indeterminate.

False Results
    Individuals who have been vaccinated against HIV or influenzamay have false positive test results.

COLLECTION/STORAGE INFORMATION

- Store up to 18 months between 2°C and 8°C, per individual test instructions.

LOINC CODES

- Code: 22358-6 (*Short Name* - HIV2 Ab Ser-aCnc)
- Code: 5223-3 (*Short Name* - HIV1+2 Ab Ser EIA-aCnc)
- Code: 22356-0 (*Short Name* - HIV 1 Ab Ser-aCnc)
- Code: 22357-8 (*Short Name* - HIV 1+2 Ab Ser-aCnc)
- Code: 5224-1 (*Short Name* - HIV 2 Ab Ser EIA-aCnc)
- Code: 5220-9 (*Short Name* - HIV 1 Ab Ser EIA-aCnc)

Human papillomavirus DNA detection

TEST DEFINITION

DNA testing to detect high-risk (oncologic) human papillomavirus (HPV) types in cervical specimens

SYNONYMS

- HPV DNA detection

REFERENCE RANGE

- Negative

Please refer to your institution's reference ranges as lab normals may vary.

INDICATIONS

Suspected human papillomavirus (HPV) infection in women with atypical squamous cells of undetermined significance (ASCUS)

> **Strength of Recommendation:** Class I
> **Strength of Evidence:** Category A
> **Results Interpretation:**
> **HPV - Human papillomavirus test positive**
>> The human papillomavirus (HPV) DNA test distinguishes between two HPV DNA groups: low-risk HPV 6, 11, 42, 43, 44 and high-risk HPV 16, 18, 31, 33, 35, 39, 45, 51, 52, 56, 58, 59, 68.
>> Overall, 30% to 60% of women with atypical squamous cells will have high-risk HPV types identified on DNA testing. All women with atypical squamous cells of undetermined significance (ASCUS) who test positive for HPV DNA initially or on repeat testing should be referred for colposcopic examination.
> **HPV - Human papillomavirus test negative**
>> Women with atypical squamous cells who test negative for human papillomavirus DNA can be followed up with repeat cytologic testing in 12 months.
> **Frequency of Monitoring**
>> Repeat human papillomavirus (HPV) DNA testing at 12 months is an acceptable management option for women with atypical squamous cells (ASC) who test positive for high-risk types of HPV but who do not have biopsy-confirmed cervical intraepithelial neoplasia (CIN). Patients should be referred for colposcopy if testing is positive.

Primary screening for human papillomavirus (HPV) as an adjunct to cytology for cervical cancer screening in women

> **Results Interpretation:**
> **HPV - Human papillomavirus test positive**
>> The human papillomavirus (HPV) DNA test distinguishes between two HPV DNA groups: low-risk HPV 6, 11, 42, 43, 44 and high-risk (oncologic) HPV 16, 18, 31, 33, 35, 39, 45, 51, 52, 56, 58, 59, 68.
>> Women whose HPV DNA test detects high-risk viral types but have a negative cytology result are at relatively low risk of having high-grade cervical intraepithelial neoplasia.
>> Overall, 30% to 60% of women with atypical squamous cells will have high-risk HPV types identified on DNA testing. All women with atypical squamous cells of undetermined significance (ASCUS) who test positive for HPV DNA initially or on repeat testing should be referred for colposcopic examination.
> **HPV - Human papillomavirus test negative**
>> Women whose screening human papillomavirus (HPV) DNA and cervical cytology tests are both negative are at very low risk of having unidentified cervical intraepithelial neoplasia (CIN)-2 or CIN-3 or cervical cancer.
> **Frequency of Monitoring**
>> Women aged 30 years and older who have negative concurrent human papillomavirus (HPV) DNA and cytology test results should undergo cervical screening no more often than every 3 years.

Women whose HPV DNA test detects high-risk viral types but who have a negative cytology result should undergo repeat HPV and cytology testing in 6 to 12 months, and if either test result if abnormal, colposcopy should be performed.

COLLECTION/STORAGE INFORMATION
- Specimen Collection and Handling:
  - Submit specimen using either the HPV collection kit (supplied by manufacturer) or liquid-based cytology preservative.
  - Collect cervical cells from exocervix and endocervical canal using sampling brush in collection kit and place brush in transport tube for shipment to laboratory.
  - When cytology preservative is used, collect samples with a cervical broom and place in liquid-based cytology fixative.

Huntington disease DNA test

TEST DEFINITION
Direct gene evaluation of DNA to predict or confirm Huntington disease

REFERENCE RANGE
- Adults and Children: ≤26 cytosine-adenine-guanine (CAG) repeat lengths
  Please refer to your institution's reference ranges as lab normals may vary.

INDICATIONS
Suspected Huntington disease
> **Strength of Recommendation:** Class IIa
> **Strength of Evidence:** Category B
> **Results Interpretation:**
> **Huntington disease DNA test positive**
>> A cytosine-adenine-guanine (CAG) repeat length of greater than 40 appears to be diagnostic for Huntington disease (HD). Thirty-six to 39 CAG repeat lengths have been associated with both clinically affected and unaffected individuals. A diagnosis of HD is unlikely with repeat lengths between 27 and 35, but transmission of this allele may expand into an HD allele in offspring, depending on several factors including the sex of the transmitting individual and the size of the allele. A CAG repeat length of equal to or less than 26 excludes the diagnosis of HD.
>> Longer CAG expansion lengths are associated with an earlier age of onset of HD and with a greater decline in neurologic and cognitive function.
>> A range of CAG repeats between 30 and 70 indicates an individual affected by HD, while a range between 9 and 34 indicates a normal individual.

CLINICAL NOTES
The American College of Medical Genetics recommends that predictive testing be offered only to those who are at least 18 years of age and be accompanied by genetic counseling. The Southern blot may be superior in diagnosing juvenile-onset Huntington disease due to its ability to amplify large expansions.

COLLECTION/STORAGE INFORMATION
- Specimen Collection and Handling:
  - Obtain whole blood sample.
  - Anticoagulate sample with EDTA or acid citrate dextrose (ACD).
  - Store sample at 4°C.
  - Store cells at −20°C or below if not possible to extract nucleic acids instantly.

LOINC CODES
- Code: 21763-8 (*Short Name* - HD Gene CAG Repeats QI)

Hydrogen breath test

TEST DEFINITION
Measurement of hydrogen from expired air following oral consumption of a sugar load for the evaluation and management of certain intestinal disorders

SYNONYMS
- H2BT - Hydrogen breath test
- H-BT - Hydrogen breath test

REFERENCE RANGE
- Adults (bacterial overgrowth): Increase of <12 ppm to 20 ppm from baseline
- Adults (lactose intolerant): Increase of <20 ppm above baseline
  Please refer to your institution's reference ranges as lab normals may vary.

INDICATIONS
Suspected bacterial overgrowth syndrome
> **Results Interpretation:**
> **Positive laboratory findings**
> > Breath tests for carbohydrate are based on the principle of bacterial degradation of non-absorbable carbohydrates. Bacteria break down the carbohydrates to hydrogen which is absorbed and exhaled in the breath. If a non-absorbable sugar is chosen (eg, lactulose) the hydrogen peak reflects either bacterial overgrowth in the small bowel or transit to the cecum.
> > If an absorbable sugar (eg, lactose) is given, an early hydrogen peak (30 to 75 minutes) suggests bacterial degradation of the carbohydrate marker in the small intestine from bacterial contamination; a later peak of hydrogen reflects transit of the sugar to the colon and defines carbohydrate malabsorption (ie, lactose intolerance).

Suspected lactose intolerance
> > **Strength of Recommendation:** Class IIa
> > **Strength of Evidence:** Category C
> **Results Interpretation:**
> **Increased level (laboratory finding)**
> > An increase in breath hydrogen concentration of greater than 20 ppm above baseline is suggestive of lactose intolerance. In children, some investigators recommend a cutoff of 10 ppm.

> **False Results**
- Results decreased in:
- Diarrhea
- Enema, recent
- Hydrogen-producing bacteria absent (up to 10% patients)
- Results increased in:
- Exercise
- Smoking
> **Frequency of Monitoring**
> Testing may take 2 to 6 hours, with samples taken at intervals of 15 to 60 minutes.

ABNORMAL RESULTS
- Methane producers

Contraindications
The test should not be done in infants and very young children because the large lactose load could cause diarrhea and dehydration if lactose intolerance is present.

COLLECTION/STORAGE INFORMATION
- Eat a low-fiber diet the day before the test
- May analyze sample immediately or store in glass syringe for 12 to 24 hours, in evacuated rubber-stoppered tube for 3 weeks, or in a laminated foil bag for 7 weeks

LOINC CODES

- Code: 16994-6 (*Short Name* - Breath H2 Test 5H)
- Code: 16989-6 (*Short Name* - Breath H2 Test 3.5H)
- Code: 16995-3 (*Short Name* - Breath H2 Test 6H)
- Code: 16988-8 (*Short Name* - Breath H2 Test 2H)
- Code: 16997-9 (*Short Name* - Breath H2 Test p glucose)

Hydroxyproline measurement

TEST DEFINITION

Measurement of alanine in plasma or serum for detection of acquired and hereditary amino acid disorders.

REFERENCE RANGE

- Premature neonate, 1 day: 0.52 ± 0.52 mg/dL (40 ± 40 micromol/L)
- Male child 6 to 18 years: <0.66 mg/dL (<50 micromol/L)
- Female child 6 to 18 years: <0.58 mg/dL (<44 micromol/L)
- Adult male: <0.55 mg/dL (<42 micromol/L)
- Adult female: <0.45 mg/dL (<34 micromol/L)
  Please refer to your institution's reference ranges as lab normals may vary.

INDICATIONS

Suspected inborn error of metabolism
    Strength of Recommendation: Class IIa
    Strength of Evidence: Category C
    Results Interpretation:
    Increased amino acid
    Inherited amino acid disorders are directly related to the absence of an enzyme involved in the metabolism of one or more amino acids; therefore, an elevated plasma level of a particular amino acid is highly suggestive of an inherited metabolic defect. In the majority of cases amino acid and organic acid analysis together permit diagnostic confirmation in infants. Immediate treatment should be initiated when an inborn error of metabolism is suspected, even if a definitive diagnosis has not yet been determined.

COLLECTION/STORAGE INFORMATION

- Specimen Collection and Handling:
  - Immediately place sample in ice water.
  - Isolate plasma sample and freeze it within 1 hour; sample stable for 1 week at -20°C.
  - Sample should be deproteinized and stored at -70°C for protracted periods of usage.

LOINC CODES

- Code: 26596-7 (*Short Name* - OH-Proline CSF-sCnc)
- Code: 2445-5 (*Short Name* - OH-Proline SerPl Ql)
- Code: 32250-3 (*Short Name* - OH-Proline Vitf-sCnc)
- Code: 13401-5 (*Short Name* - OH-Proline Amn-mCnc)
- Code: 2448-9 (*Short Name* - OH-Proline Free SerPl-mCnc)
- Code: 13374-4 (*Short Name* - OH-Proline CSF-mCnc)
- Code: 20647-4 (*Short Name* - OH-Proline SerPl-sCnc)
- Code: 32249-5 (*Short Name* - OH-Proline Fld-sCnc)
- Code: 27181-7 (*Short Name* - OH-Proline Amn-sCnc)
- Code: 2446-3 (*Short Name* - OH-Proline SerPl-mCnc)

Immunofixation electrophoresis, Cerebrospinal fluid, Serum

TEST DEFINITION
Qualitative determination of cerebrospinal fluid and serum to detect oligoclonal bands for the evaluation of neurologic disorders

SYNONYMS
- IFE
- Immunoelectrophoresis

REFERENCE RANGE
- Adults, serum: Negative
Please refer to your institution's reference ranges as lab normals may vary.

INDICATIONS
Suspected multiple sclerosis
> **Strength of Recommendation:** Class IIa
> **Strength of Evidence:** Category C
Results Interpretation:
Positive laboratory findings
> The presence of oligoclonal bands in cereborspinal fluid (CSF) by isoelectric focusing (IEF) is highly suggestive of multiple sclerosis. The significance of individual bands in CSF fluid must be interpreted in parallel with the serum specimen.
Timing of Monitoring
> The cerebrospinal fluid sample needs to be run simultaneously with the serum sample for direct comparison.

COLLECTION/STORAGE INFORMATION
- Collect serum and CSF simultaneously.
- Collect serum in marbled tube, and CSF in glass or plastic tube.

Immunoglobulin M measurement

TEST DEFINITION
Measurement of immunoglobulin M (IgM) in cerebrospinal fluid for the evaluation and management of multiple sclerosis

SYNONYMS
- Immunoglobulin M level

REFERENCE RANGE
- Adults, 21-40 years: 0.016 ± 0.003 mg/dL (0.16 ± 0.03 mg/L)
- Adults, 41-60 years: 0.017 ± 0.004 mg/dL (0.17 ± 0.04 mg/L)
- Adults, 61-87 years: 0.017 ± 0.005 mg/dL (0.17 ± 0.05 mg/L)
- Adolescence, 15 years and older: 0.02 ± 0.0009 mg/dL (0.2 ± 0.09 mg/L)
Please refer to your institution's reference ranges as lab normals may vary.

INDICATIONS
Multiple sclerosis
> **Strength of Recommendation:** Class IIa
> **Strength of Evidence:** Category B
Results Interpretation:
Immunoglobulin level - finding
> Intrathecal IgM synthesis supports a worsened prognosis in multiple sclerosis.

COLLECTION/STORAGE INFORMATION
- Specimen Collection and Handling:
  - Centrifuge
  - Analyze fresh or store at 4°C if longer than 72 hours
  - May store frozen at -20 °C for 6 months or at -70 °C indefinitely
  - Do not contaminate with blood

LOINC CODES
- Code: 26958-9 (*Short Name* - IgM 24H Ur-mCnc)
- Code: 14002-0 (*Short Name* - IgM BldCo-aCnc)
- Code: 17009-2 (*Short Name* - IgM Ser Ql)
- Code: 30142-4 (*Short Name* - IgM 24H Ur Ql IEP)
- Code: 18304-6 (*Short Name* - IgM Ur Ql IFE)
- Code: 6784-3 (*Short Name* - IgM Ur EIA-mCnc)
- Code: 25446-6 (*Short Name* - IgM Ur Ql IEP)
- Code: 2472-9 (*Short Name* - IgM Ser-mCnc)
- Code: 2471-1 (*Short Name* - IgM CSF-mCnc)
- Code: 15186-0 (*Short Name* - IgM Ser Ql IEP)
- Code: 6783-5 (*Short Name* - IgM Ur Elph-mCnc)
- Code: 18303-8 (*Short Name* - IgM Ser Ql IFE)
- Code: 13313-2 (*Short Name* - IgM SerPl-aCnc)
- Code: 21351-2 (*Short Name* - IgM CSF Ql IFE)
- Code: 15185-2 (*Short Name* - IgM Fld-mCnc)

Indirect Coombs test

TEST DEFINITION
Indirect antiglobulin (Coombs) test used for identification of antibodies to erythrocytes

SYNONYMS
- IAGT - Indirect antiglobulin test
- IAT - Indirect antiglobulin test
- Indirect antiglobulin test

REFERENCE RANGE
- Adults and Children: Negative
  Please refer to your institution's reference ranges as lab normals may vary.

INDICATIONS
Screen for suspected ABO incompatibility
Results Interpretation:
Indirect Coombs test positive
The indirect anti-human globulin (Coombs) test is used to detect antibodies in patient serum as a part of red cell compatibility testing including type, screen and crossmatching.
A positive indirect Coombs test in a crossmatch indicates ABO or other blood group incompatibility, and that blood unit should not be transfused.

Screen for suspected Rh incompatibility during pregnancy
Strength of Recommendation: Class I
Strength of Evidence: Category B
Results Interpretation:
Indirect Coombs test positive
A positive indirect Coombs screen in pregnancy suggests alloimmunization against fetal red blood cell antigens.
Titers can indicate the degree of alloimmunization. In most centers, a titer between 8 and 32 suggests a significant risk for fetal hydrops.

Frequency of Monitoring

If a positive indirect Coombs test is found at the first obstetric visit, titers should be repeated at 20 weeks' gestation and every four weeks thereafter.

Pregnancies subsequent to those with a positive indirect Coombs test should have repeat titers monthly for 6 months and every two weeks thereafter.

Timing of Monitoring

An indirect Coombs should be done at the first obstetric visit, and at 28 weeks. Indirect Coombs should be done at time of abortion if not previously done.

COMMON PANELS

• Hemolysis panel

COLLECTION/STORAGE INFORMATION

• Specimen Collection and Handling:
    • Collect serum or plasma in an EDTA (lavender top) tube.
    • Separate serum or plasma from red cells promptly.
    • Serum or plasma sample must be less than 48 hours old.
    • Store the sample at 4°C for a week or at -30°C for longer time.

LOINC CODES

• Code: 1005-8 (*Short Name* - IAT IgG-Sp Reag SerPl Ql)
• Code: 1008-2 (*Short Name* - IDAT Poly-Sp Reag SerPl Ql)
• Code: 1003-3 (*Short Name* - IAT Comp-Sp Reag SerPl Ql)

Influenza virus A AND B antibody assay

TEST DEFINITION

Detection of antibodies to influenza A and B in serum for the diagnosis of acute influenza infection or confirmation of immunity

REFERENCE RANGE

• Adults and children: Negative (less than a 4-fold increase in serum antibody titer)
Please refer to your institution's reference ranges as lab normals may vary.

INDICATIONS

Suspected influenza
   Strength of Recommendation: Class IIb
   Strength of Evidence: Category B
   Results Interpretation:
   Serology positive
   Serologic tests for influenza have been used primarily in epidemiologic investigations of outbreaks to determine which strain is prevalent in the community; they have also been used to assess immunity.

A 4-fold elevation in influenza A or B antibody titer (measured between acute and convalescent phase specimens) indicates influenza infection.

Virus-specific IgM generally appears in the blood during the first week of acute infection and becomes undetectable within 1 to 3 months. IgG appears within 2 weeks of acute infection, peaks at 4 to 8 weeks, then decreases while remaining at detectable levels for an indefinite length of time. Antibody titers measured by the hemagglutination inhibition assay rise approximately 7 days after initial infection and plateau within 2 to 4 weeks.

Because of the time frame required for serologic testing, antibody titers are not useful for acute diagnosis or management.

CLINICAL NOTES

The hemagglutination inhibition assay is considered more sensitive for influenza A, complement fixation more sensitive for influenza B, and the enzyme-linked immunosorbent assay (ELISA) equally sensitive for both A and B viruses.

COLLECTION/STORAGE INFORMATION
- Specimen Collection and Handling:
  - Collect serum in red-top tube up to 7 days post-infection and again in 14 to 60 days
  - May store at 4° C

LOINC CODES
- Code: 7930-1 (*Short Name* - Influe A+B Ab Ser-aCnc)
- Code: 22366-9 (*Short Name* - FLU A+B Ab Titr Ser)
- Code: 17013-4 (*Short Name* - Influe A+B Ab Ser IF-aCnc)
- Code: 6434-5 (*Short Name* - FLU A+B Ab Titr Ser IF)

Insulin C-peptide measurement

TEST DEFINITION
Measurement of C-peptide in blood for the evaluation and treatment of disorders related to abnormal insulin levels, such as diabetes, hypoglycemia, and insulinoma

SYNONYMS
- Connecting peptide insulin measurement
- C-peptide level
- C-peptide measurement
- Proinsulin C-peptide measurement

REFERENCE RANGE
- Adults: 0.5 - 2.0 ng/mL (0.17 - 0.66 nmol/L)
  Please refer to your institution's reference ranges as lab normals may vary.

INDICATIONS
Determination of etiology of acute or recurrent hypoglycemia
> **Strength of Recommendation:** Class IIa
> **Strength of Evidence:** Category C
> **Results Interpretation:**
> **Abnormal laboratory findings**
>> C-peptide is useful as a marker of endogenous insulin production.
>>
>> Decreased C-peptide levels of 2 ng/mL or less associated with high insulin levels in patients experiencing hypoglycemia suggest exogenous (factitious) hyperinsulinism.
>>
>> Decreased C-peptide with low insulin and low glucose levels is associated with non-insulin-mediated hypoglycemias from liver disease, ethanol hypoglycemia, or adrenal insufficiency.
>>
>> Increased C-peptide levels greater than 2 ng/mL, with elevated insulin and proinsulin levels, are usually seen in patients with insulinomas or hypoglycemia secondary to oral hypoglycemic (e.g., sulfonylureas) use.
>>
>> Patients with reactive (alimentary) hypoglycemia often present with high insulin levels; the insulin to C-peptide molar ratio will also be disproportionately high.
>
> **Frequency of Monitoring**
>> During a 72-hour inpatient fast, C-peptide levels should be monitored in conjunction with plasma glucose and proinsulin every 6 hours until the glucose level is equal to or less than 60 mg/dL. Thereafter, levels should be checked every 1 to 2 hours.

Distinguishes type 1 from type 2 diabetes mellitus
> **Strength of Recommendation:** Class IIb
> **Strength of Evidence:** Category C
> **Results Interpretation:**
> **Abnormal laboratory findings**
>> C-peptide is useful as a marker of endogenous insulin production, and assists in the evaluation of residual beta cell function in type 2 diabetics to determine the appropriate time to begin exogenous insulin administration.
>>
>> Decreased C-peptide and insulin levels associated with islet cell antibodies suggest type 1 diabetes.
>>
>> Elevated C-peptide and insulin levels without autoimmune markers suggest type 2 diabetes.

Suspected insulinoma
    Strength of Recommendation: Class IIa
    Strength of Evidence: Category C
    Results Interpretation:
    Increased level (laboratory finding)
        C-peptide is useful as a marker of endogenous insulin production.
        Increased C-peptide, insulin, and proinsulin levels with low beta hydroxybutyrate serum concentrations is suggestive of insulinoma.
        C-peptide levels of 2 nmol/L or greater usually indicate insulinoma. The diagnosis of insulinoma is usually made during a prolonged fast using the clinical findings of Whipple's triad: symptomatic patients with serum glucose levels less than 45 mg/dL, symptoms of hypoglycemia while fasting, and relief of symptoms following administration of glucose.
    Frequency of Monitoring
        For a 72-hour inpatient fast, C-peptide levels should be monitored in conjunction with plasma glucose and proinsulin every 6 hours until the glucose level is equal to or less than 60 mg/dL, following which levels should be checked every 1 to 2 hours.

COLLECTION/STORAGE INFORMATION
- Patient must be fasting before sample collection.
- Collect sample in a marbled top tube.
- Store sample at $-70°C$; serum is stable for 30 days when frozen.

LOINC CODES
- Code: 25872-3 (*Short Name* - C Peptide 24H Ur-sCnc)
- Code: 1987-7 (*Short Name* - C Peptide Ur-mCnc)
- Code: 27944-8 (*Short Name* - C Peptide 24H Ur-mRate)
- Code: 25358-3 (*Short Name* - C Peptide 24H Ur-sRate)

Insulin antibody measurement

TEST DEFINITION
Measurement of insulin antibodies in serum

REFERENCE RANGE
- Negative
- <3% binding of labeled human, beef, or pork insulin by patient's serum
  Please refer to your institution's reference ranges as lab normals may vary.

INDICATIONS
Suspected insulin resistance in diabetics due to insulin antibodies
    Strength of Recommendation: Class IIb
    Strength of Evidence: Category B
    Results Interpretation:
    Antibody studies abnormal
        Elevated insulin antibodies may be associated with decreased control of diabetes mellitus and/or increased insulin requirement.
        Insulin antibodies are produced in almost all diabetics treated with exogenous beef or pork insulin. Human insulin and higher purity animal insulins have reduced the development of antibodies.
        Indiscriminate use of insulin may also result in the development of insulin antibodies.
        The most common insulin antibody is IgG, but IgA, IgD, and IgE have been reported. Most of these insulin antibodies do not cause clinical problems because of their low affinity; however, they can complicate most insulin immunoassays. In these cases and where there is indiscriminate use of insulin, C-peptide measurement is recommended.

CLINICAL NOTES
Radioimmunoprecipitation assay cannot differentiate insulin antibodies occurring spontaneously or as a result of insulin therapy. Data may vary between laboratories. Antibody binding to labeled insulin may be inhibited by

endogenous or exogenous unlabeled insulin. Since the half-life of circulating insulin is prolonged in the presence of insulin antibody, fasting or waiting more than 12 hours after an insulin injection is inadequate to assay sera.

COLLECTION/STORAGE INFORMATION
- Specimen Collection and Handling:
  - Collect blood in marble or red top tube.
  - Separate serum from cells.
  - Freeze the sample.
  - Do not use plasma.

LOINC CODES
- Code: 2481-0 (*Short Name* - Insulin Ab Ser QI)
- Code: 11087-4 (*Short Name* - Insulin Ab Titr Ser)
- Code: 5232-4 (*Short Name* - Insulin Ab Ser RIA-aCnc)
- Code: 2482-8 (*Short Name* - Insulin Ab Ser-mCnc)

International normalized ratio

TEST DEFINITION
Calculation of international normalized ratio (INR), a standardized measurement of prothrombin time (PT) of plasma, to monitor blood coagulation time in patients receiving oral anticoagulant therapy (OAT) (ie, warfarin or other vitamin K antagonists)

SYNONYMS
- INR - International normalized ratio

REFERENCE RANGE
- Therapeutic Range:
- Prevention of venous thromboembolism (VTE): 2-3
- Treatment of VTE, pulmonary embolus, valvular heart disease: 2-3
- Treatment of arterial thromboembolism, mechanical heart valves, recurrent systemic embolism: 3-4.5
  Please refer to your institution's reference ranges as lab normals may vary.

INDICATIONS
Monitoring of international normalized ratio (INR) to assess anticoagulation status in patients receiving oral anticoagulant therapy (OAT) for atrial fibrillation
   Strength of Recommendation: Class I
   Strength of Evidence: Category A
   Results Interpretation:
   Laboratory test finding
   The recommended target INR level for patients with atrial fibrillation (AF) receiving anticoagulant therapy is 2.5 with a therapeutic range of 2 to 3.
   In AF patients who have a stroke, there is better short-term survival when their INR is maintained at a level of greater than or equal to 2.
   The optimal INR level is one that minimizes both the risk of emboli-related ischemic stroke and the risk of major hemorrhage.
   Patients with INR levels above their therapeutic range are at increased risk for bleeding. For AF patients with bleeding events, their INR range may be reduced to 1.5 to 2.
   Patients with AF and INR levels greater than 3 have an increased risk of major hemorrhage, including intracranial hemorrhage (ICH), and the risk of ICH is strongly related to INR levels greater than 4.
   The risk of ischemic stroke in AF patients increases with INR levels below 2. The risk of stroke may double with a level of 1.7 and triple with a level of 1.5 compared to a level of 2. At a level below 2 there is also marked increase in the risk of severe or fatal stroke.
   Frequency of Monitoring
   Prothrombin time monitoring for INR is generally performed daily until the patient reaches the appropriate therapeutic range and maintains that level for 2 consecutive days. It is then monitored 2 to 3 times per

week for 1 to 2 weeks, and then less often (the frequency then depends on the stability of the levels). Elderly patients may need to be monitored more frequently as they may be more likely to have additional factors affecting INR stability.

Timing of Monitoring

Two measurements of INR, at least 24 hours apart, that are within the appropriate therapeutic range are required before stopping heparin on anticoagulated patients.

Monitoring of international normalized ratio (INR) to assess anticoagulation status in patients with a history of venous thromboembolism (VTE) who receive oral anticoagulant therapy (OAT) (ie, warfarin or other vitamin K antagonists)

Strength of Recommendation: Class I

Strength of Evidence: Category A

Results Interpretation:

Laboratory test finding

The recommended target INR value for patients receiving ongoing oral anticoagulation therapy (OAT) for acute treatment or prophylaxis of venous thromboembolism (VTE) is 2.5 with a range of 2 to 3.

Monitoring of INR during treatment of acute venous thrombosis is done when the patient is on heparin and started on OAT (ie, vitamin K antagonists). When the INR is stable and in a therapeutic range (greater than 2), heparin may be discontinued.

The seventh American College of Chest Physicians (ACCP) conference recommends against using high-intensity OAT that results in an INR range of 3.1 to 4.

The risk of bleeding while on OAT significantly increases with INR levels greater than 5.

The seventh ACCP conference recommends against using low-intensity OAT that results in an INR range of 1.5 to 1.9.

Frequency of Monitoring

Prothrombin time monitoring for INR is generally performed daily until the patient reaches the appropriate therapeutic range and maintains that level for 2 consecutive days. It is then monitored 2 to 3 times per week for 1 to 2 weeks, and then less often (the frequency then depends on the stability of the levels). Elderly patients may need to be monitored more frequently as they may be more likely to have additional factors affecting INR stability.

Daily INR monitoring should be done during acute deep venous thromboembolism (DVT) treatment with heparin and oral anticoagulant therapy (OAT) to determine when the INR has reached a stable therapeutic target level. Thereafter, it should be monitored weekly until control is stable.

Two measurements of INR, at least 24 hours apart, that are within the appropriate therapeutic range are required before stopping heparin on anticoagulated patients.

The optimal frequency for on-going, long-term monitoring of INR will be affected by a multitude of factors: patient compliance, changes in comorbidities, medication changes, dietary changes, demonstration of stable dose-responses. Patients receiving a stable dose of OAT should have an INR level done at least every 4 weeks.

There is approximately a 3-day lag between changes made in OAT dosage and the corresponding INR value.

Timing of Monitoring

During OAT initiation, the prothrombin time (PT) draw for the INR should be done in the morning to monitor for excessive hypoprothrombinemia, and thereafter at the same time of the day, as PT values fluctuate (higher in the AM, lower in the PM).

Monitoring of international normalized ratio (INR) to assess anticoagulation status in patients with antiphospholipid syndrome (eg, presence of cardiolipin or lupus anticoagulant antibodies) who receive oral anticoagulant therapy (OAT)

Strength of Recommendation: Class I

Strength of Evidence: Category A

Results Interpretation:

Laboratory test finding

The general suggested therapeutic INR range for patients with antiphospholipid syndrome is 2.5 to 3.5.

For patients with antiphospholipid syndrome having appropriate response to warfarin and no additional risk factors, the suggested INR target is 2.5 with a range of 2 to 3.

For patients with antiphospholipid syndrome who have had recurrent thromboembolic events with therapeutic INR, or with other additional risks for thromboembolic events, the suggested INR target is 3 with a range of 2.5 to 3.5.

Because antiphospholipid antibodies may interfere with prothrombin time determinations, resulting in falsely-high INR levels, the College of American Pathologists recommends alternative tests to monitor those patients.

Monitoring of international normalized ratio (INR) to assess anticoagulation status in patients with inherited thrombophilia disorders (eg, deficiencies of antithrombin III, protein C or protein S, or presence of factor V Leiden mutation or prothrombin 20210) who receive oral anticoagulant therapy (OAT)
> **Strength of Recommendation:** Class I
> **Strength of Evidence:** Category A

Results Interpretation:

Laboratory test finding

The recommended INR target level is 2.5 with a range of 2 to 3 for long-term treatment of patients with first-episode deep vein thrombosis (DVT) associated with prothrombic genotype or a prognostic marker for an increased risk of recurrent thromboembolism (eg, deficiencies of antithrombin III, protein C or protein S), or with a prothrombotic gene mutation (eg, factor V Leiden or prothrombin 20210).

The use of low-intensity warfarin therapy (INR target range of 1.5 to 1.9) may reduce the risk of recurrent thrombosis by approximately 75%, while conventional-intensity warfarin therapy (INR target range 2 to 3) may reduce the risk by over 90%.

Extended long-term treatment for 2 years with low-intensity warfarin therapy (INR target range of 1.5 to 1.9) in patients with factor V Leiden or prothrombin 20210A gene mutations may result in a 6.4% absolute risk reduction in the annual incidence of recurrent venous thromboembolism (VTE).

Monitoring of international normalized ratio (INR) to assess anticoagulation status in patients with prosthetic heart valves who receive oral anticoagulant therapy (OAT)
> **Strength of Recommendation:** Class I
> **Strength of Evidence:** Category A

Results Interpretation:

Laboratory test finding

The seventh American College of Chest Physicians (ACCP) conference recommends that children with mechanical and biological prosthetic heart valves follow adult guidelines for INR levels.
- Mechanical valves:
  - St. Jude Medical® bileaflet valve in the aortic position: recommended INR target of 2.5 with a range of 2 to 3
  - CarboMedics® bileaflet valve, Medtronic Hall™ tilting disk valve in the aortic position with normal left atrium size and patient in sinus rhythm: recommended INR target of 2.5 with a range of 2 to 3
  - Tilting disk valves, bileaflet mechanical valves in the mitral position: recommended INR target of 3 with a range of 2.5 to 3.5
  - Patients with mechanical valves plus additional risk factors (eg, atrial fibrillation [AF], myocardial infarction, endocardial damage, left atrial enlargement, low ejection fraction): recommended INR target of 3 with a range of 2.5 to 3.5
  - Caged ball valves, caged disk valves: suggested INR target of 3 with a range of 2.5 to 3.5
- Bioprosthetic valves:
  - Bioprosthetic valves in the mitral position: recommended INR target of 2.5 with a range of 2 to 3, for the first 3 months after valve insertion
  - Bioprosthetic valves in the aortic position: suggested INR target of 2.5 with a range of 2 to 3, for the first 3 months after valve insertion
  - Bioprosthetic valves in patients with AF: recommended INR target of 2.5 with a range of 2 to 3, with long-term anticoagulant therapy

Patients with St. Jude valves in the mitral position have higher rates of thromboembolism at the same INR level compared to those with the valve in the aortic position.

Patients with INR levels above their therapeutic range are at increased risk for bleeding. Patients with bleeding events should be maintained at the lower end of their therapeutic INR range.

The risk of bleeding while on oral anticoagulant therapy (OAT) significantly increases with INR levels greater than 5.

Frequency of Monitoring

Prothrombin time monitoring for INR is generally performed daily until the patient reaches the appropriate therapeutic range and maintains that level for 2 consecutive days. It is then monitored 2 to 3 times per week for 1 to 2 weeks, and then less often (the frequency then depends on the stability of the levels). Elderly patients may need to be monitored more frequently as they may be more likely to have additional factors affecting INR stability.

Timing of Monitoring

Two measurements of INR, at least 24 hours apart, that are within the appropriate therapeutic range are required before stopping heparin on anticoagulated patients who also receive oral anticoagulant therapy (OAT).

COMMON PANELS
• Transplant panel

CLINICAL NOTES
The international normalized ratio (INR) was developed for use in patients with stable anticoagulation therapy. The mathematical foundation of the INR formula was designed only for such patients; it should not be used in patients with unstable anticoagulation therapy or in patients with other hemostasis problems.

Use of INR is not appropriate for monitoring patients during oral anticoagulant therapy (OAT) initiation, during discontinuation of OAT, or for patients with liver disease or vitamin K deficiency.

A variety of factors can affect INR levels, including changes in medications, diet or disease state. Any addition or discontinuation of medication or herbal supplements is an indication for additional INR levels to be checked.

The accuracy of INR can be affected by reagents of different sensitivities. Separate prothrombin time (PT) reagents have separate sensitivities to clotting factor deficiencies.

Point of care (POC) testing may be available to patients to perform their own INR testing (after appropriate instruction and monitoring).

COLLECTION/STORAGE INFORMATION
• Collect blood for prothrombin time (PT) in a blue-top sodium citrate tube.
• Draw the PT/INR last to avoid contamination with tissue thromboplastin, if multiple types of tube specimens are being collected at one blood draw.
• Draw 1 to 2 ml of blood first and discard before collecting the specimen, if only the PT/INR is being collected by venipuncture.
• Draw 10 to 15 ml of blood first and discard before collecting the specimen, if the PT/INR is being collected from an arterial or other indwelling line.
• Promptly invert the specimen tube 3 to 4 times after collection, to ensure adequate mixing of the blood with the sodium citrate anticoagulant.
• Avoid traumatic venipuncture as it may activate coagulation factors, leading to a shorter PT.
• Fill pediatric blood collection tubes at least 90% to ensure accurate results.
• Specimens are stable at room temperature for 2 hours or at 4°C for 4 hours.

LOINC CODES
• Code: 6301-6 (*Short Name* - INR PPP Qn)
• Code: 34714-6 (*Short Name* - INR Bld Qn)

Intrinsic factor antibody measurement

TEST DEFINITION
Measurement of intrinsic factor antibody type I (blocking) or type II (binding) to detect vitamin B_{12} deficiency

SYNONYMS
• Intrinsic factor antibody level
• Intrinsic factor blocking antibody measurement

REFERENCE RANGE
• Negative
  Please refer to your institution's reference ranges as lab normals may vary.

INDICATIONS
Suspected pernicious anemia
   Strength of Recommendation: Class IIa
   Strength of Evidence: Category C
   Results Interpretation:
   Autoantibody titer positive
   The presence of intrinsic factor antibody type II in patients with low serum vitamin B_{12} levels may indicate pernicious anemia with more accuracy than measuring type I antibodies alone.

Suspected vitamin B$_{12}$ (cobalamin) malabsorption and deficiency
    Strength of Recommendation: Class IIa
    Strength of Evidence: Category C
Results Interpretation:
Autoantibody titer positive
    The presence of serum IFAB may detect vitamin B$_{12}$ malabsorption and deficiency in patients with a normal serum vitamin B$_{12}$ level.

ABNORMAL RESULTS

- Present in:
    - Hyperthyroidism
    - Insulin-dependent diabetes

COLLECTION/STORAGE INFORMATION

- Patient preparation:
    - Avoid taking vitamin B$_{12}$ for 48 hours prior to blood draw
- Specimen Collection and Handling:
    - Collect serum or plasma in a lavender top (EDTA) tube
    - Specimen is stable for 4 hours at room temperature or for 3 days if refrigerated. For longer storage, freeze at -20° C

LOINC CODES

- Code: 31443-5 (*Short Name* - IF Block Ab Ser-aCnc)
- Code: 5233-2 (*Short Name* - IF Ab Ser QI RIA)
- Code: 2489-3 (*Short Name* - IF Block Ab Titr Ser)
- Code: 11564-2 (*Short Name* - IF Ab Ser-aCnc)
- Code: 31445-0 (*Short Name* - IF Block IgG Ser-aCnc)
- Code: 26892-0 (*Short Name* - IF Block IgG Ser RIA-aCnc)

Islet cell antibody measurement

TEST DEFINITION

Measurement of islet cell antibodies in serum for the evaluation and management of endocrine disorders

SYNONYMS

- ICA
- Islet cell cytoplasma antibody

REFERENCE RANGE

- Negative
    Please refer to your institution's reference ranges as lab normals may vary.

INDICATIONS

Suspected type 1 diabetes mellitus
    Strength of Recommendation: Class IIb
    Strength of Evidence: Category B
Results Interpretation:
Antibody development
    A positive result on islet cell antibody assays may predict type 1 diabetes mellitus, particularly in combination with low insulin and C-peptide levels.

COLLECTION/STORAGE INFORMATION

- Specimen Collection and Handling:
    - Collect serum in a marble topped tube.
    - Store serum at -20°C.

LOINC CODES

- Code: 5265-4 (*Short Name* - Panc Islet Cell Ab Ser Ql IF)
- Code: 31547-3 (*Short Name* - Panc Islet Cell Ab Ser Ql)
- Code: 13927-9 (*Short Name* - Panc Islet Cell Ab Titr Ser)
- Code: 8086-1 (*Short Name* - Panc Islet Cell Ab Ser-aCnc)

Isoleucine measurement

TEST DEFINITION

Measurement of isoleucine in plasma or serum for detection of acquired and hereditary amino acid disorders

REFERENCE RANGE

- Premature neonate, 1 day: 0.52 ± 0.26 mg/dL (40 ± 20 micromol/L)
- Neonate, 1 day: 0.35-0.69 mg/dL (27-53 micromol/L)
- Infants 1 to 3 months: 0.77 ± 0.18 mg/dL (59 ± 14 micromol/L)
- Infants 2 to 6 months: 0.50-1.61 mg/dL (38-123 micromol/L)
- Infants 9 to 24 months: 0.34-1.23 mg/dL (26-94 micromol/L)
- Children 3 to 10 years: 0.37-1.10 mg/dL (28-84 micromol/L)
- Children 6 to 18 years: 0.50-1.24 mg/dL (38-95 micromol/L)
- Adults: 0.48-1.28 mg/dL (37-98 micromol/L)

Please refer to your institution's reference ranges as lab normals may vary.

INDICATIONS

Suspected inborn error of metabolism

> **Strength of Recommendation:** Class IIa
> **Strength of Evidence:** Category C
> **Results Interpretation:**
> **Increased amino acid**

Inherited amino acid disorders are directly related to the absence of an enzyme involved in the metabolism of one or more amino acids; therefore, an elevated plasma level of a particular amino acid is highly suggestive of an inherited metabolic defect. In the majority of cases amino acid and organic acid analysis together permit diagnostic confirmation in infants. Immediate treatment should be initiated when an inborn error of metabolism is suspected, even if a definitive diagnosis has not yet been determined.

During acute attacks, maple syrup urine disease (MSUD) is associated with elevated blood levels of leucine, isoleucine, alloisoleucine, valine and related ketoacids.

COLLECTION/STORAGE INFORMATION

- Specimen Collection and Handling:
  - Immediately place sample in ice water.
  - Isolate plasma sample and freeze it within 1 hour; sample stable for 1 week at -20°C.
  - Sample should be deproteinized and stored at -70°C for protracted periods of usage.

LOINC CODES

- Code: 26730-2 (*Short Name* - Isoleucine Amn-sCnc)
- Code: 2510-6 (*Short Name* - Isoleucine 24H Ur-mRate)
- Code: 17029-0 (*Short Name* - Isoleucine Ur Ql)
- Code: 22659-7 (*Short Name* - Isoleucine CSF-sCnc)
- Code: 32252-9 (*Short Name* - Isoleucine Vitf-sCnc)
- Code: 26965-4 (*Short Name* - Isoleucine Ur-sCnc)
- Code: 9743-6 (*Short Name* - Isoleucine CSF-mCnc)
- Code: 2509-8 (*Short Name* - Isoleucine Ur-mCnc)
- Code: 32251-1 (*Short Name* - Isoleucine Fld-sCnc)
- Code: 25938-2 (*Short Name* - Isoleucine 24H Ur-sCnc)
- Code: 13402-3 (*Short Name* - Isoleucine Amn-mCnc)
- Code: 22714-0 (*Short Name* - Isoleucine XXX-sCnc)
- Code: 25450-8 (*Short Name* - Isoleucine 24H Ur-sRate)

Kleihauer-Betke test

TEST DEFINITION
Detection and quantitation of fetal cells in maternal circulation

SYNONYMS
- Fetal RBC determination
- Fetomaternal haemorrhage calculation, Kleihauer-Betke method
- Fetomaternal hemorrhage calculation, Kleihauer-Betke method
- Haemoglobin F cytochemical demonstration test
- Hemoglobin F cytochemical demonstration test

INDICATIONS
Prediction of pregnancy complications following maternal trauma
   Strength of Recommendation: Class IIb
   Strength of Evidence: Category B
   Results Interpretation:
   Kleihauer test abnormal
      While some findings suggest that a positive Kleihauer-Betke (KB) test may help predict pregnancy complications following maternal trauma, the studies that have been performed demonstrate highly variable accuracy, and the results of the test rarely affect clinical management. Routine use of the KB test is not indicated in an emergency department setting, although its use may be considered in cases of significant trauma when the mother is Rh-negative.

COLLECTION/STORAGE INFORMATION
- Specimen Collection and Handling:
   - Collect whole blood specimen in tube containing EDTA or heparin.
   - May store at 4°C for up to 10 days
   - Notify lab of suspected diagnosis.

LOINC CODES
- Code: 32140-6 (*Short Name* - Hgb F Bld Ql Kleih Betke)
- Code: 4633-4 (*Short Name* - Hgb F % Bld Kleih Betke)
- Code: 14276-0 (*Short Name* - Hgb F Dist Bld Kleih Betke-Imp)

Lactate dehydrogenase measurement, cerebrospinal fluid

TEST DEFINITION
Measurement of lactate dehydrogenase (LDH) in cerebrospinal fluid to evaluate acute brain cell damage

REFERENCE RANGE
- Adults: <20 units/L
- Neonates (full term):
- Ages 1-4 weeks: 50.48 +/- 6.04 units/L
- Ages 5-8 weeks: 35.46 +/- 5.45 units/L
   Please refer to your institution's reference ranges as lab normals may vary.

INDICATIONS
Suspected CNS involvement secondary to hematologic cancers
   Strength of Recommendation: Class IIa
   Strength of Evidence: Category B

Results Interpretation:
Abnormal cytological findings in CSF
CSF LDH isoenzyme measurement may be helpful in assessing hematologic cancer patients for CNS metastasis. LDH5 is present in CNS tumor tissue, and CSF isoenzyme evaluation may augment CSF cytology study findings.

Suspected Jakob-Creutzfeldt disease (JCD)
    Strength of Recommendation: Class IIa
    Strength of Evidence: Category B
Results Interpretation:
Abnormal cytological findings in CSF
Measuring CSF LDH and isoenzyme levels may help differentiate JCD from other causes of dementia.

CLINICAL NOTES
Reference ranges are highly method dependent.

COLLECTION/STORAGE INFORMATION
* Store specimen at room temperature

LOINC CODES
* Code: 2528-8 (*Short Name* - LDH CSF-cCnc)

Lactic acid measurement

TEST DEFINITION
Measurement of lactate (lactic acid) in whole blood or plasma for the evaluation of lactic acidosis

SYNONYMS
* Lactate measurement

REFERENCE RANGE
* Adults (plasma/venous): 5-15 mg/dL (0.6-1.7 mmol/L)
  Please refer to your institution's reference ranges as lab normals may vary.

INDICATIONS
Critical illness
    Strength of Recommendation: Class IIb
    Strength of Evidence: Category B
Results Interpretation:
Increased lactic acid level
Hyperlactatemia is defined as a persistent modest increase in blood lactate (2 to 5 mmol/L) without accompanying metabolic acidosis.

A lactate concentration from 5 to 6 mEq/L indicates severe lactic acidosis.

A lactate concentration less than 2 mEq/L can be considered normal in critically ill patients, and lactate concentrations of 2 to 5 mEq/L represent a gray area of questionable significance.

A number of studies have demonstrated an inverse relationship between hyperlactatemia and survival. Increased blood lactate concentrations are a prognostic indicator in ICU patients. Since lactate is an end product of glucose metabolism, it will be increased when aerobic metabolism changes to anaerobic metabolism. Increased circulating lactate concentrations may reflect a sicker population.

When tissue hypoperfusion is present, elevated lactate levels may predict a worsened prognosis. In critically ill patients, higher mortality rates have been reported with lactate levels ranging from greater than 2.5 mmol/L to 8 mmol/L.

In general, the prognosis is fairly good if the lactate level falls 5% to 10% within an hour of starting resuscitation.

Cyanide poisoning
    Strength of Recommendation: Class IIb
    Strength of Evidence: Category B

Results Interpretation:
Increased lactic acid level
   The results of a small retrospective chart review suggest that elevated lactate levels may be predictive of cyanide toxicity in the setting of known cyanide exposure. The specificity of an elevated lactate for cyanide poisoning may be higher in patients not receiving catecholamine infusions.

Hantavirus pulmonary syndrome
   Results Interpretation:
   Increased lactic acid level
   Metabolic acidosis with lactic acidemia and a decreased bicarbonate level are seen in severe hantavirus pulmonary syndrome (HPS).
   Prognosis is poorest in HPS patients with shock and severe lactic acidosis.
   Peak lactate levels greater than 4 mmol/L are associated with a fatal outcome in HPS.

HIV infection
   Strength of Recommendation: Class IIb
   Strength of Evidence: Category B
   Results Interpretation:
   Increased lactic acid level
   Elevated lactate levels may be found in a significant percentage of HIV patients and appear to be most strongly associated with stavudine use. In a few cases, symptomatic hyperlactatemia has resolved with stopping stavudine.

Reye's syndrome
   Results Interpretation:
   Increased lactic acid level
   An elevation ranging from 2 to 15 mEq/L may be noted in most patients with Reye's syndrome. There appears to be a direct correlation between the lactate level and the stage of coma.
   In critically ill patients, as well as hospitalized normotensive patients, a blood lactate concentration greater than 4 mmol/L may reflect a poor prognosis.

Suspected acute mesenteric ischemia
   Strength of Recommendation: Class IIa
   Strength of Evidence: Category B
   Results Interpretation:
   Increased lactic acid level
   Increased lactic acid levels may be a late finding in patients with established bowel infarction.
   In a retrospective series of 121 patients with mesenteric infarction, an elevated lactate level was the only significant predictor of mortality.
   Lab. test result normal
   Because lower sensitivities have been reported, a normal lactate concentration does not rule out acute mesenteric ischemia.

Suspected acute myocardial infarction
   Strength of Recommendation: Class IIb
   Strength of Evidence: Category B
   Results Interpretation:
   Increased lactic acid level
   An elevated venous lactate level appears to moderately sensitive, but poorly specific, for diagnosing acute myocardial infarction in patients with chest pain. In one study, the sensitivity was higher for lactate than for creatine kinase or cardiac troponin T. Elevated lactate levels may also be predictive of increased cardiac morbidity and mortality in patients with chest pain.

Suspected and known alcoholic ketoacidosis
   Strength of Recommendation: Class IIb
   Strength of Evidence: Category B
   Results Interpretation:
   Increased lactic acid level
   Lactic acid levels are increased in alcoholic ketoacidosis (AKA) with an increased lactate/pyruvate ratio due to the altered redox state. This may contribute to the metabolic acidosis but to a significantly lesser degree compared with beta hydroxybutyric acid and acetoacetic acid.

Most patients with AKA have minor or modest elevations of blood lactate (2 to 4 mmol/L). However, severe lactic acidosis may occur with serious concomitant illnesses, such as convulsive seizures, pneumonia with hypoxia, gastrointestinal bleeding, and thiamine deficiency.

Suspected fetal hypoxia
    Strength of Recommendation: Class IIa
    Strength of Evidence: Category B
    Results Interpretation:
    Increased lactic acid level
    Some data suggest that a fetal lactate measurement may be a better predictor of severe neonatal morbidity due to hypoxia than a fetal pH measurement.
    Clinical guidelines for fetal scalp blood pH and lactate (using Lactate Pro®):

Fetal scalp blood	pH	Lactate (mmol/L)
Normal	>7.25	<4.2
Pre-acidemia/pre-lactemia	7.20-7.25	4.2-4.8
Acidemia/lactemia	<7.20	>4.8

Suspected or known cardiogenic shock
    Results Interpretation:
    Increased lactic acid level
    Low central venous oxygen saturation levels in conjunction with high lactic acid levels are indicative of severe decompensated heart failure and patients with this presentation are likely to benefit from aggressive therapy. Ongoing monitoring is valuable in assessing response to therapeutic interventions.
    In cardiogenic or septic shock when cardiac output is high, lactic acid levels may be elevated. In primary lactic acidosis (eg, nitroprusside toxicity) patients may have elevated lactate levels in the absence of heart failure.

Suspected or known lactic acidosis
    Strength of Recommendation: Class IIa
    Strength of Evidence: Category B
    Results Interpretation:
    Increased lactic acid level
    A lactic acid level greater than 2 mEq/L supports a diagnosis of lactic acidosis.
    A lactate concentration less than 2 mEq/L can be considered normal in critically ill patients; lactate concentrations of 2 to 5 mEq/L are of indeterminate clinical significance. A lactate concentration of 5 to 6 mEq/L or greater indicates severe lactic acidosis.
    Blood lactate levels above 4 mEq/L and 4 mmol/L have been associated with a poorer prognosis. Blood lactate concentrations greater than 4 mmol/L are uncommon and require further evaluation; survival is unlikely in patients with levels above 25 mEq/L. In general, the prognosis improves if the lactate level falls 5% to 10% within an hour of starting resuscitation.
    Lactate production increases during cellular hypoxia and as a result of a primary abnormality in glycolysis. Lactacidemia is not a reliable indicator of tissue perfusion or oxygen debt because multiple mechanisms contribute to the lactate level including hypoxia, increased aerobic metabolism, endotoxins, and catecholamines.

ABNORMAL RESULTS
Values may be increased during exercise, hyperventilation, or after meals

CLINICAL NOTES
Arterial measurement of lactic acid has traditionally been regarded as superior to venous measurement as an indicator of systemic hypoperfusion although some data suggests that venous measurement may be an acceptable substitute.
    Blood collection tubes with sodium citrate as anticoagulant yield lower lactate concentrations than tubes utilizing heparin or EDTA. Plasma and serum samples yield higher lactate levels than the original whole blood.
    Results from handheld bedside blood lactate analyzers correlate well with central laboratory values, providing rapid data for the critical care setting.

COLLECTION/STORAGE INFORMATION

Patient should be at complete rest when blood sample is collected. Do not use a tourniquet. Patient should not clench hand when collecting specimen. Transport sample to lab immediately.

LOINC CODES

- Code: 2523-9 (*Short Name* - Lactate Prt-sCnc)
- Code: 29246-6 (*Short Name* - Lactate Fld-mCnc)
- Code: 30241-4 (*Short Name* - Lactate BldV-mCnc)
- Code: 27955-4 (*Short Name* - Lactate 2H p chal Bld-mCnc)
- Code: 27949-7 (*Short Name* - Lactate 4H p chal Bld-mCnc)
- Code: 27961-2 (*Short Name* - Lactate 3H p chal Bld-mCnc)
- Code: 2526-2 (*Short Name* - Lactate 24H Ur-mRate)
- Code: 27946-3 (*Short Name* - Lactate 1H p chal Bld-mCnc)
- Code: 2525-4 (*Short Name* - Lactate Snv-sCnc)
- Code: 2519-7 (*Short Name* - Lactate BldV-sCnc)
- Code: 27976-0 (*Short Name* - Lactate p fast Bld-mCnc)
- Code: 19240-1 (*Short Name* - Lactate BldMV-sCnc)
- Code: 15078-9 (*Short Name* - Lactate 24H Ur-sRate)
- Code: 19239-3 (*Short Name* - Lactate BldC-sCnc)
- Code: 14165-5 (*Short Name* - Lactate Fld-sCnc)

Lactose tolerance test

TEST DEFINITION

Measurement of fasting blood glucose levels after an oral lactose load to determine lactose absorption.

SYNONYMS

- Lactose challenge test
- LTT - Lactose tolerance test

REFERENCE RANGE

- Adults and Children: Rise in blood glucose levels of >20-30 mg/dL (1.1-1.7 mmol/L) above fasting level
  Please refer to your institution's reference ranges as lab normals may vary.

INDICATIONS

Suspected lactose intolerance
>   **Strength of Recommendation:** Class IIb
>   **Strength of Evidence:** Category C
>   **Results Interpretation:**
>   **Abnormal laboratory findings**
>   A rise in blood glucose level of less than 20 to 30 mg/dL (1.1 to 1.7 mmol/L) above the fasting level following lactose ingestion in patients with intestinal symptoms indicates lactose intolerance.
>
>   **False Results**
>   In a study of 20 patients with irritable bowel syndrome comparing the efficacy of the lactose tolerance test with the hydrogen breath test, three false-positives occurred using the lactose tolerance test.
>   Delayed gastric emptying can cause false positive results of 23% to 30%.
>   **Frequency of Monitoring**
>   In patient with a negative test, the test should be repeated within two days, with the most normal results used for interpretation.

Contraindications

Large lactose loads may be dangerous in lactose intolerant infants and very young children due to diarrhea and resulting dehydration.

LOINC CODES

- Code: 1582-6 (*Short Name* - Lactose 1H p 50 g Lac PO Ser-mCnc)
- Code: 1583-4 (*Short Name* - Lactose 2H p 50 g Lac PO Ser-mCnc)

- Code: 19249-2 (*Short Name* - Lactose 3H p 50 g Lac PO Ser-mCnc)

Lead measurement, quantitative, blood

Test Definition
Measurement of blood lead level for diagnosing lead poisoning or monitoring for lead exposure.

Reference Range
- Adults: Less than 10-20 mcg/dL (less than 0.5-1 micromol/L)
- Children: Less than 10 mcg/dL; however, no threshold level has been determined to be safe
  Please refer to your institution's reference ranges as lab normals may vary.

Indications
Suspected chronic renal disease in chronic lead poisoning
> **Strength of Recommendation:** Class IIb
> **Strength of Evidence:** Category C
> **Results Interpretation:**
> **Increased lead level**
> A serum lead level of 2.5 mg/dL or greater may help to identify persons at risk for chronic lead exposure and warrant further clinical evaluation and testing.

Suspected lead poisoning
> **Strength of Recommendation:** Class I
> **Strength of Evidence:** Category C
> **Results Interpretation:**
> **Increased lead level**
> A blood lead level (BLL) of 10 mcg/dL or higher in children is considered an elevated level by the Centers for Disease Control (CDC).
> - The American Academy of Pediatrics recommends the following clinical management for elevated BLLs in children
>   - 10 to 14 mcg/dL: Obtain a confirmatory venous BLL in 1 month; if still elevated, provide education to decrease lead exposure; repeat BLL in 3 months
>   - 15 to 19 mcg/dL: Obtain a confirmatory venous BLL in 1 month; if still elevated, conduct a thorough environmental history and provide education; repeat BLL within 2 months
>   - 20 to 44 mcg/dL: Obtain a confirmatory venous BLL within 1 week; conduct a complete medical history and physical exam. If BLL greater than 25 mcg/dL, consider chelation and consult a clinical expert
>   - 45 to 69 mcg/dL: Obtain a confirmatory venous BLL within 2 days; begin chelation therapy after consultation with a clinical expert
>   - 70 mcg/dL or higher: Hospitalize and begin immediate chelation therapy; consult with a toxicologist.
> Although no threshold for the toxic effects of lead has been identified, the effects of lead exposure on cognition in young children at BLLs of greater than 10 mcg/dL have been well defined. It has been estimated that the effects of lead exposure result in a 2- to 3-point decline in IQ with BLLs of 20 mcg/dL, as compared with BLLs of 10 mcg/dL.
> For adults in an occupational setting, OSHA (Occupational Health and Safety Administration) recommends that an individual with a BLL of 50 mcg/dL be removed from the workplace. A BLL of 20 mcg/dL or higher in an adult suggests that lead exposure is present, and the source should be determined.
> Ingestion of a lead-containing foreign body generally does not produce lead toxicity unless it is not eliminated within 2 weeks of the ingestion; however, acute elevations of BLL (up to 89 mcg/dL 48 hours post ingestion) have occurred, especially when the foreign body remained in the stomach.

Suspected lead poisoning in iron-deficient children
> **Strength of Recommendation:** Class IIa
> **Strength of Evidence:** Category B
> **Results Interpretation:**
> **Increased blood lead level**
> A blood level level of 10 mcg/dL or higher may be associated with both decreased dietary iron and decreased baseline iron stores in young children.

COLLECTION/STORAGE INFORMATION
- Specimen Collection and Handling:
    - Collect blood sample via venipuncture (preferred) or fingerstick
    - Collect specimen in metal-free container; avoid contamination by environmental lead
    - Refrigerate blood sample

LOINC CODES
- Code: 14807-2 (*Short Name* - Lead Bld-sCnc)
- Code: 32325-3 (*Short Name* - Lead RBC-sCnc)
- Code: 10368-9 (*Short Name* - Lead BldC-mCnc)
- Code: 10912-4 (*Short Name* - Lead SerPl-mCnc)

Lead mobilization test

TEST DEFINITION
Measurement of lead in urine for evaluation and management of suspected lead poisoning

REFERENCE RANGE
- Index value: <1 (ratio of mcg of lead excreted to mg of edetate calcium disodium given)
  Please refer to your institution's reference ranges as lab normals may vary.

INDICATIONS
Suspected lead poisoning
   Strength of Recommendation: Class IIa
   Strength of Evidence: Category B
   Results Interpretation:
   Increased lead level
   The outcome of the lead mobilization test (LMT) is ascertained by the amount of lead (Pb) excreted per dose of calcium disodium ($CaNa_2$) EDTA.
   A lead excretion ratio of greater than 1 micromoles of urinary Pb excretion to millimoles of $CaNa_2$ EDTA administered corresponds to a cutoff value for 24-hour unstimulated urinary Pb excretion of 10.4 mcg.
   An 8-hour LMT is considered positive if the Pb urinary excretion ratio is more than 0.6, although some consider 0.5 as the cutoff point.
   An LMT result of greater than 1.5 mcg Pb/mg $CaNa_2$ EDTA administered or an LMT total urinary Pb excretion of greater than 200 mcg indicates that chelation therapy should be initiated.
   Urine collection is finished when 24-hour creatinine clearance is at least 90 mL/min/1.73 m^2.
   An LMT confirms Pb poisoning but should not be used in children with blood Pb levels greater than 55 mcg/dL.

ABNORMAL RESULTS
- Decreased results:
    - Low iron levels
    - Renal disorders
- Increased results:
    - Repeated lead mobilization tests in patients with normal lead levels

CLINICAL NOTES
   Lead mobilization test is primarily used for asymptomatic patients and not in children with blood lead levels greater than 55 micrograms/dL.

COLLECTION/STORAGE INFORMATION
- Begin 24 hour urine collection after drug dose.
- Collect at least 100 mL of urine for accurate test results.

LOINC CODES
- Code: 1586-7 (*Short Name* - Lead p EDTA Ur-mCnc)

Lead screening, urine

TEST DEFINITION
Measurement of lead levels in urine for the evaluation and management of lead poisoning

REFERENCE RANGE
- Adults and Children: <80 mcg/L (<0.39 micromol/L)
- Occupational exposure: <120 mcg/L (<0.58 micromol/L)
  Please refer to your institution's reference ranges as lab normals may vary.

INDICATIONS
Suspected lead poisoning
> **Strength of Recommendation:** Class IIb
> **Strength of Evidence:** Category C
> **Results Interpretation:**
> **Increased lead level**
>> A urine lead level greater than 80 mcg/L indicates lead poisoning, except for those with occupational exposure for whom the normal range cutoff is 120 mcg/L. A mobilization test is often used as a confirmation test for lead poisoning.

COMMON PANELS
- Heavy metal screen, urine

CLINICAL NOTES
A 24-hour urine is preferred, but the test may be run on a random urine collection of at least 100 mL in an emergency situation.

COLLECTION/STORAGE INFORMATION
- Collect a 24-hour urine in a lead-free container that has been washed with nitric acid.
- Refrigerate specimen during and after 24-hour urine collection.
- Urine should be voided directly into collection bottle, not obtained from catheter or measuring devices.
- Specimen remains stable for 1 week at 4°C.

Legionella antibody assay

TEST DEFINITION
Serologic test for detection of antibody against *Legionella pneumophila*

SYNONYMS
- Serologic test for Legionella

REFERENCE RANGE
- IgM titer: ≤1:64
- Combined IgG/IgA/Igm titer: <1:128 (<4-fold increase in antibody titer)
  Please refer to your institution's reference ranges as lab normals may vary.

INDICATIONS
Suspected legionellosis
> **Strength of Recommendation:** Class IIb
> **Strength of Evidence:** Category B
> **Results Interpretation:**
> **Legionella antibody positive**
>> A 4-fold increase in *Legionella pneumophila* antibody titer suggests legionellosis. A single acute titer has no diagnostic meaning due to the prevalence of antibodies in the general public.

False Results
- False positives may occur with:
- *Yersinia pestis*
- *Francisella tularensis*
- *Bacteroides fragilis*
- *Mycoplasma pneumoniae*
- *Leptospira interrogans*
- Campylobacter serotypes

Frequency of Monitoring

An acute serum sample should be collected at onset of disease and a convalescent sample 4 to 6 weeks later.

CLINICAL NOTES

Serologic tests for *Legionella* infection are most useful for epidemiologic purposes because results do not isolate an organism nor are they available within a clinically useful time frame. In addition, there is a 20% seroconversion failure rate. In most cases, the best diagnostic combination consists of urinary antigen testing plus sputum culture.

COLLECTION/STORAGE INFORMATION

- Collect specimen in marble top (tiger top) tube

LOINC CODES

- Code: 30143-2 (*Short Name* - Legionella Ab #1 Ser QI)
- Code: 30144-0 (*Short Name* - Legionella Ab sp2 Ser QI)
- Code: 26633-8 (*Short Name* - L bozemaniae Ab Ser QI)
- Code: 7957-4 (*Short Name* - Legionella Ab Ser-aCnc)
- Code: 22399-0 (*Short Name* - Legionella Ab Titr Ser)
- Code: 26628-8 (*Short Name* - Legionella Polyval B Ab Ser QI)
- Code: 26629-6 (*Short Name* - Legionella Polyval C Ab Ser QI)
- Code: 26635-3 (*Short Name* - L micdadei Ab Ser QI)
- Code: 26632-0 (*Short Name* - L dumoffii Ab Ser QI)
- Code: 26627-0 (*Short Name* - Legionella Polyval A Ab Ser QI)
- Code: 6450-1 (*Short Name* - Legionella Ab Titr Ser IF)

Legionella immunofluorescence

TEST DEFINITION

Detection of *Legionella* species in respiratory tract secretions

REFERENCE RANGE

- Adults and Children: Negative

Please refer to your institution's reference ranges as lab normals may vary.

INDICATIONS

Suspected Legionnaire disease (legionellosis)

Strength of Recommendation: Class IIb

Strength of Evidence: Category B

Results Interpretation:

Legionella antibody positive

Presence of 1 or more fluorescent organisms on a minimum of 3 smear, or a minimum of 5 organisms on a single smear, is diagnostic of *Legionella pneumophila*.

CLINICAL NOTES

Sputum provides the optimum specimen for examination by direct fluorescent antibody (DFA) stain.

Monoclonal antibody DFA reagent is superior in accuracy to polyclonal reagents, due to the monoclonal reagent's ability to minimize background fluorescence. Additionally, monoclonal reagents suppress false-positive results arising from cross-reactivity with non-Legionella organisms.

Legionella species culture

TEST DEFINITION
Culture of body fluids and tissue for the isolation and identification of *Legionella pneumophila*

REFERENCE RANGE
• Negative culture (no growth)
  Please refer to your institution's reference ranges as lab normals may vary.

INDICATIONS
Suspected atypical pneumonia
    Strength of Recommendation: Class IIb
    Strength of Evidence: Category B
    Results Interpretation:
    Positive microbiology findings
        A positive sputum culture test (the presence of *Legionella* colonies) is diagnostic of *Legionella* pneumonia.
        A negative culture does not rule out the diagnosis of *Legionella* pneumonia, due to the low sensitivity of present culture methodology. The testing combination of respiratory tract secretion culture in conjunction with either urine antigen or direct fluorescent antibody testing is recommended for the majority of atypical pneumonia cases suspected of arising from *Legionella pneumophila* infection.
    Timing of Monitoring
        Isolate samples should be obtained prior to initiating antimicrobial therapy.

Suspected Legionnaire's disease
    Strength of Recommendation: Class IIa
    Strength of Evidence: Category B
    Results Interpretation:
    Positive microbiology findings
        A positive culture test (the presence of *Legionella* colonies) is diagnostic of Legionnaire's disease.
        A negative culture does not rule out the diagnosis of Legionnaire's disease, due to the low sensitivity of present culture methodology. The testing combination of respiratory tract secretion culture in conjunction with either urine antigen or direct fluorescent antibody testing is recommended for the majority of suspected cases of *Legionella pneumophila* infection.
    Timing of Monitoring
        Isolate samples should be obtained prior to initiating antimicrobial therapy.

CLINICAL NOTES
Lower respiratory tract secretions (bronchoscopy-obtained or expectorated) are the preferred samples for *Legionella* culture, and bronchoscopic samples are more likely produce a diagnostic yield of *Legionella* compared with expectorated secretions. *Legionella* colony growth generally requires 3 to 5 days of incubation

The relatively low sensitivity of *Legionella* species culture mandates concurrent testing with the direct fluorescent antibody assay (DFA) in order to maximize diagnostic yield; a negative culture cannot rule out a diagnosis of *Legionella* infection.

COLLECTION/STORAGE INFORMATION
• Specimen Collection and Handling:
    • Store all body fluid samples at 4°C, tissue samples at −20°C
    • Attempt to isolate organisms during acute phase of disease

LOINC CODES
• Code: 589-2 (*Short Name* - Legionella Bro Cult)

Legionella urine antigen

TEST DEFINITION
Detection of *Legionella* species antigen in urine

SYNONYMS
- Legionella antigen assay, urine

REFERENCE RANGE
- Negative
  Please refer to your institution's reference ranges as lab normals may vary.

INDICATIONS
Suspected *Legionella* **infection**
> **Strength of Recommendation:** Class IIa
> **Strength of Evidence:** Category B
> **Results Interpretation:**
> **Positive laboratory findings**
>> A positive antigen test is diagnostic for *Legionella pneumophila* infection and appears to be moderately sensitive. The test is a useful screening tool for investigating outbreaks of Legionnaire disease.
>> Diagnostic tests for *Legionella* either lack sensitivity for detecting all clinically important *Legionella* species or are unable to provide results within a clinically useful time frame. In most cases, the best diagnostic combination is the use of both the urinary antigen test and sputum culture. Urinary antigen detection provides an early diagnosis (within 15 minutes with an immunochromatographic assay) and is particularly valuable in areas where *L pneumophila* serogroup 1 is the most common cause of the disease.
>> The utility of urinary antigen testing for *Legionella* infection declines in direct proportion to the prevalence of *L pneumophila* serotype 1.
>> Antigenuria may persist for a prolonged period following acute infection.
>> Urinary antigen testing may be more sensitive for *Legionella pneumophila* arising from travel-associated and community-acquired sources compared with nosocomial infections, although there is conflicting data regarding this distinction.

LOINC CODES
- Code: 32781-7 (*Short Name* - Legionella Ag Ur Ql)

Leishmaniasis screening

TEST DEFINITION
Detection of *Leishmania* antigens and antibodies for the diagnosis of leishmaniasis

REFERENCE RANGE
- Negative
  Please refer to your institution's reference ranges as lab normals may vary.

INDICATIONS
Suspected cutaneous and mucocutaneous leishmaniasis
> **Strength of Recommendation:** Class IIb
> **Strength of Evidence:** Category B
> **Results Interpretation:**
> **Serology positive**
>> A positive serology test for leishmaniasis in patients with the appropriate clinical presentation suggests cutaneous leishmaniasis (CL).
>> A positive serology result should be confirmed by identification of the parasite.
>> Antibody titers may be low or undetectable in CL, thus a negative test does not rule out disease.
>> Mucocutaneous leishmaniasis is a metastatic complication of New World cutaneous leishmaniasis, and serological tests are more likely to be positive than for cutaneous leishmaniasis.

> **False Results**
>> The presence of trypanosomal disease may cause a false positive serology result for leishmaniasis.

Suspected visceral leishmaniasis
> **Strength of Recommendation:** Class IIb
> **Strength of Evidence:** Category B

Results Interpretation:
Serology positive
A positive serology test for leishmaniasis in conjunction with the appropriate clinical presentation is presumptive evidence for a diagnosis of visceral leishmaniasis. However, a positive test does not distinguish between active and past infection.

A positive serology result should be confirmed by identification of the parasite in tissue or fluid.

High levels of antileishmanial antibodies may be found during the acute illness and for years thereafter.

Antibody titers to *Leishmania donovani* greater than or equal to 1:8 are considered positive for kala-azar (visceral leishmaniasis).

False Results
The presence of trypanosomal disease may cause a false positive antibody titers to *Leishmania donovani*.

If HIV infection preceded the diagnosis of visceral leishmaniasis, antibodies to *Leishmania donovani* may not be detectable

CLINICAL NOTES
Leishmaniasis serology is used to screen for *Leishmania* infection. Definitive diagnosis is made by demonstrating the parasite in body fluids and tissues.

COLLECTION/STORAGE INFORMATION
• Specimen Collection and Handling:
  • Collect in serum separator tube; if any delay, freeze specimen.
  • Test is generally available in specialized laboratories only.

Leptospira antibody assay

TEST DEFINITION
Measurement of antibodies in serum for evaluation of leptospirosis

SYNONYMS
• Serologic test for Leptospira

REFERENCE RANGE
• Negative
Please refer to your institution's reference ranges as lab normals may vary.

INDICATIONS
Suspected leptospirosis
  Strength of Recommendation: Class IIa
  Strength of Evidence: Category C
  Results Interpretation:
  Parasite antibody titer - finding
  Febrile illness and a single elevated titer suggest acute leptospirotic infection. Although the Centers for Disease Control defines a titer of greater than or equal to 200 as probable leptospirosis, titer level is dependent on level of exposure and seroprevalence. In areas where leptospirosis is endemic, a single titer of greater than or equal to 800 with correlating symptoms is indicative of leptospirosis. A fourfold or greater rise in titer between paired sera and correlating clinical presentation, regardless of the interval between samples, confirms the diagnosis of leptospirosis.

  Antibodies appear within 5 to 7 days after symptom onset in leptospirosis and are detectable for many months. Leptospiral IgM is detectable approximately five days from onset of symptoms using the most sensitive methods available.

  Titers rise in the second or third week of illness and may be extremely high (greater than or equal to 25,000). Levels may take months or years to fall to low levels.

  In patients with previous leptospirosis infection, the initial rise in antibody titer is often in response to the infecting serovar from the prior exposure. Identifying the serovar or serogroup responsible for the present infection evolves over time as the titer or specific antibody rises.

Timing of Monitoring

Serum sample for leptospira antibody levels should be drawn at onset of illness and again 2 to 3 weeks later (antibody titers increase in the second to third week of illness).

CLINICAL NOTES

The microscopic agglutination test (MAT) is the gold standard serodiagnostic method for leptospirosis, but is inherently complex, limiting its use to experienced laboratory personnel. Other disadvantages include high cost, maintenance of live strains of serovars, and the requirement of paired serum samples that may delay diagnosis. Results are interpreted subjectively and there may be difficulty ensuring standardization between laboratories.

The MAT can be applied to sera from any animal species, and the range of antigens used can be increased or decreased as needed. However, identification of infecting serovars with MAT cannot be done without isolates, offering only a general impression of the serogroups present within a population.

Enzyme-linked immunosorbent assay (ELISA) may be more sensitive for detection of IgM antibodies than agglutinating antibodies.

COLLECTION/STORAGE INFORMATION

• Draw serum blood sample in red-topped tube.

LOINC CODES

• Code: 23168-8 (*Short Name* - L borgp Ball Ab Ser Ql Aggl)
• Code: 27093-4 (*Short Name* - Leptospira IgG CSF EIA-aCnc)
• Code: 23199-3 (*Short Name* - Leptospira IgG Ser Ql EIA)
• Code: 23167-0 (*Short Name* - L borgp Ball Ab Ser Ql)
• Code: 31485-6 (*Short Name* - Leptospira IgG Ser-aCnc)
• Code: 23193-6 (*Short Name* - L borgp Sej Ab Ser Ql)
• Code: 23194-4 (*Short Name* - L borgp Sej Ab Ser Ql Aggl)
• Code: 23200-9 (*Short Name* - Leptospira IgG Ser Ql)
• Code: 23197-7 (*Short Name* - Leptospira Ab Ser Ql Aggl)
• Code: 23198-5 (*Short Name* - Leptospira Ab Titr Ser Aggl)
• Code: 23196-9 (*Short Name* - Leptospira Ab Ser Ql)
• Code: 31483-1 (*Short Name* - Leptospira Ab Ser-aCnc)
• Code: 25866-5 (*Short Name* - L borgp Sej Ab Titr Ser)
• Code: 31484-9 (*Short Name* - Leptospira IgG CSF-aCnc)
• Code: 5239-9 (*Short Name* - Leptospira Ab Titr Ser LA)
• Code: 25940-8 (*Short Name* - L borgp Sej Ab Titr Ser CF)
• Code: 31476-5 (*Short Name* - L borgp Sej Ab Ser-aCnc)
• Code: 23195-1 (*Short Name* - Leptospira Ab Ser Ql EIA)
• Code: 7959-0 (*Short Name* - Leptospira Ab Titr Ser)

Leptospira species culture, Blood, Urine, Cerebrospinal fluid

TEST DEFINITION

Culture of *Leptospira* species from blood, urine, and cerebrospinal fluid to facilitate diagnosis and treatment of leptospirosis

REFERENCE RANGE

• Normal results: negative culture
Please refer to your institution's reference ranges as lab normals may vary.

INDICATIONS

Suspected leptospirosis

        Strength of Recommendation: Class IIb
        Strength of Evidence: Category C

Results Interpretation:
Abnormal laboratory findings

A positive culture strongly supports the diagnosis of leptospirosis. However, because *Leptospira* are fastidious, culture is time consuming, technically challenging, and relatively insensitive. Advances in serologic and molecular diagnostic techniques are enabling earlier diagnosis and treatment.

CLINICAL NOTES

Success of blood culture is dependent on successful isolation of *Leptospira* during the acute bacteremic phase of infection. After the first week of infection, cultures from urine, and possibly cerebrospinal fluid, may support growth.

COLLECTION/STORAGE INFORMATION

- Incubate aerobic culture at 28°C to 30°C, in dark, up to 4 months.
- Maintain culture pH between 7.2 and 7.6.
- Examine weekly, by dark field microscopy, for evidence of growth.
- Addition of 5-fluorouracil, or other antibiotics, to media may suppress growth of microbial contaminants.

LOINC CODES

- Code: 6455-0 (*Short Name* - Leptospira Ur Cult)
- Code: 20869-4 (*Short Name* - Leptospira Tiss Ql Cult)
- Code: 594-2 (*Short Name* - Leptospira XXX Cult)
- Code: 6453-5 (*Short Name* - Leptospira Bld Cult)
- Code: 6454-3 (*Short Name* - Leptospira CSF Cult)
- Code: 23599-4 (*Short Name* - Leptospira Tiss Cult)

Leucine measurement

TEST DEFINITION

Measurement of leucine in plasma or serum for detection of acquired and hereditary amino acid disorders

SYNONYMS

- Leucine level

REFERENCE RANGE

- Premature neonate, 1 day: 0.92 ± 0.33 mg/dL (70 ± 25 micromol/L)
- Neonate, 1 day: 0.62-1.43 mg/dL (47-109 micromol/L)
- Infants 1 to 3 months: 1.36 ± 0.39 mg/dL (104 ± 30 micromol/L)
- Infants 9 to 24 months: 0.59-2.03 mg/dL (45-155 micromol/L)
- Children 3 to 10 years: 0.73-2.33 mg/dL (56-178 micromol/L)
- Children 6 to 18 years: 1.03-2.28 mg/dL (79-174 micromol/L)
- Adults: 0.98-2.29 mg/dL (75-175 micromol/L)
  Please refer to your institution's reference ranges as lab normals may vary.

INDICATIONS

Suspected inborn error of metabolism
> **Strength of Recommendation:** Class IIa
> **Strength of Evidence:** Category C
Results Interpretation:
Increased amino acid

A blood leucine measurement of 4 mg/dL (300 micromol/L) or greater in a newborn necessitates an urgent clinical examination. If any signs or symptoms of encephalopathy are present, a further workup and immediate cessation of all protein intake is required.

Inherited amino acid disorders are directly related to the absence of an enzyme involved in the metabolism of one or more amino acids; therefore, an elevated plasma level of a particular amino acid is highly suggestive of an inherited metabolic defect. In the majority of cases amino acid and organic acid analysis together permit diagnostic confirmation in infants. Immediate treatment should be initiated when an inborn error of metabolism is suspected, even if a definitive diagnosis has not yet been determined.

During acute attacks, maple syrup urine disease (MSUD) is associated with elevated blood levels of leucine, isoleucine, alloisoleucine, valine and related ketoacids. A confirmatory diagnosis of MSUD requires a finding of deficient enzyme activity of the branched-chain alpha-ketoacid dehydrogenase in cultured fibroblasts or lymphoblasts.

COLLECTION/STORAGE INFORMATION
- Specimen Collection and Handling:
  - Immediately place sample in ice water.
  - Isolate plasma sample and freeze it within 1 hour; sample stable for 1 week at -20°C.
  - Sample should be deproteinized and stored at -70°C for protracted periods of usage.

LOINC CODES
- Code: 9412-8 (*Short Name* - Leucine CSF-sCnc)
- Code: 2561-9 (*Short Name* - Leucine Ur-mCnc)
- Code: 25941-6 (*Short Name* - Leucine 24H Ur-sCnc)
- Code: 2562-7 (*Short Name* - Leucine 24H Ur-mRate)
- Code: 13768-7 (*Short Name* - Leucine/creat Ur-mRto)
- Code: 22693-6 (*Short Name* - Leucine/creat Ur-sRto)
- Code: 29293-8 (*Short Name* - Leucine Bld-mCnc)
- Code: 26710-4 (*Short Name* - Leucine Amn-sCnc)
- Code: 32254-5 (*Short Name* - Leucine Fld-sCnc)
- Code: 30053-3 (*Short Name* - Leucine/creat Ur-Rto)
- Code: 25460-7 (*Short Name* - Leucine 24H Ur-sRate)
- Code: 22719-9 (*Short Name* - Leucine XXX-sCnc)
- Code: 27323-5 (*Short Name* - Leucine Ur-sCnc)
- Code: 32253-7 (*Short Name* - Leucine Vitf-sCnc)
- Code: 25942-4 (*Short Name* - Leucine/creat 24H Ur-sRto)
- Code: 29284-7 (*Short Name* - Leucine Bld QI)
- Code: 13403-1 (*Short Name* - Leucine Amn-mCnc)

Lipoprotein-associated phospholipase A2 measurement

TEST DEFINITION
Measurement of lipoprotein-associated phospholipase A_2 in plasma for predicting a cardiac event or stroke

SYNONYMS
- Lp-PLA2 measurement

REFERENCE RANGE
Reference range data is laboratory-dependent
Please refer to your institution's reference ranges as lab normals may vary.

INDICATIONS
To assess risk of cerebrovascular accident
    Strength of Recommendation: Class IIa
    Strength of Evidence: Category B
    Results Interpretation:
    Increased level (laboratory finding)
        Elevated lipoprotein-associated phospholipase A_2 (Lp-PLA$_2$) is associated with an increased risk for stroke.

To assess risk of coronary artery disease
    Strength of Recommendation: Class IIa
    Strength of Evidence: Category B

Results Interpretation:
Increased level (laboratory finding)
   Elevated lipoprotein-associated phospholipase A$_2$ (Lp-PLA$_2$) is a strong indicator for increased risk of a coronary event.
   Lp-PLA$_2$ activity was higher in men than in women.
   Lipoprotein-associated phospholipase A$_2$ is not used as a stand-alone test for predicting coronary artery disease; rather, results must be interpreted in light of other tests, specifically CRP and the low density lipoprotein (LDL) cholesterol test per recommendation of the Food and Drug Administration (FDA) 2003.

CLINICAL NOTES
   Lp-PLA$_2$ as a marker for coronary heart disease, has been found to be independent of age, diastolic blood pressure, diabetes, smoking, and C-reactive protein (CRP); it is an independent predictor of coronary heart disease.

COLLECTION/STORAGE INFORMATION
- Specimen Collection and Handling:
  - Collect a non-fasting venous blood sample.
  - Store at -70°C until analysis.

Low density lipoprotein measurement

TEST DEFINITION
   Measurement of low-density lipoprotein cholesterol (LDL) in serum or plasma for the assessment and management of coronary heart disease and dyslipidemia

REFERENCE RANGE
- Adults, optimal level: <100 mg/dL (<2.59 mmol/L)
- Adults, near or above normal: 100-129 mg/dL (2.59-3.34 mmol/L)
- Adults, borderline high: 130-159 mg/dL (3.36-4.11 mmol/L)
- Adults, high: 160-189 mg/dL (4.13-4.88 mmol/L)
- Adults, very high: ≥190 mg/dL (≥4.91 mmol/L)
  Please refer to your institution's reference ranges as lab normals may vary.

INDICATIONS
Screening and prevention of coronary heart disease
   Strength of Recommendation: Class I
   Strength of Evidence: Category A
   Results Interpretation:
   Increased LDL level
   An LDL level under 100 mg/dL is considered optimal. LDL levels between 100 and 129 mg/dL are considered near optimal. LDL levels between 130 and 159 mg/dL are considered borderline high and are suggestive of hyperlipidemia. LDL levels between 160 and 189 mg/dL are considered high and levels exceeding 189 mg/dL are considered very high. All levels above 100 mg/dL suggest atherogenesis, particularly in the presence of multiple risk factors. LDL levels of 160 mg/dL or greater cause rapid progression of atherosclerosis, and can lead to premature CHD when other risk factors are present. Premature CHD can occur in those with levels above 190 mg/dL, irrespective of whether or not other risk factors are present.
   Management goals for patients with elevated LDL levels are based on the patient's level of risk for CHD. In persons who are at increased risk of CHD due to multiple risk factors, the LDL goal should be less than 130 mg/dL and therapeutic lifestyle changes should be initiated. Other researchers have suggested that a goal of less than 100 mg/dL is a reasonable alternative based on more current research. Persons with multiple risk factors whose 10-year risk is less than 10% (low to moderate) should not receive LDL-lowering drugs if their LDL level is borderline (130 to 150 mg/dL), although drug therapy should be considered when LDL levels are 160 mg/dL or higher. For persons with a higher 10-year risk (10% to 20%), LDL-lowering drugs should be considered when an LDL of less than 130 mg/dL cannot be obtained by lifestyle changes alone. Those at highest risk (10-year risk greater than 20%) should strive to attain an even lower LDL of less than 100 mg/dL, while a goal of less than 70 mg/dL has been proposed as an alternative therapeutic option. Consideration should be given to simultaneous drug therapy and therapeutic lifestyle changes when LDL levels are 130 mg/dL or higher.

For those at low risk (0 to 1 risk factor), the LDL goal is less than 160 mg/dL and therapeutic lifestyle changes should be emphasized when LDL is 130 mg/dL to 159 mg/dL. Drug therapy is generally not recommended in these individuals, but should be considered when lifestyle changes cannot reduce the LDL to less than 160 mg/dL, and is strongly recommended with LDL levels of 190 mg/dL or higher.

Therapeutic lifestyle changes are recommended for young adults (20 years or older) with LDL cholesterol between 100 and 120 mg/dL. Clinical monitoring and oversight of lifestyle changes is recommended when LDL is borderline high (130 to 150 mg/dL) or high (160 to 189 mg/dL). LDL-lowering therapy should be considered in those with high LDL levels that do not respond to therapeutic lifestyle interventions, particularly when LDL is 190 mg/dL or higher.

Lowering LDL should be the primary target of cholesterol-lowering therapy. Recommendations published subsequent to the National Cholesterol Education Program (NCEP) Expert Panel guidelines recommend that drug therapy lower LDL levels by a minimum of 30% to 40% in moderately high-risk and high-risk persons.

The frequency of follow-up testing for those with CHD who have achieved their LDL target goal is based on their risk level, LDL goal, and observed LDL level as follows:

Risk Level	LDL Goal (mg/dL)	LDL Observed (mg/dL)	Repeat lipoprotein testing
CHD or CHD risk equivalents	<100	<100	<1 year
2+ risk factors	<130	<130	≤2 years
0-1 risk factor	<160	130-159	≤2 years
0-1 risk factor	<160	<130	≤5 years

Decreased LDL level
Low density lipoprotein (LDL) cholesterol levels begin to decrease several hours after an acute coronary event, drop substantially after 24 to 48 hours, and remain low for weeks. Values obtained on admission may therefore not accurately reflect the patient's true baseline.

Timing of Monitoring
Patients admitted to the hospital with suspected acute coronary syndrome or for coronary procedures should have lipid measurements obtained on admission or within 24 hours of admission.

COMMON PANELS
- Diabetic management panel
- General health panel
- Lipid profile

CLINICAL NOTES
Friedewald's formula is not accurate for patients with triglyceride values greater than 400 mg/dL; ultracentrifugation is recommended in those instances. Results from plasma samples are approximately 3% lower than serum samples.

COLLECTION/STORAGE INFORMATION
- Instruct the patients to fast for 9 to 12 hours before the test.
- Collect sample in yellow-top, red-top, or serum separator tube. Do not use oxalate, citrate, heparin, or fluoride tubes.
- Store up to 3 days at 4°C; frozen samples may be stored at -70°C after the addition of hypertonic sucrose.

LOINC CODES
- Code: 9346-8 (*Short Name* - B-Lipoprotein SerPl Calc-mCnc)
- Code: 17083-7 (*Short Name* - B-LP Fld-mCnc)
- Code: 9620-6 (*Short Name* - B-Lipoprotein Plr-mCnc)
- Code: 14815-5 (*Short Name* - B-LP SerPl Calc-sCnc)
- Code: 2574-2 (*Short Name* - B-Lipoprotein SerPl-mCnc)
- Code: 14814-8 (*Short Name* - B-Lipoprotein SerPl Elph-sCnc)
- Code: 17846-7 (*Short Name* - B-Lipoprotein SerPl Ql)
- Code: 26821-9 (*Short Name* - B-Lipoprotein Fld Ql)

Lymphocyte count

TEST DEFINITION
Measurement of lymphocytes in blood for the evaluation and management of immunologic, hematologic, and neoplastic disorders

REFERENCE RANGE
- Adults:
- Absolute: 1.5-4 X 10^3 cells/microL
- Relative: 22%-44%
- Adults, 21 years:
- Absolute: 1-4.8 X 10^3 cells/microL
- Relative: 34%
- Neonates, 0 to 2 days:
- Absolute: 1.6-7.4 X 10^3 cells/microL
- Neonates, 4 days:
- Absolute: 1.6-6 X 10^3 cells/microL
- Neonates, 5 to 28 days:
- Absolute: 2.8-9 X 10^3 cells/microL
- Infants, 1 to 4 weeks:
- Absolute: 2.9-9.1 X 10^3 cells/microL
- Infants, 6 months:
- Absolute: 4-13.5 X 10^3 cells/microL
- Children, 1 year:
- Absolute: 4-10.5 X 10^3 cells/microL
- Relative: 61%
- Children, 2 years:
- Absolute: 3-9.5 X 10^3 cells/microL
- Children, 4 years:
- Absolute: 2-8 X 10^3 cells/microL
- Relative: 50%
- Children, 6 years:
- Absolute: 1.5-7 X 10^3 cells/microL
- Relative: 42%
- Children, 10 years:
- Absolute: 1.5-6.5 X 10^3 cells/microL
- Relative: 38%
  Please refer to your institution's reference ranges as lab normals may vary.

INDICATIONS
Suspected bacteremia
    Strength of Recommendation: Class IIa
    Strength of Evidence: Category B
Results Interpretation:
Decreased lymphocyte production
    Lymphopenia may suggest bacteremia, with extreme lymphopenia (count less than 0.25 x 10^9 /L) indicating the highest risk for bacteremia.

Suspected chronic lymphocytic leukemia
    Strength of Recommendation: Class I
    Strength of Evidence: Category C
Results Interpretation:
Increased lymphocyte production
    An absolute lymphocyte count greater than 5 x 10^9 /L without known cause suggests early stage chronic lymphocytic leukemia; however, many other disorders causing a proliferation of lymphocytes must be ruled out.

Suspected cytomegalovirus (CMV) infection
    Strength of Recommendation: Class IIb
    Strength of Evidence: Category C

Results Interpretation:
Increased lymphocyte production

Absolute lymphocytosis is a common finding in cytomegalovirus (CMV) infection, with at least 20% of the leukocyte count composed of atypical lymphocytes.

In pregnant women, increased lymphocyte production (40% or above) may differentiate primary CMV from recurrent and nonactive CMV.

Suspected immunocompromised state
Strength of Recommendation: Class IIb
Strength of Evidence: Category B
Results Interpretation:
Decreased lymphocyte production

An absolute lymphocyte count (ALC) less than 1,000 cells/mm$_3$ is suggestive of a CD4 count less than 200 cells/mm^3, while an ALC greater than 2,000 cells/mm^3 is suggestive of a CD4 count greater than 200 cells/mm^3.

Suspected infectious mononucleosis
Strength of Recommendation: Class IIa
Strength of Evidence: Category C
Results Interpretation:
Lymphocyte abnormality

At presentation, 70% to 75% of patients with infectious mononucleosis have a relative and absolute lymphocytosis (at least 50% lymphocytes, with total leukocyte count greater than 10,000/mm^3) and usually have at least an atypical lymphocytes of at least 10%. Even with a negative heterophile antibody test, an atypical lymphocytosis of at least 20%, or an atypical lymphocytosis of at least 10% plus a lymphocytosis of 50% or greater, strongly supports the diagnosis.

The diagnosis rarely confirmed serologically when atypical lymphocytosis is present without other suggestive signs and symptoms (eg, splenomegaly, pharyngitis, adenopathy)

A lower relative percent of atypical lymphocytes may be noted in children younger than 4 years of age, compared with that of older children and young adults.

Suspected lymphocytosis
Strength of Recommendation: Class IIa
Strength of Evidence: Category B
Results Interpretation:
Increased lymphocyte production

Lymphocytosis (counts greater than 1.5 to 4 x 10^9/L in adults and 1.5 to 8.8 x 10^9/L in children) may indicate a variety of conditions, particularly viral infections and hematologic disorders..

Acute stressful events such as trauma, cardiac emergency, or surgery may be accompanied by a transient increase of lymphocytes (4,000 to 10,400/microL), which typically resolves within 24 to 48 hours.

Suspected lymphopenia
Strength of Recommendation: Class IIa
Strength of Evidence: Category B
Results Interpretation:
Decreased lymphocyte production

Low lymphocyte count (less than 1.5 x 10^9/L in adults and less than 3 x 10^9/L in children) underlies a variety of disease processes, including immunologic and hematologic disorders, renal failure, carcinoma,, and the development of febrile neutropenia after chemotherapy.

Suspected severe acute respiratory syndrome (SARS)
Strength of Recommendation: Class IIa
Strength of Evidence: Category B
Results Interpretation:
Decreased lymphocyte production

Severe lymphopenia (less than 1 x 10^9 cells/L) is a hallmark laboratory indicator of severe acute respiratory syndrome (SARS), noted in up to 70% of cases.

Progressive lymphopenia (absolute count less than 1,000/mm^3) may be present in the early stages of SARS, reaching a low point during the second week and recovering during the third week.

COMMON PANELS
• Complete blood count with automated differential

CLINICAL NOTES
Depending on methodology, false-positive and false-negative detection of immature cells may occur.

COLLECTION/STORAGE INFORMATION
* Specimen Collection and Handling:
  * Collect whole blood in purple top tube (EDTA).
  * Do not use heparin.
  * Specimen is stable for 24 hours at 23°C and for 48 hours at 4°C.

LOINC CODES
* Code: 731-0 (*Short Name* - Lymphocytes # Bld Auto)
* Code: 30181-2 (*Short Name* - Fiss Lymphs # Bld Manual)
* Code: 30364-4 (*Short Name* - Lymphocytes # Bld FC)
* Code: 30418-8 (*Short Name* - Fiss Lymphs # Bld)
* Code: 26474-7 (*Short Name* - Lymphocytes # Bld)
* Code: 30412-1 (*Short Name* - Abnormal Lymphs # Bld)
* Code: 732-8 (*Short Name* - Lymphocytes # Bld Manual)
* Code: 14106-9 (*Short Name* - Lymphocytes # CSF Manual)
* Code: 29262-3 (*Short Name* - Abnormal Lymphs # Bld Manual)
* Code: 20585-6 (*Short Name* - Lymphocytes # XXX Auto)
* Code: 6744-7 (*Short Name* - Lymphocytes # Fld Manual)

Lysergic acid diethylamide measurement

TEST DEFINITION
Measurement of lysergic acid diethylamide (LSD) and its metabolites in urine for suspected hallucinogen abuse assessment.

SYNONYMS
* LSD measurement

REFERENCE RANGE
* Negative
  Please refer to your institution's reference ranges as lab normals may vary.

INDICATIONS
Suspected lysergic acid diethylamide (LSD) ingestion
> **Strength of Recommendation:** Class IIb
> **Strength of Evidence:** Category C
> **Results Interpretation:**
> **Positive laboratory findings**
> A positive test suggests recent LSD use (within the last 12 to 22 hours). The metabolite 2-oxo-3-hydroxy-LSD is present in the urine in much higher concentrations than LSD itself, and maybe detected for a longer time period..

COMMON PANELS
* Drugs of abuse testing, urine

CLINICAL NOTES
Lysergic acid diethylamide (LSD) is not detected on most toxicology screens. Urine LSD levels are not useful other than to establish the diagnosis of LSD abuse and underlying organic disorders.

COLLECTION/STORAGE INFORMATION
* Specimen Collection and Handling:
  * Obtain random urine sample
  * Store specimen at 8°C

LOINC CODES
- Code: 3732-5 (*Short Name* - LSD Ur QI)
- Code: 3730-9 (*Short Name* - LSD SerPl QI)
- Code: 16214-9 (*Short Name* - LSD Ur QI Cnfrn)
- Code: 19528-9 (*Short Name* - LSD Ur QI Scn)
- Code: 3731-7 (*Short Name* - LSD SerPl-mCnc)
- Code: 20542-7 (*Short Name* - LSD Ur Cnfrn-mCnc)
- Code: 5678-8 (*Short Name* - LSD SerPl RIA-mCnc)
- Code: 19531-3 (*Short Name* - LSD CtO Ur Cfm-mCnc)
- Code: 19530-5 (*Short Name* - LSD CtOff Ur Scn-mCnc)
- Code: 5679-6 (*Short Name* - LSD Ur-mCnc)

Lysine measurement

TEST DEFINITION
Measurement of lysine in plasma or serum for detection of acquired and hereditary amino acid disorders

REFERENCE RANGE
- Premature neonate, 1 day: 2.77 ± 0.88 mg/dL (190 ± 60 micromol/L)
- Neonate, 1 day: 1.66-3.93 mg/dL (114-269 micromol/L)
- Infants 1 to 3 months: 1.5 ± 0.48 mg/dL (103 ± 33 micromol/L)
- Infants 9 to 24 months: 0.66-2.10 mg/dL (45-144 micromol/L)
- Children 3 to 10 years: 1.04-2.2 mg/dL (71-151 micromol/L)
- Children 6 to 18 years: 1.58-3.4 mg/dL (108-233 micromol/L)
- Adults: 1.21-3.47 mg/dL (83-238 micromol/L)
  Please refer to your institution's reference ranges as lab normals may vary.

INDICATIONS
Suspected inborn error of metabolism
> **Strength of Recommendation:** Class IIa
> **Strength of Evidence:** Category C
> **Results Interpretation:**
> **Increased amino acid**
>
> Inherited amino acid disorders are directly related to the absence of an enzyme involved in the metabolism of one or more amino acids; therefore, an elevated plasma level of a particular amino acid is highly suggestive of an inherited metabolic defect. In the majority of cases amino acid and organic acid analysis together permit diagnostic confirmation in infants. Immediate treatment should be initiated when an inborn error of metabolism is suspected, even if a definitive diagnosis has not yet been determined.
>
> Carbamoyl phosphate synthetase deficiency is associated with increased alanine, glutamine, glycine and lysine, and low or undetectable arginine and citrulline levels.

COLLECTION/STORAGE INFORMATION
- Specimen Collection and Handling:
  - Immediately place sample in ice water.
  - Isolate plasma sample and freeze it within 1 hour; sample stable for 1 week at -20°C.
  - Sample should be deproteinized and stored at -70°C for protracted periods of usage.

LOINC CODES
- Code: 30048-3 (*Short Name* - Lysine/creat Ur-Rto)
- Code: 22651-4 (*Short Name* - Lysine CSF-sCnc)
- Code: 32256-0 (*Short Name* - Lysine Fld-sCnc)
- Code: 32255-2 (*Short Name* - Lysine Vitf-sCnc)
- Code: 22713-2 (*Short Name* - Lysine XXX-sCnc)
- Code: 13375-1 (*Short Name* - Lysine CSF-mCnc)
- Code: 27304-5 (*Short Name* - Lysine Ur-sCnc)
- Code: 27107-2 (*Short Name* - Lysine Amn-sCnc)
- Code: 25953-1 (*Short Name* - Lysine/creat 24H Ur-sRto)
- Code: 25952-3 (*Short Name* - Lysine 24H Ur-sCnc)

- Code: 13769-5 (*Short Name* - Lysine/creat Ur-mRto)
- Code: 13404-9 (*Short Name* - Lysine Amn-mCnc)

MS alpha-fetoprotein level

TEST DEFINITION
The measurement of maternal alpha-fetoprotein (MSAFP) levels in serum for the evaluation of pregnancy complications

SYNONYMS
- Maternal serum alpha fetoprotein level
- MSAFP level

REFERENCE RANGE
- Adults: <15 ng/mL (<15 mcg/L)
- Black adults: 10% to 15% higher than Caucasian
  Please refer to your institution's reference ranges as lab normals may vary.

INDICATIONS
Prenatal screening for possible neural tube defects and other fetal congenital anomalies
  Strength of Recommendation: Class I
  Strength of Evidence: Category A
  Results Interpretation:
  Abnormal laboratory findings
    Laboratories establish their own cutoff for multiples of the median (MoM) values, usually at 2 to 2.5 times the median value when compared to normal controls at the same week of gestation. A positive screen is not diagnostic, but indicates an elevated risk that warrants further testing.
    MSAFP levels in serum increase at 15% to 20% per week between 16 and 22 weeks gestation. MSAFP levels are approximately 100 times lower than AFP levels in amniotic fluid.
    A decreased level of MSAFP at 0.8 MoM for normal control pregnancies is associated with an increased risk of Down syndrome.
  Timing of Monitoring
    The optimal gestation age for maternal serum alpha-fetoprotein testing is between 16 and 18 weeks, when the test is most accurate. Earlier or later screening decreases sensitivity.

COMMON PANELS
- Maternal serum quadruple screen
- Maternal serum triple screen

COLLECTION/STORAGE INFORMATION
- Specimen Collection and Handling:
  - Collect blood sample in a marbled top tube.
  - Store sample at 2°C to 8°C if assay is to be performed within 24 hours of collection, otherwise store at -20°C.

Magnesium measurement, serum

TEST DEFINITION
Measurement of magnesium in serum for the evaluation and management of conditions that affect magnesium metabolism

REFERENCE RANGE
- Adults: 1.8 mg/dL-3 mg/dL (0.8 mmol/L-1.2 mmol/L)
  Please refer to your institution's reference ranges as lab normals may vary.

INDICATIONS

Diabetic ketoacidosis
Results Interpretation:
Hypomagnesemia
Chronic magnesium deficiency has been well described in diabetes; urinary losses of magnesium during diabetic ketoacidosis (DKA) may exacerbate the severity of the problem. Urinary losses of up to 23 mEq of magnesium have been reported during the initial treatment phase.

Heart failure
Strength of Recommendation: Class IIa
Strength of Evidence: Category B
Results Interpretation:
Hypomagnesemia
Low magnesium levels may predict increased arrhythmias and mortality rates in patients with congestive heart failure. Low potassium, phosphate, and calcium levels may coexist in these patients, particularly in those taking diuretics.
Hypermagnesemia
High magnesium levels may predict increased mortality rates in patients with CHF. This outcome may not be a direct result of magnesium, given the lower rates of arrhythmias and sudden death, but may be secondary to more comorbidities.
Timing of Monitoring
Electrolytes, including magnesium and calcium, should be ordered in the initial evaluation of patients with suspected heart failure and monitored regularly in patients with known heart failure.

Hypocalcemia
Strength of Recommendation: Class IIa
Strength of Evidence: Category C
Results Interpretation:
Hypomagnesemia
Hypocalcemia should not be attributed to hypomagnesemia if the serum magnesium level is greater than 1.2 mg/dL, as mild hypomagnesemia (1.2 mg/dL to 1.8 mg/dL) may stimulate secretion of parathyroid hormone.
Overt hypomagnesemia is present in about 22% of patients with hypocalcemia; however, because less than 1% of total body magnesium is in extracellular fluid, patients with hypocalcemia may be magnesium-deficient despite normal serum magnesium concentrations.
Significantly lower mononuclear cell magnesium contents have been found in hypocalcemic patients than in normocalcemic patients, which suggests that intracellular magnesium content may be more important than serum magnesium level in diagnosing hypomagnesemia in these patients.
Measurement of serum magnesium is important in patients with ionized hypocalcemia because magnesium replacement may be sufficient to correct hypocalcemia. Following magnesium replacement, calcium may rise rapidly.

Hypokalemia
Strength of Recommendation: Class IIa
Strength of Evidence: Category C
Results Interpretation:
Hypomagnesemia
Hypomagnesemia may be found in up to 40% of patients with hypokalemia.

Peripheral vascular disease
Strength of Recommendation: Class IIb
Strength of Evidence: Category B
Results Interpretation:
Hypomagnesemia
Low serum magnesium levels may be predictive of future stroke or carotid artery intervention in patients with pre-existing peripheral vascular disease. Hypomagnesemia does not appear to predict death or future cardiac events in these patients. Further studies are needed to verify these findings.

Seizure disorder
Results Interpretation:
Hypomagnesemia
Magnesium levels less than 1.3 mEq/L are often associated with neurologic symptoms.

Magnesium may act as a physiologic calcium channel blocker affecting calcium influx. The resulting neurochemical changes can enhance the propensity for seizure activity.

Hypomagnesemia may lower the seizure threshold in alcohol withdrawal syndrome.

Severe head injury
Strength of Recommendation: Class IIb
Strength of Evidence: Category B
Results Interpretation:
Hypomagnesemia
Patients with severe head injury may be at increased risk for hypomagnesemia.

Status post total thyroidectomy
Strength of Recommendation: Class IIa
Strength of Evidence: Category C
Results Interpretation:
Hypomagnesemia
Patients who undergo total thyroidectomy, particularly if they also undergo neck dissection or receive a large volume of intravenous fluids following surgery, seem to be at increased risk for hypomagnesemia.

Suspected alcohol withdrawal
Results Interpretation:
Hypomagnesemia
Mean levels of magnesium in patients withdrawing from alcohol range from 0.7 mEq/L to 1.4 mEq/L.

Suspected and known atrial fibrillation
Results Interpretation:
Hypomagnesemia
Low magnesium levels can contribute to the development of atrial fibrillation.

Suspected and known Wernicke-Korsakoff syndrome
Results Interpretation:
Hypomagnesemia
Thiamine, in the form of thiamine pyrophosphate, requires magnesium as a cofactor for its role in glucose metabolism (eg, Krebs cycle) and other metabolic functions. Patients with hypomagnesemia may be at an increased risk for developing Wernicke-Korsakoff syndrome, especially in the situation of thiamine deficiency.

Suspected hypermagnesemia
Strength of Recommendation: Class I
Strength of Evidence: Category C
Results Interpretation:
Hypermagnesemia
- Magnesium levels above 1.9 mEq/L are abnormal; however, symptoms typically do not occur until the magnesium level is greater than 4 mEq/L:
  - >4 mEq/L: Diminished deep tendon reflexes
  - 4 to 5 mEq/L: Bradycardia, hypotension
  - 4 to 7 mEq/L: Somnolence
  - 5 to 10 mEq/L: Prolonged PR, QRS, and QT intervals on ECG
  - >10 mEq/L: Flaccid paralysis, respiratory depression, apnea
  - >15 mEq/L: Complete heart block, asystole

Suspected hypomagnesemia
Strength of Recommendation: Class I
Strength of Evidence: Category C
Results Interpretation:
Hypomagnesemia
Hypomagnesemia is defined as a serum magnesium level less than 1.3 mEq/L; however, a serum magnesium level less than 0.5 mEq/L probably is needed before manifestations become present. Even with severe hypomagnesemia, signs and symptoms associated with magnesium deficiency may be absent.

Some patients with a serum magnesium concentration within normal limits may have a total body magnesium deficit, particularly those patients with a chronic negative magnesium balance, as serum levels may be supported by magnesium from other tissue pools. Conversely, a lower serum magnesium concentration with a normal total body magnesium content also may occur.

Timing of Monitoring

Physicians should not wait for signs and symptoms of magnesium deficiency prior to ordering a serum magnesium concentration.

Suspected porphyria
Results Interpretation:
Decreased level (laboratory finding)

Hypomagnesemia severe enough to cause frank tetany is frequently observed in conjunction with hyponatremia during acute porphyria attacks.

Thermal burn.
Results Interpretation:
Hypomagnesemia

Hypomagnesemia occurs in up to 40% of patients with severe burns during the early recovery period. The low magnesium appears to be primarily due to cutaneous exudative losses.

Ventricular tachyarrhythmias
Strength of Recommendation: Class IIa
Strength of Evidence: Category B
Results Interpretation:
Hypomagnesemia

Because magnesium may play a critical role in the pathogenesis of cardiac arrhythmia associated with hypokalemia, the monitoring of serum magnesium is recommended in hypokalemic patients.

COMMON PANELS
- Enteral/Parenteral nutritional management panel
- Parathyroid panel
- Renal panel
- Transplant panel

COLLECTION/STORAGE INFORMATION
- Collect serum in marbled tube
- May refrigerate for several days

LOINC CODES
- Code: 19123-9 (*Short Name* - Magnesium SerPl-mCnc)
- Code: 2600-5 (*Short Name* - Magnesium Free SerPl-sCnc)
- Code: 2601-3 (*Short Name* - Magnesium SerPl-sCnc)

Manganese measurement, serum

TEST DEFINITION
Measurement of manganese in serum or blood to detect manganese toxicity

SYNONYMS
- Blood manganese level
- Serum manganese level #1

REFERENCE RANGE
- Adults and Children:
- Whole blood: 10.9 ± 0.6 mcg/L (198 ± 11 nmol/L)
- Serum: 0.59 ± 0.16 mcg/L (10.7 ± nmol/L)
  Please refer to your institution's reference ranges as lab normals may vary.

INDICATIONS

Suspected manganese toxicity
    Strength of Recommendation: Class IIa
    Strength of Evidence: Category B
    Results Interpretation:
    Increased level (laboratory finding)
        Because magnesium (Mn) is rapidly cleared from the body, whole blood Mn levels correlate with current but not past exposure. Mean blood Mn levels reflect the total body burden on a group, but not an individual basis, especially after exposure ceases.

        Mn miners exposed to high levels of Mn in dust and well water have increased whole blood Mn levels and increased respiratory impairment.

        Whole blood Mn levels may be elevated in patients with primary biliary cirrhosis or cirrhosis; increased levels correlate with abnormal brain MRI findings.

        The concentration of manganese in whole blood that results in neurotoxicity has not been clearly defined. Susceptibility to Mn toxicity is variable and Mn blood concentrations do not accurately predict the likelihood of neurotoxicity.

CLINICAL NOTES

Approximately 85% of manganese (Mn) is bound to hemoglobin in erythrocytes; serum Mn levels are generally much lower than whole blood Mn levels.

COLLECTION/STORAGE INFORMATION

- Collect specimen in a metal-free container.
- Whole blood sample is stable for 7 days at room temperature.

LOINC CODES

- Code: 5683-8 (*Short Name* - Manganese SerPl-mCnc)
- Code: 25467-2 (*Short Name* - Manganese SerPl-sCnc)

Manganese measurement, urine

TEST DEFINITION

Measurement of manganese in urine for evaluation of suspected manganese exposure or toxicity

REFERENCE RANGE

- Adults: <10 mcg/L (<0.18 micromol/L)
Please refer to your institution's reference ranges as lab normals may vary.

INDICATIONS

Suspected exposure to manganese
    Strength of Recommendation: Class IIa
    Strength of Evidence: Category C
    Results Interpretation:
    Abnormal urine levels, non-medicinal sources
        An elevated urine manganese level may be useful as a screening test for acute occupational or environmental manganese exposure.

        Urine manganese can be used for monitoring acute exposure to manganese, but there is no correlation between increased urine manganese levels and prior manganese exposure or chronic manganese poisoning. Increased levels of urinary manganese do not correlate well with the severity of symptoms.

COLLECTION/STORAGE INFORMATION

- Collect a random urine specimen in a plastic container.

LOINC CODES

- Code: 29935-4 (*Short Name* - Manganese/creat 24H Ur-mRto)
- Code: 8203-2 (*Short Name* - Manganese 24H Ur-mRate)

Mean corpuscular hemoglobin concentration determination

TEST DEFINITION
Measurement of the average concentration of hemoglobin in whole blood for evaluation and management of hematologic disorders

SYNONYMS
- MCHC determination
- MCHC - Mean cell haemoglobin concentration
- MCHC - Mean cell hemoglobin concentration
- Mean corpuscular haemoglobin concentration determination

REFERENCE RANGE
- Adults: 31-37 g/dL (310-370 g/L)
- Fetal blood:
- 18 to 20 weeks' gestation: 32 +/- 2.3 g/dL (320 ± 24 g/L)
- 21 to 22 weeks' gestation: 31.7 +/- 2.78 g/dL (317 ± 28 g/L)
- 23 to 25 weeks' gestation: 32.1 +/- 3.2 g/dL (321 ± 32 g/L)
- 26 to 30 weeks' gestation: 32.1 +/- 3.6 g/dL (321 ± 36 g/L)
- Neonates (cord blood): 30-36 g/dL
- Neonates, 2 weeks: 28-35 g/dL (280-350 g/L)
- Infants, 1 month: 28-36 g/dL (280-360 g/L)
- Infants, 2 months: 28-35 g/dL (280-350 g/L)
- Infants, 4 months: 29-37 g/dL (290-370 g/L)
- Children, 6 months to 17 years: 32-37 g/dL (320-370 g/L)
  Please refer to your institution's reference ranges as lab normals may vary.

INDICATIONS
Suspected hereditary spherocytosis
> **Strength of Recommendation:** Class I
> **Strength of Evidence:** Category B
> **Results Interpretation:**
> **MCHC - raised**
> Mean corpuscular Hgb concentration (MCHC) values may be increased with hereditary spherocytosis (HS), but rarely over 38 g/dL.

COMMON PANELS
- Anemia panel
- Complete blood count

ABNORMAL RESULTS
- Results increased in:
  - Autoagglutination
  - Cellular dehydration
  - Hemolysis
  - Lipemia
  - Xerocytosis
- Results decreased in:
  - High WBC

CLINICAL NOTES
Mean corpuscular hemoglobin concentration results may be erroneous after administration of blood substitutes.

COLLECTION/STORAGE INFORMATION
- Collect 5 mL of whole blood in a lavender top (EDTA) tube
- May store specimen at 25°C for up to 6 hours or at 4°C for up to 24 hours
- Fetal blood: Collect by percutaneous umbilical blood sampling

LOINC CODES
- Code: 28540-3 (*Short Name* - MCHC RBC-mCnc)
- Code: 786-4 (*Short Name* - MCHC RBC Auto-mCnc)

Mean corpuscular hemoglobin determination

TEST DEFINITION
Mean corpuscular hemoglobin, also called mean cell hemoglobin (MCH), is the calculated mass of hemoglobin (Hb) per average red blood cell (RBC) and useful in the evaluation abnormalities effecting either Hb content or RBC volume.

SYNONYMS
- MCH determination
- MCH - Mean cell haemoglobin
- MCH - Mean cell hemoglobin
- MCH - Mean corpuscular haemoglobin
- MCH - Mean corpuscular hemoglobin
- Mean cell haemoglobin
- Mean cell hemoglobin
- Mean corpuscular haemoglobin determination

REFERENCE RANGE
- Adults: 26-34 pg/cell
  Please refer to your institution's reference ranges as lab normals may vary.

INDICATIONS
Mean corpuscular hemoglobin may be useful in the differential diagnosis of anemia
  Results Interpretation:
  A low mean corpuscular hemoglobin (MCH) is consistent with anemia due to either iron deficiency or impaired hemoglobin synthesis. An elevated MCH is consistent with conditions related to iron overload such as hemochromatosis.

COMMON PANELS
- Anemia panel
- Complete blood count
- Complete blood count with automated differential
- Disseminated intravascular coagulopathy panel
- Enteral/Parenteral nutritional management panel
- General health panel
- Hemolysis panel
- Human immunodeficiency virus panel
- Prenatal screening panel
- Transplant panel

COLLECTION/STORAGE INFORMATION
Specimen Collection and Handling
- Collect whole blood in an EDTA (pink) tube
- Specimen is stable at 25°C up to 6 hours and at 4°C up to 24 hours

LOINC CODES
- Code: 785-6 (*Short Name* - MCH RBC Qn Auto)

Measles antibody level

TEST DEFINITION
Serologic diagnosis of measles virus infection or assessment of measles immune status

REFERENCE RANGE
• Adult and Children: Negative
Please refer to your institution's reference ranges as lab normals may vary.

INDICATIONS
Determination of measles immune status
      Strength of Recommendation: Class IIa
      Strength of Evidence: Category C
Results Interpretation:
Serology positive
    The measles vaccine produces a mild or inapparent, non-communicable infection and antibodies develop in approximately 95% of susceptible children vaccinated at about 15 months of age. Immune individuals usually have titers of 4 or greater.
    Studies suggest that vaccine-induced antibody titers confer disease protection, although the titers are lower than those following natural disease exposure. In some individuals, asymptomatic reinfection with measles virus from vaccination or natural disease can occur in those with prior positive antibody levels.
    The hemagglutination inhibition (HI) assay is sensitive and may be used to measure immunity; enzyme immunoassay (EIA) is also commonly used and is technically easier to perform. Routine screening to assess immunity is not recommended.

Suspected or known measles exposure
      Strength of Recommendation: Class IIa
      Strength of Evidence: Category B
Results Interpretation:
Serology positive
    Positive results may indicate recent vaccination or exposure to disease. IgM enzyme immunoassays (EIAs) are the preferred method to diagnose measles. Recent infection can also be diagnosed by a 4-fold rise in titer between acute and convalescent sera.
    IgM antibody may not be detectable with some assays until at least 72 hours after the onset of rash. However, antibody levels can be detectable at the onset of rash, peak approximately 10 days later, and are usually undetectable 30 to 60 days after the onset of rash.
    Correct interpretation depends on the timing of specimen collection in relation to rash onset and on the characteristics of the immunoassay used.
    To evaluate potential disease exposure an accurate history of vaccination is necessary. IgM antibody response may persist for up to 8 weeks or more after immunization whereas, the IgG antibody remains positive indefinitely.

False Results
    False positive results can occur in the presence of rheumatoid factor and occur more frequently with indirect IgM assays. Sera from patients with Epstein-Barr virus, cytomegalovirus, human herpesvirus 6, and mycoplasma have also produced false positive or equivocal results. Attempts to remove these immune complexes have not been successful.
    False positive results can also occur more frequently when disease prevalence is low. To resolve potential issues surrounding positive IgM results in isolated suspected measle cases, laboratories can use the results generated from IgG EIAs along with IgM results.
    False negative results have also been reported with IgM assays if the serum sample is collected too early after the first appearance of a clinically suspicious rash.

CLINICAL NOTES
    Immunoglobulin M (IgM) EIAs are the preferred laboratory assay to confirm the clinical diagnosis of measles. Most EIAs can be done with a single serum specimen and require approximately 20 mL of serum. Acute measles infection can be diagnosed from the time of rash onset until greater than or equal to 4 weeks after the onset of rash.

As the incidence of measles declines in the United States and in some countries throughout the world, clinical experience with the illness is also in decline. As a result, laboratory confirmation has become an important part of diagnosis.

In general, confirmation of suspected measle cases is recommended by a measles-specific IgM assay especially in areas where the incidence of disease is low.

COLLECTION/STORAGE INFORMATION
- Collect serum specimen by venipuncture or finger/heel stick into a serum-gel separator tube.
- Obtain specimen as soon as possible after the onset of rash, and 2 to 4 weeks later to evaluate acute and chronic titers.
- Freeze specimen if unable to test immediately.

LOINC CODES
- Code: 22498-0 (*Short Name* - MeV Ab Titr CSF)
- Code: 9565-3 (*Short Name* - MeV Ab Titr CSF CF)
- Code: 5242-3 (*Short Name* - MeV Ab Ser EIA-aCnc)
- Code: 7961-6 (*Short Name* - MeV Ab Ser-aCnc)
- Code: 5243-1 (*Short Name* - MeV Ab Titr Ser CF)
- Code: 22499-8 (*Short Name* - MeV Ab Titr Ser)
- Code: 17553-9 (*Short Name* - MeV Ab CSF-aCnc)

Measurement of feces pH

TEST DEFINITION
Measurement of stool pH for the evaluation of disorders associated with carbohydrate malabsorption

SYNONYMS
- Faeces pH
- Feces pH
- Measurement of faeces pH

REFERENCE RANGE
- Adults and Children: 7-7.5
- Neonates: 5-7
  Please refer to your institution's reference ranges as lab normals may vary.

INDICATIONS
Assessment of diarrhea secondary to suspected carbohydrate malabsorption
> **Strength of Recommendation:** Class IIb
> **Strength of Evidence:** Category C
> **Results Interpretation:**
> **Decreased level (laboratory finding)**
- Carbohydrate intolerance: pH <5.3
- Disaccharidase deficiency: pH <5.5
> **Increased level (laboratory finding)**
- Cholerheic enteropathy (bile acid diarrhea) after intestinal resection: pH >6.8
  An increase in pH does not exclude the diagnosis of disaccharidase deficiency

Suspected lactose intolerance.
> **Strength of Recommendation:** Class IIb
> **Strength of Evidence:** Category C
> **Results Interpretation:**
> **Decreased level (laboratory finding)**
- Adults: pH <5.3 is suggestive of carbohydrate malabsorption
- Children: pH <6 is typical result for lactase deficiency

ABNORMAL RESULTS
- Results increased in:
  - Colitis
  - Villous adenoma
- Results decreased in:
  - Decreased fat absorption

COLLECTION/STORAGE INFORMATION
- Refrigerate sample until analysis

LOINC CODES
- Code: 2755-7 (*Short Name* - pH Stl-sCnc)

Mercury measurement, urine

TEST DEFINITION
Measurement of mercury in urine for evaluation of exposure and toxicity

SYNONYMS
- Urine mercury
- Urine mercury level

REFERENCE RANGE
- Adults: <20 mcg/L (<99.8 nmol/L)
  Please refer to your institution's reference ranges as lab normals may vary.

INDICATIONS
Suspected mercury exposure
> **Strength of Recommendation:** Class IIb
> **Strength of Evidence:** Category C
> **Results Interpretation:**
> **Increased level (laboratory finding)**

Signs and symptoms of toxicity may begin to occur at urinary mercury concentrations between 20 and 100 mcg/L. Clinical disorders are commonly seen at mercury levels greater than 100 mcg/L. Renal disease is unlikely at mercury excretion levels below 50 mcg/g creatinine.

Urinary mercury is the best biological marker for chronic elemental or inorganic mercury exposure. However, levels often do not correlate with clinical signs and symptoms of toxicity. There is a high degree of intraindividual variation in urine mercury levels suggesting that averaging of several urinary mercury determinations may be required.

Spot urine collections can be used to approximate the 24-hour sample. The interpretation of these levels is most accurate when samples are taken at the same time of day and are corrected for specific gravity or, more preferably, creatinine.

Urinary mercury levels are not useful in determining methylmercury exposure due to fish or seafood ingestion since approximately 90% of methylmercury is excreted via the bile into the feces.

CLINICAL NOTES
Blood mercury concentration is a better determinant of total body methylmercury, whereas urinary mercury is the best biological marker for chronic elemental or inorganic mercury exposure.

COLLECTION/STORAGE INFORMATION
- Specimen Collection and Handling:
  - Collect specimen in metal-free container.
  - Acidify specimen with nitric acid to a pH of 2.
  - May be left at room temperature.

LOINC CODES

- Code: 19056-1 (*Short Name* - Mercury Ur QI)
- Code: 13961-8 (*Short Name* - Mercury 24H Ur QI)
- Code: 5689-5 (*Short Name* - Mercury Ur-mCnc)
- Code: 5688-7 (*Short Name* - Mercury Ur QI Visual.Reinsch)
- Code: 6693-6 (*Short Name* - Mercury 24H Ur-mRate)
- Code: 22680-3 (*Short Name* - Mercury/creat Ur-sRto)
- Code: 13465-0 (*Short Name* - Mercury/creat Ur-mRto)
- Code: 30921-1 (*Short Name* - Mercury ?Tm Ur-mCnc)

Metanephrines measurement, total, urine

TEST DEFINITION

Measurement of metanephrine levels in urine for the evaluation of pheochromocytoma

SYNONYMS

- Urine metanephrin
- Urine metanephrin level

REFERENCE RANGE

- Adults: 0.05-1.2 mcg/mg creatinine (0.03-0.69 mmol/mol creatinine)
- Infants, 0-1 year: 0.001-4.60 mcg/mg creatinine (0.0006-2.64 mmol/mol creatinine)
- Children, 1-2 years: 0.27-5.38 mcg/mg creatinine (0.15-3.09 mmol/mol creatinine)
- Children, 2-5 years: 0.35-2.99 mcg/mg creatinine (0.21-1.72 mmol/mol creatinine)
- Children, 5-10 years: 0.43-2.7 mcg/mg creatinine (0.25-1.55 mmol/mol creatinine)
- Children and Adolescents, 10-15 years: 0.001-1.87 mcg/mg creatinine (0.0006-1.07 mmol/mol creatinine)
- Adolescents, 15-18 years: 0.001-0.67 mcg/mg creatinine (0.0006-0.38 mmol/mol creatinine)
  Please refer to your institution's reference ranges as lab normals may vary.

INDICATIONS

Suspected pheochromocytoma
    Strength of Recommendation: Class IIa
    Strength of Evidence: Category B
    Results Interpretation:
    Raised biochemistry findings
    Elevated 24-hour urine total metanephrines measurement is highly suggestive of pheochromocytoma in patients with hypertension.
    Normal biochemistry findings
    A normal 24-hour urine total metanephrines level does not rule out pheochromocytoma since some tumors do not secrete enough catecholamine to produce positive test results; also, pheochromocytomas often secrete catecholamines and metabolites episodically.

COMMON PANELS

- Hypertension panel

CLINICAL NOTES

Twenty-four hour urine tests are superior to plasma tests in the diagnosis of pheochromocytoma, because these tumors often secrete catecholamines intermittently.

COLLECTION/STORAGE INFORMATION

- Patient Preparation
  - Avoid dietary intake of chocolate, coffee, bananas, vanilla and nuts shortly before and for the duration of the test.
  - Collect specimen when patient is stress free, medically stable and free of catecholamine containing or stimulating medications.
- Specimen Collection and Handling:

- Discard the first morning specimen, then collect all urine, including the final voided specimen, at the end of the 24-hour period.
- Utilize glacial acetic acid (15 mL) as a preservative in collection container.
- Deliver specimen to lab within 1 hour of collection.
- Specimen stable for several weeks at 4°C

LOINC CODES

- Code: 2609-6 (*Short Name* - MetanephS 24H Ur-mRate)
- Code: 14832-0 (*Short Name* - MetanephS Ur-sCnc)
- Code: 21422-1 (*Short Name* - Normetanephrine 24H Ur-mCnc)
- Code: 25964-8 (*Short Name* - Normetanephrine 24H Ur-sCnc)
- Code: 15083-9 (*Short Name* - Normetanephrine 24H Ur-sRate)
- Code: 14833-8 (*Short Name* - MetanephS 24H Ur-sRate)
- Code: 11139-3 (*Short Name* - Metaneph Ur-mCnc)
- Code: 13771-1 (*Short Name* - Metanephrines/creat Ur-mRto)
- Code: 9645-3 (*Short Name* - Metaneph/creat Ur-mRto)
- Code: 27978-6 (*Short Name* - Metanephrines/creat 24H Ur-sRto)
- Code: 21019-5 (*Short Name* - Metaneph 24H Ur-mCnc)
- Code: 19050-4 (*Short Name* - Metanephrines 24H Ur-mCnc)
- Code: 25955-6 (*Short Name* - Metaneph 24H Ur-sCnc)
- Code: 19049-6 (*Short Name* - Metaneph 24H Ur-mRate)
- Code: 2608-8 (*Short Name* - Metanephrines Ur-mCnc)

Methemoglobin measurement, quantitative

TEST DEFINITION

Measurement of methemoglobin in whole blood for the evaluation and management of methemoglobinemia

SYNONYMS

- Methaemoglobin measurement, quantitative

REFERENCE RANGE

- Adults and Children: <1% of total hemoglobin
  Please refer to your institution's reference ranges as lab normals may vary.

INDICATIONS

Suspected acquired methemoglobinemia
    Strength of Recommendation: Class I
    Strength of Evidence: Category C
    Results Interpretation:
    Increased methemoglobin
- Methemoglobin levels (% of total hemoglobin):
  - <3%: No signs or symptoms
  - 15% to 30%: Cyanosis, chocolate brown blood
  - 30% to 50%: Dyspnea, dizziness, nausea, anxiety, chest pain; headache, fatigue, syncope, weakness, pulse oximetry reading at about 85%
  - 50% to 70%: Tachypnea, metabolic acidosis, dysrhythmias, seizures, central nervous system depression, coma
  - >70%: Severe hypoxia, death

    Patients with anemia, heart disease, or other conditions that could make them more susceptible to hypoxia may become symptomatic at lower levels.

    Patients who have had chronic exposure to a methemoglobinemia-inducing substance usually have levels under 20%.

    Treatment should usually be initiated at methemoglobin levels of 20% in symptomatic patients and at levels of 30% in asymptomatic patients.

Suspected congenital methemoglobinemia
>**Strength of Recommendation:** Class I
>**Strength of Evidence:** Category C

Results Interpretation:
Increased methemoglobin

In patients with hemoglobin M (HbM) variants (a group of abnormal hemoglobins amino acid substitutions near the heme iron resulting in facilitated oxidation of the hemoglobin to methemoglobin), co-oximetry may yield falsely normal methemoglobin fractions. Because of this, spectral characterization and ratios or electrophoresis should be utilized if an HbM variant is suspected.

Homozygotes for enzymopenic hereditary methemoglobinemia usually have methemoglobin levels greater than 10% and are typically asymptomatic unless the methemoglobin level rises above 25%.

COLLECTION/STORAGE INFORMATION

- Specimen Collection and Handling:
  - Collect venous or arterial blood in sodium fluoride tube.
  - Keep sample on ice and send to laboratory for immediate analysis as methemoglobin is highly unstable.

LOINC CODES

- Code: 15082-1 (*Short Name* - MetHgb Bld-mCnc)

Methionine measurement

TEST DEFINITION

Measurement of methionine in plasma or serum for detection of acquired and hereditary amino acid disorders

SYNONYMS

- Methionine level

REFERENCE RANGE

- Premature neonate, 1 day: 0.52 ± 0.07 mg/dL (35 ± 5 micromol/L)
- Neonate, 1 day: 0.13-0.61 mg/dL (9-41 micromol/L)
- Infants 1 to 3 months: 0.31 ± 0.13 mg/dL (21 ± 9 micromol/L)
- Infants 9 to 24 months: 0.04-0.43 mg/dL (3-29 micromol/L)
- Children 3 to 10 years: 0.16-0.24 mg/dL (11-16 micromol/L)
- Children 6 to 18 years: 0.24-0.55 mg/dL (16-37 micromol/L)
- Adults: 0.09-0.6 mg/dL (6-40 micromol/L)
  Please refer to your institution's reference ranges as lab normals may vary.

INDICATIONS

Suspected inborn error of metabolism
>**Strength of Recommendation:** Class IIa
>**Strength of Evidence:** Category C

Results Interpretation:
Increased amino acid

The diagnostic criteria for homocystinuria secondary to cystathionine-beta-synthase (CBS) deficiency include a methionine level greater than 100 micromol/L, the presence of free homocystine, reduced cystine, and a total plasma homocystine level of greater than 25 micromol/L. Other forms of homocystinuria do not cause elevated methionine levels. Elevated methionine levels are also associated with galactosemia and tyrosinemiaand false positives can result from high protein intake, liver disease and variations in enzymes associated with demethylation of methionine to homocysteine. Because methionine levels rise slowly and inconsistently in newborns, initial screening results may be negative. Routine retesting can identify additional cases of CBS.

Inherited amino acid disorders are directly related to the absence of an enzyme involved in the metabolism of one or more amino acids; therefore, an elevated plasma level of a particular amino acid is highly suggestive of an inherited metabolic defect. In the majority of cases amino acid and organic acid analysis together permit diagnostic confirmation in infants. Immediate treatment should be initiated when an inborn error of metabolism is suspected, even if a definitive diagnosis has not yet been determined.

Collection/Storage Information
- Specimen Collection and Handling:
  - Immediately place sample in ice water.
  - Isolate plasma sample and freeze it within 1 hour; sample stable for 1 week at -20°C.
  - Sample should be deproteinized and stored at -70°C for protracted periods of usage.

LOINC Codes
- Code: 13376-9 (*Short Name* - Methionine CSF-mCnc)
- Code: 25476-3 (*Short Name* - Methionine 24H Ur-sRate)
- Code: 30063-2 (*Short Name* - Methionine/creat Ur-Rto)
- Code: 13405-6 (*Short Name* - Methionine Amn-mCnc)
- Code: 22681-1 (*Short Name* - Methionine/creat Ur-sRto)
- Code: 25957-2 (*Short Name* - MSO 24H Ur-sCnc)
- Code: 32258-6 (*Short Name* - Methionine Fld-sCnc)
- Code: 25477-1 (*Short Name* - MSO 24H Ur-sRate)
- Code: 22648-0 (*Short Name* - Methionine CSF-sCnc)
- Code: 22716-5 (*Short Name* - Methionine XXX-sCnc)
- Code: 26844-1 (*Short Name* - Methionine Amn-sCnc)
- Code: 2623-7 (*Short Name* - Methionine Ur-mCnc)
- Code: 27098-3 (*Short Name* - Methionine 24H Ur Ql)
- Code: 2624-5 (*Short Name* - Methionine 24H Ur-mRate)
- Code: 25959-8 (*Short Name* - Methionine/creat 24H Ur-sRto)
- Code: 13772-9 (*Short Name* - Methionine/creat Ur-mRto)
- Code: 25956-4 (*Short Name* - Methionine 24H Ur-sCnc)
- Code: 26963-9 (*Short Name* - Methionine Ur-sCnc)
- Code: 32257-8 (*Short Name* - Methionine Vitf-sCnc)
- Code: 17264-3 (*Short Name* - Methionine Ur Ql)
- Code: 25958-0 (*Short Name* - MSO/creat 24H Ur-sRto)
- Code: 2620-3 (*Short Name* - Methionine Bld Ql)

Metyrapone test

Test Definition
Measurement of 11-deoxycortisol, cortisol, and adrenocorticotrophic hormone (ACTH) in plasma and their metabolites in urine after the administration of metyrapone, for the evaluation of pituitary ACTH reserve

Synonyms
- Metopirone stimulation test
- Metyrapone panel
- Metyrapone stimulation test

Reference Range
Normal levels are indication specific, patient specific and technique specific.
Please refer to your institution's reference ranges as lab normals may vary.

Indications
Suspected adrenal insufficiency
   Strength of Recommendation: Class IIb
   Strength of Evidence: Category B
   Results Interpretation:
   Abnormal laboratory findings
   Levels of 11-deoxycortisol and cortisol less than 200 nmoL/L suggest an abnormal metyrapone test.
   Post metyrapone administration plasma adrenocorticotrophic hormone (ACTH) levels in secondary adrenal failure can discriminate between normal (ACTH greater than 100 ng/L), diminished (ACTH below 100 ng/L), and absent (ACTH below 20 to 40 ng/L) ACTH reserve.

Suspected Cushing's syndrome
    Strength of Recommendation: Class IIb
    Strength of Evidence: Category B
Results Interpretation:
Abnormal laboratory findings
    Maximum levels of 17-oxogenic steroids of 200% or more above baseline after giving metyrapone are considered abnormal. A majority of patients with Cushing's syndrome will exhibit an abnormal rise in 11-deoxycortisol levels. A 1-fold increase in 11-deoxycortisol in response to a metyrapone test may indicate Cushing's syndrome. The mean adrenocorticotrophic hormone (ACTH) concentration in pituitary-dependent Cushing's syndrome is 300 ng/L while undetectable levels suggest a primary adrenal origin. However, because an abnormal rise in plasma ACTH (greater than 200% increase from baseline) also occurs in patients with ACTH-secreting tumors, and ACTH responses are highly variable, the metyrapone test has limited value in identifying the source of ACTH.

Suspected ectopic adrenocorticotrophic hormone (ACTH)-producing tumor
    Strength of Recommendation: Class IIb
    Strength of Evidence: Category B
Results Interpretation:
Abnormal laboratory findings
    An abnormal rise in plasma adrenocorticotrophic hormone (ACTH) levels of greater than 200% from baseline is suggestive of ACTH-secreting tumors. However, elevated ACTH levels are also seen in Cushing's syndrome, and because ACTH responses are highly variable, the metyrapone test has limited value in identifying the source of ACTH.

Microalbumin measurement, 24H urine

TEST DEFINITION
    Measurement of albumin in 24-hour urine sample for evaluation of renal disorders associated with microalbuminuria

REFERENCE RANGE
- <30 mg/24 hours
    Please refer to your institution's reference ranges as lab normals may vary.

INDICATIONS
Suspected microalbuminuric diabetic nephropathy
    Strength of Recommendation: Class IIb
    Strength of Evidence: Category B
Results Interpretation:
Increased albumin
    The spot urine sample is preferred over the 24-hour urine collection method for microalbuminuria screening for diabetic nephropathy.
    Persistent microalbuminuria (30 to 299 mg/24 hours) occurs in the earliest stage of diabetic nephropathy in type 1 diabetes, and is a marker for the development of nephropathy in type 2 diabetes.
    Macroalbuminuria is defined as greater than or equal to 300 mg/24 hours. Diabetics who proceed from microalbuminuria to macroalbuminuria are at increased risk of developing end-stage renal disease during the course of their disease.
Frequency of Monitoring
    Presence of microalbuminuria should be confirmed with repeated testing. At least 2 of 3 abnormal tests within a 3- to 6-month period is recommended to confirm the diagnosis of microalbuminuria or macroalbuminuria.

Suspected renal disease in patients with hypertension
    Strength of Recommendation: Class IIa
    Strength of Evidence: Category C

Results Interpretation:
Microalbuminuria

Microalbuminuria is defined as a urine albumin excretion of 30 to 300 mg/24 hours. The presence of microalbuminuria is a sensitive indicator of kidney disease in patients with hypertension. Increased urine albumin appears before other measurable changes in renal function and is indicative of small blood vessel disease in the kidney.

Frequency of Monitoring

The National Kidney Foundation recommends a confirmation test within 3 months of initial detection of microalbuminuria. Patients at risk for renal dysfunction (eg, diabetics, hypertensives) should be monitored annually for microalbuminuria.

ABNORMAL RESULTS

- Transient albuminuria can occur in:
  - Decompensated heart failure
  - Fever
  - Urinary tract infection
  - Strenuous exercise
  - Marked hyperglycemia
  - Sleep apnea

COLLECTION/STORAGE INFORMATION

- Collect a 24-hour urine without use of preservatives.
- Store at 2°C to 4°C; freeze for longer storage.

LOINC CODES

- Code: 30003-8 (*Short Name* - Microalbumin 24H Cnc Ur)
- Code: 14956-7 (*Short Name* - Microalbumin 24H rate Ur)

Microbial culture of sputum

TEST DEFINITION

Culture of sputum to diagnose etiology of lower respiratory tract infections

REFERENCE RANGE

Adults and Children: Negative
Please refer to your institution's reference ranges as lab normals may vary.

INDICATIONS

Patients with aspiration pneumonitis and a suspected secondary bacterial infection
Results Interpretation:
Positive microbiology findings

A sputum culture may be necessary for patients with aspiration pneumonitis when pathogenic organisms invade the injured lung and produce a secondary infection.

Patients hospitalized for community-acquired pneumonia
Strength of Recommendation: Class IIb
Strength of Evidence: Category B
Results Interpretation:
Positive microbiology findings

The utility of sputum culture in the treatment of community-acquired pneumonia remains controversial due to the difficulty in obtaining a good quality sputum specimen (ie, absence [or minimum] of contamination of specimen with upper airway flora). Inadequate sputum samples (ie, predominantly upper respiratory or contained oropharyngeal flora) were reported in 46% of samples. The regular contamination of specimens by the resident oropharyngeal commensal flora, and the fact that the identity of the organism is not often determined using standard culture techniques, limits the usefulness of testing.

Patients hospitalized for pneumonia should have an expectorated sputum Gram stain and culture. A deep-cough specimen should be obtained before antibiotic treatment and rapidly processed within a few hours of collection.

Bacterial pathogens that have been cultured in sputum specimens of patients with bacterial respiratory infection have included *Haemophilus influenzae, Streptococcus pneumoniae, Moraxella catarrhalis, Staphylococcus aureus, Klebsiella pneumoniae, Streptococcus viridans, Escherichia coli, Neisseria meningitidis, Enterobacteria, Pseudomonas aeruginosa,* and *Pasteurella multocida.*

Etiologic diagnosis is probable with a compatible clinical syndrome combined with detection by culture of a likely pulmonary pathogen in respiratory secretions (eg, expectorated sputum). There should be significant growth with quantitative culture or moderate or heavy growth with semiquantitative culture.

Timing of Monitoring

Expectorated sputum specimen should be a deep-cough specimen obtained before antibiotic treatment and should be processed within a few hours of collection.

Suspected acute chest syndrome
   Results Interpretation:
   Abnormal laboratory findings

Culture findings include Streptococcus pneumoniae, Haemophilus influenzae, Salmonella species, Staphylococcus aureus, Escherichia coli, and Mycoplasma pneumoniae.

Suspected plague
   Results Interpretation:
   Positive microbiology findings

It takes about 48 hours before colonies can be seen on plain agar.
The colonies are small and grayish.

Suspected sepsis
   Strength of Recommendation: Class IIb
   Strength of Evidence: Category C
   Results Interpretation:
   Positive microbiology findings

Sputum cultures should be obtained as part of the diagnostic work up of sepsis.

CLINICAL NOTES

Specimens can easily be contaminated with saliva (greater than 25 squamous epithelial cell per low power field); these samples are rejected for bacterial culture in some laboratories.

COLLECTION/STORAGE INFORMATION

- Specimen Collection and Handling:
    - Collect expectorated or induced sputum sample.
    - Instruct patient to rinse mouth and gargle with water and to cough deeply and expectorate sputum (preferably 5 to 10 mL) into sterile container. For patients with a non-productive cough, have patient breathe aerosolized droplets of a solution of 15% sodium chloride and 10% glycerin for about 10 minutes to induce cough reflex.
    - Collect lower respiratory secretions via a tracheal aspirate in patients with a tracheostomy and place in a Lukens trap.
    - Collect early morning sample.
    - Transport specimen to lab immediately (less than one hour) or refrigerate.

LOINC CODES

- Code: 17893-9 (*Short Name* - Spt Aerobe Cult org #2)
- Code: 17896-2 (*Short Name* - Spt Aerobe Cult org #5)
- Code: 17895-4 (*Short Name* - Spt Aerobe Cult org #4)
- Code: 6460-0 (*Short Name* - Spt Routine Cult)
- Code: 17894-7 (*Short Name* - Spt Aerobe Cult org #3)
- Code: 622-1 (*Short Name* - Spt Aerobe Cult)
- Code: 624-7 (*Short Name* - Spt Resp Cult)

Microbial identification kit, rapid strep method

TEST DEFINITION

Rapid detection of streptococcal antigen from throat smears for the identification of group A beta-hemolytic streptococcal infection

SYNONYMS

- Streptococcus screening test, direct

REFERENCE RANGE

- Negative
  Please refer to your institution's reference ranges as lab normals may vary.

INDICATIONS

Suspected group A beta-hemolytic streptococcal throat infection
> **Strength of Recommendation:** Class IIa
> **Strength of Evidence:** Category B
> **Results Interpretation:**
> **Positive microbiology findings**
>> A positive result on a rapid antigen detection test (RADT) in the presence of 2 or more clinical criteria for streptococcal pharyngitis may be sufficient to diagnose and treat group A beta-hemolytic streptococcus (GAS) infection.
>
> **Negative microbiology findings**
>> Some advisory groups recommend that a negative rapid antigen detection test (RADT) be confirmed by culture.

COLLECTION/STORAGE INFORMATION

- Adequately swab both tonsils, initiating at the most inflamed spots.
- May store at 4°C.

Microbial ova-parasite examination, fecal

TEST DEFINITION

Detection of ova or parasites in stool for suspected intestinal parasitic infection.

SYNONYMS

- Microbial ova-parasite examination, faecal

REFERENCE RANGE

- Negative
  Please refer to your institution's reference ranges as lab normals may vary.

INDICATIONS

Chronic diarrhea of more than 4 weeks with suspected intestinal parasitic infection
> **Strength of Recommendation:** Class I
> **Strength of Evidence:** Category B
> **Results Interpretation:**
> **Feces: parasite present**
>> The finding of ova or parasites in stool in association with patient history and comorbidities may likely confirm the etiology of chronic organic diarrhea.

Frequency of Monitoring

For direct stool observation, following fixation and staining, the classical recommendation is that three sequential samples must be observed for maximal detection; however, other studies indicate that, in most instances, a single pooled specimen has adequate sensitivity to support a diagnosis. Notable exceptions include *Entamoeba histolytica*, *G lambia*, and hookworms, where as many as four observations may be necessary to provide a 5% false negative rate.

COLLECTION/STORAGE INFORMATION

* Patient Preparation:
  * Maintain patients on a lactose-free diet for several days prior to evaluation.
  * Avoid antimicrobial therapy capable of affecting gastrointestinal flora for one week prior to obtaining sample.
  * Avoid antidiarrheal medication, oily laxatives, antacids, and barium contrast studies for one week prior to evaluation.
* Specimen Collection and Handling:
  * Collect fresh stool sample in wax paper or dry plastic container taking care to avoid contamination with water or urine.
  * If using a commercial kit, follow the manufacturer's directions.
  * Transport specimen immediately to lab.
  * If lab analysis can not be performed within 30 to 60 minutes, add appropriate (lab specified) preservative to specimen.

LOINC CODES

* Code: 18493-7 (*Short Name* - O+P sp3 Stl Conc)
* Code: 18307-9 (*Short Name* - O+P Stl IH Stn)
* Code: 18496-0 (*Short Name* - O+P #2 Stl Tri Stn)
* Code: 13319-9 (*Short Name* - O&P Prep #2 Stl)
* Code: 10704-5 (*Short Name* - O+P Stl Micro)
* Code: 13320-7 (*Short Name* - O&P Prep #3 Stl)
* Code: 18495-2 (*Short Name* - O+P sp3 Stl Tri Stn)
* Code: 10701-1 (*Short Name* - O+P Stl Conc)
* Code: 18494-5 (*Short Name* - O+P #2 Stl Conc)
* Code: 20925-4 (*Short Name* - O+P Stl McMaster Conc)
* Code: 9785-7 (*Short Name* - O+P Prep Stl)
* Code: 20924-7 (*Short Name* - O+P Stl Sedimentation)
* Code: 32357-6 (*Short Name* - O+P Stl)
* Code: 10702-9 (*Short Name* - O+P Stl ImStn)
* Code: 10703-7 (*Short Name* - O+P Stl KH Stn)

Microbial ova-parasite examination, urine

TEST DEFINITION

Detection of ova or parasites in urine for evaluation of suspected parasitic infection

REFERENCE RANGE

* Negative
Please refer to your institution's reference ranges as lab normals may vary.

INDICATIONS

Suspected schistosomiasis
  Strength of Recommendation: Class IIa
  Strength of Evidence: Category A
  Results Interpretation:
  Presence of ova cysts and parasites - finding
    The number of eggs per 10 mL of urine, as detected by microscopic direct examination, indicates infection severity and may reflect total body worm burden in schistosomiasis. However, one-point excretion counts are not reliable, and multiple daily measurements are required for accurate diagnosis.

Both circulating anodic antigens (CAA) assays and circulating cathodic antigens (CCA) assays are a measure of worm load; however, they may not reflect tissue egg load. The diagnostic utility of urine CCA assays increases when parallel serum CAA measurements are performed.

Genital schistosomiasis in women may occur in the absence of egg excretion in urine.

COLLECTION/STORAGE INFORMATION

- Collect last 10 to 20 mL of passed urine, or collect terminal urine specimens for 24 hours. Urine collected near midday has highest yield.
- Collect urine for microscopy for 2 to 3 consecutive days.
- Centrifuge urine for direct wet mount preparation.
- Add 0.5 mL of 10% formalin to specimen if examination is delayed.

Microhemagglutination test for antibody to syphilis

TEST DEFINITION

Detection of antibodies to *Treponema pallidum* in serum for the presumptive diagnosis of syphilis

REFERENCE RANGE

- Adults and children: nonreactive
  Please refer to your institution's reference ranges as lab normals may vary.

INDICATIONS

Suspected syphilis
   Results Interpretation:
   Positive laboratory findings
      A positive nontreponemal test followed by a positive microhemagglutination test is suggestive of syphilis.
      Up to 85% of patients who undergo treatment for syphilis will remain seropositive indefinitely regardless of disease state or treatment rendered, while the remaining 15% to 25% of patients will return to seronegative status in 2 to 3 years.
      Inconclusive microhemagglutination test results have been observed in patients with infectious mononucleosis who have high heterophil antibody levels.

CLINICAL NOTES

Because no relationship between titer levels and disease progression or treatment response has been established, results are reported qualitatively, rather than quantitatively.

LOINC CODES

- Code: 8041-6 (*Short Name* - T pallidum Ab Ser Ql IHA)
- Code: 26009-1 (*Short Name* - T pallidum Ab Titr Ser IHA)

Microscopy (acid fast bacilli)

TEST DEFINITION

Microscopic examination of tissue or fluid specimen stained smear for detection of acid-fast bacilli (AFB) and management of mycobacterial infections

REFERENCE RANGE

- Negative
  Please refer to your institution's reference ranges as lab normals may vary.

INDICATIONS

Suspected atypical mycobacterial infection
Strength of Recommendation: Class IIa
Strength of Evidence: Category C
Results Interpretation:
Positive microbiology findings

In developing countries, *Mycobacterium tuberculosis* is the primary mycobacterium detected in sputum by smear microscopy. Atypical nontuberculosis mycobacteria (NTM) mainly infect immunocompromised patients; however, these infections are not as easily diagnosed by the acid-fast sputum smear.

AFB smears cannot distinguish between *M. tuberculosis* and nontuberculosis mycobacteria infections. The NTM *M. bovis* may cause up to 6.2% of all tuberculosis cases.

Suspected tuberculosis
Strength of Recommendation: Class I
Strength of Evidence: Category C
Results Interpretation:
Positive microbiology findings

The detection of *M. tuberculosis* AFB in stained smears provides preliminary confirmation of tuberculosis (TB) diagnosis. Quantitation of AFB positive smears is necessary and if each specimen only has 1 or 2 bacilli upon microscopic examination, a repeat specimen collection is recommended. A minimum of 5,000 to 10,000 organisms/mL in sputum must be present for a positive acid-fast bacilli (AFB) smear test.

In the setting of high clinical suspicion for TB, a positive AFB test is sufficient to prompt the initiation of treatment while waiting for culture results. If suspicion for active TB is minimal and AFB smears are negative, treatment can be delayed until culture results are available.

Unconcentrated AFB sputum smears accurately reflect infectivity status. Patients with positive smears are the most infectious. Patients with positive cultures and negative sputum smears are less contagious.

Although the detection of mycobacteria in cerebrospinal fluid (CSF) by AFB smear staining is diagnostic for TB meningitis, AFB-CSF positivity rates are low because patients have typically been on antibiotic therapy prior to hospital admission, resulting in poor CSF mycobacteria yields.

Variations in AFB smear positivity rates occur in relation to tissue specimen histological category. In necrotizing granuloma specimens, the AFB test with auramine-rhodamine staining may be more sensitive than culture for bacilli.

Sixty percent to 80% of patients with minimally to moderately advanced cavitary disease may have negative AFB smears vs 5% to 10% of patients with far-advanced cavitary lesions.

HIV infection does not appear to compromise the diagnostic utility of sputum AFB smears. A presumptive diagnosis of pulmonary TB should be made in HIV patients with positive AFB sputum smears.

AFB smears may remain positive longer than cultures in patients who have received chemotherapy; however, AFB sputum stains do not distinguish viable from nonviable bacilli.

Patients with AFB-positive smears should be reported promptly to the public health department; the CDC recommends that positive respiratory specimen test results be reported within 24 hours.

A decrease in the number of *M tuberculosis* bacilli in sputum indicates a favorable response to treatment. Repeat positive AFB smears or a return of positive smears after a period of negative smears suggests a poor response to treatment. A positive AFB sputum in cases of treatment failure indicates the need for an empirical retreatment regimen until susceptibility tests are available. In a retreatment program, AFB rapidly disappear from sputum during or after the first phase of short-course chemotherapy.

Negative microbiology findings

Twenty percent to 60% of patients with positive *M tuberculosis* cultures will have negative AFB smears. Therefore, a negative AFB smear does not rule out active pulmonary TB.

Frequency of Monitoring

In TB positive patients receiving treatment, monthly AFB smears and cultures should be obtained until 2 consecutive specimen cultures are negative. Additional AFB smears may be indicated in order to assess early response to treatment.

CLINICAL NOTES

The CDC recommends the fluorochrome smear staining method (auramine-rhodamine) for detection of acid-fast bacilli (AFB) because it is more accurate than carbol fuchsin staining.

Inexperienced or poorly trained lab personnel can reduce AFB smear test accuracy.

The anatomical specimen for the AFB smear test and culture should be the same.

Bronchoalveolar lavage can be used if patients are unable to produce an adequate sputum sample.

COLLECTION/STORAGE INFORMATION

- Specimen Collection and Handling:
    - Refrigerate specimens from contaminated sites (eg, sputum, respiratory and gastric secretions, urine, and feces) if unable to process immediately.
    - If gastric lavage specimen processing is delayed, add 10% sodium hydroxide to the sample until the pH is neutral.
    - Collect early morning sputum and voided urine specimens on 3 consecutive days.

Microsomal thyroid antibody measurement

TEST DEFINITION

Measurement of anti-microsomal antibodies, particularly thyroid peroxidase antibodies, in serum for the evaluation of thyroid disease

REFERENCE RANGE

- Adults and Children:
- Thyroid microsomal antibodies :
- Hemagglutination: Nondetectable
- Complement fixation antibody: <1:100
- Competitive protein binding radioassay: ≤25 units/mL (≤25 kilounits/L)
- Immunoradiometric assay: 280 ± 60 units/mL (280 ± 60 kilounits/L)
- Thyroid peroxidase antibodies (immunometric): 69 ± 15 units/mL (69 ± 15 kilounits/L)
    Please refer to your institution's reference ranges as lab normals may vary.

INDICATIONS

Suspected autoimmune thyroiditis
   Strength of Recommendation: Class IIa
   Strength of Evidence: Category B
   Results Interpretation:
   Autoantibody titer positive
      Elevated anti-microsomal antibodies are found in autoimmune thyroiditis. They are markers for subclinical thyroid disease and of increased risk for progression to hypothyroidism.
      Positive anti-microsomal antibody titers occur in greater than 90% of patients with Hashimoto's thyroiditis, the most common form of autoimmune thyroiditis.

Suspected Graves' disease
   Strength of Recommendation: Class IIa
   Strength of Evidence: Category B
   Results Interpretation:
   Autoantibody titer positive
      Elevated anti-thyroid peroxidase antibodies (TPOAb) are found in approximately 75% of patients with Graves' disease, and their presence may be helpful in confirming an otherwise unclear diagnosis.
      High titers of anti-microsomal antibodies indicate Graves' disease in patients presenting with clinical and biochemical evidence of hyperthyroidism.

Thyroid cancer
   Strength of Recommendation: Class IIb
   Strength of Evidence: Category B
   Results Interpretation:
   Autoantibody titer positive
      Anti-thyroid peroxidase antibodies (TPOAb) occur more frequently in patients with differentiated thyroid carcinoma than in the general population, and levels appear to decline following treatment.

ABNORMAL RESULTS

- During pregnancy, titers gradually decrease, followed by a transient increase postpartum.

CLINICAL NOTES

Anti-thyroid peroxidase antibody (TPOAb) is the primary, if not the only, anti-microsomal antibody, and assays for TPOAb are more sensitive and specific than hemagglutination tests for anti-microsomal antibodies. TPOAb is more significantly associated with thyroid disease than is anti-thyroglobulin antibody.

COLLECTION/STORAGE INFORMATION

• Draw blood for a serum specimen.

LOINC CODES

• Code: 5382-7 (*Short Name* - TPO Ab Ser RIA-aCnc)
• Code: 11574-1 (*Short Name* - TPO Ab Ser-aCnc)
• Code: 32042-4 (*Short Name* - TPO Ab Ser QI)
• Code: 5383-5 (*Short Name* - TPO Ab Titr Ser LA)
• Code: 17706-3 (*Short Name* - TPO Ab Titr CSF LA)

Monocyte count

TEST DEFINITION

Measurement of monocytes in blood for the evaluation and management of immunologic, hematologic, and neoplastic disorders

SYNONYMS

• Monocyte count - observation

REFERENCE RANGE

• Adults:
• Absolute: 0.2-0.95 x 10^3 cells/microL
• Relative: 4%-11%
• Adults, 21 years:
• Absolute: 0-0.8 x 10^3 cells/microL
• Relative: 4%
• Neonates, Birth to 2 days
• Absolute: 0-2 x 10^3 cells/microL
• Neonates, 4 days to 28 days:
• Absolute: 0-1.7 x 10^3 cells/microL
• Infants, 1 to 4 weeks:
• Absolute: 0.7 x 10^3 cells/microL
• Infants, 6 months to 1 year:
• Absolute: 0.6 x 10^3 cells/microL
• Infants, 1 year:
• Relative: 4.8%
• Children, 2 years:
• Absolute: 0-1 x 10^3 cells/microL
• Children, 4 to 10 years:
• Absolute: 0-0.8 x 10^3 cells/microL
• Relative: 4.3%-5%
   Please refer to your institution's reference ranges as lab normals may vary.

INDICATIONS

Assessment of risk for complications following acute myocardial infarction
   Strength of Recommendation: Class IIb
   Strength of Evidence: Category B
   Results Interpretation:
   Monocytosis
   The peripheral monocytosis that occurs 2 to 3 days after acute myocardial infarction (AMI) reflects infiltration of monocytes and macrophages into the necrotic myocardium. A peak monocytosis, at or above 900/mm^3, is associated with complications of left ventricular dysfunction and left ventricular aneurysm, and suggests a possible role of monocytes in left ventricular remodeling following reperfusion AMI.

Daily monitoring of peripheral blood monocyte counts may have prognostic value in patients with acute myocardial infarction.

Suspected brucellosis
Strength of Recommendation: Class IIa
Strength of Evidence: Category C
Results Interpretation:
Monocyte count raised
Monocytosis and mild anemia are common children with brucellosis, whereas thrombocytopenia, leukocytosis, and leukopenia are uncommon.

Suspected monocytic leukemia
Strength of Recommendation: Class I
Strength of Evidence: Category B
Results Interpretation:
Monocyte count raised
Acute monocytic, chronic monocytic, acute myelomonocytic, and chronic myelomonocytic leukemia may be associated with markedly increased numbers of monoblasts and/or monocytes in the peripheral blood and bone marrow. In patients with typical bone marrow findings of acute myelomonocytic leukemia, peripheral monocytosis (equal to or greater than 5×10^9 /L) is common.

Typical peripheral blood findings in chronic myelomonocytic leukemia (CMML) include persistent monocytosis (greater than 1×10^9 /L), neutrophilia with morphologic abnormalities, and less than 5% blasts. Adults with CMML have monocytosis, whether they have features of myeloproliferative disorders (neutrophilia, splenomegaly) or of myelodysplastic disorders (normal or low neutrophil counts, no organomegaly).

Suspected monocytopenia
Strength of Recommendation: Class IIb
Strength of Evidence: Category B
Results Interpretation:
Monocyte count abnormal
If the total leukocyte count is normal or increased, a low percent (eg, 0%) differential monocyte count may suggest an absolute monocytosis, but the diagnosis requires an automated count of many more cells (eg, 10,000) to document absolute (vs relative) monocytopenia (ie, monocytes concentration below the 95% confidence interval).

Monocytopenia refers to a concentration of circulating monocytes below the lower reference value for the method used.

Because large numbers of counted cells are required in a differential to obtain reliable counts, few studies addressed monocytopenia prior to the availability of automated blood counting methods. Monocytopenia has been associated with hairy cell leukemia and brief transient monocytopenia with prednisone therapy.

Suspected monocytosis
Results Interpretation:
Monocytosis
Monocytosis is an increased concentration (vs percentage) of monocytes above the upper reference value. Pathologic (disease-related) monocytosis is associated with brucellosis, some drugs, Hodgkin's disease, leukemia, and tuberculosis. Monocytosis during the recovery stage of acute infection is a favorable prognostic sign, whereas monocytosis in tuberculosis is an unfavorable prognostic sign.

Monocytosis is sometimes a clue to a specific disease. In a case series of 11 AIDS patients with *Mycobacterium fortuitum* infection, 7 patients had relative and 4 patients had absolute monocytosis.

Hematologic diseases (leukemia, lymphoma [typically Hodgkin's disease], multiple myeloma, myeloproliferative disorders) are relatively common causes of monocytosis. In a study of 160 patients with absolute monocytosis, 53% had hematologic disease, 10% had connective tissue disease, 8% had nonhematologic malignancy, and only 6% had infectious disease.

COMMON PANELS
• Complete blood count with automated differential

CLINICAL NOTES
The percentage of monocytes in a differential count is relative to other leukocytes, not the concentration in blood. Thus, if the total leukocyte count is low, a normal percentage of monocytes indicates an absolute decrease in concentration of monocytes.

Relative monocyte counts percentage are included in differential leukocyte counts, but absolute monocyte counts are used to define monocytosis and monocytopenia. The absolute count (concentration) is the percentage of monocytes times the total leukocyte count.

Normal ranges for monocyte counts depend on the automated technique used, with automated methods reporting higher monocyte counts than manual methods.

The reproducibility of 100-cell manual leukocyte differentials is poor.

An automated differential that classifies 10,000 leukocytes has a much narrower range of normal (95% confidence interval) than a manual differential that classifies 100 leukocytes, with the automated differential permitting detection of monocytopenia and abnormal changes in monocyte counts that are unappreciated when using manual 100-leukocyte differentials

COLLECTION/STORAGE INFORMATION
- Specimen Collection and Handling:
  - Collect 7 mL of venous blood in lavender top (EDTA) tube
  - Do not use heparin
  - Stable for 24 hours at 23°C; 48 hours at 4°C

LOINC CODES
- Code: 30440-2 (*Short Name* - Abn Monocytes # Bld)
- Code: 29260-7 (*Short Name* - Abn Monocytes # Bld Manual)
- Code: 26484-6 (*Short Name* - Monocytes # Bld)

Mumps Virus antibody assay

TEST DEFINITION
Measurement of antibody to the mumps virus to confirm diagnosis or assess immune status

SYNONYMS
- Serologic test for Mumps virus

REFERENCE RANGE
- Adults and children: Less than a four-fold increase between acute and convalescent titers
  Please refer to your institution's reference ranges as lab normals may vary.

INDICATIONS
Suspected mumps exposure; determination of immunity to mumps
    Strength of Recommendation: Class IIb
    Strength of Evidence: Category C
    Results Interpretation:
    Serology positive
        A positive test can diagnose recent illness or previous infection. A four-fold rise in antibody titer between acute and convalescent titers (approximately 2 weeks apart) can confirm recent viral exposure.
        Antibody titers rise following vaccination, and seroconversion can be evaluated by obtaining baseline and post-vaccination titers.

CLINICAL NOTES
Enzyme immunoassay and neutralization test are the most sensitive assays.

COLLECTION/STORAGE INFORMATION
- Specimen Collection and Handling:
  - Collect serum samples at onset of disease and 2 to 4 weeks later to determine acute and convalescent titers; freeze samples if not tested immediately.
  - Specimen collection may include serum or CSF.

LOINC CODES
- Code: 30146-5 (*Short Name* - MuV Ab sp2 Ser Ql)
- Code: 17293-2 (*Short Name* - MuV IgG+IgM Ser-aCnc)

Mumps virus culture

TEST DEFINITION
Detection of the mumps virus for the evaluation and diagnosis of parotitis

REFERENCE RANGE
- Adults and children: No growth
  Please refer to your institution's reference ranges as lab normals may vary.

INDICATIONS
Suspected mumps
> **Strength of Recommendation:** Class IIb
> **Strength of Evidence:** Category B
> **Results Interpretation:**
> **Positive microbiology findings**
> While the diagnosis of mumps is usually made clinically, positive tissue cultures can confirm the diagnosis of mumps and may be available within a week. The shell vial method is a rapid and specific culture; results are usually available in 2 to 3 days or longer.
> Throat swabs and urine samples have similar efficacy when obtained during the first 7 to 10 days after symptoms appear; however, urine testing may be more helpful after this period because the virus can be detected for up to 2 weeks.

COLLECTION/STORAGE INFORMATION
- Use a sterile culture swab for obtaining specimens (eg, saliva, throat) and place in virus transport medium; transport all specimens immediately to lab.
- Body fluid specimens should be held at 4°C or, if delay in processing, frozen at -70°C.
- CSF samples may be incubated at 37°C; do not refrigerate.

LOINC CODES
- Code: 13921-2 (*Short Name - MuV XXX QI Cult*)

Myoglobin measurement, urine

TEST DEFINITION
Detection of myoglobin in urine as a marker of cardiac or skeletal muscle damage

REFERENCE RANGE
- By Method:
- Ammonium sulfate solubility: Negative
- Colorimetric: Greater than 0.85 A_{600}/A_{580} (sensitive to a myoglobin concentration of 30 mg/dL)
- Complement fixation (CF), nephelom, precipitin: <0.1-0.2 mg/dL (<1-2 mg/L) (sensitivity 1 mcg/L)
- Electrophoresis (EP): Negative
- Hemagglutination: Negative (sensitivity 1 mcg/mL)
- Isoelectric focusing (IEF): Negative
- Orthotoludidine: Negative
- Radial immunodiffusion (RID): <5 mg/dL (<50 mg/L) (sensitivity 15 mcg/mL)
- Radioimmunoassay (RIA): 0.4 - 4 mcg/day (sensitivity 0.5 mcg/L)
- Ultrafiltration: Absence of heme protein
  Please refer to your institution's reference ranges as lab normals may vary.

INDICATIONS
Suspected neuroleptic malignant syndrome
> **Results Interpretation:**
> **Myoglobinuria**
> Myoglobinuria, present in about two thirds of patients, reflects severe myonecrosis and enhances the risk of acute renal failure.

Suspected rhabdomyolysis
> **Strength of Recommendation:** Class IIa
> **Strength of Evidence:** Category C
Results Interpretation:
Myoglobinuria
> Myoglobin concentration in the urine is dependent on renal function. It is noted in urine if plasma concentration exceeds 0.5 to 1.5 mg/dL, but only becomes visible when urine myoglobin is greater than 100 mg/dL.
> Myoglobin is present if urine dipstick is positive for blood, despite the absence of erythrocytes on microscopic examination.
> * Results:
>   * Visual presentation: Pigmented red-brown (tea-colored) urine with occasional dense brown casts. Myoglobin may be present without appreciable color change, resembling concentrated urine specimen.
>   * Microscopic evaluation:
>   * Erythrocytes: present occasionally
>   * Protein: present or absent

> **False Results**
> In one study, 18% of patients with rhabdomyolysis had a negative orthotoluidine test for myoglobin.

CLINICAL NOTES
Lysis of as little as 200 g of skeletal muscle may result in myoglobinuria.

COLLECTION/STORAGE INFORMATION
* Specimen Collection and Handling:
  * Use fresh urine or urine adjusted to pH 7 with 0.1 mol/L sodium hydroxide
  * Observe color promptly since myoglobin will change from red to brown upon standing
  * May freeze at -25° C for up to 2 years

LOINC CODES
* Code: 32197-6 (*Short Name* - Myoglobin 24H Ur-mCnc)
* Code: 2641-9 (*Short Name* - Myoglobin Ur-mCnc)
* Code: 2642-7 (*Short Name* - Myoglobin 24H Ur-mRate)
* Code: 11147-6 (*Short Name* - Myoglobin/creat Ur-mRto)

Nasopharyngeal culture

TEST DEFINITION
Detection and screening via culture of nasopharyngeal specimens to assess for the carrier state of *S aureus* or for suspected infection (eg, B *pertussis*)

SYNONYMS
* Nasopharynx culture

REFERENCE RANGE
* Adults and Children: Negative
Please refer to your institution's reference ranges as lab normals may vary.

INDICATIONS
Suspected meningococcal disease in patients with prior antibiotic treatment
> **Results Interpretation:**
> **Positive microbiology findings**
> In about 50% of patients with systemic disease, meningococci can be isolated from the posterior pharyngeal wall, preferably accessed through the mouth (or through the nose if the patient is unconscious or delirious). When meningococcal disease is confirmed by culture, meningococci isolated from the nasopharynx are indistinguishable from strains obtained from the patient's blood or cerebrospinal fluid.
> Cultures are particularly valuable if antibiotics have been given before admission since, unlike blood and cerebrospinal fluid cultures, nasopharyngeal cultures are not affected by prior antibiotic treatment.

Oro- or nasopharyngeal cultures are not helpful in determining the need for chemoprophylaxis in patient contacts.

Negative microbiology findings

A single negative throat swab is unreliable in predicting noncarriers of meningococci. Awaiting culture results may unnecessarily delay the institution of chemoprophylaxis. The risk of disease is highest during the 2 to 3 days it takes to obtain the culture results.

Suspected respiratory tract infection due to pertussis
>   **Strength of Recommendation:** Class IIa
>   **Strength of Evidence:** Category C
> **Results Interpretation:**
> **Nose swab culture positive**

A positive culture in a symptomatic patient is diagnostically specific for pertussis. The highest predictive value of positive culture results is associated with age less than 5 years, acute symptoms of spasmodic cough, and lymphocytosis (WBC greater than 10,000/mm(3)).

Cultures are likely to be positive in 50% to 60% of patients during the first 2 weeks of illness, decrease to 30% to 40% in the following 2 weeks, and usually are not positive after 6 weeks. In addition, cultures are likely to be positive in patients in whom specimens are collected less than 21 days after onset of cough, who are not receiving erythromycin/sulfamethoxazole prior to culture, who have had less than 3 doses of pertussis vaccine, and whose specimen got to the laboratory in less than 4 days. Inadequate specimen collection may decrease sensitivity.

Failure to isolate *B pertussis* does not exclude the diagnosis. Organisms grow slowly; it may take 4 to 5 days for culture results to become positive. Reliance on culture alone for diagnosis can result in underdiagnosis and misdiagnosis. Extending the incubation period of cultures up to 12 days improves recovery rates for both *B pertussis* and *B parapertussis*.

CLINICAL NOTES

Nasopharyngeal aspirates are preferred to nasopharyngeal swabs in the diagnosis of pertussis.

COLLECTION/STORAGE INFORMATION
- Specimen Collection and Handling:
  - Insert swab approximately one inch into nose and rotate against nasal mucosa.
  - Collect specimen in sterile transport system.
  - Transport specimen immediately to lab.

Neisseria gonorrheae culture

TEST DEFINITION

Detection by culture of *Neisseria gonorrhoeae* in purulent discharge from endocervix, vagina, urethra, rectum, oropharynx, or conjunctiva, and, if disseminated infection is suspected, from skin lesions, blood, or synovial fluid

SYNONYMS
- Neisseria gonorrhoeae culture

REFERENCE RANGE
- No growth
  Please refer to your institution's reference ranges as lab normals may vary.

INDICATIONS

Suspected *Neisseria gonorrhoeae* infection
>   **Strength of Recommendation:** Class IIa
>   **Strength of Evidence:** Category C
> **Results Interpretation:**
> **Positive microbiology findings**

A minimum of 24 to 72 hours is required from specimen collection to definitive culture results. A positive culture confirms an isolate as *Neisseria gonorrhoeae*.

Patients with symptoms persisting after treatment should be evaluated by culture and antimicrobial susceptibility testing.

False Results
    Delayed plating of 12 to 48 hours must be avoided, as it may cause a 25% loss of positive results.

COMMON PANELS

- Prenatal screening panel

CLINICAL NOTES

Clinicians are strongly encouraged to report all positive *Neisseria gonorrhoeae* cultures to their local or state health department.

COLLECTION/STORAGE INFORMATION

- Specimen Collection and Handling:
    - Obtain gonococcal culture prior to Papanicolaou smear
    - Collect endocervical, vaginal, and rectal specimens under direct visualization using a speculum. Obtain urethral specimens with a smaller gauge sterile calcium alginate swab
    - Draw at least 10 mL for blood cultures
    - Obtain skin lesion specimens from scrapings of individual lesions
    - Incubate specimens at 35°C to 36.5° C in a CO_2 -enriched atmosphere
- Specimen Collection and Handling in Child Sexual Abuse:
    - Obtain specimens from the following sites:
        - Pharynx and anus in both boys and girls
        - Vagina in girls
        - Urethra in boys
        - For boys with a urethral discharge, a meatal discharge specimen is an adequate substitute for an intraurethral swab specimen.
    - Cervical specimens are not recommended for prepubertal girls.

LOINC CODES

- Code: 695-7 (*Short Name* - N gonorrhoea Snv QI Cult)
- Code: 688-2 (*Short Name* - N gonorrhoea Cvx QI Cult)
- Code: 691-6 (*Short Name* - N gonorrhoea Gen QI Cult)
- Code: 696-5 (*Short Name* - N gonorrhoea Thrt QI Cult)
- Code: 30099-6 (*Short Name* - N gonorrhoea Cnjt Cult-aCnc)
- Code: 690-8 (*Short Name* - N gonorrhoea Endm QI Cult)
- Code: 693-2 (*Short Name* - N gonorrhoea GenV QI Cult)
- Code: 694-0 (*Short Name* - N gonorrhoea Smn QI Cult)
- Code: 692-4 (*Short Name* - N gonorrhoea GenL QI Cult)
- Code: 697-3 (*Short Name* - N gonorrhoea Urth QI Cult)
- Code: 14127-5 (*Short Name* - N gonorrhoea Anal QI Cult)
- Code: 698-1 (*Short Name* - N gonorrhoea XXX QI Cult)

Neisseria gonorrheae nucleic acid amplification test

TEST DEFINITION

Amplification and detection of *Neisseria gonorrhoeae* -specific DNA or RNA sequences in clinical specimens

SYNONYMS

- Neisseria gonorrhoeae nucleic acid amplification test

REFERENCE RANGE

- Negative
    Please refer to your institution's reference ranges as lab normals may vary.

INDICATIONS

Suspected urogenital *Neisseria gonorrhoeae* **infection**
Strength of Recommendation: Class IIa
Strength of Evidence: Category A
Results Interpretation:
Positive laboratory findings
Nucleic acid amplification assays have moderate sensitivity and high specificity for the detection of urogenital gonorrhea infections.
Additional testing should be considered in a low prevalence setting.
Nucleic acid amplification tests may provide accurate and rapid diagnosis of gonorrheal infections in urogenital samples.

False Results
False-positive results may occur secondary to cross-reactivity with nongonococcal pathogenic and nonpathogenic *Neisseria*.

CLINICAL NOTES

Nucleic acid amplification testing (NAAT) may yield a positive result in the presence of very little target DNA or RNA.
NAAT may be helpful in settings that are not conducive to culture.
The ligase chain reaction assay for *Neisseria gonorrhoeae* (LCx®) is no longer commercially available.

COLLECTION/STORAGE INFORMATION

• Specimen Collection and Handling:
    • Urine specimen
        • Obtain first-catch urine (first 10 to 30 mLs voided after initiating stream) approximately 1 hour after last void.
        • Store urine for up to 24 hours at room temperature or at 2°C to 8°C for up to 5 days.
    • Endocervical and urethral specimen
        • Endocervical specimen: Remove all secretions and discharge from cervical os. Insert manufacturer-supplied swab 1 to 2 cm into endocervical canal, rotate 2 or more times, and withdraw without touching vaginal walls.
        • Urethral specimen: Insert urogenital swab gently into the urethra (females, 1 to 2 cm; males, 2 to 4 cm) and rotate in one direction for one or more revolutions and withdraw. In the presence of urethral discharge, exudate collected from the meatus is sufficient.
        • Immerse swab in manufacturer-supplied or isolation transport medium.
        • Store swab at 2°C to 27°C for up to 5 days or at 2°C to 8°C for up to 7 days.

Neisseria gonorrheae nucleic acid hybridization test

TEST DEFINITION

Detection of nucleotide sequences for the diagnosis of *Neisseria gonorrhoeae* infection

SYNONYMS

• Neisseria gonorrhoeae nucleic acid hybridization test

REFERENCE RANGE

• Negative
Please refer to your institution's reference ranges as lab normals may vary.

INDICATIONS

Suspected *Neisseria gonorrhoeae* **infection**
Strength of Recommendation: Class IIa
Strength of Evidence: Category B

Results Interpretation:
Positive biochemistry findings

A positive nucleic acid hybridization test should be considered presumptive evidence of *Neisseria gonorrhoeae* infection. Additional testing may be indicated in low-prevalence populations.

Culture may be preferred if antibiotic sensitivities are desired.

When using a nucleic acid hybridization test that will exhibit a positive result in the presence of either *Neisseria gonorrhoeae* or *Chlamydia trachomatis*, additional testing should be done to identify the causative organism(s).

COLLECTION/STORAGE INFORMATION

- Specimen Collection and Handling:
  - Endocervical specimen: Insert manufacturer-provided swab 1 to 2 cm into endocervical canal and rotate 2 or more times. Withdraw swab without touching any vaginal surface.
  - Urethral specimen: Collect fluid from discharge with manufacturer-provided swab. If no discharge is present, insert swab into urethra (males, 2 to 4 cm; females, 1 to 2 cm) 1 or more hours after voiding, and gently rotate several times in one direction.
  - Immerse swab in manufacturer-supplied medium.
  - Transport specimen within 7 days at 2°C to 25°C.
  - Freeze specimen at -20°C or below.
  - Specimen can be tested up to 60 days after collection.

Neuron-specific enolase measurement

TEST DEFINITION

Measurement of neuron-specific enolase, an enzyme primarily found in neurons, peripheral neuroendocrine tissue, and some tumors, used as a marker in certain diseases and injuries

SYNONYMS

- NSE measurement
- S-NSE measurement

REFERENCE RANGE

- Adults: Less than 12.5 mcg/L
  Please refer to your institution's reference ranges as lab normals may vary.

INDICATIONS

Acute cerebrovascular accident (CVA)
Strength of Recommendation: Class IIb
Strength of Evidence: Category B
Results Interpretation:
Increased level (laboratory finding)

Elevated NSE levels have been shown to correlate with size of infarction and with severity of symptoms in patients with acute anterior circulation stroke.

The ratio of NSE to carnosine may help to differentiate ischemic from hemorrhagic stroke in the absence of neuroimaging, with the highest ratios seen in patients with primary intracerebral hemorrhage. The NSE:carnosine ratio was significantly associated with 90-day outcome, with patients who died or were institutionalized having higher ratios than those who were discharged home.

Neuroblastoma
Strength of Recommendation: Class IIa
Strength of Evidence: Category B
Results Interpretation:
Increased level (laboratory finding)

Elevated serum levels of NSE correlate with stage of neuroblastoma, with higher levels generally corresponding to more advanced stages of the disease. NSE can be used as a marker for recurrence; in the majority of cases, elevated levels of NSE will either precede or rise concomitantly with a relapse.

Post-anoxic coma following cardiopulmonary resuscitation (CPR)
  Strength of Recommendation: Class IIb
  Strength of Evidence: Category B
  Results Interpretation:
  Increased level (laboratory finding)
    In the setting of post-anoxic coma, NSE serum levels greater than 25 mcg/L at 48 hours after admission may be predictive of the failure to regain consciousness. Validation in a prospective study of this retrospectively determined cutoff value is warranted.

Severe traumatic brain injury
  Strength of Recommendation: Class IIb
  Strength of Evidence: Category B
  Results Interpretation:
  Increased level (laboratory finding)
    Serum neuron-specific enolase (NSE) levels above 21.7 mcg/L may predict death or poor outcome within 6 months of traumatic brain injury (TBI). More data validating this model is needed prior to implementing routine clinical use of NSE in the setting of TBI.
    In children with inflicted TBI, a second peak in cerebral spinal fluid NSE levels may reflect delayed neuronal death and aid in establishing time of injury.
  Timing of Monitoring
    Some data suggest that variations in serum neuron-specific enolase values occur depending on how much time has lapsed between traumatic brain injury and blood draw.

Small cell lung cancer (SCLC)
  Strength of Recommendation: Class IIb
  Strength of Evidence: Category B
  Results Interpretation:
  Increased level (laboratory finding)
    An elevated NSE level appears to be fairly specific for SCLC and may indicate disease extent and progression. An elevated NSE level has been found to correlate with prognosis for SCLC. Further prospective studies may be helpful in establishing the clinical utility of this test.

COLLECTION/STORAGE INFORMATION
- Obtain venous or arterial blood sample
- Store sample at -70° C to 20° C until ready for assay

LOINC CODES
- Code: 10477-8 (*Short Name* - NSE Ag Tiss Ql ImStn)
- Code: 2225-1 (*Short Name* - NSE SerPl-cCnc)
- Code: 15060-7 (*Short Name* - NSE SerPl-mCnc)
- Code: 19193-2 (*Short Name* - NSE SerPl-aCnc)
- Code: 19194-0 (*Short Name* - NSE Plr-aCnc)

Neutrophil count

TEST DEFINITION
Measurement of neutrophils in blood for the evaluation and management of immunologic, hematologic, and neoplastic disorders

REFERENCE RANGE
- Adults:
- Relative: 40%-70%
- Absolute: 1.8-7.7 X 10^3 cells/microL
- Neonates, 0 to 11 hours:
- Absolute: 2-6 X 10^3 cells/microL
- Neonates, 12 hours:
- Absolute: 8-14 X 10^3 cells/microL
- Neonates, 1 day:
- Absolute: 7-13 X 10^3 cells/microL

- Neonates, 2 days:
- Absolute: 3.5-7.5 X 10^3 cells/microL
- Neonates, 4 days:
- Absolute: 1.8-6.5 X 10^3 cells/microL
- Neonates, 5 days to 4 weeks:
- Absolute: 1.8-5.4 X 10^3 cells/microL
- Infants, 6 months:
- Absolute: 1-8.5 X 10^3 cells/microL
- Children, 1 to 4 years:
- Absolute: 1.5-8.5 X 10^3 cells/microL
- Children, 6 years:
- Absolute: 1.5-8 X 10^3 cells/microL
- Children, 10 years:
- Absolute: 1.8-8 X 10^3 cells/microL
- Black or African Americans:
- Absolute: 1000-1400 cells/mm^3

Please refer to your institution's reference ranges as lab normals may vary.

INDICATIONS

Psoriasis
Strength of Recommendation: Class IIb
Strength of Evidence: Category C
Results Interpretation:
Increased level (laboratory finding)
In patients with psoriasis, an elevated neutrophil count may correlate with disease severity.

Suspected chronic benign neutropenia
Strength of Recommendation: Class I
Strength of Evidence: Category C
Results Interpretation:
Neutropenia
Chronic benign neutropenia (CBN) in infancy and childhood is typically first diagnosed at an age of less than 14 months with neutrophil counts dropping below 200/mm^3 and is usually accompanied by normal bone marrow with a low risk of severe bacterial infection. When an absolute neutrophil count (ANC) remains below 500 to 1000/mm^3 for 3 to 4 months without clinical indicators such as serious infection, a diagnosis of CBN may be established.

Although the severity of neutropenia often varies from case to case in childhood, an ANC less than 500/mm^3 may suggest CBN. Additionally, ANC values may fluctuate between zero and normal; therefore, during an acute infection, a patient with CBN may exhibit a rise in ANC to what is otherwise a normal value.

Neutrophil counts below 1.5 X 10^9 /L (in adults and children over 1 year) may be seen in certain ethnic groups (eg, blacks and Middle Eastern) when the patient is otherwise healthy and without repeated infections.

Suspected cyclic neutropenia
Strength of Recommendation: Class I
Strength of Evidence: Category C
Results Interpretation:
Neutropenia
A neutrophil count less than 200/mm^3 every 21 days is consistent with cyclic neutropenia.

Most patients (70%) with cyclic neutropenia experience repetitive infectious complications every 21 days in conjunction with regularly occurring neutropenic episodes that may persist for 3 to 10 days.
Frequency of Monitoring
Obtain neutrophil blood counts 2 to 3 times per week for up to 8 weeks to identify the 21-day cycle typifying cyclic neutropenia and to identify nadirs lasting 3 to 5 days.

Suspected drug-induced neutropenia
Strength of Recommendation: Class IIa
Strength of Evidence: Category B
Results Interpretation:
Neutropenia
Medications account for about 70% of all cases of neutropenia and are associated with mortality of up to 25%.

A severe decline of neutrophils in patients receiving antithyroid medications, antibiotics, anticonvulsants, or clozapine may indicate drug-induced neutropenia and is associated with a high incidence of infection.

Suspected febrile neutropenia in cancer patients
> **Strength of Recommendation:** Class I
> **Strength of Evidence:** Category C
Results Interpretation:
Neutropenia
- Neutropenia severity scales according to the National Cancer Institute (NCI):
  - Mild neutropenia: <1500/mm^3
  - Moderate neutropenia: <1500-1000/mm^3
  - Severe neutropenia: <1000-500/mm^3
  - Life-threatening or disabling neutropenia: <500/mm^3
- Cancer patients with severe neutropenia (less than 0.1 X 10^9/L) and no sign of fever or infection should be considered at high risk for developing fever, infection, and serious complications.
- Neutropenia of less than 7 days' duration or that is expected to resolve within 10 days is a low risk finding for severe infection in febrile neutropenic cancer patients.
- Infectious Diseases Society of America (IDSA) guidelines state that neutrophil counts are critical for determining the discontinuation of antibiotic therapy in cancer patients. When a neutrophil count reaches 500 cells/mm^3 or greater for 3 consecutive days and the patient is afebrile for 48 hours or more, antibiotic therapy may be safely discontinued.
- In a study of patients with small-cell lung cancer, the probability of developing fever was approximately 10% per day for each day that patients had a neutrophil count of less than 0.5 X 10^9/L.
- A patient's risk for developing fever and infection after chemotherapy is directly related to the severity and duration of neutropenia. One of the most important prognostic factors in these patients is the recovery of the neutrophil count. Neutropenia also may exacerbate the adverse effects of chemotherapy.

Suspected neonatal congenital neutropenia
> **Strength of Recommendation:** Class I
> **Strength of Evidence:** Category C
Results Interpretation:
Neutropenia
In neonates from birth to 5 days, a neutrophil count equal to or less than 500/microL may indicate a type of congenital neutropenia resulting from pregnancy-induced hypertension. Typically, this type of neutropenia resolves within 72 hours to 5 days.

Suspected neutropenia
> **Strength of Recommendation:** Class I
> **Strength of Evidence:** Category B
Results Interpretation:
Neutropenia
Neutropenia may be classified as mild (1-1.5 X 10^3/microL), moderate (0.5-1 X 10^3/microL), or severe (less than 0.2-0.5 X 10^3/microL).

Normal neutrophil counts vary in certain ethnic groups. Reportedly, 25% to 50% of individuals of blacks have a normal neutrophil count that is lower than the standard normal of 1.5 X 10^3/microL. Similar findings have been noted in individuals of Middle Eastern descent.

Transient instances of neutropenia in infants and children that resolves spontaneously within 2 weeks are rarely associated with clinical problems. Chronic neutropenia may be considered in the same population when neutrophil counts remain abnormally low for more than 6 months.

COMMON PANELS
- Complete blood count with automated differential

COLLECTION/STORAGE INFORMATION
- Specimen Collection and Handling:
  - Collect whole blood in purple top tube (EDTA)
  - Do not use heparin
  - Specimen is stable for 24 hours at 23°C and for 48 hours at 4°C

LOINC CODES

- Code: 759-1 (*Short Name* - Neutrophils # Prt Manual)
- Code: 17359-1 (*Short Name* - Neutrophils # Smn Manual)
- Code: 760-9 (*Short Name* - Neutrophils # Snv Manual)
- Code: 757-5 (*Short Name* - Neutrophils # Plr Manual)
- Code: 26504-1 (*Short Name* - Neutrophils # Snv)
- Code: 26503-3 (*Short Name* - Neutrophils # Smn)
- Code: 753-4 (*Short Name* - Neutrophils # Bld Manual)
- Code: 26502-5 (*Short Name* - Neutrophils # Prt)
- Code: 26499-4 (*Short Name* - Neutrophils # Bld)
- Code: 762-5 (*Short Name* - Neutrophils # Ur Manual)
- Code: 26501-7 (*Short Name* - Neutrophils # Plr)
- Code: 755-9 (*Short Name* - Neutrophils # CSF Manual)
- Code: 30448-5 (*Short Name* - Neutrophils # Ur)
- Code: 16290-9 (*Short Name* - Neutrophils Stl Ql)

Nortriptyline measurement

TEST DEFINITION

Measurement of nortriptyline in serum or plasma for therapeutic monitoring or suspected toxicity

SYNONYMS

- Nortryptyline measurement

REFERENCE RANGE

- Therapeutic Range: 50 - 170 ng/mL (190 - 646 nmol/L)
- Toxic Level: >500 ng/mL (>1.9 micromol/L)
  Please refer to your institution's reference ranges as lab normals may vary.

INDICATIONS

Suspected nortriptyline toxicity
> **Strength of Recommendation:** Class IIa
> **Strength of Evidence:** Category C
Results Interpretation:
Abnormal biochemistry findings
   Tricyclic serum or plasma levels are useful in initial assessment of suspected nortriptyline toxicity to confirm a history of ingestion. Monitor cardiac rhythm and obtain serial ECGs. Electrolytes, renal function, CPK and ABG levels should be followed as clinically indicated.

Therapeutic nortriptyline drug monitoring
> **Strength of Recommendation:** Class IIa
> **Strength of Evidence:** Category C
Results Interpretation:
Abnormal biochemistry findings
   Low nortriptyline levels may be due to insufficient dosage, noncompliance, or rapid metabolization of the drug. It may take several weeks to achieve therapeutic levels; dose adjustment should be considered in patients who do not reach therapeutic range within 2 to 4 weeks after medication is initiated. Fast metabolism of the drug may be idiosyncratic or caused by substances that promote the production of hepatic enzymes such as oral contraceptives, barbiturates or chloral hydrate..
   Plasma levels that are too high are due to too high a dose, slow drug metabolism, or noncompliance. Slow metabolism can be idiosyncratic or caused by concomitant administration of antipsychotics, cimetidine or fluoxetine. The elderly (over the age of 56 to 60) and those with comorbidities are at greater risk for developing high levels, and subsequent toxic effects, with therapeutic doses and therefore require more careful monitoring. Weight loss and different brands of medication may also impact plasma levels..
   Substantial variations in plasma levels can occur between different individuals receiving the same dose, and high levels of nortriptyline are not necessarily correlated with toxicity.

Timing of Monitoring
The ideal timing for specimen collection to determine steady-state levels is 10 to 14 hours after the last dose of medication for patients taking once-daily dosing, and just before the morning dose for patients who are on a divided-dosing schedule. To determine whether a patient is a slow, normal, or fast metabolizer, draw a sample after 5 days of continuous same-dose administration. If the laboratory has the ability to measure low plasma concentrations precisely, one level drawn 24 to 36 hours after a single dose of medication can also be used to evaluate the efficacy of a given dose.

CLINICAL NOTES
Reference methods for tricyclic antidepressants have not been determined. Intermethod variability is substantial and large coefficients of variation of methods exist. In addition, because of their relatively low therapeutic concentrations, tricyclic antidepressants are difficult to reliably analyze.

COLLECTION/STORAGE INFORMATION
Collection tubes containing gel separator are not suitable for tricyclic antidepressant specimen collection. The stoppers in vacuum blood collection systems must be free of tris-butoxyethyl phosphate which causes specimen contamination. Glass syringes are generally acceptable.
Specimens are stable at room temperature for 5 days and may be frozen up to 1 year. Specimens should be centrifuged as quickly as possible after collection.

LOINC CODES
- Code: 3874-5 (*Short Name* - Nortrip Ur Ql)
- Code: 3875-2 (*Short Name* - Nortrip Ur-mCnc)
- Code: 29407-4 (*Short Name* - Nortrip Gast-mCnc)

Ocular cytology

TEST DEFINITION
Evaluation of ocular cytology for rapid diagnosis of anterior segment eye disorders

REFERENCE RANGE
- Negative cytological examination
Please refer to your institution's reference ranges as lab normals may vary.

INDICATIONS
Morphologic determination of suspected ocular inflammation in the conjunctiva
Strength of Recommendation: Class IIb
Strength of Evidence: Category C
Results Interpretation:
Abnormal cytology findings
Conjunctival brush cytology (CBC) identifies abnormal cell populations including keratinized, elongated, and goblet cells in ocular specimens versus impression cytology where all 3 cell types are often not obtained, making CBC more reliable for indicating conjunctival inflammation and other ocular surface disorders.

Suspected intraocular (bacterial, viral, or fungal) infections
Results Interpretation:
Abnormal cytology findings
Intraocular infections are characterized by a preponderance of particular cell types such as polymorphonuclear leukocytes in bacterial infections, lymphocytes, monocytes and inclusion bodies in viral infections, and positive Giemsa staining specimens in the detection of fungal infections.
Ocular cytology findings may reveal abnormal cell populations during morphology examination which may definitively diagnose bacterial, viral or fungal infections.

Suspected neoplasms of the eye and surrounding tissues
Strength of Recommendation: Class I
Strength of Evidence: Category C

Results Interpretation:
Abnormal cytology findings
   Ocular cytology by fine-needle aspiration in conjunction with expert pathology appears to be a reliable test in the diagnosis of ocular malignancies and malignancy type including carcinoma, lymphoma, melanoma, retinoblastoma, and sarcoma.

Contraindications
   Ocular cytology scraping is contraindicated in patients where the corneal epithelium is intact and the disease state is deep in the cornea.

COLLECTION/STORAGE INFORMATION
- Specimen Collection and Handling:
   - Ocular Smear Cytology:
      - Requires sterile technique
      - Loop will be applied to conjunctiva, moistened or dry swab will be applied to lid margins, dry swab will be applied to meibomian and canalicular secretions
      - Collect specimen from the involved site (eg, purulent processes)
   - Ocular Scrape Techniques (Kimura spatula or small cytology brush):
      - Requires sterile technique
      - Make two or three passes across affected site in the same direction
      - Do not apply excessive pressure when obtaining specimen (to avoid hemorrhages or corneal injury)
      - Use the Cytobrush (small) for conjunctival brush cytology (CBC)
      - Apply a topical anesthetic to the eye prior to CBC
      - Scrape the temporal bulbar conjunctiva several times in the same direction under biomicroscopic observation to avoid unnecessary pressure on the conjunctiva
      - Following CBC, place the brush in 2 mL of Hank's buffered solution and shake, detaching the cells from the brush and filter suspended cells using the Millipore filter technique
   - Ocular Impression Cytology:
      - Requires sterile technique
      - 1 or 2 drops of proparacaine hydrochloride 0.5% improves patient cooperation with impression cytology
      - Use half-section cellulose acetate filter paper glossy side up, to the inflamed site
      - Apply filter paper with the blunt end of a glass rod for several seconds and remove with forceps and mount on glass slide with double-sided tape
   - Fixation Techniques:
      - Regardless of collection technique, specimen must be fixed to slide immediately
      - May use 95% ethanol, 95% methanol, absolute ethanol, or absolute methanol as the fixative
   - Staining Techniques:
      - Use Gram's stain for microbiological evaluation
      - Use Giemsa stain for cytological evaluation

Ornithine measurement

TEST DEFINITION
   Measurement of ornithine in plasma or serum for detection of acquired and hereditary amino acid disorders

REFERENCE RANGE
- Premature neonate, 1 day: 1.1 ± 0.26 mg/dL (90 ± 20 micromol/L)
- Neonate, 1 day: 0.65-1.99 mg/dL (49-151 micromol/L)
- Infants 1 to 3 months: 0.95 ± 0.3 mg/dL (72 ± 23 micromol/L)
- Infants 9 to 24 months: 0.13-1.41 mg/dL (10-107 micromol/L)
- Children 3 to 10 years: 0.36-1.13 mg/dL (27-86 micromol/L)
- Children 6 to 18 years: 0.25-1.07 mg/dL (19-81 micromol/L)
- Adults: 0.4-1.4 mg/dL (30-106 micromol/L)
   Please refer to your institution's reference ranges as lab normals may vary.

INDICATIONS

Suspected inborn error of metabolism
   Strength of Recommendation: Class IIa
   Strength of Evidence: Category C
   Results Interpretation:
   Increased amino acid
      Inherited amino acid disorders are directly related to the absence of an enzyme involved in the metabolism of one or more amino acids; therefore, an elevated plasma level of a particular amino acid is highly suggestive of an inherited metabolic defect. In the majority of cases amino acid and organic acid analysis together permit diagnostic confirmation in infants. Immediate treatment should be initiated when an inborn error of metabolism is suspected, even if a definitive diagnosis has not yet been determined.
      Hyperornithinemia-hyperammonemia-homocitrullinuria (HHH) syndrome is associated with an increased ornithine blood level.

COLLECTION/STORAGE INFORMATION
* Specimen Collection and Handling:
   * Immediately place sample in ice water.
   * Isolate plasma sample and freeze it within 1 hour; sample stable for 1 week at -20°C.
   * Sample should be deproteinized and stored at -70°C for protracted periods of usage.

LOINC CODES
* Code: 25966-3 (*Short Name* - Ornithine/creat 24H Ur-sRto)
* Code: 22647-2 (*Short Name* - Ornithine CSF-sCnc)
* Code: 2681-5 (*Short Name* - Ornithine 24H Ur-mRate)
* Code: 25491-2 (*Short Name* - Ornithine 24H Ur-sRate)
* Code: 22682-9 (*Short Name* - Ornithine/creat Ur-sRto)
* Code: 32260-2 (*Short Name* - Ornithine Fld-sCnc)
* Code: 17389-8 (*Short Name* - Ornithine Ur QI)
* Code: 25965-5 (*Short Name* - Ornithine 24H Ur-sCnc)
* Code: 13786-9 (*Short Name* - Ornithine/creat Ur-mRto)
* Code: 27219-5 (*Short Name* - Ornithine Amn-sCnc)
* Code: 22725-6 (*Short Name* - Ornithine XXX-sCnc)
* Code: 30049-1 (*Short Name* - Ornithine/creat Ur-Rto)
* Code: 2680-7 (*Short Name* - Ornithine Ur-mCnc)
* Code: 32261-0 (*Short Name* - Ornithine Vitf-sCnc)
* Code: 13379-3 (*Short Name* - Ornithine CSF-mCnc)

Osmotic fragility

TEST DEFINITION
   Determination of osmotic fragility for the evaluation and management of erythrocyte membrane disorders

SYNONYMS
* RBC osmotic fragility

REFERENCE RANGE
* No increased hemolysis as compared with normal control
   Please refer to your institution's reference ranges as lab normals may vary.

INDICATIONS

Suspected erythrocyte membrane disorder
      Strength of Recommendation: Class IIa
      Strength of Evidence: Category B
   Results Interpretation:
   Abnormal laboratory findings
      In laboratories not equipped with osmotic gradient ektacytometry, osmotic fragility testing remains the laboratory test of choice for screening RBC surface area deficiencies including hereditary spherocytosis and thalassemia anemias.

Osmotic fragility is typically increased in hereditary spherocytosis and decreased in thalassemia and microcytic anemias.

Serial osmotic fragility testing may play a role in the determination of cell age.

ABNORMAL RESULTS
- Results decreased in:
  - Hypochromic, microcytic anemias
  - Asplenia

CLINICAL NOTES
Osmotic fragility testing may be normal initially, even in the presence of RBC membrane defects; therefore, the test is incubated at 37°C for 24 hours to increase sensitivity.

Osmotic gradient ektacytometry is the state-of-the-art method for determining RBC membrane status and is preferred to osmotic fragility testing when available.

COLLECTION/STORAGE INFORMATION
- Collect 7 mL of venous blood sample and anticoagulate with heparin

LOINC CODES
- Code: 23912-9 (*Short Name* - OF 0.35% NaCl % RBC)
- Code: 4667-2 (*Short Name* - OF % RBC)
- Code: 23919-4 (*Short Name* - OF.65% NaCl % RBC)
- Code: 23914-5 (*Short Name* - OF 0.45% NaCl % RBC)
- Code: 23911-1 (*Short Name* - OF 0.30% NaCl % RBC)
- Code: 23913-7 (*Short Name* - OF.40% NaCl % RBC)
- Code: 23917-8 (*Short Name* - OF.60% NaCl % RBC)
- Code: 23915-2 (*Short Name* - OF 0.50% NaCl % RBC)
- Code: 23916-0 (*Short Name* - OF 0.55% NaCl % RBC)
- Code: 23922-8 (*Short Name* - OF 0.75% NaCl % RBC)
- Code: 23910-3 (*Short Name* - OF 0% NaCl % RBC)

Osteocalcin measurement

TEST DEFINITION
Measurement of osteocalcin in serum for the evaluation of bone formation disorders

SYNONYMS
- Bone g1a protein measurement

REFERENCE RANGE
- Adult male: 3-13 nanograms/mL (3-13 micrograms/L)
- Adult premenopausal female: 0.4-8.2 nanograms/mL (0.4-8.2 micrograms/L)
- Adult postmenopausal female: 1.5-11 nanograms/mL (1.5-11 micrograms/L)
- Children, 2 to 17 years: 2.8-41 nanograms/mL (2.8-41 micrograms/L)
- Neonates: 20-40 nanograms/L (20-40 micrograms/L)
- In adult males, circadian variations result in a 5- to 10-nanograms/mL fluctuation in osteocalcin levels over a 24-hour period. Circulating levels are lowest in late afternoon and peak nocturnally.
- Serum osteocalcin (OC) assays lack standardization because different assays recognize different molecular fragments. OC levels on the same serum sample, measured at different laboratories, can vary by more than 4 fold. More consistent results can be obtained if the OC level is expressed as a percentage of serum OC in normal individuals.

  Please refer to your institution's reference ranges as lab normals may vary.

INDICATIONS
Postmenopausal women at risk for osteoporosis
> **Strength of Recommendation:** Class III
> **Strength of Evidence:** Category B

Results Interpretation:
Increased level (laboratory finding)
Increased levels of osteocalcin suggest high bone turnover.

Bone formation and reabsorption remains relatively stable in postmenopausal women. The majority of women with high bone turnover at baseline (early menopause) had high bone turnover at 4-year follow-up..

Suspected secondary malignant neoplasm of bone
Strength of Recommendation: Class IIb
Strength of Evidence: Category B
Results Interpretation:
Increased level (laboratory finding)
The clinical utility of elevated serum osteocalcin (OC) levels in patients with bone metastasis has not been established.

COMMON PANELS
- Bone and joint panel

ABNORMAL RESULTS
- Results increased in:
  - Adolescent growth spurts (range 40-80 nanograms/mL in boys)
  - Chronic renal failure
  - Hyperthyroidism
- Results decreased in:
  - Pregnancy
  - Cirrhosis

CLINICAL NOTES
Assays for serum osteocalcin (OC) levels are not standardized and are characterized by wide variability.

COLLECTION/STORAGE INFORMATION
- Specimen Collection and Handling:
  - Freeze specimen immediately upon collection; specimen is stable at –20 °C for 14 months.
  - Collect specimens at the same time of day to reduce variability of results due to circadian variations.
- Patient Preparation: Instruct patient to fast prior to blood test.

LOINC CODES
- Code: 15084-7 (*Short Name* - Osteocalcin Ser-sCnc)
- Code: 2697-1 (*Short Name* - Osteocalcin Ser-mCnc)

P-ANCA measurement

TEST DEFINITION
Measurement of perinuclear antineutrophil cytoplasmic antibodies (p-ANCA) in serum, generally used in the evaluation of systemic vasculitis.

REFERENCE RANGE
- Adults:
- Qualitative: Negative
- Quantitative: Less than 1.4 units/mL (less than 1.4 kilounits/L)
  Please refer to your institution's reference ranges as lab normals may vary.

INDICATIONS
Suspected Churg-Strauss syndrome
Strength of Recommendation: Class IIa
Strength of Evidence: Category B

Results Interpretation:
p-Antineutrophil cytoplasmic antibody positive
> Patients with active Churg-Strauss syndrome are more likely to test positive for perinuclear antineutrophil cytoplasmic antibody (p-ANCA) than patients with inactive disease.

Suspected idiopathic pauci-immune necrotizing crescentic glomerulonephritis
> **Strength of Recommendation:** Class IIa
> **Strength of Evidence:** Category B
> **Results Interpretation:**
> **p-Antineutrophil cytoplasmic antibody positive**
>> A majority of patients with pauci-immune necrotizing and crescentic glomerulonephritis will test positive for antineutrophil cytoplasmic antibodies (ANCA). Perinuclear-ANCA, particularly when associated with myeloperoxidase, appears to be more common in patients with renal-limited disease.
>> Perinuclear-ANCA has a greater than 80% association with pauci-immune glomerulonephritis.

Suspected microscopic polyangiitis (MPA)
> **Strength of Recommendation:** Class IIb
> **Strength of Evidence:** Category B
> **Results Interpretation:**
> **p-Antineutrophil cytoplasmic antibody positive**
>> A positive perinuclear antineutrophil cytoplasmic antibody (p-ANCA) by indirect immunofluorescence (IF) alone may be seen in many different disorders, including multiple connective tissue diseases. In conjunction with antibodies to myeloperoxidase (MPO) by ELISA, however, there is a strong association with vasculitides, including microscopic polyangiitis..

COMMON PANELS
- Collagen/Lupus panel

ABNORMAL RESULTS
- Results increased in:
  - Ulcerative colitis
  - High antinuclear antibody (ANA) titers

CLINICAL NOTES
Assays are not standardized in the United States, and different assays may have varying sensitivities and specificities. While immunofluorescence is considered the 'gold standard,' results are subjective and not consistently reproducible even when the test is performed by experienced personnel. Additional antigen-specific enzyme-linked immunosorbent assay (ELISA) testing for anti-myeloperoxidase (MPO) will improve specificity.
Quantitative testing is used to follow disease progression.

COLLECTION/STORAGE INFORMATION
- Collect 7 mL blood serum sample in red-topped tube
- Store sample at -20°C

LOINC CODES
- Code: 14278-6 (*Short Name* - P-ANCA Titr Ser IF)

PCR test for Helicobacter pylori

TEST DEFINITION
Detection of *Helicobacter pylori* by polymerase chain reaction (PCR)

REFERENCE RANGE
- Negative
Please refer to your institution's reference ranges as lab normals may vary.

INDICATIONS

Suspected *Helicobacter pylori* **gastrointestinal tract infection**

   Strength of Recommendation: Class IIb
   Strength of Evidence: Category B
Results Interpretation:
Positive laboratory findings

   The specificity of a polymerase chain reaction (PCR) assay for *Helicobacter pylori* in stool is decreased one month following treatment, suggesting that a longer follow-up period may be necessary for the accurate interpretation of this test.

   The sensitivity of PCR for *H pylori* is fairly high, but specificity varies widely.

CLINICAL NOTES

   Polymerase chain reaction (PCR) testing may be done on a biopsy obtained during endoscopy (invasive) or on a saliva or feces sample (non-invasive).

COLLECTION/STORAGE INFORMATION

- Specimen Collection and Handling:
    - Avoid contamination with extraneous DNA, RNA, and heme
    - Avoid heparin
    - Store nucleic acids frozen at -20°C or below

PCR test for Treponema pallidum

TEST DEFINITION

   Molecular identification of *Treponema pallidum* in tissues, body fluids or lesions for the detection of syphilis.

SYNONYMS

- PCR test for syphilis

REFERENCE RANGE

- Adults and children: negative
   Please refer to your institution's reference ranges as lab normals may vary.

INDICATIONS

Suspected syphilis

   Strength of Recommendation: Class IIa
   Strength of Evidence: Category B
Results Interpretation:
Positive microbiology findings

   Molecular detection of *T. pallidum* by polymerase chain reaction (PCR) is consistent with a diagnosis of syphilis. Reverse transcriptase polymerase chain reaction (RT-PCR) is not able to differentiate *T. pallidum* subspecies *pallidum* from *T. pallidum* subspecies *pertenue*.

PCR test for avian influenza A

TEST DEFINITION

   Detection of influenza A RNA in respiratory specimens for the presumptive diagnosis of avian influenza A.

REFERENCE RANGE

- Adults and children: negative
   Please refer to your institution's reference ranges as lab normals may vary.

INDICATIONS

Suspected avian influenza A

    Strength of Recommendation: Class IIa

    Strength of Evidence: Category C

    Results Interpretation:

    Positive laboratory findings

Positive specimens should be forwarded to the Centers for Disease Control (CDC) for confirmatory testing under heightened Biosafety Level 3 (BSL-3) conditions. The CDC Director's Emergency Operations Center should be immediately informed. Original clinical material should be sent to avoid possible pre-analytical contamination. All laboratory results must be evaluated in the context of clinical and epidemiological findings in consultation with influenza surveillance experts. Negative test results do not rule out diagnosis.

    False Results

False-negatives results occur from inappropriate collection, handling and shipping of specimens causing viral RNA degradation. Appropriate application of extraction and inhibition assay controls can help prevent false negatives by identifying poor-quality samples. Cross-contamination during shipping can cause reverse transcriptase polymerase chain reaction (RT-PCR) false positives. False positive results can be prevented by utilizing multiple negative control samples in each assay as well as employing confirmatory testing of positive samples.

    Timing of Monitoring

Respiratory samples should be collected during the first 4 days of illness.

CLINICAL NOTES

The decision to test for avian influenza A should be made in consultation with local or state health departments. Clinicians should contact their local or state health departments in all cases of suspected infection with any novel influenza A virus; state and local health departments should in turn contact the Centers for Disease Control (CDC) Emergency Response Hotline. The use of reverse transcriptase polymerase chain reaction (RT-PCR) to identify and subtype avian influenza viruses is limited to laboratories with biosafety level-2 (BSL-2) capabilities using approved reagents provided by the CDC. Any specimen testing positive and suspected of avian influenza infection should have further testing by a designated WHO H5 reference laboratory to verify results.

COLLECTION/STORAGE INFORMATION

Meticulous collection, handling, and shipping of specimens is imperative to prevent false-negative results.

Serial specimen collection over several days is optimal; specimens collected within the first 3 days of illness onset are more likely to detect the virus.

Oropharyngeal swab specimens and lower respiratory tract specimens, such as bronchoalveolar lavage and tracheal aspirates, are preferred because they appear to contain more virus; nasal and nasopharyngeal swab specimens are less optimal because they may contain a lower viral count.

To obtain a nasopharyngeal aspirate/wash, instill 1 ml to 1.5 ml nonbacteriostatic saline (pH) into one nostril. Flush a plastic catheter or tubing with 2 ml to 3 ml of saline. Insert tubing into nostril parallel to the palate and aspirate nasopharyngeal secretions. Repeat procedure with second nostril.

To obtain a nasopharyngeal or oropharyngeal swab insert a swab into the nostril parallel to the palate. Leave the swab in place for a few seconds to absorb secretions. Repeat with second nostril. All swabs used for specimen collection should have an aluminum or plastic shaft and a Dacron tip. Calcium alginate swabs, cotton-tipped swabs, or swabs with wooden shafts should not be used for specimen collection. Place specimen at 4°C immediately after collection.

To collect sputum, have patient rinse mouth with water then expectorate deep cough sputum directly into a sterile screw-cap sputum collection cup or sterile dry container. Use cold packs to keep sample at 4°C for domestic shipping. For international shipping pack in dry ice.

During bronchoalveolar lavage or tracheal aspirate, use a double-tube system to maximize shielding from oropharyngeal secretions; bronchoalveolar lavage is a high-risk, aerosol generating procedure. Centrifuge half of the specimen and fix the cell pellet in formalin. Place the remaining unspun fluid in sterile vials with external caps and internal O-rings. If no O-rings are available, seal tightly with available cap and secure with Parafilm®. Label each specimen with patient's ID and collection date. For domestic shipping use cold packs to keep sample at 4°C. For international shipping, ship fixed cells at room temperature and unfixed cells frozen.

Contact the Centers for Disease Control (CDC) Emergency Response Hotline before shipping influenza A specimens. Specimens should be sent Priority Overnight Shipping for receipt within 24 hours. Follow approved CDC protocols for standard interstate shipping of etiologic agents.

Nucleic acid extraction lysis buffer can be added to specimens to inactivate virus and stabilize RNA, after which specimens can be stored and shipped at 4°C. If buffer is not added, specimens should be frozen at −70°C and shipped on dry ice. Avoid repeated freeze/thaw cycles.

LOINC CODES
• Code: 34487-9 (*Short Name* - Avian FLU RNA XXX Ql PCR)

PCR test for herpesvirus 6

TEST DEFINITION
Detection of human herpesvirus 6 (HHV-6) DNA in plasma and other body fluids for the diagnosis and management of HHV-6 infection

SYNONYMS
• Herpesvirus 6 DNA detection
• Polymerase chain reaction test for herpesvirus 6

REFERENCE RANGE
• Adults and children: negative
  Please refer to your institution's reference ranges as lab normals may vary.

INDICATIONS
Suspected roseola infantum (exanthem subitum) in children
    Strength of Recommendation: Class IIa
    Strength of Evidence: Category B
    Results Interpretation:
    Positive biochemistry findings
    The presence of human herpesvirus 6 (HHV-6) by polymerase chain reaction (PCR) is diagnostic of exanthem subitum in children. HHV-7 antibodies have been found in patients with exanthem subitum, suggesting HHV-7 may also be a causative organism. The finding of HHV-6 viral DNA in saliva suggests previous infection.

Known and suspected human herpesvirus 6 infection
    Strength of Recommendation: Class IIa
    Strength of Evidence: Category B
    Results Interpretation:
    Positive biochemistry findings
    Detection of human herpesvirus 6 (HHV-6) DNA in plasma by polymerase chain reaction (PCR) in the presence of serum HHV-6 IgM may reliably predict acute HHV-6 infection in the immunosuppressed patient.
    Qualitative DNA PCR using serum, plasma or other body fluids cannot differentiate between latent and active HHV-6 infection. More sensitive quantitative methods have been described. The combinations of both blood and saliva PCR, and blood PCR and IgG testing, have been suggested to improve the test sensitivity for acute infection. Although HHV-6 is present in 90% of children by 2 years of age, healthy adults have no detectable viral load.

CLINICAL NOTES
The higher viral load in whole blood relative to plasma may influence the sensitivity of polymerase chain reaction (PCR) for detecting the presence of human herpesvirus 6 DNA.

COLLECTION/STORAGE INFORMATION
• Specimen Collection and Handling:
  • Obtain specimen during acute phase of illness.
  • Transport specimen in viral transport medium.
  • Store all specimens except blood samples at 4°C until processed.

LOINC CODES
• Code: 29495-9 (*Short Name* - HHV6 DNA XXX Ql PCR)
• Code: 33940-8 (*Short Name* - HHV6 DNA Tiss Ql PCR)
• Code: 33941-6 (*Short Name* - HHV6 DNA Bld Ql PCR)
• Code: 33942-4 (*Short Name* - HHV6 DNA CSF Ql PCR)

PCR test for herpesvirus 8

TEST DEFINITION
Detection of human herpesvirus 8 (HHV-8) in biological samples for the evaluation and management of immunological disorders

SYNONYMS
- Polymerase chain reaction test for herpesvirus 8

REFERENCE RANGE
- Negative
  Please refer to your institution's reference ranges as lab normals may vary.

INDICATIONS
Suspected angiofollicular lymph node hyperplasia (multicentric Castleman's disease) as a result of human herpesvirus 8 (HHV-8) infection
> **Strength of Recommendation:** Class I
> **Strength of Evidence:** Category B
> **Results Interpretation:**
> **Positive laboratory findings**
>> A positive result on a polymerase chain reaction (PCR) test for human herpesvirus 8 (HHV-8) may indicate multicentric Castleman's disease.
>> As human immunodeficiency virus (HIV) ribonucleic acid (RNA) plasma levels increase, levels of HHV-8 viral load also rise.

Suspected Kaposi's sarcoma as a result of human herpesvirus 8 (HHV-8) infection
> **Strength of Recommendation:** Class I
> **Strength of Evidence:** Category B
> **Results Interpretation:**
> **Positive laboratory findings**
>> A positive result on a polymerase chain reaction (PCR) test for human herpesvirus 8 (HHV-8) occurs in greater than 90% of patients with Kaposi's sarcoma.
>> HHV-8 is less easily detectable after commencement of retroviral treatment and may become undetectable after eradication of Kaposi's sarcoma.

Suspected primary effusion lymphoma (PEL) as a result of human herpesvirus 8 (HHV-8) infection
> **Strength of Recommendation:** Class I
> **Strength of Evidence:** Category B
> **Results Interpretation:**
> **Positive laboratory findings**
>> A positive result on a polymerase chain reaction (PCR) test for human herpesvirus 8 (HHV-8) is invariably present in patients with primary effusion lymphoma.
>> As human immunodeficiency virus (HIV) ribonucleic acid (RNA) plasma levels increase, levels of HHV-8 viral load also rise.

CLINICAL NOTES
Rigorous control over procedure is essential to avoid false-positive results.

COLLECTION/STORAGE INFORMATION
- Store tissue at -20°C or below and body fluids at 4°C.

LOINC CODES
- Code: 32364-2 (*Short Name* - HHV 8 DNA Ser Ql PCR)

Pancreatic polypeptide measurement

TEST DEFINITION
Tumor marker for diagnosis and monitoring of pancreatic endocrine tumor.

SYNONYMS
- Human pancreatic polypeptide measurement
- Pancreatic polypeptide level

REFERENCE RANGE
- Adults 20 to 29 years: 26-158 ng/L (26-158 pg/mL).
- Adults 30 to 39 years: 55-284 ng/L (55-284 pg/mL).
- Adults 40 to 49 years: 64-243 ng/L (64-243 pg/mL).
- Adults ≥ 50 years: 51-326 ng/L (51-326 pg/mL).
  Please refer to your institution's reference ranges as lab normals may vary.

INDICATIONS
Pancreatic islet cell tumors in multiple endocrine neoplasia type 1 (MEN 1).
    Strength of Recommendation: Class IIb
    Strength of Evidence: Category B
    Results Interpretation:
    Increased polypeptide hormone level
    A fasting plasma pancreatic polypeptide level greater than 3 times the normal age-specific range in individuals with MEN 1 is indicative of pancreatic islet cell tumor.

Suspected pancreatic endocrine tumor.
    Strength of Recommendation: Class IIa
    Strength of Evidence: Category C
    Results Interpretation:
    Increased polypeptide hormone level
    Pancreatic polypeptide measurement is a useful diagnostic test for pancreatic endocrine tumors. Fasting plasma concentrations of pancreatic polypeptide above 300 pmol/L are considered abnormal.
    Frequency of Monitoring
    Serial pancreatic polypeptide measurement is an acceptable option for evaluating tumor growth.

CLINICAL NOTES
Age and gender-related variations should be considered when evaluating fasting pancreatic polypeptide measurements.

COLLECTION/STORAGE INFORMATION
- Specimen Collection and Handling:
  - Have patient fast for 8 hours prior to testing
  - Discontinue antacids which may affect insulin levels prior to testing
  - Collect specimen in a red top tube or lavender top EDTA tube
  - Freeze specimen immediately after collection

Parainfluenza virus antibody level

TEST DEFINITION
Detection of antibody to parainfluenza virus in serum for the evaluation of respiratory viral infection

REFERENCE RANGE
- Adults and children: Negative
  Please refer to your institution's reference ranges as lab normals may vary.

INDICATIONS

Suspected parainfluenza
> **Strength of Recommendation:** Class IIb
> **Strength of Evidence:** Category C

Results Interpretation:

Serology positive
> A positive serology test is defined as a fourfold increase in titer between acute and convalescent stages and is diagnostic of parainfluenza.

Timing of Monitoring
> Specimens should be collected during the acute phase and again during the convalescent period, approximately 14 days after primary infection.

ABNORMAL RESULTS

- Results increased in:
  - Other viral infections such as mumps

COLLECTION/STORAGE INFORMATION

- Specimen Collection and Handling:
  - Collect specimen in a red top tube.
  - Keep specimen at room temperature.
  - Transport specimen to laboratory immediately upon collection.

LOINC CODES

- Code: 31555-6 (*Short Name* - Parainflu Ab Ser-aCnc)
- Code: 26855-7 (*Short Name* - Parainflu Ab Titr Ser IF)

Parathyroid hormone measurement

TEST DEFINITION

Measurement of parathyroid hormone (PTH) in serum or plasma for the evaluation and management of thyroid and kidney disorders

SYNONYMS

- Immunoreactive PTH measurement
- Parathormone measurement
- PTH measurement
- PTH - Parathyroid hormone level

REFERENCE RANGE

- Adults (serum):
- C-terminal and midmolecule: 50-330 pg/mL (50-330 ng/L)
- N-terminal: 8-24 pg/mL (8-24 ng/L)
- Intact molecule: 10-65 pg/mL (10-65 ng/L)
- Adults (plasma):
- C-terminal and midmolecule: <50 microLEq/mL (<50 mLEq/L)
- N-terminal: <6.1 pmol/L
- Intact molecule: 1-5 pmol/L
- Pediatrics:
- C-terminal and midmolecule (ages 1-16): 51-217 pg/mL (51-217 ng/L)
- N-terminal (ages 2-13): 14-21 pg/mL (14-21 ng/L)
- Intact molecule (ages 2-20): 9-52 pg/mL (9-52 ng/L)
  Please refer to your institution's reference ranges as lab normals may vary.

INDICATIONS

Parathyroidectomy in patients with primary hyperparathyroidism
> **Strength of Recommendation:** Class IIa
> **Strength of Evidence:** Category B

Results Interpretation:
Decreased level (laboratory finding)

An intraoperative drop in parathyroid hormone (PTH) of greater than 50% immediately following resection has been described as curative. Surgical cure has also been defined as a serum calcium level of less than 10.2 mg/dL within 6 months following parathyroidectomy.

Frequency of Monitoring

In one study, intraoperative parathyroid hormone (ioPTH) levels were drawn just before the surgical incision and again at 5, 10, and 15 minutes after resection.

Hypocalcemia secondary to thyroidectomy

Strength of Recommendation: Class IIa
Strength of Evidence: Category B
Results Interpretation:
Hypoparathyroidism

A single intraoperative or postoperative intact parathyroid hormone (iPTH) measurement may predict the development of symptomatic postoperative hypocalcemia in thyroidectomy patients, and may predict the need for vitamin D supplementation.

Suspected hypercalcemia due to hyperparathyroidism

Strength of Recommendation: Class IIa
Strength of Evidence: Category C
Results Interpretation:
Abnormal biochemistry findings

In the presence of normal renal function, persistently mild hypercalcemia and elevated intact parathyroid hormone (iPTH) levels at the upper end of the normal range are findings consistent with a diagnosis of primary hyperparathyroidism. Normal changes in parathyroid hormone (PTH) secretion occur over a very narrow range of serum calcium concentrations. Maximal suppression of PTH occurs at a serum calcium level of 11 to 12 mg/dL or greater; maximal secretion of PTH is stimulated with a serum calcium level of 7 to 8 mg/dL or lower.

A decreased PTH level is common in most nonparathyroid hypercalcemic disorders without renal failure, including hypercalcemia related to malignancy.

Chronic kidney disease

Strength of Recommendation: Class IIa
Strength of Evidence: Category C
Results Interpretation:
Hyperparathyroidism due to renal insufficiency

An elevated parathyroid hormone (PTH) level in conjunction with secondary hyperparathyroidism is common in patients with chronic kidney disease (CKD), particularly in stage 3 patients with glomerular filtration rates (GFR) less than 60 mL/min/1.73 m^2. Hyperparathyroid bone disease is found in a majority of these patients. Treatment with small doses of vitamin D sterols improves bone mineral density without negatively impacting kidney function.

- Target ranges for patients with CKD are different than those with normal kidney function since some assays may incorrectly detect inactive fragments of PTH in CKD patients. The target ranges of plasma intact parathyroid hormone (iPTH) by stage of CKD are as follows:
  - Stage 3: 35-70 pg/mL (3.85-7.7 pmol/L)
  - Stage 4: 70-110 pg/mL (7.7-12.1 pmol/L)
  - Stage 5: 150-300 pg/mL (16.5 to 33 pmol/L)
- Dietary phosphorus should be limited to between 800 and 1,000 mg/day when iPTH levels are above the target range for the patient's CKD stage. Phosphate binders are recommended if dietary restrictions do not maintain iPTH and phosphorus levels within the target ranges. When CKD patients stages 3 and 4 present with iPTH levels above the target range for their CKD stage, serum 25-hydroxyvitamin D should be measured promptly, and repeated annually if normal. If the iPTH is above the target range and the 25-hydroxyvitamin D level is less than 30 ng/mL, vitamin D$_2$ supplementation is recommended. If the iPTH is above the target range and the 25-hydroxyvitamin D level is above 30 ng/mL, the administration of active oral vitamin D sterol may be appropriate for some patients. Patients with CKD stage 5 who have iPTH levels above the target range should be treated with vitamin D sterol until the PTH returns to the target range.
  An iPTH of less than 400 pg/mL in the presence of low or normal serum calcium levels is consistent with mild hyperparathyroidism. iPTH above 500 to 600 pg/mL suggests moderate or severe hyperparathyroidism. Parathyroidectomy may be appropriate in hypercalcemic and/or hyperphosphatemic patients with repeated iPTH levels above 800 pg/mL who do not respond to standard medical interventions.

Frequency of Monitoring

Serum phosphorus, calcium and intact parathyroid hormone (iPTH) should be monitored in all chronic kidney disease (CKD) patients with a glomerular filtration rate (GFR) below 60 mL/min/1.73 m^2. Patients with CKD stage 3 with a GFR of 30 to 59 mL/min/1.73 m^2 should have their parathyroid hormone (PTH) levels measured every 12 months. Patients with CKD stage 4 with a GFR of 15 to 29 mL/min/1.73 m ^{2} should have their PTH levels measured every 3 months. CKD stage 5 patients undergoing dialysis or with a GFR less than 15 mL/min/1.73 m should have their PTH levels tested every 3 months. Less frequent monitoring may be appropriate for patients with PTH levels at the low end of the target values. More frequent monitoring may be necessary in transplant patients.

Patients with CKD stages 3 or 4 who are undergoing therapy with vitamin D sterols should have their plasma PTH levels measured at least every 3 months for 6 months, and every 3 months thereafter. Patients with CKD stage 5 receiving vitamin D sterols should have plasma PTH levels drawn monthly for a minimum of 3 months when therapy is initiated or the dose is increased, then every 3 months once target PTH levels are reached.

Hypocalcemia
Results Interpretation:
Raised biochemistry findings

Elevated parathyroid hormone (PTH) may be found in hypocalcemia due to intestinal malabsorption, vitamin D deficiency, renal failure, and hereditary vitamin D resistance. Additionally, if PTH levels are not elevated in untreated patients with these disorders, then primary parathyroid failure should be considered as an additional diagnosis.

Lowered biochemistry findings

Parathyroid hormone may be decreased or absent in hypocalcemia due to either medical or surgical causes of parathyroid insufficiency.

Suspected or known bone disease
Strength of Recommendation: Class IIa
Strength of Evidence: Category B
Results Interpretation:
Raised biochemistry findings

Elevated parathyroid hormone (PTH) levels are associated with hyperparathyroid bone disease. PTH levels 2 to 3 times normal are considered necessary in order to sustain normal bone formation and to prevent adynamic bone disease in chronic kidney disease patients.

COMMON PANELS
- Parathyroid panel

ABNORMAL RESULTS
- Results decreased in young adults
- Results increased in African-Americans

COLLECTION/STORAGE INFORMATION
- Draw fasting morning sample in red-top or serum separator tube and then freeze immediately.
- Draw plasma samples in EDTA tube.
- Store at -20°C and -70°C.

LOINC CODES
- Code: 16164-6 (*Short Name* - PTH-Intact 2H p chal SerPl-mCnc)
- Code: 2731-8 (*Short Name* - PTH-Intact SerPl-mCnc)
- Code: 14866-8 (*Short Name* - PTH-Intact SerPl-sCnc)
- Code: 16163-8 (*Short Name* - PTH-Intact 1H p chal SerPl-mCnc)
- Code: 14865-0 (*Short Name* - PTH SerPl-Imp)
- Code: 32045-7 (*Short Name* - PTH-Biointact SerPl-mCnc)

Parathyroid related protein measurement

TEST DEFINITION

Measurement of parathyroid hormone-related protein (PTHrP) in serum or plasma for the assessment of malignancy-related hypercalcemia

REFERENCE RANGE

- Adults: <1.3 pmol/L
  Please refer to your institution's reference ranges as lab normals may vary.

INDICATIONS

Suspected or known hypercalcemia secondary to malignancy
    Strength of Recommendation: Class IIb
    Strength of Evidence: Category B
    Results Interpretation:
    Raised biochemistry findings
       In the presence of elevated calcium levels, detectable parathyroid hormone related peptide (PTHrP) is suggestive of hypercalcemia-related malignancy. The relationship between elevated PTHrP levels and prognosis is not clear.

COLLECTION/STORAGE INFORMATION

- Draw sample in tube containing protease inhibitors and place sample on ice immediately.
- Store at -20°C in plastic vial.

LOINC CODES

- Code: 15087-0 (*Short Name* - PTH Related Prot SerPl-sCnc)
- Code: 2729-2 (*Short Name* - PTH Related Prot SerPl-mCnc)

Partial pressure arterial oxygen/fraction inspired oxygen ratio

TEST DEFINITION

Calculation of the ratio of partial pressure arterial oxygen content to fraction of inspired oxygen (PaO_2/FiO_2) for purposes of quantifying the degree of pulmonary impairment

SYNONYMS

- PaO2/FiO2 ratio

REFERENCE RANGE

- Adults: Room air partial pressure arterial oxygen (PaO_2) 80-100 mmHg (11-13 kPa)
- Fraction inspired oxygen (FiO_2) in air: 21%
- Normal range (PaO_2/FiO_2): $\geq$ 400
  Please refer to your institution's reference ranges as lab normals may vary.

INDICATIONS

Acute respiratory distress syndrome (ARDS)
    Results Interpretation:
    Hematology finding
       According to the American-European Consensus Conference on Acute Respiratory Distress Syndrome (ARDS), a stable or improving PaO2/FiO_2 ratio at a constant level of positive end-expiratory pressure (PEEP) for 24 hours is indicative of the stabilization of acute lung injury (ALI). Continued improvement of oxygenation over the subsequent 24 hours is indicative of the resolution of ALI.

Transfusion related acute lung injury (TRALI)
    Results Interpretation:
    Respiratory depression
        A partial pressure arterial oxygen to fraction inspired oxygen ratio (PaO_2 /FiO_2) less than or equal to 300 mmHg is consistent with a diagnosis of transfusion related acute lung injury (TRALI).
        A partial pressure arterial oxygen to fraction inspired oxygen ratio (PaO_2 /FiO_2) less than 400 is abnormal.

ABNORMAL RESULTS
- Results increased in:
  - Oxygen enriched air
  - Exercise
  - Angiomas of the brain
- Results decreased in:
  - Advancing age
  - High altitude (eg, hypoxemia)
  - Decreased cardiac output
  - Carbon monoxide poisoning
  - Anesthesia
  - Near drowning

CLINICAL NOTES
Partial pressure of arterial oxygen (PaO_2) is dependent upon fraction inspired oxygen (FiO_2), pulmonary function, hemoglobin concentration, and cardiac output.

COLLECTION/STORAGE INFORMATION
- Specimen Collection and Handling:
  - Collect arterial blood gas in an anaerobic, sealed, heparinized tube.
  - Place tube on ice and transport to the lab for immediate analysis.

Partial thromboplastin time, activated

TEST DEFINITION
Measurement of clotting time in plasma for evaluation of bleeding or thrombotic disorders and monitoring of heparin therapy

SYNONYMS
- APTT
- APTT - Activated partial thromboplastin time
- PTT, activated
- PTT assay
- PTT - Partial thromboplastin time

REFERENCE RANGE
- Adults: 22.1-35.1 seconds
  Please refer to your institution's reference ranges as lab normals may vary.

INDICATIONS
Acute lower gastrointestinal bleeding to determine coagulation status
    Strength of Recommendation: Class IIa
    Strength of Evidence: Category C
    Results Interpretation:
    Increased level (laboratory finding)
        Obtain partial thromboplastin time in all patients with lower gastrointestinal bleeding to determine coagulation status and need for clotting factors, particularly in patients with a history of liver disease or those on anticoagulant medication.

Hantavirus pulmonary syndrome
Strength of Recommendation: Class IIa
Strength of Evidence: Category C
Results Interpretation:
Increased partial thromboplastin time

Prolonged PT is a common finding in hantavirus pulmonary syndrome. In one series, PTT was prolonged (median peak PTT was 54.4 [range, 31 to 150 seconds]) in two thirds of patients at the time of admission and in about 80% subsequently.

Prolonged PTT, when combined with other laboratory tests, is a strong predictor of mortality in hantavirus pulmonary syndrome.

Monitoring heparin therapy
Strength of Recommendation: Class I
Strength of Evidence: Category B
Results Interpretation:
Increased partial thromboplastin time

Activated partial thromboplastin time (aPTT) should be maintained at 1.5 to 2.5 times the levels of normal controls, or maintain an aPTT prolongation corresponding to plasma heparin levels of 0.3 to 0.7 International Units/mL anti-Xa activity by the amidolytic assay. Analytic techniques (ie, reagent and coagulometers) and tissue extracts, however, will vary between institutions resulting in different therapeutic ranges to achieve equal degrees of anticoagulation.

The risk of recurrence of venous thromboembolism is decreased when a therapeutic aPTT target (ie, 1.5 to 2.5 times control) is achieved.

Reye's syndrome
Strength of Recommendation: Class IIa
Strength of Evidence: Category C
Results Interpretation:
Increased partial thromboplastin time

Partial thromboplastin time may be prolonged to 2 times normal secondary to hypofibrinogenemia and decreased levels of liver-dependent coagulation factors. Prolonged levels are indicative of severe disease and the probability of progression.

Suspected blood coagulation disorder in patients with liver disease
Results Interpretation:
Increased partial thromboplastin time

End stage liver disease provokes multifactorial and potentially profound hemostatic failure that involves clotting factors, platelets, and the fibrinolytic system, which can result in a prolonged prothrombin time (PT) and activated partial thromboplastin time (aPTT).

Suspected DIC
Strength of Recommendation: Class IIa
Strength of Evidence: Category B
Results Interpretation:
Activated partial thromboplastin time abnormal

Partial thromboplastin time (PTT) is used primarily to evaluate coagulation abnormalities in the intrinsic pathway, as well as severe functional deficiencies in factors II, V, X or fibrinogen. PTT does not measure activation of the procoagulant system, but rather reflects the late consumptive stage of DIC when prolonged. PTT is also affected by therapeutic anticoagulant use.

Suspected heat stroke
Results Interpretation:
Increased partial thromboplastin time

A prolonged activated partial thromboplastin time (PTT) is commonly seen in severe cases of heat stroke, secondary to direct thermal damage to all clotting factors.

Clotting dysfunction peaks at 18 to 36 hours after the acute phase of heat stroke.

Suspected hemophilia A or B
Results Interpretation:
Increased partial thromboplastin time

Activated partial thromboplastin time (aPTT) can be normal or near normal in mild hemophilia A or B but prolonged in moderate to severe hemophilia A and B.

Suspect hemophilia with an inhibitor, if an aPTT done with 1 part patient's plasma to 1 part normal plasma and incubated for 1 to 2 hours fails to shorten.

Suspected hereditary factor XI deficiency
Results Interpretation:
Increased partial thromboplastin time
The diagnosis of hereditary factor XI deficiency should be suspected in a patient with an isolated prolonged activated partial thromboplastin time and a family history of a mild to moderate bleeding tendency with an autosomal inheritance pattern. Confirmation of the diagnosis requires a specific factor XI assay.

Suspected meningococcemia
Results Interpretation:
Increased partial thromboplastin time
A partial thromboplastin time greater than 50 seconds appears to predict poor outcome in children with purpuric sepsis syndrome.

Suspected or known hemolytic uremic syndrome (HUS)
Results Interpretation:
Normal hematology findings
In postdiarrheal hemolytic uremic syndrome (HUS), the partial thromboplastin time (PTT) is usually normal.

Suspected sepsis
Strength of Recommendation: Class IIa
Strength of Evidence: Category C
Results Interpretation:
Increased prothrombin time
Prolongation of the activated partial thromboplastin time is common in sepsis, even in the absence of overt DIC.
Timing of Monitoring
A baseline activated partial thromboplastin time should be obtained.

Suspected vitamin K deficiency
Results Interpretation:
Increased partial thromboplastin time
Activated partial thromboplastin time and prothrombin time are both prolonged in vitamin K-dependent deficiencies such as poor nutrition, obstructive jaundice, some drug therapies, and ingestion of rodenticides. In the absence of other hemostatic defects, the thrombin time, fibrinogen and platelet count are normal.

COMMON PANELS
- Disseminated intravascular coagulation screen
- Disseminated intravascular coagulopathy panel
- Transplant panel

DRUG/LAB INTERACTIONS
- Drotrecogin Alfa - inaccurate activated partial thromboplastin time (APTT) serum assay results

CLINICAL NOTES
Reference ranges can vary with the reagent used. The sensitivity of the method is dependent on the type and concentration of the activator and phospholipid used.

COLLECTION/STORAGE INFORMATION
- Specimen Collection and Handling:
  - Collect sample in sodium citrate (blue-top) tube.
  - Sample is stable for 1 hour at 4°C and for 28 days if frozen.

LOINC CODES
- Code: 3173-2 (*Short Name* - aPTT Bld Qn)
- Code: 13060-9 (*Short Name* - aPTT sp4 PPP Qn)
- Code: 5899-0 (*Short Name* - aPTT Inv Ratio PPP Qn Coag)

- Code: 12185-5 (*Short Name* - aPTT Bld Cont Qn)
- Code: 14979-9 (*Short Name* - aPTT PPP Qn Coag)

Peripheral blood buffy coat smear interpretation

TEST DEFINITION

Microscopic examination of a stained buffy-coat (leukocyte layer) smear, obtained from centrifuged blood, for the early identification of bacteremia

REFERENCE RANGE

- Adults and Children: Negative
Please refer to your institution's reference ranges as lab normals may vary.

INDICATIONS

Suspected bacterial septicemia
    Strength of Recommendation: Class IIb
    Strength of Evidence: Category B
    Results Interpretation:
Positive microbiology findings

Buffy-coat smears may detect bacterial pathogens in blood, depending on the bacterial load and the skill of the reviewer. The test is limited by low sensitivity.

Occasionally, reported low-level bacterial detections occur with a buffy coat smear. Eg, Gram-stained *Staphylococcus aureus* results were positive with as few as 50 colony-forming units (CFU)/mL blood, the generally-reported limit for Gram stain detection is greater than or equal to 10^5 CFU/mL, and for acridine-orange stained buffy coat smears, it is 10^4 CFU/mL. In several studies, the quantity of bacteria required for detection (either intracellular or extracellular) was so great as to make this test of greater use for predicting mortality rather than determining treatment.

Buffy coat smear results may be useful in guiding antibiotic therapy.

As with blood culture, specimen contamination during collection may be a problem.

While buffy-coat smear may identify bacteria in blood, blood culture is the diagnostic reference standard.

- Detectable Gram-positive organisms by buffy-coat smear:
  - *Staphylococcus aureus*
  - *Staphylococcus albus*
  - *Streptococcus pneumoniae*
  - *Streptococcus faecalis*
  - *Clostridium perfringens*
- Detectable Gram-negative organisms by buffy-coat smear:
  - *Neisseria meningitidis* (meningococcus)
  - *Pseudomonas aeruginosa*
  - *Salmonella*, including *S typhi*
  - *Coliform bacteria*
  - *Klebsiella pneumoniae*
  - *Proteus mirabelis*
  - *Serratia marcescens*

Negative microbiology findings

A negative buffy-coat smear finding does not rule out septicemia.

Suspected malaria
    Results Interpretation:
    Hematology finding

Quantitative Buffy Coat malaria test is a sensitive but nonspecific test for malaria and should only be used as a screening tool. It does not detect the sexual stages of the disease.

CLINICAL NOTES

The potential advantage of this method is the faster turnaround time for buffy-coat smear results compared to blood culture.

COLLECTION/STORAGE INFORMATION
• Collect venous or capillary blood in a lavender-top EDTA tube.

LOINC CODES
• Code: 33270-0 (*Short Name* - Micro Buffy Coat)

pH measurement, pleural fluid

TEST DEFINITION
Measurement of pH in pleural fluid for evaluation and management of parapneumonic effusions

REFERENCE RANGE
• Adults:
• Transudates: 7.4-7.5
• Exudates: 7.35-7.45
Please refer to your institution's reference ranges as lab normals may vary.

INDICATIONS
Suspected neoplasm of lung
　　Strength of Recommendation: Class IIa
　　Strength of Evidence: Category C
Results Interpretation:
Abnormal biochemistry findings
Lower pleural fluid pH in the presence of large or massive pleural effusion suggests malignancy..
Lower pleural fluid pH increase need for pleural drainage (specific pH cutoffs have not been established) and signal more extensive pleural involvement.
Low pleural fluid pH (less than 7), low pleural fluid glucose (less than 40 mg/dL or positive Gram stain or culture), and high pleural fluid LDH often indicate complicated parapneumonic effusion and need for chest tube insertion. Pleural fluid pH less than 7.2 requires urgent drainage.
Higher pleural fluid pH levels indicate medical management of effusion is adequate (specific pH cutoffs have not been established).

False Results
Pleural fluid pH can be invalid in conditions such as systemic acidosis and local anesthetics prepared in acid solutions that enter the pleural space.

Suspected or known esophagal perforation or rupture with esophageal leakage into the thoracic cavity
Results Interpretation:
pH - finding
The pleural fluid in esophageal rupture is usually <7.30. (The low pH pleural effusion is primarily related to generation of acid from polymorphonuclear cell metabolism). Esophageal rupture is particularly suspect when the pleural fluid pH is <6.5.
Other conditions associated with a low pleural fluid pH are empyema, malignancy, collagen vascular disease, tuberculosis, and hemothorax..

CLINICAL NOTES
Use of litmus paper to determine pleural fluid pH is unreliable and should not be considered an acceptable alternative to the arterial blood gas analyzer.

COLLECTION/STORAGE INFORMATION
• Specimen Collection and Handling:
　• Collect pleural fluid in heparinized syringe
　• Maintain strict anaerobic conditions
　• Transport on ice and measure within 6 hours

LOINC CODES
• Code: 2750-8 (*Short Name* - pH Plr-sCnc)

Phenothiazine measurement

TEST DEFINITION

Measurement of plasma or serum level of the phenothiazine drug class

REFERENCE RANGE

It is difficult to establish ranges for normal serum levels of this class of drugs due to the large number of metabolites for each drug as a result of extensive liver metabolism.

Please refer to your institution's reference ranges as lab normals may vary.

INDICATIONS

Measurement of phenothiazines in serum for therapeutic monitoring

Strength of Recommendation: Class IIb

Strength of Evidence: Category C

Results Interpretation:

Blood drug levels - finding

Monitoring of therapeutic phenothiazine levels may have clinical application in improving patient therapy by determining patient compliance and drug bioavailability.

The significance of any level measured is confounded by the ability of some metabolites to undergo conversion back to the parent compound.

CLINICAL NOTES

The significance of any level measured is confounded by the ability of some metabolites to undergo conversion back to the parent compound. This has been demonstrated with the inactive metabolite, chlorpromazine N-oxide's ability to convert back to the active parent compound.

Phenylalanine measurement

TEST DEFINITION

Measurement of phenylalanine in plasma, serum or whole blood for detection of acquired and hereditary amino acid disorders.

SYNONYMS

- Guthrie test
- Phenylalanine screening test, blood

REFERENCE RANGE

- Guthrie bacterial inhibition assay (whole blood):
- Newborn, 2 to 5 days: ≤2 mg/dL (≤121 micromol/L)
- Fluorometry:
- Low-birth weight or premature neonate: 2-7.5 mg/dL (121-454 micromol/L)
- Fluorometry:
- Newborn, full-term and normal weight: 1.2-3.4 mg/dL (73-206 micromol/L)
- Fluorometry:
- Phenylketonuric, 2 to 3 days after birth: >4.5 mg/dL (>272 micromol/L)
- Phenylketonuric, untreated at 10 days: 15-30 mg/dL (907-1,815 micromol/L)
- Fluorometry:
- Adults: 0.8-1.8 mg/dL (48-109 micromol/L)
- Ion-exchange chromatography:
- Premature neonate: 1.49 ± 0.33 mg/dL (90 ± 20 micromol/L)
- Ion-exchange chromatography:
- Neonate, 1 day: 0.69-1.82 mg/dL (42-110 micromol/L)
- Ion-exchange chromatography:
- Infants 1 to 3 months: 0.86 ± 0.23 mg/dL (52 ± 14 micromol/L)
- Ion-exchange chromatography:
- Infants 2 to 6 months: 0.86-1.6 mg/dL (52-97 micromol/L)

- Ion-exchange chromatography:
- Infants 9 to 24 months: 0.38-1.14 mg/dL (23-69 micromol/L)
- Ion-exchange chromatography:
- Children 3 to 10 years: 0.43-1.01 mg/dL (26-61 micromol/L)
- Ion-exchange chromatography:
- Children 6 to 18 years: 0.64-1.26 mg/dL (39-76 micromol/L)
- Ion-exchange chromatography:
- Adults: 0.61-1.45 mg/dL (37-88 micromol/L)
  Please refer to your institution's reference ranges as lab normals may vary.

INDICATIONS
Suspected hyperphenylalaninemia
> **Strength of Recommendation:** Class IIa
> **Strength of Evidence:** Category C

Results Interpretation:
Increased amino acid
Blood phenylalanine (Phe) levels above 20 mg/dL, along with the presence of phenylketones, are often seen in patients with phenylketonuria (PKU). Non-PKU hyperphenylalaninemia will result in a lower Phe level without phenylketone accumulation. Infants with Phe levels above 10 mg/dL should have medical nutritional therapy initiated as soon as possible, but no later than 7 to 10 days after birth. The goal of therapy is to obtain therapeutic Phe levels within the first 2 to 3 weeks of life. Tetrahydrobiopterin deficiency must be excluded before therapy is begun. In the majority of cases amino acid and organic acid analysis together permit diagnostic confirmation in infants.

In newborn screening, Phe levels of 2 to 4 mg/dL are considered borderline and may indicate PKU, hyperphenylalaninemia, or another metabolic condition. Phe levels of greater than 4 mg/dL in newborns are considered abnormal and are suggestive of probable PKU, hyperphenylalaninemia, PKU in the mother, or another metabolic condition. Elevated levels could also be due to false positive results.

Discussion is ongoing regarding the ideal blood Phe level in PKU, and guidelines vary by country. British policy recommends a range of 2 to 6 mg/dL in infants and young children. The German Working Group for Metabolic Diseases suggests a range of 0.7 to 4 mg/dL from birth to 10 years of age, 0.7 to 15 mg/dL between 10 and 15 years of age and 0.7 to 20 mg/dL after 15 years. The NIH PKU Consensus Statement recommends blood Phe levels of 2 to 6 mg/mL for neonates through age 12, and 2 to 15 mg/dL for patients over 12 years of age, although a tighter range of 2 to 10 mg/dL is suggested during adolescence. The United States Maternal Phenylketonuria Collaborative Study recommends a maternal range of 2 to 6 mg/dL during pregnancy while British and German recommendations suggest a target maternal range of 1 to 4 mg/dL. A level of less than 6 mg/dL is recommended for at least 3 months prior to conception. Because adults with PKU have displayed diminished cognitive function, lifelong Phe monitoring and diet restriction is recommended.

Frequency of Monitoring
In patients with phenylketonuria (PKU), phenylalanine testing is recommended weekly during the first year of life, twice monthly from 1 to 12 years of age, monthly after 12 years of age, and twice weekly during pregnancy for women with PKU.

Timing of Monitoring
Phenylketonuria (PKU) screening is recommended within 48 hours of birth.

COLLECTION/STORAGE INFORMATION
- Specimen Collection and Handling:
  - Immediately place sample in ice water.
  - Isolate plasma sample and freeze it within 1 hour; sample stable for 1 week at -20°C.
  - Plasma or serum sample should be deproteinized and stored at -70°C for protracted periods of usage.
  - Guthrie bacterial inhibition assay sample is stable for 10 days at 30°C or for 2 months at 4°C.
  - Two days of protein feeding is suggested before specimen is collected; inadequate protein intake may cause a false-negative result.
  - All positive results must be confirmed with quantitative testing or by chromatography.
  - Antibiotics will interfere with results interpretation.
  - Diurnal variations are normal in healthy newborns with peak levels occurring in the evening.

LOINC CODES
- Code: 32264-4 (*Short Name* - Phenylalanine Vitf-sCnc)
- Code: 22646-4 (*Short Name* - Phe CSF-sCnc)
- Code: 2766-4 (*Short Name* - Phe Ur-mCnc)
- Code: 25495-3 (*Short Name* - Phe 24H Ur-sRate)

- Code: 2763-1 (*Short Name* - Phe CSF-mCnc)
- Code: 22737-1 (*Short Name* - Phe XXX-sCnc)
- Code: 2767-2 (*Short Name* - Phe 24H Ur-mRate)
- Code: 30055-8 (*Short Name* - Phenylalanine/creat Ur-Rto)
- Code: 32263-6 (*Short Name* - Phe Fld-sCnc)
- Code: 25969-7 (*Short Name* - Phe 24H Ur-sCnc)
- Code: 13893-3 (*Short Name* - Phe Ur Ql)
- Code: 25970-5 (*Short Name* - Phe/creat 24H Ur-sRto)
- Code: 26967-0 (*Short Name* - Phe Ur-sCnc)
- Code: 26981-1 (*Short Name* - Phenylalanine Amn-sCnc)
- Code: 2762-3 (*Short Name* - Phenylalanine Bld-mCnc)

Phenylketonuria screening

TEST DEFINITION
Measurement of phenylalanine in plasma to screen for phenylketonuria, most commonly in newborns

REFERENCE RANGE
- Newborns: ≤2 mg/dL (≤121 micromol/L)
  Please refer to your institution's reference ranges as lab normals may vary.

INDICATIONS
Screening for phenylketonuria (PKU) in neonates
> **Strength of Recommendation:** Class I
> **Strength of Evidence:** Category C
> **Results Interpretation:**
> **Phenylalanine level - finding**
>> Cutoff levels vary from state to state, from 2 mg/dL to greater than 4 mg/dL.
>> Further confirmatory testing should be performed on all patients with a positive phenylketonuria screen.
> **Timing of Monitoring**
>> Blood should be collected in the neonatal period between 24 hours of life and 7 days. If blood is collected before 24 hours, the test should be repeated at 2 weeks of age.
>> A phenylketonuria screen should be administered at any age for individuals with unexplained mental retardation and/or severe behavioral disturbances.

ABNORMAL RESULTS
- Results increased in:
  - Premature infants with immature livers
- Results decreased in:
  - Insufficient protein intake

COLLECTION/STORAGE INFORMATION
- Specimen Collection and Handling:
  - Collect whole blood on filter paper
  - May store at 30° C for 10 days or at 4° C for 2 months

Phenytoin measurement

TEST DEFINITION
Measurement of total phenytoin in serum or plasma for therapeutic drug monitoring and suspected toxicity.

SYNONYMS
- Dilantin measurement
- Diphenylhydantoin measurement

REFERENCE RANGE
- Adults, therapeutic level: 10-20 mcg/mL (40-79 micromol/L)
- Adults, toxic level: >20 mcg/mL (>79 micromol/L)
  Please refer to your institution's reference ranges as lab normals may vary.

INDICATIONS
Suspected phenytoin toxicity
>**Strength of Recommendation:** Class IIa
>**Strength of Evidence:** Category C
>**Results Interpretation:**
>**Phenytoin level - finding**
>>Toxicity is rare at levels below 20 mcg/mL. Toxic effects such as nystagmus, ataxia, and mental changes are usually seen at levels greater than 20 mcg/mL, 30 mcg/mL, and 40 mcg/mL, respectively. Signs and symptoms of toxicity may persist for up to 7 to 10 days.
>>Although the risk of toxicity increases at levels above 80 micromols/L, and is expected at levels above 100 micromols/L, toxicity cannot be ruled out at levels below 80 micromols/L and a trial reduction in dosage may be indicated if toxicity is suspected.
>
>**Frequency of Monitoring**
>>In acute oral overdose, a minimum of 2 serial levels are recommended due to delayed absorption, even if initial levels are negligible.

Therapeutic monitoring of phenytoin levels
>**Strength of Recommendation:** Class I
>**Strength of Evidence:** Category C
>**Results Interpretation:**
>**Phenytoin level - finding**
>>The upper limit for therapeutic serum phenytoin is generally considered to be 20 mcg/mL. Small changes in dosage can result in marked changes in blood levels. The correct therapeutic dose of phenytoin should be determined by seizure control and clinical toxicity, not by serum drug levels. Supratherapeutic levels are required to control seizures in some cases.
>
>**Frequency of Monitoring**
>>A serum phenytoin level is recommended several days after starting drug therapy, and again after 2 to 3 weeks to evaluate for delayed toxicity. Phenytoin levels should be drawn before the first oral dose, and 1 to 4 hours post-intravenous loading dose. For patients on fosphenytoin, recommended sample timing is at least 2 hours post-intravenous dose or 4 hours post-intramuscular dose. Ongoing measurement of drug levels is not necessary for patients whose seizures are controlled on well tolerated dosages.

DRUG/LAB INTERACTIONS
- Clove - a false increase in phenytoin levels

CLINICAL NOTES
Differences in formulation between brand names and generic equivalents can result in altered bioavailability, causing toxicity or the development of subtherapeutic levels; switching brands should be undertaken with caution.

COLLECTION/STORAGE INFORMATION

LOINC CODES
- Code: 29224-3 (*Short Name* - Phenytoin Fld-mCnc)
- Code: 12310-9 (*Short Name* - Phenytoin Ur Ql)
- Code: 17444-1 (*Short Name* - Phenytoin Ur-mCnc)

Phosphate measurement

Test Definition
Measurement of phosphate level in blood to evaluate the effects of certain disease states on phosphate levels including: abnormalities in calcium homeostasis (eg, parathyroid disease), acute alterations of intracellular metabolic requirements (eg, refeeding after starvation or thyrotoxicosis), cell lysis (eg, tumor lysis syndrome, rhabdomyolysis), primary or secondary disorders effecting gastrointestinal phosphate absorption, inappropriate nutritional supplementation, or abnormal renal function (eg, renal insufficiency, renal failure)

Synonyms
- Phosphate level

Reference Range
- Adults: 3-4.5 mg/dL (1-1.4 mmol/L)
- Menopause: levels increased approximately 0.2 mg/dL (0.06 mmol/L) during first ten years
- Premature neonates: 5.4-10.9 mg/dL (1.74-3.52 mmol/L)
- Neonates: 4.5-9 mg/dL (1.45-2.91 mmol/L)
- Infants: 4.5-5.5 mg/dL (1.45-1.78 mmol/L)
- Children (24 months to 12 years): 4.5-5.5 mg/dL (1.45-1.78 mmol/L)
  Please refer to your institution's reference ranges as lab normals may vary.

Indications
Patients hospitalized for community acquired pneumonia
Results Interpretation:
Hypophosphatemia
The combination of hypophosphatemia, hypocalcemia, hypokalemia, and alkalosis in hospitalized patients with bacterial pneumonia may be a predictor of illness severity. The presence of hypophosphatemia is associated with prolonged hospitalization and increased mortality.

A diagnosis of Legionnaires disease should be strongly considered in patients with hypophosphatemia, as a low phosphate level is found in 50% of these patients; however, pneumonia of other etiologies can also cause hypophosphatemia.

Another study comparing Legionnaire's disease with other bacterial etiologies of community acquired pneumonia showed no difference in the degree of hypophosphatemia.

Diagnosis and monitoring of tumor lysis syndrome
Results Interpretation:
Hyperphosphatemia
Hyperphosphatemia results from the rapid release of phosphate by fragmented tumor nuclei in quantities that exceed the excretory capacity of the kidneys. Hyperphosphatemia is associated with an LDH level greater than 1500 international units/L.

Dialysis should be considered if the phosphorus level is greater than 10 mg/dL (phosphate greater than 3.2 mmol/L) or rising rapidly.
Timing of Monitoring
In tumor lysis syndrome, hyperphosphatemia develops 24 to 48 hours after cytotoxic therapy is begun.

Initial evaluation and monitoring of diabetic ketoacidosis
Results Interpretation:
Hyperphosphatemia
Despite total-body phosphate depletion averaging approximately 1 mmol/kg in diabetic ketoacidosis (DKA), serum phosphate levels are often normal or increased at presentation.

The hyperphosphatemia usually observed with diabetic ketoacidosis (DKA) is primarily insulin mediated. Specifically, a lack of insulin or insulin resistance impairs cellular uptake of both carbohydrates and phosphate, leading to increased serum levels. Critically, the catabolic cascade associated with DKA results in depletion of total body phosphate. The treatment of DKA with insulin and rehydration can result in symptomatic hypophosphatemia due to intracellular phosphate shifts and the hemodilution of circulating phosphate.
Hypophosphatemia
Serum phosphate levels decrease with insulin therapy during treatment for DKA as phosphate re-enters the intracellular compartment.

Frequency of Monitoring

Phosphate levels should be obtained every 2 to 4 hours during the treatment.

Known chronic kidney disease

Strength of Recommendation: Class I
Strength of Evidence: Category C
Results Interpretation:
Renal failure-associated hyperphosphatemia

- Selected National Kidney Foundation recommendations for using serum phosphorus measurements in the prevention and management of chronic kidney disease (CKD)-related metabolic bone disease:
  - The calcium malabsorption associated with severe renal failure (GFR <30) requires prescribing oral calcium with meals if the serum phosphorus is high, or at night if the phosphorus is normal.
  - Neither calcitriol (vitamin D) nor calcium carbonate administration is recommended in the presence of an elevated calcium phosphorus product (ie, ≥75).
  - In Stages 3 and 4 CKD patients, the serum level of phosphorus should be maintained between 2.7 mg/dL (0.87 mmol/L) and 4.6 mg/dL (1.49 mmol/L).
  - Dietary phosphorus should be restricted to 800 to 1,000 mg/day (adjusted for dietary protein needs) when the serum phosphorus levels are elevated, ie, >4.6 mg/dL (1.49 mmol/L) in Stages 3 and 4 of CKD, and >5.5 mg/dL (1.78 mmol/L) in Stage 5 (kidney failure)
  - Dietary phosphorus should be restricted to 800 to 1,000 mg/day (adjusted to dietary protein needs) when the plasma levels of intact parathyroid hormone (iPTH) are above the target range of the CKD Stage.
  - If the serum phosphorus exceeds 4.6 mg/dL on vitamin D therapy, a phosphate binder should be added or the dose increased. If hyperphosphatemia persists, vitamin D therapy should be discontinued.
  - Treatment with an active vitamin D sterol should be undertaken only in patients with serum levels of corrected total calcium <9.5 mg/dL (2.37 mmol/L) and serum phosphorus <4.6 mg/dL (1.49 mmol/L).

Frequency of Monitoring

The serum phosphorus (phosphate) levels should be monitored monthly following the initiation of dietary phosphorus restriction

After starting vitamin D therapy, serum levels of calcium and phosphorus should be monitored at least monthly for the first 3 months, then every 3 months thereafter.

Timing of Monitoring

Serum levels of calcium, phosphorus, and intact plasma parathyroid hormone (iPTH) should be measured in all patients with chronic kidney disease (CKD) and GFR <60 mL/minute/1.73 m^2.

Metabolic acidosis

Strength of Recommendation: Class IIa
Strength of Evidence: Category C
Results Interpretation:
Hyperphosphatemia

The effect of metabolic acidosis on phosphate levels does not appear directly related to a pH phenomenon.

The specific pathophysiology underlying the hyperphosphatemia of lactic acidosis is unclear. However, it may be due to intracellular phosphate leakage resulting from hypoxia.

Suspected and known alcoholic ketoacidosis

Results Interpretation:
Lowered biochemistry findings

Serum phosphate is commonly depressed in alcoholics.

Suspected and known hypocalcemia

Results Interpretation:
Hyperphosphatemia

Hyperphosphatemia is a finding in renal failure, primary hypoparathyroidism, and pseudohypoparathyroidism.

Hypophosphatemia

Hypophosphatemia is found in hypovitaminosis D, malabsorption syndromes, chronic alcohol abuse, and hyperalimentation, as well as in patients receiving loop diuretics.

Suspected hypercalcemia
Results Interpretation:
Decreased level (laboratory finding)
Serum phosphorus level may be decreased in patients with hypercalcemia of malignancy.
Increased level (laboratory finding)
An increased serum phosphorus level with hypercalcemia may occur in hypervitaminosis D or granulomatous disease.

Suspected hyperphosphatemia
Strength of Recommendation: Class I
Strength of Evidence: Category C
Results Interpretation:
Hyperphosphatemia
Hyperphosphatemia can result from exogenous phosphate overload, hypoparathyroid disease, acute cell lysis (eg, tumor lysis syndrome or rhabdomyolysis), metabolic acidosis, impaired renal excretion, or increased renal phosphate resorption.

Suspected hyperventilation
Results Interpretation:
Decreased level (laboratory finding)
The phosphate level can decline during hyperventilation, and remain low following the cessation of hyperventilation.
A decline in phosphate may manifest as malaise, dizziness, paresthesias, disorientation, and a decrease in attention span, which are also common symptoms of hyperventilation syndrome.

Suspected hypophosphatemia
Strength of Recommendation: Class IIa
Strength of Evidence: Category C
Results Interpretation:
Hypophosphatemia
Hypophosphatemia can result from acute increases in intracellular energy requirements as observed in refeeding after starvation, nutritional deficiency, thyrotoxicosis, gastrointestinal absorptive impairment, hyperparathyroid disease, hypercalcemia, or phosphaturia due to impaired renal phosphate absorption. Identification of a definitive etiology requires additional testing.

Suspected rhabdomyolysis
Results Interpretation:
Hyperphosphatemia
Muscle necrosis may cause release of phosphates from hydrolyzed nonregenerated adenosine 5'-triphosphate (ATP) into the extracellular fluid with resultant hyperphosphatemia. Serum phosphate level correlates best with serum anion gap and inversely with bicarbonate concentration.
Hypophosphatemia
Hypophosphatemia is seen in 40% of patients with rhabdomyolysis. This may be an initial finding or develop after therapy begins. Patients with levels greater than 5 mg/dL on admission have a higher frequency of hypophosphatemia later in their hospitalization.

Suspected sepsis
Strength of Recommendation: Class IIb
Strength of Evidence: Category C
Results Interpretation:
Hypophosphatemia
Hypophosphatemia has been associated with septic shock and poor prognosis.

Thermal burn
Results Interpretation:
Decreased phosphate level
Hypophosphatemia is common with major burns and may itself be severe. Major phosphate loss appears to be urinary with exudative losses being less important.
Phosphate shifting occurs during refeeding as phosphate enters the cells with glucose.

Common Panels
- Bone and joint panel
- Enteral/Parenteral nutritional management panel
- Parathyroid panel
- Renal panel
- Transplant panel

Abnormal Results
- Results increased in:
  - May and June
  - With bed rest
- Results decreased in:
  - Winter

Clinical Notes
- Phosphate levels follow diurnal variation; nadir prior to noon and peak prior to midnight

Collection/Storage Information
Specimen Collection and Handling:
- Patients should be instructed to fast (overnight) prior to test
- Collect 5 mL of venous blood in heparinized tube
- Separate from erythrocytes within 1 hour of collection to avoid spurious results
- Store at 4°C for several days or frozen for several months

LOINC Codes
- Code: 22733-0 (*Short Name* - Phosphate XXX-sCnc)
- Code: 25501-8 (*Short Name* - Phosphate Fld-sCnc)
- Code: 14407-1 (*Short Name* - Phosphate Gast-mCnc)
- Code: 14879-1 (*Short Name* - Phosphate SerPl-sCnc)
- Code: 14408-9 (*Short Name* - Phosphate Amn-mCnc)
- Code: 2774-8 (*Short Name* - Phosphate Bld-mCnc)
- Code: 2780-5 (*Short Name* - Phosphate Ur Ql)
- Code: 2777-1 (*Short Name* - Phosphate SerPl-mCnc)
- Code: 12242-4 (*Short Name* - Phosphate Fld-mCnc)
- Code: 24519-1 (*Short Name* - Phosphate Bld-sCnc)
- Code: 14404-8 (*Short Name* - Phosphate Plr-mCnc)
- Code: 13542-6 (*Short Name* - Phosphate CSF-mCnc)
- Code: 10884-5 (*Short Name* - Phosphate Stl-mCnt)
- Code: 2775-5 (*Short Name* - Phosphate Diaf-mCnc)
- Code: 13539-2 (*Short Name* - Phosphate Ur-sCnc)
- Code: 2778-9 (*Short Name* - Phosphate Ur-mCnc)
- Code: 27123-9 (*Short Name* - Phosphate RBC-mCnt)
- Code: 14405-5 (*Short Name* - Phosphate Prt-mCnc)
- Code: 14406-3 (*Short Name* - Phosphate Snv-mCnc)

Phosphatidylglycerol measurement, semi-quantitative, amniotic fluid

Test Definition
Measurement of phosphatidylglycerol levels in amniotic fluid for the evaluation and management of fetal lung maturity

Reference Range
- Pregnant women (3rd trimester):
- Thin-layer chromatography
- Absent: Fetal lung immaturity

- Slide-agglutination test
- Negative: <0.5 mg/L
- Enzymatic assay: 19-83 mg/L
  Please refer to your institution's reference ranges as lab normals may vary.

INDICATIONS
Prediction of fetal lung maturity in high-risk pregnancies
   Strength of Recommendation: Class IIa
   Strength of Evidence: Category C
   Results Interpretation:
   Fetal lung development
   Phosphatidylglycerol (PG) is a minor component of surfactant that usually appears in sufficient quantity to be measured around 34 to 37 weeks gestation. Its absence indicates a significant risk of fetal lung immaturity and respiratory distress syndrome (RDS).
   If PG is present by thin-layer chromatography, the probability of RDS is approximately 1%, although the absence of PG does not always mean that RDS is inevitable.
   In the slide agglutination method, negative results (less than 0.5 mg/L) are a poor predictor of fetal lung maturity and may need to be verified by thin-layer chromatography or other methods or tests. High-positive results are generally greater than 2 mg/L with low-positive results greater than 0.5 mg/L.

   False Results
   In women with poorly controlled diabetes, phosphatidylglycerol (PG) levels may be absent as late as 38 to 39 weeks' gestation and may require a different approach in assessing fetal maturity. The Amniostat-FLM® rapid slide agglutination test may be recommended to rule out false predictions of fetal lung maturity obtained by other rapid tests. A high positive result (greater than 2 mg/L) is used by some clinicians to predict fetal lung maturity in cases of maternal diabetes.
   Timing of Monitoring
   Phosphatidylglycerol (PG) determination is usually performed between 34 and 37 weeks' gestation. It is rarely performed prior to 33 weeks, when fetal lung maturity is unlikely, or later than 37 weeks, when the incidence of respiratory distress syndrome is less than 1%.

CLINICAL NOTES
   An advantage of phosphatidylglycerol determination is that it is not affected by contaminants (eg, blood, meconium).
   Determination of phosphatidylglycerol is often done in conjunction with the lecithin-sphingomyelin ratio.

COLLECTION/STORAGE INFORMATION
- Specimen Collection and Handling:
  - A minimum of 3 to 4 mL of amniotic fluid is required; 10 mL is preferred.
  - Sterile specimens are obtained by amniocentesis; nonsterile specimens may be collected following rupture of membranes from the free flow of fluid in the vagina, although this method is discouraged.
  - Centrifuge upon receipt of specimen; do not freeze prior to centrifugation.
  - If the test is delayed, refrigerate sterile specimens (obtained from amniocentesis); freeze contaminated specimens (obtained from vaginal pooling).

LOINC CODES
- Code: 2786-2 (*Short Name* - PG Amn-mCnc)
- Code: 27420-9 (*Short Name* - PG Amn-aCnc)

Phosphorus measurement, urine

TEST DEFINITION
   Measurement of phosphorus in urine for causative identification of nephrolithiasis

REFERENCE RANGE
   Adults (varies with intake): 400 -1300 mg/24 hours (12.9-42 mmol/24 hours)
   Please refer to your institution's reference ranges as lab normals may vary.

INDICATIONS

Kidney stones
>**Strength of Recommendation:** Class IIb
>**Strength of Evidence:** Category B
>**Results Interpretation:**
>**Abnormal biochemistry findings**
>>Urinary phosphorus levels are correlated with the risk of stone formation. Stone formers have lower concentrations of urinary phosphorus than healthy controls.
>>Urine phosphorus excretion has significant diurnal variation with values highest in the afternoon. Urine phosphorous excretion also varies depending on diet.
>>A creatinine clearance greater than 40 to 50 mL/min is required for accurate interpretation of results.

Suspected hyperphosphaturia
>**Strength of Recommendation:** Class IIa
>**Strength of Evidence:** Category C
>**Results Interpretation:**
>**Hyperphosphaturia**
>>Elevated urine phosphorus level is a diagnostic aid in the evaluation of a number of systemic and endocrine disease processes.

COLLECTION/STORAGE INFORMATION
- Collect 24-hour urine in acid-washed, detergent-free container.
- Sample stable for 6 months.

LOINC CODES
- Code: 25127-2 (*Short Name* - Phosphorus/creat 24H Ur-sRto)

Pinworm slide

TEST DEFINITION
Detection of *Enterobius vermicularis* by recovery of pinworm ova or adult worm from anal verge

REFERENCE RANGE
- No worms or ova present
  Please refer to your institution's reference ranges as lab normals may vary.

INDICATIONS
Suspected enterobiasis
>**Strength of Recommendation:** Class I
>**Strength of Evidence:** Category C
>**Results Interpretation:**
>**Presence of ova cysts and parasites - finding**
>>The positive presence of worms or ova is diagnostic. Adult male worms measure 2 to 5 mm; adult female worms measure 8 to 13 mm.

LOINC CODES
- Code: 675-9 (*Short Name* - Pinworm Exam XXX)
- Code: 6676-1 (*Short Name* - Pinworm Exam Tiss)

Plasma activated protein C resistance

TEST DEFINITION
Screening test for factor V Leiden mutation and subsequent risk for venous thrombosis

REFERENCE RANGE
• Adults: Ratio >2.1
Please refer to your institution's reference ranges as lab normals may vary.

INDICATIONS
Suspected factor V Leiden mutation
   Strength of Recommendation: Class IIa
   Strength of Evidence: Category A
   Results Interpretation:
   Positive laboratory findings
      Factor V Leiden mutation and resistance to activated protein C are independent risk factors for venous thromboembolism.
      Factor V Leiden is associated with about a 7-fold risk for thrombosis in heterozygote carriers and an 80-fold risk in homozygote carriers.
      Factor V Leiden is found in about 5% of healthy persons of northern European ancestry and in 30% to 50% of persons investigated for thrombophilia.
      The definitive diagnosis of factor V Leiden mutation requires molecular methods, such as polymerase chain reaction DNA amplification.

   False Results
      A positive activated protein C resistance assay is predictive of factor V Leiden mutation, but false-positive results can occur for various reasons including high factor VIII activity and oral contraceptive use.

Suspected risk for venous thromboembolism in pregnancy secondary to personal or family history of venous thromboembolism
   Strength of Recommendation: Class IIa
   Strength of Evidence: Category B
   Results Interpretation:
   Positive laboratory findings
      Activated protein C resistance (APCR) testing currently is recommended only for pregnant women who have a personal history of venous thromboembolism or a family history of factor V Leiden mutation.
      Women with a positive activated protein C resistance assay should undergo DNA-based genetic testing to definitively confirm or exclude factor V Leiden mutation.
      Although about 23% to 60% of women who develop deep venous thrombosis (DVT) during pregnancy have factor V mutation, the absolute risk of DVT is low. DVT occurs in about one in 1500 pregnancies overall; among factor V Leiden-positive women, DVT occurs in about one in 400 to 500 pregnancies.
      Routine screening of pregnant women for factor V Leiden is not recommended, because of the relatively low absolute risk of deep venous thrombosis (DVT), uncertainties about management of DVT during pregnancy, and the potential harm from unnecessary interventions (eg, with antithrombotics).

Suspected venous thromboembolism with a known family history of thrombosis
   Strength of Recommendation: Class IIa
   Strength of Evidence: Category A
   Results Interpretation:
   Positive laboratory findings
      Activated protein C (APC) inhibits coagulation by proteolytically inactivating coagulation factors Va and VIIIa. Resistance to APC (APCR) is usually caused by factor V Leiden mutation but, even in the absence of factor V Leiden, APCR is an independent risk factor for venous thromboembolism.
      A point mutation of clotting factor V (factor V Leiden mutation) leading to activated protein C resistance is the most common inherited factor predisposing to venous thromboembolism in white persons. Factor V Leiden is present in 3% to 7% of white persons, but is rare in blacks and Asians.
      Patients with factor V Leiden are twice as likely to present with deep venous thrombosis (DVT) without pulmonary embolism (PE) symptoms than with isolated PE, possibly because the DVT is distal (not ilio-femoral) and associated with smaller thrombi.
   Timing of Monitoring
      Generally, hypercoagulable state testing should be delayed up to 6 months after an acute thrombotic event. The modified activated protein C resistance assay and DNA-based gene mutation assays are not affected by anticoagulant therapy, but anticoagulants and acute thrombosis per se commonly affect other assays.

Thromboembolic stroke secondary to suspected hypercoagulable state
    Strength of Recommendation: Class IIb
    Strength of Evidence: Category C
Results Interpretation:
Positive laboratory findings
    The clinical relevance of activated protein C resistance or factor V Leiden mutation in thromboembolic stroke is unclear, and should be considered in the context of multiple factors that can contribute to the development of thromboemboli in stroke.

- Arterial thrombosis:
  - Data supporting a role of activated protein C resistance is much more convincing in venous than in arterial thromboembolic disease.
  - Genetic markers other than homocysteine levels and anticardiolipin antibodies have not been convincingly shown to be associated with arterial thrombosis.
- Factor V Leiden mutation:
  - The most relevant inherited coagulation defect associated with cerebral venous thrombosis; present in 10% to 20% of cases.
  - A particularly important contributing factor in childhood strokes, increasing the risk for stroke 5-fold in this population.
  - May be an important contributor to arterial strokes in young women with this mutation and an additional prothrombotic state (eg, homocystinemia), as well as non-factor V Leiden-related activated protein C resistance in certain ethnic populations (eg, Hispanics).
- Activated protein C resistance (APCR) has been associated with:
  - Increased risk of cerebrovascular disease, including nonfatal thromboembolic stroke, independent of the factor V Leiden mutation.
  - Thromboembolism in children with underlying cardiac disease.
  - An almost 10% incidence in Hispanics with ischemic stroke.

COMMON PANELS
- Hypercoagulation panel

CLINICAL NOTES
A positive activated protein C resistance assay strongly suggests factor V Leiden mutation, but DNA analysis is required to confirm the diagnosis.

COLLECTION/STORAGE INFORMATION
- Collect venous blood in blue top (sodium citrate) tube.

LOINC CODES
- Code: 13590-5 (*Short Name* - APCr PPP)

Plasma aldosterone level

TEST DEFINITION
Measurement of aldosterone in serum for evaluation of adrenal dysfunction

REFERENCE RANGE
- Adults:
- Supine, normal-sodium diet: 2-9 ng/dL (55-250 pmol/L)
- Upright, normal-sodium diet: 2 to 5 times supine value with normal-sodium diet
- Supine, low-sodium diet: 2 to 5 times supine value with normal-sodium diet
- Adrenal vein: 200-800 ng/dL (5.54-22.16 nmol/L)
  Please refer to your institution's reference ranges as lab normals may vary.

INDICATIONS
Suspected aldosteronism due to adrenal cortical tumor in hypertensive patients
    Strength of Recommendation: Class IIa
    Strength of Evidence: Category C

Results Interpretation:
Increased aldosterone level

Plasma aldosterone is one of several sequential tests used to diagnose aldosteronism due to an adrenal cortical tumor.

- Primary aldosteronism:
  - Plasma aldosterone concentration (PAC) in upright position >20 ng/dL, confirmed by a PAC >10 ng/dL after a saline infusion test
  - PAC to plasma renin activity (PRA) ratio >30 with PAC ≥15 ng/dL and PRA ≤ 1 ng/mL/hour
  - PAC < 8.5 ng/dL (240 pmol/L) after a saline infusion performed in the morning excludes primary aldosteronism
- In differentiation between aldosterone-producing adenomas (APA) and idiopathic hyperaldosteronism, the following suggest APA:
  - A postural test in which the plasma aldosterone level either decreases or remains the same
  - An aldosterone level unaffected by salt loading
  - Higher plasma aldosterone concentrations (greater than 25 ng/dL or 700 pmol/L)

Suspected aldosteronism in hypertensive patients
  Strength of Recommendation: Class IIa
  Strength of Evidence: Category B
Results Interpretation:
Increased aldosterone level

Primary aldosteronism should be suspected in patients with spontaneous hypokalemia, metabolic alkalosis, and a high serum sodium level. It is causative in about 50% of patients with hypertension and hypokalemia. Characteristically, the plasma renin activity is suppressed, whereas aldosterone levels are high.

- Primary aldosteronism:
  - Plasma aldosterone concentration (PAC) in upright position >20 ng/dL, confirmed by a PAC >10 ng/dL after a saline infusion test
  - PAC to plasma renin activity (PRA) ratio >30 with PAC ≥ 15 ng/dL and PRA ≤1 ng/mL/hour
  - PAC <8.5 ng/dL (240 pmol/L) after a saline infusion performed in the morning excludes primary aldosteronism
- Primary vs secondary aldosteronism
  - In almost all untreated patients with primary aldosteronism, PRA is decreased, but in secondary aldosteronism, PRA is high

ABNORMAL RESULTS

- Results decreased in:
  - Addison's disease
  - Diabetes mellitus
  - Acute alcoholic intoxication

CLINICAL NOTES

Hypokalemia can cause an increased aldosterone level and, therefore, needs to be corrected before the test.

The following parameters should be standardized when performing this test: the timing of the test (morning), the posture of the patient (upright), and the unit of measurement.

COLLECTION/STORAGE INFORMATION

- Patient Preparation:
  - Advise patient to discontinue diuretics, certain antihypertensives, estrogens, and progestational agents and avoid black licorice 2 weeks prior to testing
- Specimen Collection and Handling:
  - If an upright sample is needed, patient should be upright (standing or seated) for at least 2 hours
  - Collect whole blood in a tube containing either heparin or EDTA
  - Collect the blood sample in the morning
  - Separate sample into plasma or serum
  - Store frozen. In an airtight container, sample is stable up to 2 years at -20 °C

LOINC CODES

- Code: 16330-3 (*Short Name* - Aldost sp7 p chal SerPl-mCnc)
- Code: 14586-2 (*Short Name* - Aldost SerPl-sCnc)
- Code: 1763-2 (*Short Name* - Aldost SerPl-mCnc)
- Code: 16331-1 (*Short Name* - Aldost sp8 p chal SerPl-mCnc)

- Code: 16329-5 (*Short Name* - Aldost sp6 p chal SerPl-mCnc)
- Code: 16332-9 (*Short Name* - Aldost sp9 p chal SerPl-mCnc)

Plasma aspartic acid level

TEST DEFINITION
Measurement of aspartic acid in plasma for detection of acquired and hereditary amino acid disorders.

SYNONYMS
- Plasma aspartic acid measurement

REFERENCE RANGE
- Premature neonate, 1 day: 0.13 ± 0.13 mg/dL (10 ± 10 micromol/L)
- Neonate, 1 day: < 0.21 mg/dL (< 16 micromol/L)
- Infants 1 to 3 months: 0.05 ± 0.03 mg/dL (4 ± 2 micromol/L)
- Infants 9 to 24 months: < 0.12 mg/dL (< 9 micromol/L)
- Children 19 months to 10 years: < 0.27 mg/dL < 20 micromol/L)
- Children 6 to 18 years: < 0.19 mg/dL (< 14 micromol/L)
- Adults: < 0.32 mg/dL (< 24 micromol/L)
  Please refer to your institution's reference ranges as lab normals may vary.

INDICATIONS
Suspected inborn error of metabolism
  Strength of Recommendation: Class IIa
  Strength of Evidence: Category C
  Results Interpretation:
  Increased amino acid
  Inherited amino acid disorders are directly related to the absence of an enzyme involved in the metabolism of one or more amino acids; therefore, an elevated plasma level of a particular amino acid is highly suggestive of an inherited metabolic defect. In the majority of cases amino acid and organic acid analysis together permit diagnostic confirmation in infants. Immediate treatment should be initiated when an inborn error of metabolism is suspected, even if a definitive diagnosis has not yet been determined.

COLLECTION/STORAGE INFORMATION
- Specimen Collection and Handling:
  - Immediately place sample in ice water.
  - Isolate sample and freeze it within 1 hour; sample stable for 1 week at -20°C.
  - Sample should be deproteinized and stored at -70°C for protracted periods of usage.

LOINC CODES
- Code: 1912-5 (*Short Name* - Aspartate SerPl Ql)
- Code: 1913-3 (*Short Name* - Aspartate SerPl-mCnc)
- Code: 20639-1 (*Short Name* - Aspartate SerPl-sCnc)

Plasma factor XIII screening test

TEST DEFINITION
Qualitative detection of factor XIII in blood as a screening test for deficiency; correlates with clot stability

REFERENCE RANGE
- No deficiency detected
- >0.02-0.05 units/mL (20-50 units/L)
- >2%-5% (0.02-0.05) of normal concentration
  Please refer to your institution's reference ranges as lab normals may vary.

INDICATIONS
Suspected factor XIII deficiency
>**Strength of Recommendation:** Class I
>**Strength of Evidence:** Category C
>**Results Interpretation:**
>**Coag./bleeding tests abnormal**
>>Clot dissolution suggests severe (2% to 5% factor activity or less) deficiency of factor XIII.
>>Demonstrating clot solubility in both urea and monochloroacetic acid may increase the accuracy of the test for factor XIII deficiency. An abnormal factor XIII screen should be confirmed by quantitative testing (eg, quantitative enzyme assay).

COLLECTION/STORAGE INFORMATION
* Specimen Collection and Handling:
  * Collect plasma in blue top tube (citrate)
  * Specimen will remain stable for 2 hours at 4° C

Plasma fasting glucose measurement

TEST DEFINITION
Measurement of serum or plasma fasting glucose level to diagnose diabetes mellitus, prediabetes, hypoglycemia, and hyperglycemia

SYNONYMS
* Plasma fasting glucose level

REFERENCE RANGE
* Adults: 75-115 mg/dL (4.2-6.4 mmol/L)
* Adults 60 to 90 years: 82-115 mg/dL (4.6-6.4 mmol/L)
* Adults >90 years: 75-121 mg/dL (4.2-6.7 mmol/L)
* Premature neonates: 20-60 mg/dL (1.1-3.3 mmol/L)
* Neonates, cord blood: 45-96 mg/dL (2.5-5.3 mmol/L)
* Neonates, 1 day old: 40-60 mg/dL (2.2-3.3 mmol/L)
* Infants >1 day: 50-80 mg/dL (2.8-4.4 mmol/L)
* Children: 60-100 mg/dL (3.3-5.6 mmol/L)

Please refer to your institution's reference ranges as lab normals may vary.

INDICATIONS
Suspected diabetes mellitus
>**Strength of Recommendation:** Class I
>**Strength of Evidence:** Category C
>**Results Interpretation:**
>**Increased glucose level**
>>Fasting plasma glucose (FPG) levels greater than or equal to 126 mg/dL (7 mmol/L) indicate diabetes mellitus. Fasting means no caloric intake for at least 8 hours, and a subsequent FPG level must confirm abnormal test results.
>>FPG levels of 100 mg/dL to 125 mg/dL (5.6 mmol/L to 6.9 mmol/L) indicate prediabetes.

Suspected gestational diabetes mellitus (GDM)
>**Strength of Recommendation:** Class IIa
>**Strength of Evidence:** Category B
>**Results Interpretation:**
>**Increased glucose level**
>>A fasting plasma glucose (FPG) level in pregnant women equal to or greater than 126 mg/dL, confirmed on a subsequent day, meets the diagnostic threshold for gestational diabetes mellitus (GDM). If unequivocal symptoms of hyperglycemia are present, the follow up FPG measurement is not necessary to diagnose GDM.

Timing of Monitoring

After assessing risk for gestational diabetes mellitus (GDM) at the first prenatal visit, high risk pregnant women should have a fasting plasma glucose (FPG) or a casual plasma glucose level measured promptly to detect early GDM. Low risk women do not require glucose testing.

Suspected hypoglycemia
Strength of Recommendation: Class I
Strength of Evidence: Category C
Results Interpretation:
Decreased glucose level

Following a supervised 72-hour fast, fasting plasma glucose levels equal to or less than 45 mg/dL with signs and symptoms of hypoglycemia, interpreted within a group of tests including insulin levels, C peptide levels, proinsulin levels, beta-hydroxybutyrate levels, sulfonylurea levels, and plasma glucose response to intravenous glucagon can aid in diagnosing hypoglycemic disorders.

Timing of Monitoring

Draw fasting plasma glucose (FPG) levels every six hours starting from the onset of the patient's 72-hour fast, until the plasma glucose level is equal to or less than 60 mg/dL, then draw FPG levels every one to two hours. A FPG level equal to or less than 45 mg/dL or symptoms of hypoglycemia should end the fast.

Suspected impaired fasting glucose (IFG) (prediabetes)
Results Interpretation:
Impaired fasting glucose

Impaired fasting glucose (IFG) represents a metabolic state between normal glucose homeostasis and diabetes mellitus. IFG is defined as a fasting plasma glucose level of 100 to 125 mg/dL (5.6 to 6.9 mmol/L) and indicates prediabetes. Within 5 years, 10% to 15% of people with prediabetes will develop diabetes.

COMMON PANELS
- Basic metabolic panel
- Comprehensive metabolic panel
- Diabetic management panel
- Enteral/Parenteral nutritional management panel
- General health panel
- Hypertension panel
- Pancreatic panel
- Prenatal screening panel
- Transplant panel

CLINICAL NOTES

The standard sample is venous plasma glucose. Results may vary depending upon specimen type and handling.

COLLECTION/STORAGE INFORMATION
- No caloric intake for at least 8 hours prior to blood draw:
- Specimen Collection and Handling:
  - Serum:
    - Separate from cells rapidly
    - Stable for 8 hours at 25° C and 72 hours at 4° C
  - Plasma:
    - Preserve with sodium fluoride or iodoacetate
    - Stable for 24 hours at room temperature
  - Whole blood:
    - Analyze immediately or preserve with sodium fluoride
    - Anticoagulate with heparin

LOINC CODES
- Code: 1554-5 (*Short Name* - Glucose p 12H fast SerPl-mCnc)
- Code: 1493-6 (*Short Name* - Glucose 1.5H p 0.05-0.15 U/kg Ins IV p 1)
- Code: 1500-8 (*Short Name* - Glucose 1H p 0.05-0.15 U Ins/kg IV p 12H)
- Code: 14771-0 (*Short Name* - Glucose p fast SerPl-sCnc)

Plasma glutamic acid level

TEST DEFINITION
Measurement of glutamic acid in plasma for detection of acquired and hereditary amino acid disorders.

SYNONYMS
* Plasma glutamic acid measurement

REFERENCE RANGE
* Premature neonate, 1 day: 0.96 ± 0.51 mg/dL (65 ± 35 micromol/L)
* Neonate, 1 day: 0.29-1.57 mg/dL (20-107 micromol/L)
* Children 6 months to 3 years: 0.28 ± 1.47 mg/dL (19-100 micromol/L)
* Children 3 to 10 years: 0.34-3.68 mg/dL (23-250 micromol/L)
* Children 6 to 18 years: 0.1-0.96 mg/dL (7-65 micromol/L)
* Adults: 0.21-2.82 mg/dL (14-192 micromol/L)
  Please refer to your institution's reference ranges as lab normals may vary.

INDICATIONS
Suspected inborn error of metabolism
> **Strength of Recommendation:** Class IIa
> **Strength of Evidence:** Category C
> **Results Interpretation:**
> **Increased amino acid**
>> Inherited amino acid disorders are directly related to the absence of an enzyme involved in the metabolism of one or more amino acids; therefore, an elevated plasma level of a particular amino acid is highly suggestive of an inherited metabolic defect. In the majority of cases amino acid and organic acid analysis together permit diagnostic confirmation in infants. Immediate treatment should be initiated when an inborn error of metabolism is suspected even if a definitive diagnosis has not yet been determined.

COLLECTION/STORAGE INFORMATION
* Specimen Collection and Handling:
  * Immediately place sample in ice water.
  * Isolate plasma sample and freeze it within 1 hour; sample stable for 1 week at -20°C.
  * Sample should be deproteinized and stored at -70°C for protracted periods of usage.

LOINC CODES
* Code: 2363-0 (*Short Name* - Glutamate SerPl Ql)
* Code: 20642-5 (*Short Name* - Glutamate SerPl-sCnc)
* Code: 2364-8 (*Short Name* - Glutamate SerPl-mCnc)

Plasma glutamine measurement

TEST DEFINITION
Measurement of glutamine in plasma for detection of acquired and hereditary amino acid disorders.

SYNONYMS
* Plasma glutamine level

REFERENCE RANGE
* Infants 3 months to 6 years: 6.93-10.89 mg/dL (475-746 micromol/L)
* Children 6 to 18 years: 5.26-10.8 mg/dL (360-740 micromol/L)
* Adults: 5.78-10.38 mg/dL (396-711 micromol/L)
  Please refer to your institution's reference ranges as lab normals may vary.

INDICATIONS

Suspected inborn error of metabolism
> **Strength of Recommendation:** Class IIa
> **Strength of Evidence:** Category C

Results Interpretation:
Increased amino acid

Inherited amino acid disorders are directly related to the absence of an enzyme involved in the metabolism of one or more amino acids; therefore, an elevated plasma level of a particular amino acid is highly suggestive of an inherited metabolic defect. In the majority of cases amino acid and organic acid analysis together permit diagnostic confirmation in infants. Immediate treatment should be initiated when an inborn error of metabolism is suspected, even if a definitive diagnosis has not yet been determined.

Ornithine-transcarbamylase deficiency is associated with elevated plasma glutamine levels. Carbamoyl phosphate synthetase deficiency is associated with increased alanine, glutamine, glycine and lysine, and low or undetectable arginine and citrulline. N-acetylglutamic acid synthetase deficiency is associated with increased glutamine as well as low or undetectable citrulline levels.

COLLECTION/STORAGE INFORMATION

- Specimen Collection and Handling:
  - Immediately place sample in ice water.
  - Isolate plasma sample and freeze it within 1 hour; sample stable for 1 week at -20°C.
  - Sample should be deproteinized and stored at -70°C for protracted periods of usage.

LOINC CODES

- Code: 20643-3 (*Short Name* - Glutamine SerPl-sCnc)
- Code: 2372-1 (*Short Name* - Glutamine SerPl-mCnc)
- Code: 2371-3 (*Short Name* - Glutamine SerPl QI)

Plasma glycine measurement

TEST DEFINITION

Measurement of glycine levels in plasma for the evaluation of inborn errors of metabolism

SYNONYMS

- Plasma glycine level

REFERENCE RANGE

- Adults: 0.90-4.16 mg/dL (120-554 micromol/L)
- Premature neonates, birth to 1 day: 3.45 ± 2.06 mg/dL (460 ± 275 micromol/L)
- Neonates, birth to 1 day: 1.68-3.86 mg/dL (224-514 micromol/L)
- Infants, 1 to 3 months: 1.23 ± 0.22 mg/dL (164 ± 29 micromol/L)
- Infants, 2 to 6 months: 1.31-2.22 mg/dL (175-296 micromol/L)
- Infants, 9 months to 2 years: 0.42-2.31 mg/dL (56-308 micromol/L)
- Children, 3 to 10 years: 0.88-1.67 mg/dL (117-223 micromol/L)
- Children, 6 to 18 years: 1.18-2.27 mg/dL (158-302 micromol/L)
  Please refer to your institution's reference ranges as lab normals may vary.

INDICATIONS

Suspected non-ketotic hyperglycinemia
> **Strength of Recommendation:** Class IIa
> **Strength of Evidence:** Category C

Results Interpretation:
Raised biochemistry findings

In the neonatal form of non-ketotic hyperglycinemia (NKH), plasma glycine levels in untreated patients can be more markedly elevated than in NKH patients with the atypical, late-onset type.

Plasma glycine levels can be elevated 2 to 8 times the normal range in NKH; however, high plasma glycine levels are harmless.

Plasma glycine levels can be elevated in genetic disorders and clinical conditions other than NKH, and by therapeutic agents and iatrogenic and technical factors. These types of hyperglycinemia can be differentiated from NKH by the associated finding of decreased plasma levels of branched-chain amino acids and the restoration of normal glycine levels after adequate nutrition and achievement of biochemical balance.

COLLECTION/STORAGE INFORMATION
- Specimen Collection and Handling:
  - Collect specimen in EDTA or heparin-containing tube.
  - Avoid hemolysis of sample.
  - Place specimen in ice water immediately upon collection.
  - Freeze specimen within 1 hour of collection.
  - Specimen is stable for 1 week at $-20°C$; for longer periods of storage deproteinize and store at $-70°C$.
  - Collect plasma and cerebrospinal fluid simultaneously, if possible.

LOINC CODES
- Code: 2391-1 (*Short Name* - Glycine SerPl-mCnc)
- Code: 2390-3 (*Short Name* - Glycine SerPl QI)
- Code: 20644-1 (*Short Name* - Glycine SerPl-sCnc)

Plasma homocysteine measurement

TEST DEFINITION
Measurement of homocysteine levels in plasma for the evaluation of conditions that alter the function or blood concentration of the B vitamins, particularly folate and cobalamin, and/or influence renal function or enzyme activities

SYNONYMS
- Plasma homocysteine level

REFERENCE RANGE
- Adults: 0-12 micromol/L
  Please refer to your institution's reference ranges as lab normals may vary.

INDICATIONS
Cardiovascular disease related to suspected homocysteinemia.
    Strength of Recommendation: Class IIa
    Strength of Evidence: Category A
    Results Interpretation:
    Homocystinemia
    There is a significant increase in cardiovascular risk when the plasma homocysteine level is greater than 13 to 15 micromol/L; however, there is no definite set point at which a homocysteine level correlates with an increased risk of cardiovascular events. High levels of homocysteine cause damage to the arterial endothelium, leading to severe atherosclerotic lesions.
    There is a strong association between cerebral infarction and homocysteinemia. Elevated homocysteine levels are associated with the progression of aortic atheromas, an independent risk factor for stroke. Moderate increases in levels of homocysteine are associated with an increased risk of stroke in young women
    Risk for venous thrombosis in persons with hyperhomocysteinemia increases with age and is greater in women than men.
    Frequency of Monitoring
    Evaluation of serum homocysteine levels every 3 to 5 years is recommended for patients diagnosed with, or at high-risk for, cardiovascular disease A single measurement of fasting total homocysteine is sufficient for evaluation since daily disparities are insignificant.

Pregnant women with early-onset pregnancy complications, women who have previous pregnancy complications or who have had a child with birth defects, and women with known vitamin deficiency or those at risk for vitamin deficiencies
    Strength of Recommendation: Class I
    Strength of Evidence: Category C

Results Interpretation:
Homocystinemia
Elevated homocysteine levels are associated with birth defects and pregnancy complications, secondary to placental vasculopathy. Pregnancy complications include preeclampsia, recurrent early spontaneous abortions, premature delivery, low birth weight, and placental abruption or infarction. Birth defects include neural tube defects, orofacial clefts, clubfoot, and Down's syndrome.
Timing of Monitoring
Women who have had complications with their pregnancy or have had a child with birth defects should have a homocysteine measurement done 3 months postpartum.
Women with known vitamin deficiency or those at risk for vitamin deficiencies should have regular homocysteine measurements, preferably before and once during pregnancy

Suspected cobalamin or folate deficiency.
    Strength of Recommendation: Class IIa
    Strength of Evidence: Category C
Results Interpretation:
Homocystinemia
Elevated homocysteine levels are suggestive of folate or cobalamin deficiency. Diagnosis should be confirmed by serum cobalamin and serum folate measurement.

Suspected homocystinuria
    Results Interpretation:
    Homocystinemia
Homocystinuria should be suspected in individuals with a total plasma homocysteine level greater than 100 micromol/L. An increase in fasting total blood homocysteine of 40 times normal levels may be seen. Whites homozygous for this mutation having a low dietary folate intake have a 50% increase in total homocysteine level.
Close to half of untreated persons homozygous for this mutation will experience arterial or venous disorders before the age of 30 years.
Diagnosis should be confirmed with urine homocysteine measurement. There are three different homozygous homocysteinurias, all of which demonstrate high levels of homocysteine in the blood and urine.
    Normal laboratory findings
Normal basal homocysteine may be seen in persons with the heterozygous form of homocystinuria.

ABNORMAL RESULTS
- Results decreased in pregnancy, due to hemodilution
- Results increased in:
  - Males
  - Postprandial
  - Low physical activity
  - Smoking
  - Increased blood pressure
  - Increased blood cholesterol level
  - Folate, vitamin B_{12}, and/or vitamin B_6 deficiency
  - Renal impairment
  - Metabolic disease

COLLECTION/STORAGE INFORMATION
- Ideally, specimen should be drawn after a minimum 12-hour fast although specimen can be drawn fasting or nonfasting, and before or after methionine loading.
- Collect blood sample in tube containing EDTA. Centrifuge immediately. If this is not possible, chill or place specimen directly on ice or in ice water immediately and until plasma is separated. Separate plasma from red blood cells within 1 hour of collection.
- Plasma sample may be stored for up to 4 days at room temperature, for several weeks if refrigerated, or for several years at -20°C. After freezing, inhomogeneity of sample matrix may occur; thorough mixing of sample is required after thawing.

LOINC CODES
- Code: 13965-9 (*Short Name* - Homocysteine SerPl-sCnc)
- Code: 2428-1 (*Short Name* - Homocysteine SerPl-mCnc)

Plasma renin level

TEST DEFINITION
Indirectly measures renin levels, based on generation of angiotensin I in plasma, for evaluation and management of renal and adrenal disorders

REFERENCE RANGE
- Adults, normal sodium diet:
- Supine: 0.2-1.6 ng angiotensin I/mL/hour (0.2-1.6 mcg angiotensin I/L/hour)
- Standing (4 hours): 0.7-3.3 ng angiotensin I/mL/hour (0.7-3.3 mcg angiotensin I/L/hour)
- Neonates, cord blood: 4-32 ng angiotensin I/mL/hour (4-32 mcg angiotensin I/L/hour)
- Neonates 1 to 7 days: 2-35 ng angiotensin I/mL/hour (2-35 mcg angiotensin I/L/hour)
- Infants 1 to 12 months: 2.4-37 ng angiotensin I/mL/hour (2.4-37 mcg angiotensin I/L/hour)
- Children 1 to 3 years: 1.7-11.2 ng angiotensin I/mg/mL/hour (1.7-11.2 mcg angiotensin I/L/hour)
- Children 3 to 5 years: 1-6.5 ng angiotensin I/mL/hour (1-6.5 mcg angiotensin I/L/hour)
- Children 5 to 10 years: 0.5-5.9 ng angiotensin I/mL/hour (0.5-5.9 mcg angiotensin I/L/hour)
- Children 10 to 15 years: 0.5-3.3 ng angiotensin I/mL/hour (0.5-3.3 mcg angiotensin I/L/hour)
  Please refer to your institution's reference ranges as lab normals may vary.

INDICATIONS
Guide management of hypertensive crisis
> **Strength of Recommendation:** Class IIb
> **Strength of Evidence:** Category C

Results Interpretation:
Abnormal laboratory findings
- Medium to high renin state (Plasma renin activity [PRA] greater than or equal to 0.65 ng/mL/hour) indicates :
  - Malignant hypertension
  - Unilateral renovascular hypertension
  - Renal trauma
  - Renal vasculitis
  - Adrenergic crises
- Sodium-volume overload/low renin state (PRA less than 0.65 ng/mL/hour) indicates :
  - Primary aldosteronism
  - Acute tubular necrosis
  - Acute glomerulonephritis
  - Urinary tract obstruction
- Sodium-volume overload/relatively low renin state (PRA about 1 ng/mL/hour) indicates :
  - Preeclampsia/eclampsia (PRA level drops from normal pregnancy 6-10 ng/mL/hour range)

Suspected adrenal incidentaloma associated with hypertension
> **Strength of Recommendation:** Class IIa
> **Strength of Evidence:** Category C

Results Interpretation:
Lab. test result normal
All incidentally discovered adrenal masses greater than 1 cm in diameter require laboratory assessment for hormonal activity (eg, a dexamethasone suppression test and total 24-hour urine measurement of metanephrines and fractionated catecholamines).

If the patient is hypertensive, the assessment also includes a serum potassium and plasma aldosterone concentration to plasma renin activity (PRA) ratio. Adrenal incidentalomas are hormonally inactive masses (usually nonfunctioning adrenal cortical adenomas) with normal hormone measurements. A plasma aldosterone concentration (PAC) to PRA ratio of 20 or greater and a plasma aldosterone concentration of 15 ng/dL or greater suggests primary aldosteronism caused by a hormonally active adrenal adenoma.

Timing of Monitoring
Patients with apparently benign nonfunctioning adrenal cortical masses less than 4 cm in diameter should undergo repeat imaging at 3 and 12 months and repeat hormonal assessment at 12 and 24 months. If there are no imaging or hormonal changes after 24 months of follow-up, further studies are unnecessary.

Suspected primary aldosteronism
   Strength of Recommendation: Class IIa
   Strength of Evidence: Category C
Results Interpretation:
Abnormal laboratory findings
   Plasma renin activity (PRA) levels are low in primary aldosteronism, but such findings alone are too non-specific to be recommended in screening for primary aldosteronism. However, the plasma aldosterone concentration (PAC) to PRA ratio is the screening test of choice for primary aldosteronism in hypertensive patients.

Suspected renovascular hypertension
   Strength of Recommendation: Class IIb
   Strength of Evidence: Category B
Results Interpretation:
Abnormal laboratory findings
   Static plasma renin activity (PRA) assay: generally, the results are not helpful for renovascular hypertension (RV-HTN) screening. However, extreme PRA values offer some guidance: very low levels suggest RV-HTN is unlikely, whereas very high levels suggest RV-HTN is likely.
   Renal vein plasma renin activity (PRA): bilateral PRA measurements are more useful for identifying complete renal artery occlusion (and justifying nephrectomy) than for identifying renal artery occlusion amenable to revascularization. However, even at the best combined cut-off value of renal vein renin ratio (RVRR) of 1.7, the high sensitivity of 87% is associated with a false-positive rate of 22%.
   Simplified captopril-stimulation test: a plasma renin activity (PRA) level greater than 5.4 ng/mL/hour (or equivalent for given institution) is considered positive.

COMMON PANELS
* Hypertension panel

ABNORMAL RESULTS
* Results increased in:
   * Low sodium diet
   * Upright posture
   * Pregnancy
   * Luteal phase of menstrual cycle

CLINICAL NOTES
   There are two basic types of renin measurements: plasma renin activity (PRA) and plasma renin concentration. The technically less difficult PRA assay is most widely used in clinical practice. Both assays provide similar clinically relevant information.

COLLECTION/STORAGE INFORMATION
* Specimen Collection and Handling:
   * Draw blood into iced (EDTA) tubes
   * Place in ice water
   * Centrifuge at 4°C
   * Promptly separate and freeze plasma at -20°C
   * Stable for several months at -20°C

LOINC CODES
* Code: 2917-3 (*Short Name* - Renin sup Plas-mCnc)
* Code: 17516-6 (*Short Name* - Renin sup Plas-cCnc)
* Code: 30895-7 (*Short Name* - Renin SerPl-aCnc)
* Code: 17515-8 (*Short Name* - Renin BS Plas-cCnc)
* Code: 2915-7 (*Short Name* - Renin Plas-cCnc)
* Code: 13867-7 (*Short Name* - Renin 1H p 25 mg Cpl PO Plas-cCnc)
* Code: 13868-5 (*Short Name* - Renin 2H p 25 mg Cpl PO Plas-cCnc)

Plasminogen assay

TEST DEFINITION
Measurement of plasminogen in blood for the evaluation of thromboembolic disorders

REFERENCE RANGE
- Adults:
- Functional assay: 80%-130% (0.8-1.3)
- Antigenic assay: 8.4-14 mg/dL (84-140 mg/L)
- Neonates: 60% of adult value
  Please refer to your institution's reference ranges as lab normals may vary.

INDICATIONS
Suspected fibrinolytic system disorder (hypoplasminogenemia or dysplasminogenemia)
  Strength of Recommendation: Class IIb
  Strength of Evidence: Category B
  Results Interpretation:
  Hypoplasminogenemia
  Hypoplasminogenemia (type I plasminogen deficiency) is characterized by both decreased plasminogen activity and antigen level.
  While in some populations, prevalence of heterozygous plasminogen deficiency appears to be somewhat higher in persons with a history of thrombosis than in the general population, neither heterozygous nor homozygous plasminogen deficiency increases thrombosis risk.
  Hypoplasminogenemia is associated with chronic inflammatory disease of the mucous membranes, including ligneous conjunctivitis and oral lesions.
  Dysplasminogenemia
  Dysplasminogenemia (type II plasminogen deficiency) is characterized by decreased serum activity with a normal antigen level. The clinical significance is unclear; it is not associated with an increased risk of thrombosis.

Suspected ligneous conjunctivitis
  Strength of Recommendation: Class I
  Strength of Evidence: Category B
  Results Interpretation:
  Hypoplasminogenemia
  Ligneous conjunctivitis is associated with heterozygous plasminogen deficiency. In general, symptom severity appears to correlate with the degree of plasminogen deficiency.
  Dysplasminogenemia
  Dysplasminogenemia is not associated with development of mucous membrane abnormalities, including ligneous conjunctivitis.

ABNORMAL RESULTS
- Results increased in:
  - Pregnancy (peak of 165% of normal in third trimester)
  - Increased triglyceride and/or cholesterol levels
- Results decreased in:
  - Liver disease
  - Consumptive coagulopathies
  - Fibrinolytic therapy
  - DIC
  - Advanced age

COLLECTION/STORAGE INFORMATION
- Specimen Collection and Handling:
  - Collect serum in a citrate (blue top) tube.
  - Specimen is stable for 8 hours at room temperature and for 1 month at -20°C.

LOINC CODES
- Code: 5970-9 (*Short Name* - PLG PPP Chro-aCnc)

Platelet aggregation test

TEST DEFINITION

Assessment of platelet function in platelet-rich plasma (PRP) by observation of platelet response in the presence of exogenous compounds that normally induce aggregation. Aggregation agents include adenosine diphosphate (ADP), arachidonic acid, collagen, epinephrine, ristocetin, and thrombin receptor-activated peptide (TRAP-6)

SYNONYMS

- Aggregometer test
- Platelet aggregation assay

REFERENCE RANGE

Adults: >65% aggregation in response to adenosine diphosphate (ADP), arachidonic acid, collagen, epinephrine and ristocetin.

Please refer to your institution's reference ranges as lab normals may vary.

INDICATIONS

Suspected congenital platelet function disorder
    Strength of Recommendation: Class IIb
    Strength of Evidence: Category B
    Results Interpretation:
    Decreased platelet aggregation
    Decreased platelet aggregation in the presence of certain aggregation agents is consistent with, though not diagnostic of, specific types of congenital platelet function disorders (eg, Bernard-Soulier Syndrome, Glanzmann's thrombasthenia, etc). Further analysis is required for definitive diagnosis.
    Increased platelet aggregation
    Excessive platelet aggregation in platelet-rich plasma (PRP), in association with specific aggregators, is consistent with the autosomal dominant expression of sticky platelet syndrome (SPS).

Suspected drug induced platelet dysfunction
    Strength of Recommendation: Class IIb
    Strength of Evidence: Category B
    Results Interpretation:
    Decreased platelet aggregation
    Decreased platelet aggregation is consistent with, though not diagnostic of, drug induced platelet dysfunction. Further analysis is required for conclusive diagnosis.
    Nonsteroidal anti-inflammatory agents, thienopyridines, and GPIIb-IIIa receptor antagonists are commonly used inhibitors of platelet aggregation. Drugs known to interfere with platelet function do so by interference with the platelet membrane or receptor sites, through interference with prostaglandin pathways, and through interference with phosphodiesterase activity.

ABNORMAL RESULTS

- Results increased in:
  - Hemolysis
  - Lipemia
  - Nicotine

COLLECTION/STORAGE INFORMATION

- Exercise activates platelets and should be avoided 15 to 20 minutes prior to test
- Collect blood in (blue-top) tube containing citrate for centrifugation and isolation of platelet-rich plasma
- Patient must avoid aspirin for 7 to 10 days prior to test
- Test should be performed as soon as possible since specimen is only stable at room temperature for up to 3 hours

LOINC CODES

- Code: 21027-8 (*Short Name* - Platelet Agg PPP-Imp)
- Code: 13592-1 (*Short Name* - IPA XXX PRP)

Platelet count

TEST DEFINITION
Measurement of the number of platelets in whole blood for the evaluation of bleeding disorders

SYNONYMS
- Platelet count - observation
- Plt - Platelet count

REFERENCE RANGE
- Adults: 150-350 $\times$ 10^3 /mm^3 (150-350 $\times$ 10^9 /L)
  Please refer to your institution's reference ranges as lab normals may vary.

INDICATIONS
Suspected and known pediatric meningococcal disease
Results Interpretation:
Thrombocytopenia

Early severe thrombocytopenia and neutropenia identify the highest risk cases of severe meningococcal disease. The two values together predict mortality better than either count alone.

The platelet count is also highly predictive for DIC.

Platelet count, serum potassium level, base excess, and serum C-reactive protein level are significantly associated with fatal outcome in children with meningococcal septic shock.

Timing of Monitoring

A platelet count should be obtained at the time of admission on all patients with suspected meningococcal infection.

Sickle cell disease
Results Interpretation:
Thrombocytopenia

Platelet count may drop acutely during splenic sequestration crises and in association with disseminated intravascular coagulation due to bacterial sepsis. Thrombocytopenia may be severe enough to cause clinical bleeding.

Thrombocytosis

Platelet count is commonly elevated (greater than 400,000/mm^3) in sickle cell disease. Marked elevations have been associated with an increased risk of priapism in males.

Suspected and known acute coronary syndrome
Strength of Recommendation: Class I
Strength of Evidence: Category C
Results Interpretation:
Acquired thrombocytopenia

Thrombocytopenia in acute non-ST-segment coronary events and following thrombolysis is associated with a higher morbidity and mortality.

Frequency of Monitoring

Daily platelet count monitoring is indicated following thrombolytic therapy to identify patients with thrombocytopenia.

Timing of Monitoring

Platelet count should be included in the initial laboratory evaluation in all patients with suspected acute coronary syndrome.

Suspected and known avian influenza
Results Interpretation:
Thrombocytopenia

Mild-to-moderate thrombocytopenia is a common finding in avian influenza. In one series, the median platelet count was 75,000 (range 45,000 to 174,000)/mm^3.

Thrombocytopenia is associated with the development of acute respiratory distress syndrome (ARDS) and a fatal outcome.

Suspected and known community-acquired pneumonia
Results Interpretation:
Thrombocytopenia
In male patients with bacteremic community-acquired lobar pneumonia, the presence of thrombocytopenia is more suggestive of Klebsiella than of pneumococcal pneumonia.

At the peak of the respiratory illness of severe acute respiratory syndrome (SARS), 30% to 50% of patients have thrombocytopenia or low-normal platelet counts (50,000 to 150,000/microL).

Suspected and known ehrlichiosis
Results Interpretation:
Thrombocytopenia
Thrombocytopenia is a characteristic feature during the first week of illness, noted in approximately 70% of patients with human monocytic ehrlichiosis and 90% of those with human granulocytic anaplasmosis, formerly called human granulocytic ehrlichiosis. It is often present on initial evaluation and is most severe 3 to 9 days after illness onset, with a return to baseline around day 14. In severe infection, thrombocytopenia and coagulopathy may predispose to hemorrhagic complications.

Suspected and known hemolytic uremic syndrome (HUS)
Results Interpretation:
Thrombocytopenia
Although the platelet count may be normal initially, 75% of patients with hemolytic uremic syndrome (HUS) present with a platelet count of less than 50,000/mL on admission. Platelet counts less than 10,000/mL are unusual. Thrombocytopenia may not be documented in approximately 5% of cases.

The greatest degree of thrombocytopenia often occurs within several days after the diagnosis has been made. The platelet count returns to normal at a mean of 9 days. Thrombocytopenia may last 1 to 3 weeks.

The severity and duration of thrombocytopenia do not correlate with illness severity.

Suspected and known hemophilia
Results Interpretation:
Platelet count normal
No platelet abnormalities are seen in any type of hemophilia.
Thrombocytopenia
Thrombocytopenia has been in hemophiliacs with HIV infection. Thrombocytopenia is present at some time in about 20% of HIV-infected hemophiliacs and about 3% of those without HIV. The incidence of thrombocytopenia increases with age.

Suspected and known Kawasaki disease
Results Interpretation:
Thrombocytosis
Thrombocytosis is characteristic in the subacute phase of Kawasaki disease (KD), with platelet counts ranging from 500,000 to over $1,000,000/mm^3$.

The platelet count is usually normal during the acute febrile stage of KD. It rises in the second week, peaks between 500,000 and over $1,000,000/mm^3$ in the third week, and returns to normal in 4 to 8 weeks.
Thrombocytopenia
A small number of patients with KD may manifest early thrombocytopenia, which may be a sign of disseminated intravascular coagulation.

Thrombocytopenia in the acute phase of KD may be predictive of increased risk for coronary artery aneurysms and myocardial infarction.
Frequency of Monitoring
A baseline value should be obtained initially and monitored every three to four days until day 21, then weekly until the count returns to normal.

Suspected and known peripheral vascular disease
Results Interpretation:
Thrombocytosis
Thrombocytosis, either primary or secondary to stress, sepsis, occult malignancy, or following splenectomy, may predispose patients with peripheral vascular disease to arterial thrombosis or embolism.
Thrombocytopenia
Thrombocytopenia with sudden arterial embolization has been reported in patients receiving heparin therapy. This may be related to heparin-induced antibodies that cross-react with and bind platelets and should be followed in an anticipatory fashion.

An otherwise unexplained platelet count fall (usually more than 50% from a baseline/prior level, even if the platelet count nadir [lowest level] remains greater than 100,000/mm) plus the presence of HIT antibodies indicates a diagnosis of type II heparin-induced thrombocytopenia (HIT). (Skin lesions at heparin injection sites, or an acute systemic reaction following intravenous administration of a heparin bolus may also be present). The platelet counts return to normal levels within days or weeks, and the detectable pathogenic HIT antibodies disappear within a few weeks or months [3]).

Suspected and known preeclampsia
Results Interpretation:
Thrombocytopenia

An admission platelet count is an excellent predictor of subsequent thrombocytopenia; counts less than 150,000/microL at admission are associated with a 50% chance of subsequent counts less than 100,000/microL.

A platelet count less than 100,000/mm^3 alone or with evidence of microangiopathic hemolytic anemia (with increased LDH concentration) increases the certainty of a diagnosis of preeclampsia. It is a marker of severe preeclampsia.

Suspected fat embolism
Results Interpretation:
Thrombocytopenia

Thrombocytopenia with evidence of platelet activation and intravascular coagulation gives supportive evidence to the diagnosis of fat embolism. Most patients have platelet counts less than 150,000/mm^3. The cause of the thrombocytopenia is believed to be related to the coating of fat emboli by platelets.

Suspected giant cell (temporal) arteritis
Results Interpretation:
Thrombocytosis

- An elevated platelet count is a useful marker for a positive temporal artery biopsy.
- An elevated platelet count is a risk factor for visual loss in a patient with giant cell (temporal) arteritis
- Anterior ischemic optic neuropathy:
  - An elevated platelet count may help differentiate arteritic from nonarteritic anterior ischemic optic neuropathy.
  - Arteritic and nonarteritic anterior ischemic optic neuropathy are better differentiated by a platelet count than by an erythrocyte sedimentation rate.
- Platelet counts return to normal after patients with giant cell (temporal) arteritis start corticosteroid therapy.
- A computer-based decision analytic model that had not yet been clinically validated found:
  - At low pretest probabilities (ie, low disease risk), the model suggests that the absence of thrombocytosis can obviate the need for temporal artery biopsy (TAB).
  - At high pretest probabilities (ie, high disease risk), the model suggests that a normal platelet count warrants bilateral TAB to confirm or rule out disease.
  - At high pretest probabilities, the model suggests that thrombocytosis warrants treatment and a TAB is not necessary.

Suspected hantavirus pulmonary syndrome
Results Interpretation:
Thrombocytopenia

Thrombocytopenia is a characteristic laboratory abnormality, noted on admission in 70% of patients. The median lowest platelet count is 64,000/mm^3.

Evidence of thrombocytopenia may be helpful to screen for early hantavirus pulmonary syndrome (HPS) among patients with mild febrile illness who may be at risk for HPS.

Thrombocytopenia does not require treatment with a platelet transfusion; it simply mirrors the clinical course.

Suspected hemorrhagic shock
Results Interpretation:
Platelet count - finding

In hemorrhagic shock, a coagulopathy may develop that is characterized by consumption of clotting factors and platelets.

Suspected heparin-induced thrombocytopenia
    Strength of Recommendation: Class I
    Strength of Evidence: Category B
    Results Interpretation:
    Thrombocytopenia
        Heparin-induced thrombocytopenia should be suspected in patients who have decreasing platelet counts, platelet counts less than 100,000/mm^3, or new thrombotic or hemorrhagic events during heparin therapy.
        One type of heparin-induced thrombocytopenia is a result of temporary platelet aggregation, margination, and peripheral sequestration. The degree of platelet count reduction is mild and occurs 2 to 4 days after receiving heparin. This type of thrombocytopenia resolves despite the continued administration of heparin.
        The second type of heparin-induced thrombocytopenia is mediated by a heparin-dependent IgG antibody. A rapid reduction in the platelet count generally occurs on the fourth to eighth day of heparin therapy. This type of thrombocytopenia does not resolve with continued therapy and could predispose the patient to a thromboembolic event (white clot syndrome).
    Frequency of Monitoring
        Patients receiving heparin therapy should have platelet counts monitored closely for at least 20 days.
        Infants should have platelets monitored every 2 to 3 days while receiving heparin therapy.

Suspected hypothermia
    Results Interpretation:
    Decreased platelet count
        A decrease in the number of platelets secondary to splenic, liver, and intravascular sequestration occurs at 32°C and is marked at 28°C.
        Thrombocytopenia may occur after rewarming.
        Hypothermia induces a reversible platelet dysfunction.
        Thrombocytopenia is common in the elderly and neonates.

Suspected Lyme disease
    Results Interpretation:
    Thrombocytopenia
        In endemic areas, Lyme disease should be suspected in patients who present with flu-like symptoms and thrombocytopenia, particularly in absence of erythema migrans (EM).
        In one series, thrombocytopenia was present in only 1.5% of culture confirmed cases of EM.
        Case reports indicate a possible association between thrombocytopenia and Lyme disease that may be refractory to doxycycline therapy.
        The presence of thrombocytopenia also suggests coinfection with *Ehrlichia* or *Babesia*.

Suspected malaria
    Results Interpretation:
    Thrombocytopenia
        Thrombocytopenia is a common finding in malaria, but it is rapidly reversible with appropriate antimalarial therapy.
        Although severe thrombocytopenia may occur, it generally does not result in spontaneous hemorrhage and rarely requires platelet transfusion.

Suspected meningitis
    Results Interpretation:
    Thrombocytopenia
        Thrombocytopenia may be found in *Haemophilus influenzae* and meningococcal meningitis.
        H influenzae meningitis complicated by severe thrombocytopenia and unassociated with clinical or laboratory evidence of DIC has been reported. The most likely cause is the effect of *H influenzae* or one of its products (endotoxin) on platelets.
        In meningococcal meningitis, a platelet count less than 100,000/mm^3 to 150,000/mm^3 is predictive of a poor outcome.
    Thrombocytosis
        Thrombocytosis has been reported in children with *Haemophilus influenzae* meningitis, usually during the recovery phase.

Suspected or known disseminated intravascular coagulation (DIC)
Results Interpretation:
Acquired thrombocytopenia
- Thrombocytopenia appears to be an early finding in DIC. Decreased platelet counts ranging from 10,000 to 75,000/microL are present in >85% patients.
- DIC should be considered in an ICU patient with an underlying disorder know to cause DIC and thrombocytopenia (platelets <150,000/microL) or a >50,000/microL fall within 24 hours.
- Because thrombin-induced platelet aggregation is largely responsible for platelet consumption, the low platelet counts in DIC strongly correlate with markers of thrombin generation. Moreover, a rapid progressive decrease in serial platelet counts reflects both consumption and thrombin generation and, therefore, helps establish both the possible presence and the severity of DIC.
- In addition to DIC, moderate thrombocytopenia (50,000 to 100,000/microL) typically is caused by thrombotic thrombocytopenic purpura (TTP), heparin-induced thrombocytopenia (HIT), hemophagocytic syndrome, or liver disease/hypersplenism.
- Severe thrombocytopenia (<20,000/microL) typically is caused by drug-induced thrombocytopenia, immune thrombocytopenic purpura (ITP), or post-transfusion purpura, not DIC.

Suspected or known type II heparin-induced thrombocytopenia (HIT)
    Strength of Recommendation: Class I
    Strength of Evidence: Category C
Results Interpretation:
Thrombocytopenia
    A platelet count of less than 100,000/mm^3 defines thrombocytopenia. Spontaneous bleeding is unlikely with counts between 50,000 and 100,000/mm^3 but usually is a risk only when the platelet count is below 20,000/mm^3.
    Other influences, such as platelet function and vascular integrity, affect the role of platelets in hemostasis and must be considered when judging bleeding risk in thrombocytopenia.
- Diagnosis of type II heparin-induced thrombocytopenia (HIT)
  - Thrombocytopenia, defined as a fall in the platelet count greater than 50% or a count less than 100,000/mm^3, is the most common clinical manifestation of type II HIT and occurs in over 95% of patients. The thrombocytopenia nadir (ie, the lowest value) ranges between 15,000 and 100,000/mm^3 for 90% of HIT patients, and the median nadir is 50,000 to 60,000/mm^3.
  - A diagnosis of HIT should be strongly considered if the platelet count falls by greater than 50% (or to less than 100,000/mm^3) and/or a thrombotic event occurs 4 to 14 days following the initiation of heparin, even if the heparin has been discontinued.

    Type II HIT should be considered when thrombocytopenia occurs with a temporal pattern consistent with heparin-induced immunization (eg, the platelet count fall begins 5 to 10 days or thrombocytopenia occurs 7 to 14 days after starting heparin) or when sequelae of HIT (eg, thrombosis) occur in patients treated (or recently treated) with heparin. The estimated probability of HIT is also influenced by the pattern of the platelet count decline and by the likelihood of an alternative cause of the thrombocytopenia.

    False Results
    Spurious low platelet counts can be obtained when the CBC is done by electronic counter. Giant platelets, platelet clumping, and platelet adherence to leukocytes may be influenced by the test and thus give false results. A platelet count less than 50,000/mm^3 requires a repeat chamber count using phase contrast microscopy to rule out pseudothrombocytopenia.

Suspected sepsis
    Strength of Recommendation: Class I
    Strength of Evidence: Category C
Results Interpretation:
Thrombocytopenia
    Sepsis may cause a platelet count of less than 150,000/microL. A count less than 100,000/microL may be associated with organ dysfunction in severe sepsis.
    Platelets may be decreased due to DIC or, more commonly, as an isolated finding due to increased turnover.

Suspected thrombocytopenia
    Strength of Recommendation: Class I
    Strength of Evidence: Category C

Results Interpretation:
Thrombocytopenia

A platelet count of less than 150,000/mm^3 defines thrombocytopenia. Patients with platelet counts between 100,000 and 150,000/mm^3 generally do not require treatment but should be followed. Spontaneous bleeding is unlikely with counts between 50,000 and 100,000/mm^3 but usually is a risk only when the platelet count is below 20,000/mm^3.

Other influences, such as platelet function and vascular integrity, affect the role of platelets in hemostasis and must be considered when judging bleeding risk in thrombocytopenia.

False Results

Spurious low platelet counts can be obtained when the CBC is done by electronic counter. Giant platelets, platelet clumping, and platelet adherence to leukocytes may be influenced by the test and thus give false results. A platelet count less than 50,000/mm^3 requires a repeat chamber count using phase contrast microscopy to rule out pseudothrombocytopenia.

EDTA used to preserve blood samples and heparinized samples can also cause false results.

Suspected toxic shock syndrome
Results Interpretation:
Decreased platelet count

In staphylococcal toxic shock syndrome (TSS), thrombocytopenia occurs in the first week of illness, with a platelet count as low as 11,000/mm$_3$. Recovery of the platelets count occurs within 2 weeks.

A platelet count of 100,000/mm$_3$ or less is seen in patients with streptococcal TSS.

COMMON PANELS
- Complete blood count
- Disseminated intravascular coagulopathy panel

ABNORMAL RESULTS
- Results increased in:
  - High altitude
  - Strenuous exercise
- Results decreased in:
  - Menstruation
  - Pregnancy

COLLECTION/STORAGE INFORMATION
- Patient Preparation:
  - Advise patient to avoid strenuous exercise prior to test.
  - Discontinue drugs that can alter test results (aspirin, other nonsteroidal anti-inflammatory drugs).
- Specimen Collection and Handling:
  - Obtain specimen peripherally rather than through heparinized lines.
  - Collect venous blood in a lavender top EDTA tube.

LOINC CODES
- Code: 26516-5 (*Short Name* - Platelet # Plas)
- Code: 26515-7 (*Short Name* - Platelet # Bld)
- Code: 13057-5 (*Short Name* - Platelet Diaf-aCnc)

Poliovirus antibody level

TEST DEFINITION

Detection of antibodies to poliovirus serotype I, II, and III in serum for the diagnosis of poliovirus infection, or to confirm immunity

REFERENCE RANGE

Adults and Children: negative (less than 4-fold increase in immunoglobulin G antibody serum titer)
Please refer to your institution's reference ranges as lab normals may vary.

INDICATIONS

Suspected acute poliovirus infection
>   **Strength of Recommendation:** Class IIb
>   **Strength of Evidence:** Category C
>   **Results Interpretation:**
>   **Positive immunology findings**
>>   Neutralization of sera against paired antigens of the 3 poliovirus serotypes is diagnostic of infection and can also differentiate between wild-type and vaccine-strain virus.

CLINICAL NOTES

A 4-fold increase in poliovirus immunoglobulin G (IgG) antibody titer between acute and convalescent sera is considered representative of viral infection. A single positive IgM titer connotes a probable recent primary infection.

COLLECTION/STORAGE INFORMATION

- Specimen Handling and Storage:
    - Collect serum specimens at illness onset and during convalescent phase (2 to 4 weeks after acute onset).
    - Maintain specimen in viral transport medium.
    - Store and transport at 4°C for all specimens except blood,.
    - Freeze specimen at −70°C if not tested immediately.

LOINC CODES

- Code: 16284-2 (*Short Name* - PV Ab Ser-aCnc)
- Code: 27261-7 (*Short Name* - PV Ab Titr Ser CF)

Polymerase chain reaction for Bacillus anthracis

TEST DEFINITION

Detection of *Bacillus anthracis* DNA in body tissues or fluids, or from the environment, for assessment of anthrax infection or bioterrorism threat

REFERENCE RANGE

Negative
Please refer to your institution's reference ranges as lab normals may vary.

INDICATIONS

Suspected cutaneous anthrax
>   **Strength of Recommendation:** Class IIa
>   **Strength of Evidence:** Category C
>   **Results Interpretation:**
>   **Polymerase chain reaction observation**
>>   Detection of deoxyribonucleic acid (DNA) of *Bacillus anthracis* is highly suggestive of anthrax infection.
>>   *Bacillus anthracis*, a spore forming, Gram-positive bacillus, is a high-priority biological agent (category A) that poses a risk to national security because it can be easily disseminated or transmitted person-to-person; causes high mortality, with potential for major public health impact; might cause public panic and social disruption; and requires special action for public health preparedness.
>>   The World Health Organization recommends the polymerase chain reaction (PCR) technique as the standard diagnostic approach for identifying *B anthracis* ; however, the Centers for Disease Control do not consider PCR testing confirmatory.
>>   PCR-positive specimens are forwarded to one of 100 noncommercial laboratories with advanced capacity in the United States Laboratory Response Network (LRN), established by the CDC.
>>   Commercially available rapid handheld immunoassays for detection of anthrax are intended only for screening of environmental samples and should not be used to make decisions about patient management or prophylaxis.

Timing of Monitoring
The American Academy of Dermatology recommends a skin biopsy be done prior to starting antibiotics whenever cutaneous anthrax is suspected, and evaluated by IHC testing.

Suspected inhalation anthrax.
Strength of Recommendation: Class IIa
Strength of Evidence: Category C
Results Interpretation:
Polymerase chain reaction observation
Detection of deoxyribonucleic acid (DNA) by polymerase chain reaction of *Bacillus anthracis* is highly suggestive of anthrax.

Bacillus anthracis, a spore forming Gram-positive bacillus, is a high-priority biological agent (category A) that poses a risk to national security because it can be easily disseminated or transmitted person-to-person; causes high mortality, with potential for major public health impact; might cause public panic and social disruption; and requires special action for public health preparedness.

The World Health Organization recommends the polymerase chain reaction (PCR) technique as the standard diagnostic approach for identifying *B anthracis* ; however, the Centers for Disease Control do not consider PCR testing confirmatory.

PCR-positive specimens are forwarded to one of 100 non-commercial laboratories with advanced capacity in the United States Laboratory Response Network (LRN), established by the Centers for Disease Control (CDC).

Commercially available rapid handheld immunoassays for detection of anthrax are intended only for screening of environmental samples and should not be used to make decisions about patient management or prophylaxis.

COLLECTION/STORAGE INFORMATION
- Collect specimen from blood, pleural fluid, serum, cerebrospinal fluid, lung tissue and/or lymph node tissue.
- Exercise great care in handling specimens. Conduct work with immunized personnel. Handle samples in biological safety cabinets wearing gloves, gowns, and masks.
- Disinfect all work surfaces with 5% hypochlorite or 5% phenol; decontaminate all supplies, materials, and equipment.

Potassium measurement, urine

TEST DEFINITION
Measurement of potassium in urine for the evaluation of acid-base disorders

SYNONYMS
- Urine potassium
- Urine potassium level

REFERENCE RANGE
- Adults: 25 - 100 mEq/24 hr (25 - 100 mmol/24 hr)
Please refer to your institution's reference ranges as lab normals may vary.

INDICATIONS
Potassium disorder of unknown etiology
Results Interpretation:
Potassium level - finding
The expected value for a 24 hour urine potassium in hypokalemic and hyperkalemic patients is less than 10 mmol/day, and greater than 150 mmol/day, respectively. In hyperkalemia values as high as 400 mmol/day have been reported. Expected spot urine potassium values in hypokalemia are less than 20 mmol/L if due to a nonrenal cause, and greater than 20 mmol/L if due to a renal cause. The expected spot urine potassium value in hyperkalemia is undetermined.

In a hypokalemic patient, a normal urinary potassium level may not indicate renal potassium wasting unless the duration of hypokalemia has been known to be greater than 10 days. Hypokalemia must be chronic (lasting longer than a week) to be reflected as a decreased urinary potassium concentration.

Urine potassium values are directly affected by urine sodium delivery, urine volume and urine concentration. To adjust for these variables the transtubular potassium gradient (TTKG) formula may be utilized to obtain a more reliable measure of renal potassium handling.

Suspected acid-base disorder
    Strength of Recommendation: Class IIa
    Strength of Evidence: Category C
  Results Interpretation:
  Abnormal biochemistry findings
    Urine potassium levels greater than 30 mEq/day in the presence of hypokalemia indicate renal potassium wasting resulting from mineralocorticoid (eg, aldosterone) excess.
    Acidosis and increased urinary potassium suggest diabetic ketoacidosis or proximal or distal renal tubular acidosis. Acidosis in conjunction with a urinary potassium level less than 20 mEq/L is associated with diarrhea, ureterosigmoidostomy, malfunctioning ileal loop, or malabsorption. Alkalosis in conjunction with a urinary potassium level less than 20 mEq/L is associated with vomiting without bicarbonaturia.

Suspected hyperaldosteronism
    Strength of Recommendation: Class IIa
    Strength of Evidence: Category C
  Results Interpretation:
  Abnormal biochemistry findings
    High urine sodium and low urine potassium levels suggest aldosterone deficiency or resistance. Hyperaldosteronism stimulates renal reabsorption of sodium which also leads to excretion of large amounts of potassium in the urine.

Suspected hyponatremia
  Results Interpretation:
  Abnormal biochemistry findings
    A urine potassium concentration greater than 30 mEq/L may be associated with hyponatremia secondary to edematous states, or with ongoing diuretic use. The urine potassium concentration will be less than 30 mEq/L in hyponatremia due to extrarenal loss.

Suspected renal disorder
    Strength of Recommendation: Class IIb
    Strength of Evidence: Category C
  Results Interpretation:
  Abnormal biochemistry findings
    When urinary potassium greater than 20 mEq/L occurs in the presence of hypokalemia, the kidneys should be suspected as the primary source of potassium loss.

CLINICAL NOTES

    Specimen should be collected before electrolyte correction therapy is initiated, although treatment should not be postponed while test results are pending.
    Loop diuretics can cause increased renal potassium excretion.

COLLECTION/STORAGE INFORMATION

- Urine potassium can be collected as a spot specimen or a 24 hour specimen.
- Normal range varies with intake

LOINC CODES

- Code: 2828-2 (*Short Name* - Potassium Ur-sCnc)
- Code: 18372-3 (*Short Name* - Potassium 6H Ur-sRate)
- Code: 32550-6 (*Short Name* - Potassium ?Tm sub Ur Qn)
- Code: 11148-4 (*Short Name* - Potassium/creat Ur-mRto)

Pregnancy-associated protein A measurement, serum

TEST DEFINITION

    Measurement of pregnancy-associated plasma protein A (PAPP-A) in blood for the evaluation and management of pregnancy complications, and as a marker for acute coronary syndromes

SYNONYMS

- PAPP-A measurement - Pregnancy-associated plasma protein A measurement
- Pregnancy-associated plasma protein A measurement

REFERENCE RANGE

- Pregnant women:
- Maternal: <32 mg/dL
- Levels increase gradually through gestation
- Levels become undetectable within a few days to 5 weeks after birth
  Non-pregnant adults: undetectable to less than 10 milli-International Units/L
  Please refer to your institution's reference ranges as lab normals may vary.

INDICATIONS

Suspected fetal trisomy 21 (Down's syndrome) in early pregnancy
    Strength of Recommendation: Class IIb
    Strength of Evidence: Category B
    Results Interpretation:
    Decreased level (laboratory finding)
    Decreased levels of maternal serum PAPP-A may be associated with Trisomy 21 in the fetus.

    False Results
    In a multicenter screening study of 4,325 women who underwent first and second trimester testing for multiple markers, including PAPP-A in the first trimester, sequential second-trimester testing detected 98% of trisomy 21 pregnancies, though with a 38.7% false positive rate.
    In SURUSS, a control-matched prospective study of 47,053 singleton pregnancies, trisomy 21 was detected in 9 out of 10 affected pregnancies, with a false-positive rate of 1%, when the measurement of PAPP-A and nuchal translucency in the first trimester was combined with measurements of alpha-fetoprotein, free beta-HCG, unconjugated estriol and inhibin-A early in the second trimester.
    Timing of Monitoring
    Optimal time for performing the test is between 74 and 97 days of gestation.

Suspected trisomy 18 (Patau syndrome) in early pregnancy
    Strength of Recommendation: Class IIb
    Strength of Evidence: Category B
    Results Interpretation:
    Decreased level (laboratory finding)
    Decreased levels of maternal serum PAPP-A in the first trimester of pregnancy may be associated with trisomy 18 in the fetus.
    Timing of Monitoring
    Optimal timing for performing the test is at 74 to 97 days of gestation.

Suspected acute coronary syndromes
    Strength of Recommendation: Class Indeterminate
    Strength of Evidence: Category C
    Results Interpretation:
    Increased level (laboratory finding)
    Serum levels of PAPP-A greater than or equal to 10 milli-International Units/L may be a marker for acute coronary syndromes.

Suspected pregnancy complications
    Strength of Recommendation: Class IIb
    Strength of Evidence: Category B
    Results Interpretation:
    Decreased level (laboratory finding)
    Decreased pregnancy-associated plasma protein A (PAPP-A) levels in the lowest fifth percentile may be associated with pregnancy complications such as miscarriage at 24 weeks gestation or less, premature delivery, preeclampsia, low birth weight, stillbirth (from abruption or growth restriction), proteinuric pregnancy-induced hypertension, and premature rupture of membranes. Complete absence of PAPP-A suggests Cornelia de Lange syndrome.

Timing of Monitoring
Pregnancy-associated plasma protein A (PAPP-A) levels should be drawn at the end of the first trimester, 10 to 13 weeks after conception.

COLLECTION/STORAGE INFORMATION
- Specimen Collection and Handling:
    - Collect serum and analyze fresh or store at 4°C for 3 days
    - Freeze at -20° C for storage up to 6 months
    - Store indefinitely at -70° C

LOINC CODES
- Code: 32046-5 (*Short Name* - PAPP-A SerPl-aCnc)

Primidone blood measurement

TEST DEFINITION
Measurement of primidone in serum to facilitate therapeutic or toxicity monitoring

SYNONYMS
- Primidone: blood level

REFERENCE RANGE
- Adults and Children (therapeutic level): 5-12 mcg/mL (23-55 micromol/L)
  Please refer to your institution's reference ranges as lab normals may vary.

INDICATIONS
Drug monitoring of the anticonvulsant primidone
  Strength of Recommendation: Class IIa
  Strength of Evidence: Category C
  Results Interpretation:
 Blood drug levels - finding
  Serum levels of primidone and its active metabolite (phenobarbital) of greater than 15 mcg/mL (greater than 69 micromol/L) are considered toxic.
  Primidone/phenobarbital ratio greater than 1:2 suggests poor compliance.
  Concentrations of 15 mcg/mL of primidone with therapeutic concentrations of phenobarbital have been reported to be associated with ataxia and/or somnolence.
  Levels greater than 15 mcg/mL are associated with toxicity, and plasma levels exceeding 80 mcg/mL are generally associated with some degree of coma. In the absence of tolerance, plasma levels exceeding 20 to 30 mcg/dL may be associated with CNS depression.
  Levels of 70 to 80 mcg/mL have also been associated with crystalluria.
  In acute overdose, metabolites are detectable within 24 to 48 hours.

ABNORMAL RESULTS
- Results increased in:
    - Pregnancy (2nd trimester)

COLLECTION/STORAGE INFORMATION
- Specimen Collection and Handling:
    - Collect blood in heparin (green) or EDTA (lavender) tube
    - May store at room temperature for several hours or at 20° C for up to one year

Procainamide and N-acetylprocainamide measurement

TEST DEFINITION
Measurement of procainamide and N-acetylprocainamide (NAPA) levels in serum to facilitate therapeutic or toxicity monitoring

REFERENCE RANGE
- Procainamide: 4-10 mcg/mL (17-42 micromol/L)
- N-acetylprocainamide: 10-20 mg/L

Please refer to your institution's reference ranges as lab normals may vary.

INDICATIONS
Drug level monitoring during procainamide therapy
   Strength of Recommendation: Class IIa
   Strength of Evidence: Category C
Results Interpretation:
Blood drug levels - finding
   Procainamide monitoring is particularly important in patients who might be fast acetylators (60% to 70% of northern Europeans and 50% of black and white Americans) and in patients with renal impairment. N-acetylprocainamide (NAPA), the major active metabolite of procainamide resulting from hepatic conjugation, affects the excretion of procainamide and has effects that are more pronounced on the QTc interval. Fast acetylation status is defined by a measurement 3 hours after last dose that shows a NAPA concentration greater than or equal to that of procainamide.

   Serum monitoring and clinical observation should drive dosage adjustments in an effort to control cardiac arrhythmias and achieve target blood levels of procainamide. The range of safe and effective blood levels is narrow, and dosages should be titrated carefully.

   Procainamide levels greater than 10 to 12 mcg/mL (greater than 42 to 51 micromol/L) are toxic; NAPA levels greater than 40 mg/L are toxic.

   Procainamide concentrations should always be evaluated in conjunction with NAPA concentrations; increased toxicity is seen when the sum of the procainamide and NAPA concentrations is greater than 25 to 30 mcg/mL.

Timing of Monitoring
   For routine therapeutic monitoring of both procainamide and N-acetylprocainamide (NAPA), collect sample 1 hour before the next dose of procainamide is due. When trying to establish acetylation status, procainamide and NAPA levels should be measured on the same sample and drawn 3 hours after the last dose of procainamide.

CLINICAL NOTES
Procainamide and N-acetylprocainamide levels always should be measured on the same sample.

COLLECTION/STORAGE INFORMATION
- Specimen Collection and Handling:
  - Collect blood sample in a heparin (green-top), EDTA (lavender-top), or oxalate tube.
  - Store sample at 2°C to 8°C for 24 hours or at -20°C for 1 to 2 weeks.

LOINC CODES
- Code: 3983-4 (*Short Name* - Procainamide+NAPA SerPl-mCnc)

Proline measurement

TEST DEFINITION
Measurement of proline in plasma or serum for detection of acquired and hereditary amino acid disorders.

REFERENCE RANGE
- Premature neonate, 1 day: 2.64± 0.86 mg/dL (230 ± 75 micromol/L)
- Neonate, 1 day: 1.23-3.18 mg/dL (107-277 micromol/L)
- Infants 1 to 3 months: 2.31 ± 0.71 mg/dL (201 ± 62 micromol/L)
- Infants 9 to 24 months: 0.59-2.13 mg/dL (51-185 micromol/L)
- Children 3 to 10 years: 0.78-1.7 mg/dL (68-148 micromol/L)
- Children 6 to 18 years: 0.67-3.72 mg/dL (58-324 micromol/L)
- Adults: 1.17-3.86 mg/dL (102-336 micromol/L)

  Please refer to your institution's reference ranges as lab normals may vary.

INDICATIONS
Suspected inborn error of metabolism
> **Strength of Recommendation:** Class IIa
> **Strength of Evidence:** Category C
> **Results Interpretation:**
> **Increased amino acid**
>> Inherited amino acid disorders are directly related to the absence of an enzyme involved in the metabolism of one or more amino acids; therefore, an elevated plasma level of a particular amino acid is highly suggestive of an inherited metabolic defect. In the majority of cases amino acid and organic acid analysis together permit diagnostic confirmation in infants. Immediate treatment should be initiated when an inborn error of metabolism is suspected, even if a definitive diagnosis has not yet been determined.
>>
>> Mild hyperprolinemia is present is approximately 5% of healthy individuals. Proline levels are elevated 3 to 5 times normal in Type I hyperprolinemia and 10 to 15 times normal in Type II hyperprolinemia.

COLLECTION/STORAGE INFORMATION
- Specimen Collection and Handling:
  - Immediately place sample in ice water.
  - Isolate plasma sample and freeze it within 1 hour; sample stable for 1 week at -20°C.
  - Sample should be deproteinized and stored at -70°C for protracted periods of usage.

LOINC CODES
- Code: 25976-2 (*Short Name* - Proline/creat 24H Ur-sRto)
- Code: 17492-0 (*Short Name* - Proline Ur Ql)
- Code: 25975-4 (*Short Name* - Proline 24H Ur-sCnc)
- Code: 32267-7 (*Short Name* - Proline Fld-sCnc)
- Code: 30067-3 (*Short Name* - Proline/creat Ur-Rto)
- Code: 22743-9 (*Short Name* - Proline XXX-sCnc)
- Code: 13799-2 (*Short Name* - Proline/creat Ur-mRto)
- Code: 25510-9 (*Short Name* - Proline 24H Ur-sRate)
- Code: 27033-0 (*Short Name* - Proline Amn-sCnc)
- Code: 2847-2 (*Short Name* - Proline 24H Ur-mRate)
- Code: 2843-1 (*Short Name* - Proline CSF-mCnc)
- Code: 2846-4 (*Short Name* - Proline Ur-mCnc)
- Code: 13412-2 (*Short Name* - Proline Amn-mCnc)
- Code: 32266-9 (*Short Name* - Proline Vitf-sCnc)
- Code: 26726-0 (*Short Name* - Proline Ur-sCnc)
- Code: 22645-6 (*Short Name* - Proline CSF-sCnc)

Propoxyphene measurement

TEST DEFINITION
Measurement of propoxyphene in serum for therapeutic monitoring, toxicity evaluation, or drug of abuse assessment

SYNONYMS
- Darvocet measurement
- Darvon measurement

REFERENCE RANGE

- Propoxyphene, therapeutic concentration:
- Adults: 0.1-0.4 mcg/mL (0.3-1.2 micromol/L)
- Norpropoxyphene (metabolite), therapeutic concentration:
- Adults: 0.1-1.5 mcg/mL (0.3-4.6 micromol/L)
   Please refer to your institution's reference ranges as lab normals may vary.

INDICATIONS

Suspected dextropropoxyphene (propoxyphene) overdose
   Strength of Recommendation: Class III
   Strength of Evidence: Category C
   Results Interpretation:
   Increased level (laboratory finding)
- Propoxyphene, toxic concentration:
   - Adults and Children: >0.5 mcg/mL (>1.5 micromol/L)
- Norpropoxyphene (metabolite), toxic concentration:
   - Adults and Children: >2 mcg/mL (>6.1 micromol/L)
   Propoxyphene plasma concentrations may not correlate with clinical presentation following overdose. Plasma levels have reportedly overlapped between chronic therapy, nonfatal poisoning, and fatal overdose. In cases of fatal propoxyphene overdose, plasma propoxyphene and norpropoxyphene concentrations ranged from less than 0.1 to greater than 20 mcg/mL.
   The ratio of propoxyphene to norpropoxyphene may distinguish between acute or chronic overdose. Typically, norpropoxyphene exceeds propoxyphene levels during chronic propoxyphene therapy, in contrast, an elevated propoxyphene level as compared to norpropoxyphene may indicate acute poisoning.
   Because propoxyphene may be combined with other drugs, propoxyphene levels must also be evaluated in context with other potential agents ingested. Fatal cases of propoxyphene overdose have been reported with low plasma concentrations of propoxyphene following the ingestion of combination products containing propoxyphene and acetaminophen.

Therapeutic drug monitoring of propoxyphene
   Strength of Recommendation: Class III
   Strength of Evidence: Category C
   Results Interpretation:
   Laboratory test finding
   Plasma concentrations can vary widely with therapeutic use. Overlap between plasma concentrations found during chronic therapeutic use, nonfatal poisoning, and fatal overdose have been reported

LOINC CODES

- Code: 3545-1 (*Short Name* - Propoxyph Ur-mCnc)
- Code: 16242-0 (*Short Name* - Propoxyph Ur Cnfrn-mCnc)
- Code: 27067-8 (*Short Name* - Propoxyph Mec-mCnt)
- Code: 11234-2 (*Short Name* - Propoxyph Har-mCnt)
- Code: 27281-5 (*Short Name* - Propoxyph Stl-mCnt)
- Code: 9809-5 (*Short Name* - Propoxyph Gast Ql)
- Code: 32125-7 (*Short Name* - Propoxyph SerPl-sCnc)
- Code: 27190-8 (*Short Name* - Propoxyph Vitf-mCnc)
- Code: 16748-6 (*Short Name* - Propoxyph SerPl Ql Cfm)
- Code: 12357-0 (*Short Name* - Propoxyph Stl Ql)
- Code: 9737-8 (*Short Name* - Propoxyph Gast-mCnc)
- Code: 11027-0 (*Short Name* - Propoxyph Mec-mCnc)

Prostate specific antigen measurement

TEST DEFINITION

   Measurement of prostate specific antigen in serum for the detection and management of benign prostatic hyperplasia and prostate cancer.

SYNONYMS

- PSA measurement
- PSA - Prostate-specific antigen level
- PSA - Serum prostate specific antigen level
- tPSA measurement - Total prostate specific antigen measurement

REFERENCE RANGE

- Males, ≤40 years of age: 0-2 ng/mL (0-2 mcg/L):
- Males, >40 years of age: 0-4 ng/mL (0-4 mcg/L)
- Females: <0.5 ng/mL (<0.5 mcg/L):
  Please refer to your institution's reference ranges as lab normals may vary.

INDICATIONS

Post treatment monitoring of prostate cancer
> **Strength of Recommendation:** Class IIa
> **Strength of Evidence:** Category B
> **Results Interpretation:**
> **Raised prostate specific antigen**
> Because of its long half-life, it may be possible to detect prostate specific antigen (PSA) in serum for several weeks after a curative procedure. PSA should return to its baseline level by 21 days postoperatively.
> The time from recurrence of detectable serum PSA levels to clinical evidence of recurrent disease is variable. A rapid increase in serum PSA levels, defined as a doubling of PSA levels in less than 10 months, is associated with earlier clinical relapse, and higher preoperative PSA levels are associated with higher rates of postoperative recurrence. The time at which the PSA level becomes detectable postoperatively can predict eventual local vs distant recurrence. Detection of serum PSA within the first 2 years after prostatectomy is associated with distant disease, while an increase in PSA velocity of less than 0.75 ng/mL per year or a rise in PSA more than 2 years after treatment, is associated with local relapse. An elevated post prostatectomy PSA level in the presence of lymph node involvement, seminal vesicle invasion, or a Gleason score greater than 7, is suggestive of metastatic disease.
> PSA levels decrease gradually following radiation therapy and may not reach undetectable levels. The median time to nadir is 17 months. Interpretation criteria have not been clearly defined and the PSA threshold value and serum levels required for determining success or failure of radiation therapy is controversial. The American Society for Therapeutic Radiology and Oncology defines failure as 3 consecutive rises in PSA following radiation therapy. Patients with PSA levels that fall to less than 0.5 ng/mL are unlikely to have disease recurrence within 5 years of treatment.
> Following successful androgen deprivation therapy, PSA levels should fall significantly within 6 months, often to undetectable levels. A post treatment increase in levels suggest disease progression. Following androgen deprivation therapy, a post treatment reduction in serum PSA concentration correlates with improved clinical symptoms. A 50% or greater decrease in serum PSA levels has been associated with improved survival rates in patients with androgen-independent prostate cancer. The degree of PSA reduction after second-line treatment for metastatic disease is correlated with disease survival.
> **Frequency of Monitoring**
> Treatment guidelines recommend ongoing monitoring for disease recurrence, but the optimal strategy is unknown.

Screening for prostate cancer
> **Strength of Recommendation:** Class IIb
> **Strength of Evidence:** Category B
> **Results Interpretation:**
> **Raised prostate specific antigen**
> According to the American Cancer Society guidelines, if a screening PSA level obtained at age 40 is less than 1 ng/mL, no additional testing is required until age 45. If PSA is greater than 1 ng/mL but less than 2.5 ng/mL, annual testing is recommended. A PSA greater than 2.5 ng/mL necessitates further clinical evaluation and possible biopsy.

Suspected benign prostatic hyperplasia
> **Strength of Recommendation:** Class IIa
> **Strength of Evidence:** Category B

Results Interpretation:
Raised prostate specific antigen

A significant, strong correlation has been demonstrated between benign prostatic hypertrophy (BPH) and prostate specific antigen (PSA) levels of 2 to 9 ng/mL. However, PSA serum levels rise with advancing age and increased prostate size and elevated levels can be caused by infection, instrumentation, biopsy, or malignancy. Biopsy may be indicated if a diagnosis of BPH cannot be established.

PSA testing helps to differentiate between BPH and prostate cancer as the cause of new or worsening lower urinary tract symptoms. PSA testing is usually recommended for all men with suspected symptomatic BPH.

Suspected prostate cancer

Strength of Recommendation: Class IIa
Strength of Evidence: Category B
Results Interpretation:
Raised prostate specific antigen

Prostate cancer is uncommon with a prostate-specific antigen level (PSA) less than 1 ng/ml. Cancers that are present at this level are usually of minimal volume or are aggressive tumors not associated with PSA production. Unless the digital rectal exam (DRE) is suspicious, no further clinical evaluation is necessary. Cancer is uncommon with a PSA level of 1 to 2.5 ng/mL, although a DRE is recommended for all patients with a PSA level in this range. A PSA level of 2.5 to 4 ng/mL is highly suggestive of prostate cancer and the risk of a positive biopsy is about 20%. A PSA level in this range is associated with extensive, intermediate to high grade multi-focal disease; about half of cancer patients in this PSA range will be extraprostatic. The risk of a positive biopsy is about 25% with a PSA level in this range and tumors detected are usually clinically significant. The risk for prostate cancer increases dramatically with a PSA level of 10 to 20 ng/mL, and the rate of tumor metastases begins to increase above a PSA level of 10 ng/mL. With a PSA level greater than 20 ng/mL, extraprostatic metastasis is present in more than 80% of patients and the risk of positive nodes increases dramatically.

Biopsy is recommended if the PSA is greater than 4 ng/mL, if a rapid rise in PSA levels occurs with sequential testing, or if the DRE is suspicious.

- Healthy men with no evidence of disease will have increased PSA levels of approximately 3.2% per year, or 0.04 ng/mL/yr. Proposed age-specific normal ranges for healthy men are as follows:
  - Age 40-49: 0-2.5 ng/mL
  - Age 50-59: 0-3.5 ng/mL
  - Age 60-69: 0-4.5 ng/mL
  - Age 70-79: 0-6.5 ng/mL

In order to account for ethnic differences in normal ranges, and to improve test specificity, the following normal ranges for black males have been proposed:

Age (years)	Normal Range (ng/mL)	Test Specificity
40-49	0-2	93%
50-59	0-4	88%
60-69	0-4.5	81%
70-79	0-5.5	78%

DRUG/LAB INTERACTIONS

- Capromab Pendetide - falsely high prostate specific antigen levels
- Finasteride - a falsely decreased prostate-specific antigen (PSA) level

ABNORMAL RESULTS

Ejaculation and digital rectal exam can cause an insignificant rise in PSA levels while prostate biopsy and cystoscopy can cause substantial increases; PSA testing should be delayed until 3 to 4 weeks after these procedures. Exercise, infection and some medications can also cause a rise in PSA levels. Finasteride will lower PSA by approximately 50%.

COLLECTION/STORAGE INFORMATION

- Specimen stable for 24 hours at room temperature, and for 2 weeks at 2-8°C. Store at -20°C or colder for periods longer than 2 weeks. Avoid multiple freeze-thaw cycles.
- The laboratory result should include the name of the assay used and the reference range generated for the assay.

LOINC CODES
- Code: 2857-1 (*Short Name* - PSA Ser-mCnc)
- Code: 19195-7 (*Short Name* - PSA Ser-aCnc)
- Code: 19200-5 (*Short Name* - PSA Smn-sCnc)
- Code: 10508-0 (*Short Name* - PSA Tiss Ql ImStn)

Protein S assay

TEST DEFINITION
Measurement of protein S in plasma as total antigen, functional, and free antigen to assess risk factors for venous thrombosis

SYNONYMS
- Protein S level

REFERENCE RANGE
- Adults: Total, free and functional antigen, each: 70% - 140% (0.70 - 1.40)
  Please refer to your institution's reference ranges as lab normals may vary.

INDICATIONS
Suspected venous thromboembolism
> **Strength of Recommendation:** Class IIa
> **Strength of Evidence:** Category B
> **Results Interpretation:**
> **Decreased level (laboratory finding)**
> Decreased levels of free protein S are associated with an increased risk of venous thromboembolism.
> If the functional protein S assay is low and the patient does not present with any interfering factors, a free protein S antigen determination should be performed. If free protein S concentrations are low, a total protein S determination should be performed.

COMMON PANELS
- Hypercoagulation panel

ABNORMAL RESULTS
- Results decreased in:
  - Acute phase response
    - Infection
    - Factor VIII, elevated
    - Surgery
  - DIC
  - Liver disease
  - Pregnancy
  - Proteinuria
  - Vitamin K deficiency

COLLECTION/STORAGE INFORMATION
- Patient Preparation:
  - Patient must discontinue oral anticoagulants 10 days prior to testing
- Specimen Collection and Handling:
  - Collect plasma in a blue-top tube

LOINC CODES
- Code: 5893-3 (*Short Name* - PS PPP Chro-aCnc)
- Code: 31102-7 (*Short Name* - Prot S Act/Nor PPP Chro-)
- Code: 5892-5 (*Short Name* - PS PPP-aCnc)

Protein measurement, urine, quantitative 24 hour

Test Definition
Quantitative measurement of protein in urine for evaluation of renal dysfunction

Reference Range
- 24-hour urine:
- Adults: <150 mg/24 hours (less than 0.15 g/24 hours)
- Spot urine (ratio of urine protein to urine creatinine):
- Adults: <0.2
  Please refer to your institution's reference ranges as lab normals may vary.

Indications
Suspected glomerulonephritis
  Strength of Recommendation: Class I
  Strength of Evidence: Category C
  Results Interpretation:
  Proteinuria
    In acute glomerulonephritis, urinary protein excretion is usually less than 3 g/24 hours. Mild proteinuria persists in 15% at 2 years and in 2% at 10 years.
    Proteinuria is present in 80% to 90% of patients with poststreptococcal glomerulonephritis, which usually presents as acute glomerulonephritis. The degree of proteinuria varies according to the nature and severity of the underlying glomerular lesion. In most cases, protein excretion rates range from 0.2 to 3 g/24 hours, with a protein concentration of 30 to 100 mg/dL.
    Proteinuria is the most important prognostic indicator in poststreptococcal glomerulonephritis. Progressive renal disease is a rare consequence of poststreptococcal glomerulonephritis when renal function returns to normal and proteinuria is less than 500 mg/day. In some patients who require dialysis, proteinuria may persist for up to 2 years, and 20% to 50% of these patients have increased urine protein excretion for many years.
    Moderate proteinuria is usually present in rapidly progressive glomerulonephritis.
    Persistent proteinuria is a risk factor in IgA nephropathy for progression to ESRD.

Suspected hemolytic uremic syndrome (HUS)
  Results Interpretation:
  Proteinuria
    All patients with hemolytic uremic syndrome (HUS) have a nonselective proteinuria, typically 1 to 2 g/day but may be as high as 10 g/day. Occasionally, patients present with nephrotic syndrome or become nephrotic during the early recovery phase.
    Proteinuria correlates with poor outcome in typical HUS.

Suspected nephrotic syndrome
  Strength of Recommendation: Class I
  Strength of Evidence: Category C
  Results Interpretation:
  Proteinuria
    In the presence of edema, hypoalbuminemia, and hypercholesterolemia, urine protein exceeding 3 g per 24 hours (or 3.5 g per 1.73 m^2 of body-surface area per day) is diagnostic of nephrotic syndrome.

Suspected preeclampsia
  Strength of Recommendation: Class I
  Strength of Evidence: Category B
  Results Interpretation:
  Proteinuria
    Proteinuria may occur early in the course of pregnancy but is usually a later sign, occurring at 28 to 32 weeks' gestation as injury to renal vessels allows protein to spill into the urine. A protein level greater than 300 mg in a 24-hour urine specimen defines proteinuria. Proteinuria of 2 g or more in 24 hours occurring for

the first time during pregnancy increases certainty of the diagnosis of preeclampsia and should be considered as such in cases of pregnancy-induced hypertension until proven otherwise. Excretion of 5 g or more of protein in a 24-hour urine specimen is an indicator of severe preeclampsia.

The presence of proteinuria confers an increased risk to both mother and fetus; this risk is not affected by the absolute value of or an increase in urinary protein excretion. Patients with proteinuric preeclampsia have a quadrupled perinatal mortality as compared with patients with chronic hypertension and those with non-proteinuric gestational hypertension. In women with chronic hypertension, the presence of proteinuria early in pregnancy is associated with adverse neonatal outcomes, independent of the development of preeclampsia.

While the 24-hour urine collection is considered the gold standard for quantitation of urine protein, several other tests may accurately predict 24-hour protein excretion. In patients with suspected preeclampsia, timely diagnosis and treatment are important. A study of 65 patients with suspected preeclampsia found that 8- and 12-hour urine samples were useful indicators of 24-hour protein excretion. In a prospective study of 171 pregnant women with new onset hypertension, quantitative point of care measurement of the albumin/creatinine ratio was a good predictor of proteinuria greater than 300 mg/24 hours.

Suspected proteinuria
Strength of Recommendation: Class I
Strength of Evidence: Category C
Results Interpretation:
Proteinuria

The most commonly used quantitative measurement of proteinuria is determination of the protein content of a timed urine specimen, most often a 24-hour collection. Although the largest source of error with the method is the difficulty of collecting an accurately timed specimen, the expected amount of creatinine in a 24-hour urine specimen can be calculated and compared with the measured amount to confirm the completeness of the urine collection. Urine levels above 150 mg/24 hours are diagnostic of proteinuria.

Another quantitative measure of protein excretion is the ratio of the urine protein to the urine creatinine. This ratio numerically approximates the 24-hour protein excretion in grams, corrected for body surface area. For example, a ratio of 1 represents a urine protein excretion of approximately 1 g/d per 1.73 m^2 of body surface area. Thus, the normal ratio is less than 0.2, representing a protein excretion rate of less than 200 mg per 24 hours, whereas a patient with nephrotic syndrome will have a ratio of more than 3.5. This test may be useful in situations in which collection of an accurate 24-hour urine specimen is difficult.

In many proteinuric patients, measurement of postural proteinuria is indicated. This involves collection of two urine specimens, one while the patient is ambulatory and the other while the patient is recumbent. The amount of protein in each sample is extrapolated to 24 hours. In the case of true orthostatic proteinuria, the urine protein level should exceed 150 mg in the upright sample but must be normal in the recumbent sample. If the level is abnormal in both samples, even if it is greater in the upright sample, the definition of orthostatic proteinuria is not fulfilled.

Suspected proteinuric diabetic nephropathy
Strength of Recommendation: Class I
Strength of Evidence: Category C
Results Interpretation:
Urine protein abnormal

A urine albumin level greater than or equal to 30 mg/24 hours suggests microalbuminuria, which is often the first sign of renal dysfunction in diabetic patients. A urine albumin level of greater than or equal to 300 mg/24 hours suggests overt nephropathy or clinical albuminuria.

False Results
- Results increased in:
- Short-term hyperglycemia
- Exercise
- Urinary tract infections
- Marked hypertension
- Heart failure
- Acute febrile illness

Timing of Monitoring

Screening for urine protein should be conducted when diabetes is initially diagnosed. If the screen is positive, a quantitative 24-hour urine protein test should be performed. In some cases, screening may be done by collecting a 4-hour, overnight, or 24-hour urine specimen.

COMMON PANELS
• Renal panel

CLINICAL NOTES
While the 24-hour urine collection historically has been considered the gold standard for quantitative measurement of urine protein, there are problems with this test, including poor precision and variability of lab methods used for assay, unreliability of patient collection, and delay in obtaining results.

COLLECTION/STORAGE INFORMATION
• 24-hour urine collection.
• Spot urine.

LOINC CODES
• Code: 21482-5 (*Short Name* - Prot 24H Ur-mCnc)
• Code: 2889-4 (*Short Name* - Prot 24H Ur-mRate)

Prothrombin gene (20210) screen

TEST DEFINITION
Polymerase chain reaction analysis for genomic fingerprinting of prothrombin gene mutation factor II G20210A

SYNONYMS
• PCR test for Factor II G20210A mutation
• Prothrombin G20210A mutation

REFERENCE RANGE
• No mutation detected
Please refer to your institution's reference ranges as lab normals may vary.

INDICATIONS
Evaluation for presence of factor II G20210A mutation in venous thromboembolism
    Strength of Recommendation: Class IIa
    Strength of Evidence: Category C
    Results Interpretation:
    Polymerase chain reaction observation
    Prothrombin (factor II) levels are increased when factor II G20210A mutation is present, increasing venous thromboembolism (VTE) risk. Factor II G20210A mutation occurs in approximately 2% of the general population but in 6% of patients patients presenting with VTE.. Cancer patients with the mutation have a 17-fold increased VTE risk.
    Factor II G20210A mutation moderately increases VTE risk in pregnancy. Depending on history and other risk factors, anticoagulants may be recommended for VTE prophylaxis.

COLLECTION/STORAGE INFORMATION
• Specimen Collection and Handling:
    • May collect crude cell lysate, serum, or whole blood
    • Use caution to avoid contaminating with extraneous DNA or RNA
    • Avoid anticoagulants except citrate and EDTA
    • Avoid heparin and heme because they are strong inhibitors
    • Store nucleic acids frozen at -20°C or below

LOINC CODES
• Code: 24475-6 (*Short Name* - F2 Gene p.G20210a QI)

Prothrombin time

TEST DEFINITION
Measurement of plasma clotting time for the evaluation and management of coagulation disorders

SYNONYMS
- Protime
- PT assay
- PT - Prothrombin time
- Quick one stage prothrombin time

REFERENCE RANGE
- Adults: 11.1-13.1 seconds
- Neonates: Prolonged by 2-3 seconds
- Premature neonates, 1-3 days old: Prolonged by 3-5 seconds
  Please refer to your institution's reference ranges as lab normals may vary.

INDICATIONS
Monitoring of prothrombin time during anticoagulant therapy
    Strength of Recommendation: Class I
    Strength of Evidence: Category C
Results Interpretation:
Increased prothrombin time
    Monitoring of prothrombin time (PT) and INR is essential during oral anticoagulant therapy (OAT) to maintain a balance between the risks of thrombosis (inadequate levels) vs bleeding (excessive levels).
    Adjustments in OAT to achieve a therapeutic range are based on PT/INR measurements.
Frequency of Monitoring
    Therapeutic monitoring for anticoagulants should be conducted 4 to 7 times per week until a stable dose has been determined, and then at least every 4 weeks thereafter.

Suspected abnormal liver function
    Strength of Recommendation: Class IIa
    Strength of Evidence: Category B
Results Interpretation:
Increased prothrombin time
    A prolonged prothrombin time (PT) may be a sign of serious liver dysfunction.
    For persons with liver disease on oral anticoagulants, it is unknown if a particular PT or INR value represents the same level of anticoagulation as that in individuals without liver disease. However, the standard target range for PT/INR is still generally used in this setting.

Suspected and known hemophilia
Results Interpretation:
Normal laboratory findings
    Prothrombin time (PT) is normal in hemophilia A and B.

Suspected coagulopathy
    Strength of Recommendation: Class I
    Strength of Evidence: Category B
Results Interpretation:
Increased prothrombin time
    A prolonged prothrombin time (PT) may indicate deficiencies in factor II, V, VII or X.
    PT is used primarily to evaluate coagulation abnormalities in the extrinsic pathway, as well as severe functional deficiencies of the common pathway.
    A prolonged PT with a normal partial thromboplastin time (PTT) indicates a deficiency of factor VII. A normal PT with a prolonged PTT indicates a deficiency of factor VIII, IX, XI, or XII (eg, classic hemophilia or Christmas disease). When both PT and PTT are prolonged, factors in the final common pathway, such as prothrombin, fibrinogen, factor V and/or factor X, may be deficient. Examples of such disorders include vitamin K deficiency or warfarin therapy.

Due to its short half-life, factor VII may decrease quickly in the acute hospital setting from malnourishment, transient liver dysfunction, or other conditions, causing a prolonged PT. This usually does not indicate a new coagulopathy, and may be corrected with administration of vitamin K.

A normal PT in the presence of abnormal bleeding with other normal coagulation tests may indicate a factor XIII deficiency.

Suspected heat stroke
Results Interpretation:
Increased prothrombin time

A prolonged prothrombin time (PT) is commonly seen in severe cases of heat stroke, secondary to direct thermal damage to all clotting factors.

Clotting dysfunction peaks at 18 to 36 hours after the acute phase of heat stroke.

Suspected or known biliary obstruction
Results Interpretation:
Increased prothrombin time

Prothrombin time may be elevated in biliary obstruction due to vitamin K deficiency.

Suspected or known hemolytic uremic syndrome (HUS)
Results Interpretation:
Increased prothrombin time

In postdiarrheal hemolytic uremic syndrome (HUS), the prothrombin time (PT) is only slightly prolonged.

Suspected vitamin K deficiency
Strength of Recommendation: Class IIb
Strength of Evidence: Category C
Results Interpretation:
Increased prothrombin time

A prolonged prothrombin time (PT) is indicative of a deficiency in factor VII, X, or prothrombin, which may signify a vitamin K deficiency.

A prolonged PT is likely to be attributable to a vitamin K deficiency if administration of vitamin K results in a subsequently normal PT.

In treated vitamin K deficiency, the PT should correct itself within a few days, but may take longer if the vitamin K is delivered orally rather than parenterally.

Timing of Monitoring

To test whether a prolonged prothrombin time is attributable to a vitamin K deficiency, vitamin K should be administered, then a repeat PT assay should be performed within 12 to 24 hours.

COMMON PANELS
- Disseminated intravascular coagulopathy panel
- Hepatic function panel
- Transplant panel

CLINICAL NOTES
Ranges of normal limits may vary depending on the preparation and type of thromboplastin used for the test.

COLLECTION/STORAGE INFORMATION
- Draw plasma or whole blood in blue sodium citrate tube.
- Fill entire tube.
- May be stored at room temperature for up to 24 hours, but should be processed within that time frame. Do not store at 4°C for prolonged times since cold temperatures may shorten prothrombin time.

LOINC CODES
- Code: 5964-2 (*Short Name* - PT Bld Qn Coag)
- Code: 5894-1 (*Short Name* - PT Act/Nor PPP Qn Coag)
- Code: 5902-2 (*Short Name* - PT PPP Qn Coag)
- Code: 5901-4 (*Short Name* - PT PPP Cont Qn)

Prozac measurement

TEST DEFINITION
Measurement of fluoxetine levels in serum or plasma to facilitate therapeutic monitoring

SYNONYMS
- Fluoxetine measurement

REFERENCE RANGE
- The normal range of blood fluoxetine concentrations has not been defined due to the poor correlation between concentration and response.
  Please refer to your institution's reference ranges as lab normals may vary.

INDICATIONS
Drug level monitoring during fluoxetine therapy
> **Strength of Recommendation:** Class III
> **Strength of Evidence:** Category B
> **Results Interpretation:**
> **Blood drug levels - finding**
> There is a wide variation among individuals in their ability to metabolize fluoxetine; therefore, blood concentrations at a constant dose vary greatly and a dose-response correlation is unlikely. Since patients can tolerate wide ranges of SSRI blood concentrations, there does not appear to be a relationship between drug levels and adverse effects.
> Fluoxetine plasma levels are higher in children than adolescents, whose steady-state and accumulation profiles are similar to adults.

COLLECTION/STORAGE INFORMATION
- Specimen Collection and Handling:
  - Draw serum or plasma.
  - Do not use serum separator tubes (may lower estimates of fluoxetine concentrations).
  - Store up to 19 months at 4°C or at -20°C for several months.

LOINC CODES
- Code: 3645-9 (*Short Name* - Fluoxetine Ur Ql)
- Code: 12439-6 (*Short Name* - Fluoxetine Ur-mCnc)
- Code: 19471-2 (*Short Name* - Fluoxetine Ur Ql Cfm)
- Code: 29219-3 (*Short Name* - Fluoxetine Fld-mCnc)
- Code: 14728-0 (*Short Name* - Fluoxetine SerPl-sCnc)
- Code: 3643-4 (*Short Name* - Fluoxetine SerPl Ql)
- Code: 20529-4 (*Short Name* - Fluoxetine Ur Cnfrn-mCnc)
- Code: 3644-2 (*Short Name* - Fluoxetine SerPl-mCnc)
- Code: 14727-2 (*Short Name* - Fluoxetine Gast Ql)
- Code: 19470-4 (*Short Name* - Fluoxetine Ur Ql Scn)

Purkinje cells antibody assay

TEST DEFINITION
Detection of anti-Purkinje cell (anti-Yo) antibodies in serum or cerebrospinal fluid for the identification and management of paraneoplastic disorders

REFERENCE RANGE
- Adults: Negative
  Please refer to your institution's reference ranges as lab normals may vary.

INDICATIONS
Suspected paraneoplastic syndrome
> **Strength of Recommendation:** Class IIa
> **Strength of Evidence:** Category B

Results Interpretation:
Abnormal immunology findings
> A positive result on an anti-Purkinje cell (anti-Yo) antibody assay may indicate a paraneoplastic syndrome associated with breast or gynecological cancer.
>
> Titers of anti-Purkinje cell antibodies (APCAs) are frequently higher in cerebrospinal fluid than serum. The presence of paraneoplastic cerebellar degeneration is highly associated with the presence of anti-Yo antibody titers greater than 1:500 in serum or 1:50 in cerebrospinal fluid.
>
> Patients with paraneoplastic cerebellar degeneration who are positive for APCAs are less likely to show neurologic improvement after treatment than patients who are negative for APCAs.

LOINC CODES
- Code: 14250-5 (*Short Name* - Purkinje Cells IgG Ser IF-aCnc)
- Code: 14247-1 (*Short Name* - Purkinje Cells Ab CSF QI IF)
- Code: 12853-8 (*Short Name* - Purkinje Cells Ab Ser QI IB)
- Code: 31579-6 (*Short Name* - Purkinje Cells Ab CSF-aCnc)
- Code: 14249-7 (*Short Name* - Purkinje Cells Ab Ser QI IF)
- Code: 27068-6 (*Short Name* - Purkinje Cells Ab Ser-aCnc)

Pyruvate kinase measurement

TEST DEFINITION
Measurement of pyruvate kinase levels in serum or washed erythrocytes for evaluation and management of congenital or chronic hemolytic anemia

SYNONYMS
- PK - Pyruvate kinase activity
- Pyruvate kinase activity

REFERENCE RANGE
Please refer to your institution's reference ranges as lab normals may vary.

INDICATIONS
Suspected congenital hemolytic anemia secondary to pyruvate kinase (PK) deficiency
> **Strength of Recommendation:** Class IIb
> **Strength of Evidence:** Category C

Results Interpretation:
Lowered laboratory findings
> A pyruvate kinase (PK) deficiency is the most common enzyme deficiency in the glycolytic pathway and is usually caused by an inherited autosomal recessive defect. A deficiency in PK causes moderate to severe nonspherocytic hemolytic anemia.
>
> Patients with PK deficiency usually have 5% to 25% of the normal (mean) erythrocyte enzyme level while approximately half of the normal activity is found in heterozygotes.

ABNORMAL RESULTS
- Results increased in:
  - Infection
  - Pregnancy
  - Severe pyruvate kinase deficiency
  - Contamination of erythrocyte sample with leukocytes

COLLECTION/STORAGE INFORMATION
- Specimen Collection and Handling:

- Collect serum or whole blood (for washed cells) in a lavender tube EDTA tube, a green heparinized tube, or a yellow acid citrose dextrose tube, and then place on ice
- Centrifuge specimen thoroughly
- Stable for 6 hours at 4°C or 8 months at -70°C; washed erythrocytes are stable for 20 days at 4°C or 5 days at 25°C

LOINC CODES
- Code: 11227-6 (*Short Name* - Pyruvate Kinase Bld Ql)
- Code: 2913-2 (*Short Name* - Pyruvate Kinase Ser-cCnc)

Quinidine measurement

TEST DEFINITION
Measurement of quinidine in serum for the evaluation and management of suspected quinidine toxicity and to assess for therapeutic concentrations in the treatment of cardiac dysrhythmias

REFERENCE RANGE
- Adults: 2-5 mcg/mL (6-15 micromoles/L)
  Please refer to your institution's reference ranges as lab normals may vary.

INDICATIONS
Drug level monitoring during quinidine therapy.
    Strength of Recommendation: Class IIa
    Strength of Evidence: Category C
Results Interpretation:
Blood drug levels - finding
- Optimal therapeutic serum quinidine concentration by test method:
  - Double extraction fluorometric procedures: 2-5 mcg/mL (6.2-15.4 micromol/mL)
  - Enzyme immunoassay: 2-5 mcg/mL (6.2-15.4 micromol/mL)
  - Liquid chromatography: 1.5-4.5 mcg/mL (4.6-13.9 micromol/mL)
- Some authorities describe a range of 1 to 4 mcg/mL for therapeutic serum quinidine concentration. Others describe the therapeutic serum level as 2 to 8 mcg/mL although the optimal serum concentration for some individual may vary outside this range
- Peak concentrations of quinidine sulfate may be reached within 1.5 hours
- Slow-release preparations have more variable bioavailability and peak later; quinidine gluconate peaks at about 4 hours. Following oral administration of immediate-release quinidine sulfate, sympathetic activation by a low-salt diet (10 mEq/day) increases serum quinidine concentrations; however, disposition kinetics of intravenous quinidine are not affected by dietary salt
- Stressful events (myocardial infarction) can increase total serum quinidine concentration through increased protein binding; however, the amount of free quinidine may remain unaffected

Suspected quinidine toxicity
    Strength of Recommendation: Class IIa
    Strength of Evidence: Category C
Results Interpretation:
Quinidine overdose of undetermined intent
In general, toxic serum concentrations range from 5 to 15 mcg/mL. Patients may manifest toxic symptoms at serum quinidine levels above 5 mcg/mL. Cardiac toxicity is usually associated with serum levels above 14 mcg/mL. QT and QRS prolongation, however, may be observed at therapeutic quinidine serum concentrations above 2 mcg/mL.

Elderly patients can manifest signs of toxicity with low quinidine serum concentrations. In 2 case reports, male patients (aged 67 and 73 years) developed symptoms of psychosis following therapy initiation of quinidine 250 mg. The serum quinidine concentrations were 1 mg/L and 0.8 mg/L, respectively.

In one case report, a 16-year-old female survived an ingestion of 8 grams of quinidine. Her maximum serum quinidine concentration was 21 mg/L.

Chronic disease states such as hepatic failure can result in toxic levels of quinidine, even at therapeutic serum concentrations. In one case report, a 57-year-old man with hepatic failure had a serum quinidine concentration of 3.1 mcg/mL and a markedly prolonged quinidine elimination half-life that resulted in quinidine toxicity.

The relationship between quinidine serum levels and effect or toxicity vary depending on the specificity of the assay procedure and can be complicated by the presence of active metabolites and dihydroquinidine, a product impurity.

False Results

A false increase in serum quinidine concentration can occur if quinidine metabolites cross react. Although uncommon, renal patients are at an increased risk for false results.

DRUG/LAB INTERACTIONS
- Quinine - false increases in quinidine levels

ABNORMAL RESULTS
- Results increased in:
  - Advanced age
  - Hepatic disease
  - Hyperlipoproteinemia

CLINICAL NOTES

Quinidine in serum is not differentiated from dihydroquinidine by enzyme and fluorescence polarization immunoassays.

An EMIT® homogenous enzyme immunoassay is available for quantitation of quinidine in serum or plasma; the assay's range of quantitation is 0.5 to 8 mcg/mL of quinidine. Clinical studies have demonstrated good correlation of this method with high performance liquid chromatography and fluorometry techniques.

COLLECTION/STORAGE INFORMATION
- Specimen Collection and Handling:
  - Collect serum specimen at trough concentration
  - Run assay within 24 hours; freeze specimen if delayed by more than 24 hours
  - Specimen is stable for 1 month at $-5°C$
  - Avoid collecting specimen in serum separator tubes

LOINC CODES
- Code: 4015-4 (*Short Name* - Quinidine Ur Ql)
- Code: 17507-5 (*Short Name* - Quinidine Ur-mCnc)
- Code: 9779-0 (*Short Name* - Quinidine Free SerPl-mCnc)
- Code: 14899-9 (*Short Name* - Quinidine SerPl-sCnc)
- Code: 4014-7 (*Short Name* - Quinidine Bld-mCnc)
- Code: 29226-8 (*Short Name* - Quinidine Fld-mCnc)
- Code: 21483-3 (*Short Name* - Quinidine Peak SerPl-mCnc)
- Code: 4017-0 (*Short Name* - Quinidine Tr SerPl-mCnc)

RNP antibody measurement

TEST DEFINITION

Detection of anti-nuclear ribonuceloprotein (anti-RNP) antibodies in serum for the evaluation of immunological disorders

SYNONYMS
- Anti-ribonucleoprotein antibody measurement
- RNP antibody level

REFERENCE RANGE
- Adults: Negative
Please refer to your institution's reference ranges as lab normals may vary.

INDICATIONS

Suspected mixed connective tissue disease (MCTD)
    Strength of Recommendation: Class IIa
    Strength of Evidence: Category B
Results Interpretation:
Abnormal laboratory findings
    A positive titer of anti-nuclear ribonucleoproptein (anti-RNP) antibodies is essential for the diagnosis of mixed connective tissue disease (MCTD) and a negative anti-RNP antibody result practically excludes MCTD. High titers of anti-RNP antibodies are typical of patients with MCTD.

Suspected systemic lupus erythematosus
    Strength of Recommendation: Class IIb
    Strength of Evidence: Category B
Results Interpretation:
Abnormal laboratory findings
    A positive result on an anti-nuclear ribonucleoprotein (anti-RNP) test is of little benefit in the diagnosis of systemic lupus erythematosus.

    In the presence of other antinuclear antibodies, a positive anti-nuclear ribonucleoprotein (anti-RNP) test indicates a shorter period before clinical manifestations (typically a few months) than do positive tests for SS-B (anti-La) or SS-A (anti-Ro) antibodies.

    In patients with SLE and anti-RNP antibodies, higher anti-RNP titers are associated with active disease. Higher titers of anti-RNP antibodies, however, are more consistent with the diagnosis of mixed connective tissue disease.

COLLECTION/STORAGE INFORMATION

- Draw serum sample in a red marbled tube.
- Store sample at -30°C.

LOINC CODES

- Code: 17535-6 (*Short Name* - ENA RNP Ab Ser QI IF)
- Code: 31588-7 (*Short Name* - ENA RNP IgG Ser-aCnc)
- Code: 29374-6 (*Short Name* - ENA RNP Ab Ser-aCnc)
- Code: 9399-7 (*Short Name* - ENA RNP Ab Titr Ser)
- Code: 5302-5 (*Short Name* - ENA RNP Ab Ser QI ID)
- Code: 8091-1 (*Short Name* - ENA RNP Ab Ser QI)
- Code: 17536-4 (*Short Name* - ENA RNP Ab Ser IF-aCnc)
- Code: 29958-6 (*Short Name* - ENA RNP IgG Ser EIA-aCnc)
- Code: 5301-7 (*Short Name* - ENA RNP Ab Ser QI EIA)

Rapid HIV test

TEST DEFINITION

    Rapid point-of-care measurement of antibodies in serum, whole blood, or plasma for the detection of HIV-1, or HIV 1 and HIV-2 infection

REFERENCE RANGE

- Adults and children: nonreactive
Please refer to your institution's reference ranges as lab normals may vary.

INDICATIONS

Laboring women of unknown HIV status
    Strength of Recommendation: Class I
    Strength of Evidence: Category B
Results Interpretation:
Positive laboratory findings
    Laboring women with positive rapid HIV test results should be offered antiretroviral (ARV) prophylaxis immediately to reduce the risk of infant exposure. The newborn should also be started on ARV prophylaxis

while awaiting confirmatory results. Breast-feeding should be delayed until confirmatory test results are obtained. Although elective cesarean section is recommended by the Centers for Disease Control, the benefit may be limited in women with undetectable viral load.

Standard confirmatory follow-up testing should be done on all women after delivery who had positive rapid test results during labor.

Negative laboratory findings

A negative rapid HIV test result generally requires no further testing or other medical intervention. If an individual is concerned about recent exposure risk, retesting after 3 months is recommended and postpartum HIV counseling services should be arranged.

Occupational exposure to HIV

Strength of Recommendation: Class IIa

Strength of Evidence: Category C

Results Interpretation:

Positive laboratory findings

Repeatedly positive rapid HIV antibody test results are highly suggestive of infection. Confirmation of results by Western blot or immunofluorescent antibody is not required prior to making initial decisions about postexposure management.

Negative laboratory findings

A negative rapid antibody test result indicates absence of HIV infection. A seronegative HIV result in the absence of clinical symptoms or evidence of AIDS in the exposure source requires no further testing.

Testing in high-risk individuals or those suspected of HIV infection

Strength of Recommendation: Class IIa

Strength of Evidence: Category B

Results Interpretation:

Positive laboratory findings

A positive result on a rapid HIV assay suggests HIV infection and is considered preliminarily positive. Follow-up testing by Western blot or enzyme immunoassay is required to confirm a diagnosis. If the confirmatory test gives discordant results, repeat testing is recommended after 1 month.

In resource-constrained areas, a positive rapid HIV test result should be confirmed by a second rapid HIV test of sufficient sensitivity and specificity that utilizes different antigens and/or a different platform. Given the high sensitivity and specificity of rapid HIV tests, two positive rapid test results are considered confirmatory for HIV infection. An initial positive rapid test followed by a negative rapid test is considered inconclusive and repeat rapid testing in 6 weeks is recommended. If discordant results are again obtained at 6 weeks, following the same testing procedure, a specimen should be sent to an HIV referral laboratory for further testing.

Negative laboratory findings

A negative result on a rapid point-of-care HIV test subsequent to HIV exposure suggests that it may be too early to identify HIV antibodies present in the serum and indicates repeated testing at a later time. In resource-constrained areas, a negative result on a rapid test is considered a negative finding with counseling focused on risk-reduction behavior; follow-up counseling may also be indicated.

Timing of Monitoring

The World Health Organization (WHO) recommends serial testing in most resource-constrained situations. In serial testing, a second test is performed only if the first sample is positive, using either a different rapid test on the same sample, or a second finger stick if that was the method employed initially. The alternative -- parallel testing in which a single sample is tested simultaneously with two different HIV tests -- is less economically advantageous but may be appropriate in some situations. The decision to use serial vs parallel testing should be based on current scientific evidence, test performance, logistics, and economic considerations.

CLINICAL NOTES

The agglutination assays, immunofiltration devices and immunochromatographic strips can usually be processed in 10 to 60 minutes, 5 to 15 minutes, and 20 minutes or less, respectively.

COLLECTION/STORAGE INFORMATION

Serum, plasma or whole blood (finger-stick sample) may be used, depending on the type of kit used.

Most rapid tests do not require laboratory equipment and do not require specimen refrigeration. Specimens should be stored at between 2°C and 20 - 30°C, depending on the specific test kit used; extremes in temperatures decrease the shelf life of the tests. Kit shelf life is 12 months or longer.

Rapid HIV tests can be performed by health care workers with little or no laboratory experience independently of reference laboratories, assuming appropriate training and ongoing supervision is provided.

Rapid influenza test

TEST DEFINITION
Rapid detection of avian influenza A virus from respiratory samples for the presumptive diagnosis of avian influenza A infection

REFERENCE RANGE
• Adults and children: negative
Please refer to your institution's reference ranges as lab normals may vary.

INDICATIONS
Suspected avian influenza A
  Strength of Recommendation: Class IIa
  Strength of Evidence: Category C
  Results Interpretation:
  Positive laboratory findings
    Because of the variable impact of disease prevalence on test performance, and for surveillance monitoring purposes, confirmatory diagnostic testing by immunofluorescence assay (IFA), viral culture or polymerase chain reaction (PCR) should always be considered in the presence of a positive rapid influenza test result. During periods of low influenza prevalence, confirmatory testing is recommended by one the aforementioned methods. During periods of high disease prevalence confirmatory testing on every patient with positive rapid results may be impractical; as a result, clinical judgment and local surveillance data should guide treatment decisions. Rapid testing should only be performed when test results can affect timely patient management.
    In countries where disease surveillance is limited and influenza activity is not known, both positive and negative rapid test results should be confirmed by IFA, culture or PCR. If confirmatory testing is desired, specimens should be forwarded to the nearest National Influenza Center or a WHO Collaborating Center for Reference and Research of Influenza.
    A positive test result cannot differentiate between seasonal and avian influenza A infection.

  False Results
    During periods of peak influenza activity, false-negatives are more likely. When influenza activity is low, false positives are more likely. Inadequate specimen collection or handling can cause false negative results.
  Negative laboratory findings
    A negative results does not exclude an H5N1 influenza diagnosis.

  False Results
    During periods of peak influenza activity, false-negatives are more likely. When influenza activity is low, false positives are more likely. Inadequate specimen collection or handling can cause false negative results.
  Timing of Monitoring
    Rapid testing early in the course of an influenza season or outbreak may improve clinical awareness and help guide patient management. However, the optimal timing of specimen collection for human avian influenza infection is unknown. The collection of multiple respiratory specimens over several days from the same patient is recommended in countries in which influenza activity has been identified or is suspected.

Suspected influenza
  Results Interpretation:
  Presence of microbial antigen - finding
    Approximately 70% of patients with influenza of any type will have a positive test with the rapid influenza test.

False Results

In children, rapid influenza diagnostic tests appear to be moderately accurate and are more likely to produce false-negative than false-positive results. Clinicians should use clinical judgement and local surveillance data about circulation influenza viruses when interpreting test results

Clinical Notes

Rapid tests have varying degrees of complexity, therefore training on test methods and limitations is essential for anyone performing the test. The Food and Drug Administration has waived some of the simpler tests for use in the office or clinic setting, while the more complex tests must be used in the laboratory setting. Rapid tests vary by efficacy, specimen type accepted, specimen storage requirements, assay time, ease of use and ease of interpretation, and influenza type detected.

Clinicians should contact their local or state health departments in all cases of suspected infection with any novel influenza A virus; state and local health departments should in turn contact the Centers for Disease Control (CDC) Emergency Response Hotline.

Collection/Storage Information

While most tests can accommodate a variety of respiratory specimens, not all specimen types offer equivalent results, and the optimal specimen type for human avian influenza is unknown. The recommended specimen for testing of influenza A virus is a nasopharyngeal aspirate collected as close to the onset of symptoms as possible, and not longer than 4 to 5 days in adults. Specimen collection after 5 days may still yield useful results in young children, as viral shedding occurs for a longer period of time in this age group. Nasal aspirates, nasal washes, sputum and nasopharyngeal swabs containing cellular material are preferred over nasal and throat swabs.

Rapid plasma reagin test

Test Definition

Rapid detection of antibodies in plasma or serum for the presumptive diagnosis of syphilis

Synonyms

• RPR test

Reference Range

• Adults and children: nonreactive
Please refer to your institution's reference ranges as lab normals may vary.

Indications

Suspected and known syphilis.
Strength of Recommendation: Class I
Strength of Evidence: Category B
Results Interpretation:
Serology positive
A fourfold or greater rise in antibody titer is presumptive of syphilis but requires confirmatory treponemal testing by fluorescent treponemal antibody absorbed (FTA-ABS) or *T. pallidum* particle agglutination (TP-PA) assay. A reactive nontreponemal test that does not convert to nonreactive in 6 months is compatible with a diagnosis of syphilis. Results from nontreponemal tests typically correlate with a patient's current disease state; a rise in antibody titer usually indicates an increase in disease severity. A patient newly exposed to syphilis may take 4 to 8 weeks to seroconvert.
Negative laboratory findings
With treatment, most patients will convert to seronegative status and will remain nonreactive for life unless reinfected. In patients successfully treated for early syphilis, nontreponemal titers will decrease to low or undetectable levels within a year in most cases; however, some patients will have continually low titers for extended periods of time, and may remain seropositive throughout their lifetime. Titers will decline more slowly in those with longer disease duration, and patients who have syphilis for longer than a year should have repeat serologic testing 24 months after treatment. Retreatment should be considered for patients whose titers fail to drop at least fourfold within a year of treatment, or who have a sustained fourfold increase in titers.

Frequency of Monitoring

Quantitative nontreponemal testing should be performed at 6, 12, and 24 months after treatment for latent syphilis.

Suspected or known congenital syphilis.

Strength of Recommendation: Class I

Strength of Evidence: Category C

Results Interpretation:

Serology positive

No treatment is required for patients with a reactive nontreponemal test, a nonreactive treponemal test and no clinical or epidemiological evidence of syphilis, although both tests should be repeated within 4 weeks. Patients should be treated if evidence of syphilis exists or if the diagnosis cannot be ruled out. Pregnant women with a history of syphilis may have a rise in titer even in the absence of disease recurrence. This 'serofast reaction' can generally be attributed to pregnancy if previous treatment is documented, the titer increase is less than fourfold, and there is no evidence of positive lesions or recent exposure. Seropositive pregnant women should be considered infected unless an appropriate treatment history, and a sequential decline in antibody titers, has been documented

For infants born to infected mothers, a fourfold or greater rise in antibody titers over a 3 month period, and a positive confirmatory treponemal test, is compatible with congenital syphilis. Syphilis is unlikely in asymptomatic infants born to seropositive mothers treated during pregnancy when the mother had a fourfold or greater decrease in titer, and the infant's titer is fourfold or lower than the maternal titer was at the time of treatment. In infants who are seropositive at birth, or who are born to seropositive mothers, nontreponemal titers should decline by 3 months of age and be nonreactive by 6 months of age. The absence of a fourfold or greater increase in infant titer does not exclude syphilis.

With treatment, most patients will convert to seronegative status and will remain nonreactive for life unless reinfected. In patients successfully treated for congenital syphilis, nontreponemal titers will decrease to low or undetectable levels within a year in most cases; however, some patients will have continually low titers for extended periods of time, and may remain seropositive throughout their lifetime. Titers will decline more slowly in those with longer disease duration, and patients who have syphilis for longer than a year should have repeat serologic testing 24 months after treatment. Retreatment should be considered for patients whose titers fail to drop at least fourfold within a year of treatment, or who have a sustained fourfold increase in titers.

Frequency of Monitoring

All pregnant women should be tested at their first prenatal visit. In high-risk pregnancies or in areas where syphilis is endemic, additional serologic testing is recommended at 28 weeks gestation and again at delivery. All infants born to mothers with reactive nontreponemal or treponemal tests should have quantitative nontreponemal testing of infant sera; testing of cord blood can lead to false-positive results due to maternal contamination.

All seroreactive infants, and infants born to seroreactive mothers, should have nontreponemal antibody titers obtained every 2 to 3 months until the infant is seronegative or a fourfold decrease in titer is observed. All patients with congenital syphilis should have quantitative nontreponemal retesting at 3, 6, and 12 months after treatment.

Timing of Monitoring

In areas where prenatal care is not ideal, rapid plasma reagin (RPR) screening should be performed when pregnancy is first confirmed and treatment should be initiated at that time if results are positive. An RPR or VDRL test should be performed within 30 days of birth on all infants born to seropositive mothers. Infants should not be discharged from the hospital without the mother's serologic syphilis status determined at least once during pregnancy, and ideally again after delivery. All women who deliver stillborn infants should have serologic testing.

ABNORMAL RESULTS

- Acute (less than 6 months duration) false positive reactions have been observed with:
  - Pregnancy
  - Immunizations
  - Measles
  - Viral disease (particularly Epstein-Barr and hepatitis)
  - Protozoal infection
  - Mycoplasmal infection
  - Viral pneumonia
  - Chicken pox
  - Laboratory or technical error
  - Narcotic addiction

- Chronic (longer than 6 months duration) false-positive reactions have been observed with:
  - Increased age
  - Malignancy
  - Connective tissues diseases
  - Immunoglobulin abnormalities

CLINICAL NOTES
Results should be reported quantitatively.

COLLECTION/STORAGE INFORMATION
Use red marbled or serum separator tube.

Although plasma samples may be used, serum is the preferred specimen for the RPR card test. In congenital syphilis testing, maternal serum is preferred over neonatal serum and cord blood.

Because of differences in titer reactivity between nontreponemal tests, the same nontreponemal test used initially should be used throughout the course of treatment, and, preferably, should be processed by the same laboratory.

LOINC CODES
- Code: 20508-8 (*Short Name* - RPR Ser Qn)
- Code: 20507-0 (*Short Name* - RPR Ser Ql)
- Code: 31147-2 (*Short Name* - RPR Titr Ser)

Rapid urease test

TEST DEFINITION
Detection of *Helicobacter pylori* in gastric mucosal biopsy specimens for the diagnosis and management of *Helicobacter pylori* associated gastrointestinal disorders

SYNONYMS
- CLO test for helicobacter pylori
- Rapid urease test for helicobacter pylori
- Urease test

REFERENCE RANGE
- Adults: No color change
  Please refer to your institution's reference ranges as lab normals may vary.

INDICATIONS
Helicobacter pylori **-associated gastric lymphoma of mucosa-associated lymphoid tissue (MALT)**
> **Strength of Recommendation:** Class IIa
> **Strength of Evidence:** Category B
> **Results Interpretation:**
> **Helicobacter biopsy urease test results**
> Due to its high specificity, a positive biopsy urease test is conclusive evidence of *Helicobacter pylori* infection. Because false negative results occur with recent or active gastrointestinal bleeding or if patients have been taking certain medications (proton pump inhibitors, H_2 -receptor antagonists, antibiotics, or compounds containing bismuth), a negative result does not confirm absence of *Helicobacter pylori* infection.
> Eradication of *Helicobacter pylori* has been correlated with partial or complete regression of low grade, localized gastric MALT lymphoma in a majority of patients.

Suspected *Helicobacter pylori* **infection**
> **Strength of Recommendation:** Class IIb
> **Strength of Evidence:** Category B
> **Results Interpretation:**
> **Helicobacter biopsy urease test results**
> Due to its high specificity, a positive biopsy urease test can be interpreted as conclusive evidence of *Helicobacter pylori* infection. A negative urease test result does not confirm absence of *Helicobacter pylori* infection.

False Results
Because false negative results can occur with recent or active gastrointestinal bleeding or if patients have been taking certain medications (proton pump inhibitors, H_2-receptor antagonists, antibiotics, or compounds containing bismuth), a negative urease test result does not confirm absence of *Helicobacter pylori* infection

CLINICAL NOTES
The rapid urease test is performed on a biopsy specimen obtained during endoscopy. Test results may be invalidated by the effect on urease activity of blood or proton pump inhibitors. The latter is thought to decrease the density of *Helicobacter pylori* in the antrum and increase the density in the corpus of the stomach.

LOINC CODES
• Code: 32637-1 (*Short Name* - Urease Tiss Ql)

Red blood cell count

TEST DEFINITION
Measurement of total number of erythrocytes (RBCs) in whole blood for the evaluation of anemia and other RBC disorders

SYNONYMS
• RBC count
• RBC - Red blood cell count

REFERENCE RANGE
• Adult males : $4.5-5.9 \times 10^6$ /mm^3 ($4.5-5.9 \times 10^{12}$ /L)
• Adult females : $4-5.2 \times 10^6$ /mm^3 ($4-5.2 \times 10^{12}$ /L)
  Please refer to your institution's reference ranges as lab normals may vary.

INDICATIONS
Suspected anemia
    Strength of Recommendation: Class I
    Strength of Evidence: Category C
    Results Interpretation:
    Erythropenia
        A decreased RBC count indicates anemia, including iron deficiency anemia in infants and young children
    Erythrocytosis
        Although the RBC count is generally decreased in infants and young children with iron deficiency, a high RBC count also can be a feature of iron deficiency anemia, particularly in those with mild anemia and thus may not reliably differentiate these two conditions.

Suspected hypoxia
    Results Interpretation:
    Erythropenia
        A decrease in erythrocyte count can lead to tissue hypoxia due to impaired oxygen transport.
    Erythrocytosis
        An increase in erythrocyte count can occur when oxygen transport to the tissues is impaired, such as in anemia, cardiac or pulmonary disorders, and in the low oxygen tension of high altitudes.

COMMON PANELS
• Complete blood count

ABNORMAL RESULTS
• Results increased in :
    • Vigorous exercise
    • High altitude
    • Dehydration

- Results decreased in :
  - Recumbency

COLLECTION/STORAGE INFORMATION
- Advise patient to avoid stress and extensive exercise prior to testing.
- Collect sample in a lavender top tube.

LOINC CODES
- Code: 30390-9 (*Short Name* - RBC Stl-aCnc)
- Code: 793-0 (*Short Name* - RBC # Plr Manual)
- Code: 26453-1 (*Short Name* - RBC # Bld)
- Code: 26456-4 (*Short Name* - RBC # Plr)
- Code: 789-8 (*Short Name* - RBC # Bld Auto)
- Code: 790-6 (*Short Name* - RBC # Bld Manual)
- Code: 14290-1 (*Short Name* - RBC UrnS Manual-aCnc)
- Code: 19098-3 (*Short Name* - RBC Amn Ql)
- Code: 16828-6 (*Short Name* - RBC # Smpls Manual)
- Code: 26457-2 (*Short Name* - RBC # Prt)
- Code: 14331-3 (*Short Name* - RBC Stl Manual-aCnc)

Red cell mass

TEST DEFINITION
Measurement of circulating erythrocyte mass

REFERENCE RANGE
- Less than 2 standard deviations or 25% above the mean expected red cell mass for the individual (based on body surface area or height and weight).
- Red cell mass reported in mL/kg results in lower measured red cell mass for obese compared to lean individuals.
  Please refer to your institution's reference ranges as lab normals may vary.

INDICATIONS
To differentiate absolute polycythemia from apparent polycythemia
> **Strength of Recommendation:** Class IIa
> **Strength of Evidence:** Category B
> **Results Interpretation:**
> **Increased level (laboratory finding)**
> A red cell mass (RCM) greater than 2 standard deviations above the mean expected RCM for the individual is diagnostic of absolute polycythemia. Results of plasma volume determination should also be used to distinguish absolute polycythemia from apparent polycythemia.

ABNORMAL RESULTS
- Results increased in:
  - Pregnancy
  - Newborn hematocrit greater than 55%
  - High altitude
- Results decreased in:
  - Acute and chronic hemorrhage
  - Advanced age
  - Anemia
  - Bed rest
  - Chronic azotemia
  - Chronic infection
  - Obesity
  - Pheochromocytoma
  - Radiation
  - Starvation

Reducing substance measurement, stool

TEST DEFINITION
Measurement of unabsorbed sugars (reducing substances) in feces for evaluation of carbohydrate intolerance or malabsorption

SYNONYMS
- Faecal reducing substance level
- Faecal reducing substance measurement

REFERENCE RANGE
- Adults and Children:
- Normal: ≤ 0.25 g/dL
- Suspicious: 0.25-0.5 g/dL
- Abnormal: > 0.5 g/dL
  Please refer to your institution's reference ranges as lab normals may vary.

INDICATIONS
Suspected lactose intolerance
    Results Interpretation:
    Presence of fecal reducing substances - finding
       Fecal reducing substances greater than 250 mg/dL, following a lactose load, indicate an intolerance to lactose or other sugars.

Suspected necrotizing enterocolitis
    Results Interpretation:
    Increased level (laboratory finding)
       Elevated levels of reducing substances in stool may suggest carbohydrate malabsorption. Reducing substances can be measured, but the value of predicting necrotizing enterocolitis from testing these substances has not been established.

CLINICAL NOTES
- Clinitest will likely give positive results for these reducing sugars:
- Glucose
- Galactose
- Fructose
- Maltose
- Lactose
- Clinitest will likely give negative results for these non-reducing sugars or sugar alcohols:
- Sucrose
- Lactulose
- Sorbitol
- Mannitol

COLLECTION/STORAGE INFORMATION
- Specimen Collection and Handling:
  - Thoroughly mix one volume of stool to two volumes distilled water
  - Remove 15 drops of mixture and place in clean test tube
  - Add Clinitest tablet

LOINC CODES
- Code: 11060-1 (*Short Name* - Red Subs Stl Ql)
- Code: 32211-5 (*Short Name* - Red Subs Stl-mCnc)
- Code: 27319-3 (*Short Name* - Red Subs Stl Test Str-aCnc)

Reticulated platelet count

TEST DEFINITION
Measurement of reticulated platelets (newly released from bone marrow, still containing RNA) for evaluation and management of platelet disorder (eg, impaired thrombopoieses, increased destruction)

REFERENCE RANGE
- Adults:
- RP percentage: 3%-20%
- Absolute RP count: 17 +/-6.6 (10^3 /microL)
- Neonates< 30 weeks (from a study with 25 neonates in this age group) :
- RP percentage: 8.8% +/- 5.1%
- Absolute RP count: 20.3 +/- 11.8 (10^3 /microL)
- Neonate 30 to 36 weeks (from a study with 25 neonates in this age group):
- RP percentage: 4.6% +/- 1.7%
- Absolute RP count: 11.9 +/- 5 (10^3 /microL)
- Neonate >36 weeks (from a study with 39 neonates in this age group):
- RP percentage: 4% +/- 2.4%
- Absolute AP count: 10.5 +/- 8.7 (10^3 /microL)
  Please refer to your institution's reference ranges as lab normals may vary.

INDICATIONS
Suspected abnormal platelet production in thrombocytopenia
    Strength of Recommendation: Class IIb
    Strength of Evidence: Category B
    Results Interpretation:
    Increased level (laboratory finding)
    An elevated RP percentage in the setting of a low platelet count suggests a consumptive or hyperdestructive etiology.
    A rising RP percentage in the setting of chemotherapy-induced thrombocytopenia may indicate imminent platelet recovery.
    Decreased level (laboratory finding)
    A decreased RP percentage or absolute RP count in the setting of a low platelet count suggests a problem with bone marrow production. A decreased RP percentage in the setting of chemotherapy-induced thrombocytopenia suggests that platelet recovery is not imminent within the next 48 hours.
    Timing of Monitoring
    In a study of 6 term neonates there was no significant differences in the RP percentage when the sample was obtained from cord blood at the time of delivery (3.9%) as compared with when the sample was obtained from the umbilical artery during the first 6 hours of life (4.4%).

COLLECTION/STORAGE INFORMATION
- Collect blood sample in EDTA (lavender) tube

Reticulocyte count

TEST DEFINITION
Measurement of percentage of reticulocytes in peripheral blood for evaluation of erythropoietic activity and to help direct clinical management of anemia

SYNONYMS
- Reticulocyte count - observation

REFERENCE RANGE
- Adults: 0.5%-2.5% of total erythrocytes (0.005-0.025 erythrocytes)
- Infants, 1 day old: 3%-7% of total erythrocytes (0.03-0.07 erythrocytes)
- Infants, 3 days old: 1%-3% of total erythrocytes (0.01-0.03 erythrocytes)

- Infants, 7 days old: 0-1% of total erythrocytes (0.00-0.01 erythrocytes)
- Infants, 1 month old: 0.2%-2% of total erythrocytes (0.002-0.02 erythrocytes)
- Infants, 1.5 months old: 0.3%-3.5% of total erythrocytes (0.003-0.035 erythrocytes)
- Infants, 2 months old: 0.4%-4.8% of total erythrocytes (0.004-0.048 erythrocytes)
- Infants, 2.5 months old: 0.3%-4.2% of total erythrocytes (0.003-0.042 erythrocytes)
- Infants, 3 months old: 0.3%-3.6% of total erythrocytes (0.003-0.036 erythrocytes)
- Infants, 4 to 12 months old: 0.2%-2.8% of total erythrocytes (0.002-0.028 erythrocytes)
Please refer to your institution's reference ranges as lab normals may vary.

INDICATIONS

Differentiation between hyporegenerative and hyperregenerative states in unexplained anemia
Results Interpretation:
Decreased reticulocyte count
Reticulocytopenia (diminished number of reticulocytes) occurs in patients with marrow ablative disorders, impaired erythropoiesis, or decreased endogenous erythropoietin. Anemias associated with suppressed bone marrow function include aplastic anemia, aplastic crisis in sickle cell disease, pernicious anemia, pure red cell aplasia, thalassemic syndromes, and transient neonatal erythroblastopenia.

Anemias associated with bone marrow ablative/infiltration disorders include acute leukemia, lymphoma, myelodysplastic syndromes, myelofibrosis, myeloma, and metastatic carcinoma.

The reticulocyte count declines following exposure to ionizing irradiation. Absence of reticulocytes within 3 to 5 days of exposure suggests a high radiation dose.

Reticulocytosis
The erythropoietic activity of the bone marrow and the rate of cell delivery into the peripheral circulation determine the number of reticulocytes in the peripheral blood. Reticulocytosis (an increased number of peripheral blood reticulocytes) may be seen with anemia in the presence of functional bone marrow (eg, blood loss, intravascular hemolysis, polycythemia vera, exogenous erythropoietin administration, or replacement of folate or iron).

During a sickle cell aplastic crisis, the reticulocyte count is markedly depressed, yet may show a striking elevation during recovery from a crisis state. In patients with sickle cell disease, the average steady-state reticulocyte count is 12% (range of 5% to 30%; normal adult range: 0.5% to 2.5% cells).

In children having a positive sickle cell screen in the emergent setting, a high reticulocyte count alone (above 2% cells) was more sensitive in differentiating sickle cell disease from sickle cell trait.

Should be considered in all men unless there is another obvious cause of priapism
Results Interpretation:
Increased level (laboratory finding)
Patients with sickle cell anemia will often have an elevated reticulocyte count.

COMMON PANELS

- Anemia panel
- Hemolysis panel

ABNORMAL RESULTS

- Results increased in:
  - High-altitude residence
- Results decreased in:
  - Chronic renal disease

COLLECTION/STORAGE INFORMATION

- Specimen Collection and Handling:
  - Collect 5 mL of whole blood in EDTA tube, or capillary blood with direct dilution
  - Perform test within 6 hours at room temperature, or store up to 72 hours at 2° to 6° C

LOINC CODES

- Code: 14196-0 (*Short Name* - Retics # RBC)

Rheumatoid factor measurement

TEST DEFINITION

Measurement of rheumatoid factor antibody levels in serum for the evaluation and management of rheumatoid arthritis or other autoimmune diseases

REFERENCE RANGE

- Adults (nephelometry): <30 International Units/mL (<30 kiloInternational Units/L)
- Adults (latex agglutination): Negative
- Adults (sheep cell agglutination test) (SCAT): Negative (< 1:16)
- Adults (radioimmunoassay): Negative
- Adults (enzyme linked immunosorbent assay): <30 International Units/mL (<30 kiloInternational Units/L)
  Please refer to your institution's reference ranges as lab normals may vary.

INDICATIONS

Suspected rheumatoid arthritis
   Strength of Recommendation: Class I
   Strength of Evidence: Category B
   Results Interpretation:
   Rheumatoid factor positive
   A positive rheumatoid factor (RF) is part of the American College of Rheumatology criteria for rheumatoid arthritis (RA).
   Serum RF is a useful test for the diagnosis and prognosis of rheumatoid arthritis (RA), but not for screening.
   Serum RF is detected in up to 80% of patients with RA. High RA titers tend to correlate with severe articular disease although results vary and the test is not useful for diagnosing disease activity. Serum RF may not be measurable in some patients after receiving therapy.
   Of patients diagnosed with RA, 15% to 20% remain negative for RF. The RF test is most useful in patients with a high pre-test probability for RA and should never be used alone to make a diagnosis of RA. In a review of several studies, a positive RF titer at the onset of RA was associated with an increased progression of joint damage, disability, and a poor prognosis.
   In patients older than 70 years of age without RA, the positive RF rate is 10%. In younger people without RA, the rate is 5%.

COMMON PANELS

- Arthritis panel

ABNORMAL RESULTS

- Results increased in:
  - Elderly patients

COLLECTION/STORAGE INFORMATION

- Collect 7 mL of blood in a marbled serum separator tube (SST)
- Store specimen for up to 24 hours at 2°C to 8°C, or freeze at -20°C

Sampling of chorionic villus

TEST DEFINITION

First trimester analysis of chorionic villus to identify potential genetic, chromosomal, or biochemical diseases of the fetus

SYNONYMS

- CVB - Chorionic villus biopsy
- CVS - Chorionic villus sampling

REFERENCE RANGE
- Negative for chromosomal abnormality
  Please refer to your institution's reference ranges as lab normals may vary.

INDICATIONS
Prenatal screening for congenital fetal anomalies in high-risk pregnancies
>   **Strength of Recommendation:** Class IIb
>   **Strength of Evidence:** Category A
>   **Results Interpretation:**
>   **Abnormal chromosomal and genetic finding on antenatal screening of mother**
>   Although accurate, chromosome results from chorionic villus sampling have a weaker correlation with fetal karyotype than do results from amniocentesis, largely because of the identification of placental abnormalities that are not found in the fetus..
>   **Timing of Monitoring**
>   Chorionic villus sampling is performed between 10 and 12 weeks' gestation.

TEST COMPLICATIONS
- Complications include:
- Amniotic fluid leakage
- Fetal loss
- Talipes equinovarus
- Gestational hypertension and/or preeclampsia

COLLECTION/STORAGE INFORMATION
- Specimen Collection and Handling:
  - Perform during 10th to 12th week of pregnancy.
  - Remove approximately 20 cc of chorionic villi cells from placenta at attachment point on uterine wall.
  - Place specimen in sterile culture tube with sterile medium.

Schilling test

TEST DEFINITION
Estimates the body's ability to absorb vitamin B_{12} from the gastrointestinal tract and is used to confirm vitamin B_{12} deficiency

REFERENCE RANGE
- Adults (orally administered vitamin B_{12} excreted in urine): 7%-40%
  Please refer to your institution's reference ranges as lab normals may vary.

INDICATIONS
Suspected malabsorption syndrome in patients with cobalamin (vitamin B_{12}) deficiency
>   **Strength of Recommendation:** Class IIb
>   **Strength of Evidence:** Category C
>   **Results Interpretation:**
>   **Decreased level (laboratory finding)**
>   - Interpretation of Schilling Test Results in Cobalamin (vitamin B_{12}) Deficiency:
>   - Stage 1 normal:
>   - Dietary deficiency
>   - Protein-bound cobalamin malabsorption
- Hypochlorhydria
- Partial gastrectomy
>   - Congenital transcobalamin II deficiency
>   - Stage 1 abnormal; stage 2 normal:
>   - Pernicious anemia
>   - Previous gastrectomy or gastric bypass
>   - Congenital absence or dysfunction of intrinsic factor
>   - Stages 1 and 2 both abnormal:
>   - Ileal disease or resection

- Pernicious anemia with ileal dysfunction secondary to prolonged cobalamin deficiency
- Pernicious anemia with inadequate urine collection during stage 2
- Bacterial overgrowth syndromes
- Fish tapeworm infestation
- Pancreatic insufficiency

Suspected pernicious anemia
> **Strength of Recommendation:** Class IIb
> **Strength of Evidence:** Category C
> **Results Interpretation:**
> **Decreased level (laboratory finding)**
> In pernicious anemia, excreted oral radiolabeled cobalamin (Cbl) should be less than or equal to 7% of the ingested dose (stage I); excreted radiolabeled Cbl increases when vitamin B_{12} is administered with intrinsic factor (stage II).
> Stage I should always be abnormal in pernicious anemia; a normal stage II result would be confirmatory. However, there are instances where stage II is abnormal, such as when there is pernicious anemia with ileal dysfunction due to prolonged Cbl deficiency or if there is incomplete urine collection during stage II.
> Malabsorption of Cbl cannot be excluded based on a normal stage I and low serum Cbl because the radioactive Cbl used in the Schilling test is a crystalline variant; therefore, patients may have malabsorption of food-bound Cbl but not the radioactive Cbl. An egg yolk Cbl absorption test can be performed in this case.

ABNORMAL RESULTS

Incomplete urine collection may cause abnormal results.
Renal insufficiency may cause false results due to delayed excretion of labeled cobalamin (vitamin B_{12}).

CLINICAL NOTES

Bone marrow aspiration needs to be done before the Schilling test because the administered vitamin B_{12} may interfere with subsequent bone marrow examination.

COLLECTION/STORAGE INFORMATION

- Specimen Collection and Handling:
  - Collect a urine sample before the vitamin B_{12} doses are administered
  - Collect a 24-hour urine sample, starting at the time of the vitamin B_{12} injection. If creatinine clearance is less than 60 mL/min, collect a 48-hour urine sample
  - Avoid fecal contamination
- Patient Preparation:
  - Have the patient fast for 12 hours before the test and continue fasting for 3 hours after the vitamin B_{12} injection, however water is permitted during the fasting period. Food and drink are permitted after the 3 hours and encourage the patient to drink as much as tolerated during the entire test.
  - Advise the patient that laxatives need to be avoided during the test.

Sedimentation rate

TEST DEFINITION

Measurement of the distance in millimeters that erythrocytes fall from the top of a vertical tube during one hour for the evaluation and management of inflammatory states; serves as a marker of red cell aggregation.

REFERENCE RANGE

- Adult males: 0-17 mm/hour
- Adult females: 1-25 mm/hour
- Children: 0-10 mm/hour
  Please refer to your institution's reference ranges as lab normals may vary.

INDICATIONS

Suspected and known Kawasaki disease
Results Interpretation:
Increased level (laboratory finding)
The erythrocyte sedimentation rate (ESR) is generally greater than 20 mm/hour in acute Kawasaki disease, subsiding to normal 6 to 10 weeks after fever onset.

An elevated ESR greater than 40 mm/hour in so-called incomplete Kawasaki disease is a strong indication to proceed with further laboratory testing and an echocardiogram.

A marked elevation of 100 mm/hour or greater, or a persistent elevation, is consistent with active angiitis and is predictive of coronary artery involvement.
Frequency of Monitoring
ESR is obtained initially, monitored every 3 to 4 days until day 21 of the illness, then monitored weekly until the value is normal.

Suspected bursitis
Results Interpretation:
Raised hematology findings
The erythrocyte sedimentation rate (ESR) is usually elevated in acute inflammatory bursitis, but the ESR does not distinguish between infection and other causes of inflammation.

Suspected giant cell (temporal) arteritis
Strength of Recommendation: Class IIa
Strength of Evidence: Category A
Results Interpretation:
Increased level (laboratory finding)
Marked elevation of erythrocyte sedimentation rate (eg, greater than 50 mm per hour) is a hallmark finding in giant cell (temporal) arteritis.

A normal ESR level combined with low clinical suspicion reduces the probability of disease to less than 1%.

Normal ESR has been noted in up to 24% of biopsy-proven giant cell arteritis patients before steroid therapy.

Suspected gout
Results Interpretation:
Increased
An acute attack of gout is associated with fever and laboratory evidence of inflammation, such as an elevated WBC count or elevated erythrocyte sedimentation rate (ESR). The ESR often is mildly increased during gout attacks but may be as high as 2 times normal, indicating inflammation.

Suspected Lyme disease
Strength of Recommendation: Class IIb
Strength of Evidence: Category C
Results Interpretation:
ESR raised
An elevated erythrocyte sedimentation rate (ESR) (greater than 30 mm/hr may be seen in 25% to 50% of patients.

While erythema migrans (EM) was present, the ESR was found to be elevated (4 to 46 mm/hr) in a small subset of patients who subsequently developed arthritis, but it was normal in patients in whom arthritis did not develop.

The ESR in patients with chronic arthritis ranges from 4 to 54 mm/hr (median, 24 mm/hr).

In patients with cardiac involvement, the ESR ranges from 3 to 74 mm/hr (median, 47 mm/hr).

ESRs ranging from 2 to 46 mm/hr (median, 22 mm/hr) have been reported in patients with neurologic complications.

Suspected multiple myeloma
Strength of Recommendation: Class IIb
Strength of Evidence: Category C
Results Interpretation:
Erythrocyte sedimentation rate - finding
An elevated erythrocyte sedimentation rate (ESR) may raise suspicion for multiple myeloma, but is not diagnostic for the disease. Diagnosis is based on more specific criteria, such as the detection of a monoclonal spike on electrophoresis, bone marrow plasmacytosis, and lytic bone lesions on skeletal survey.

Suspected pelvic inflammatory disease
>**Results Interpretation:**
>**Erythrocyte sedimentation rate - finding**
>>An elevated erythrocyte sedimentation rate (ESR) supports the diagnosis of pelvic inflammatory disease (PID) in patients with pelvic tenderness and signs of lower genital tract inflammation, in whom no other cause(s) for the illness can be identified.
>>Patients with chlamydial PID tend to present with more highly elevated ESR (over 30 mm/hour) than those with gonococcal PID.

Suspected rheumatoid arthritis
>>**Strength of Recommendation:** Class IIa
>>**Strength of Evidence:** Category C
>**Results Interpretation:**
>**Increased level (laboratory finding)**
>>An erythrocyte sedimentation rate (ESR) should be included as part of the baseline laboratory evaluation of rheumatoid arthritis. An elevated ESR suggests poor prognosis. Periodic ESR measurements should be performed to follow the extent of disease.

Suspected septic arthritis
>>**Strength of Recommendation:** Class IIa
>>**Strength of Evidence:** Category C
>**Results Interpretation:**
>**ESR raised**
>>In a series of children with septic arthritis of the hip, the average erythrocyte sedimentation rate (ESR) was 94 mm/hour.
>>The combination of an ESR greater than 40mm/hour, fever, nonweight-bearing status, and serum WBC count greater than 12,000/mm^3 helps differentiate septic arthritis from transient synovitis of the hip in children.
>>The ESR is usually greater than 60 mm/hour in patients over 60 years of age with septic arthritis.

Suspected subacute thyroiditis
>**Results Interpretation:**
>**Increased level (laboratory finding)**
>>The erythrocyte sedimentation rate (ESR) is usually markedly elevated in subacute granulomatous thyroiditis and normal in subacute lymphocytic thyroiditis.
>>The ESR may be elevated greater than 100 mm/hour in painful thyroiditis.
>>A normal ESR excludes the diagnosis of active subacute granulomatous thyroiditis.
>>In silent thyroiditis (painless) the ESR may be normal or only slightly elevated.
>>In patients with recurrent subacute thyroiditis the ESR may be less than 40 mm/hour in up to one-third of the patients.

COMMON PANELS
- Anemia panel
- Arthritis panel
- Collagen/Lupus panel

ABNORMAL RESULTS
- Results increased in:
  - Female gender
  - Increasing age (steadily rises by 0.85 mm/hour for each 5-year increase in age)
  - Pregnancy (levels rise in the 4th month of pregnancy and peaks 1 week postpartum)
  - Diabetes mellitus
  - Hypothyroidism
  - Collagen renal failure
- Results decreased in:
  - Increased red blood cells
  - Abnormally shaped red blood cells
  - Hemolytic anemia
  - Hypofibrinogenemia
  - Pyruvate deficiency
  - Hyperproteinemia

CLINICAL NOTES
Erythrocyte sedimentation rate (ESR) should not be used as a screening test in asymptomatic patients. A low ESR has little diagnostic utility.

COLLECTION/STORAGE INFORMATION
• Specimen Collection and Handling:
    • Collect whole blood or capillary blood (suitable in pediatric patients) in EDTA (lavender top) or citrate (blue top) tube
    • May store specimen for 2 hours at 25°C or for 12 hours at 4°C

LOINC CODES
• Code: 30341-2 (*Short Name* - ESR Bld Qn)

Selenium measurement, urine

TEST DEFINITION
Measurement of selenium in urine

REFERENCE RANGE
• Adults and Children: 7-160 mcg/L (0.09-2.03 micromole/L)
  Please refer to your institution's reference ranges as lab normals may vary.

INDICATIONS
Suspected selenium deficiency
    Strength of Recommendation: Class IIa
    Strength of Evidence: Category C
    Results Interpretation:
    Decreased level (laboratory finding)
        Selenium levels less than 7 mcg/L (less than 0.09 micromol/L) may indicate a selenium deficiency.

Suspected selenium poisoning
    Strength of Recommendation: Class IIa
    Strength of Evidence: Category C
    Results Interpretation:
    Increased level (laboratory finding)
        Toxic concentrations in adults and children are usually greater than 400 mcg/L (greater than 5.08 micromol/L).

CLINICAL NOTES
The most reliable method for determining urinary selenium content is the 24-hour excretion measurement. Peak selenium excretion times cannot be established as diurnal urinary excretion varies from person to person. Because concentration of selenium is determined at the moment of voiding, a 24-hour urine specimen offers a more reliable result. Random urine samples are subject to the volume excreted, amount of food ingested, and the selenium level of the food ingested during the 24 hours preceding the sampling.

COLLECTION/STORAGE INFORMATION
• Specimen Collection and Handling:
    • Collect 24-hour urine in metal-free container.
    • Do not use any preservative.

LOINC CODES
• Code: 5727-3 (*Short Name* - Selenium 24H Ur-mRate)
• Code: 5726-5 (*Short Name* - Selenium Ur-mCnc)
• Code: 30927-8 (*Short Name* - Selenium ?Tm Ur-mCnc)
• Code: 29917-2 (*Short Name* - Selenium/creat 24H Ur-mRto)
• Code: 13467-6 (*Short Name* - Selenium/creat Ur-mRto)

Semen examination - general

TEST DEFINITION
Evaluation of various semen characteristics for the assessment of infertility

REFERENCE RANGE
- Reference values are not the minimum values required for conception; men with semen values below the reference cutoffs may be fertile:
- Liquefaction: < 60 minutes at room temperature. Usually liquefies within 15 minutes
- Appearance: Homogenous, grey-opalescence
- Volume: $\geq$2 mL
- Viscosity: Small, discrete drops, with a thread not exceeding 2 cm
- pH: $\geq$7.2
- Total sperm number: $\geq$40 x 10^6 spermatozoa per ejaculate/mL
- Sperm concentration: $\geq$20 X 10^6 spermatozoa/mL
- Sperm motility: $\geq$50% motile (grades a + b) or $\geq$25% with progressive motility (grade a) within 60 minutes of ejaculation
- Vitality: $\geq$50% live
- Leukocytes: < 1 x 10^6 /mL
- Immunobead test: <50% motile spermatozoa with beads bound
- Mixed antiglobulin reaction (MAR) test: <50% motile spermatozoa with adherent particles
- Agglutination: No agglutination or nonspecific aggregation
- Cells other than spermatozoa: <3.7 cells/unit volume examined
- Hypo-osmotic swelling test: >60% sperm tail swelling
- Calculation of indices of multiple sperm defects: Teratozoospermia index (TZI) value between 1.00 (each abnormal spermatozoon has just 1 defect) and 3.00 (each abnormal spermatozoon has head, midpiece, and tail defects)
- Sperm morphology: Head, neck, midpiece and tail are all normal. A consensus on a numeric reference value has not been established.
- Zinc: $\geq$2.4 micromols per ejaculate
- Fructose: $\geq$13 micromols per ejaculate
- Neutral alpha-glucosidase isoenzyme: $\geq$20 mU per ejaculate
- Acid phosphatase: $\geq$200 Units per ejaculate
  Please refer to your institution's reference ranges as lab normals may vary.

INDICATIONS
Suspected male infertility
> **Strength of Recommendation:** Class I
> **Strength of Evidence:** Category B
> **Results Interpretation:**
> **Abnormal laboratory findings**

.

While repeatedly abnormal semen analysis results may suggest male factor infertility, reference values recommended by the World Health Organization are not diagnostic for infertility, and definitive diagnostic reference ranges for each parameter have yet to be conclusively established. As each test contributes unique information, a combination of tests may offer an improved ability to diagnose infertility.

Men with ejaculatory duct obstruction or agenesis of the vasa deferentia and seminal vesicles will typically present with low fructose, low volume, low pH, no coagulation, and an absence of typical semen odor.

The presence of agglutination suggests an immunological cause of infertility. The type of agglutination should be reported from - (no agglutination) to +++ (severe clumping of all motile spermatozoa).

While excessive numbers of leukocytes may indicate infection and are associated with poor sperm quality, the absence of leukocytes does not rule out accessory gland infection. Men with a leukocyte count of greater than 1 million leukocytes/mL should be evaluated for genital tract infection.

Sperm may appear less opaque in the presence of low sperm concentration. A red-brown color is associated with the presence of red blood cells, and a yellow tinge may be due to jaundice or vitamin intake.

A pH of less than 7 in ejaculate that contains no spermatozoa may be due to ejaculatory duct obstruction or bilateral congenital absence of the vasa.

In the presence of a normal sperm count and density, abnormal morphology and/or abnormal motility may be due to varicocele, antisperm antibodies, leukocytospermia, bacteriospermia, or functional impairment of the prostate or seminal vesicles. Mild or moderate oligozoospermia can be caused by testicular dysfunction, mumps orchitis, environmental factors, or drug, chemical, or X-ray exposure. Although low sperm count is associated with decreased fertilization ability, oligozoospermic men can fertilize naturally. Combined, severe abnormalities of morphology, motility, and low sperm count are associated with Y chromosome microdeletions.

Azoospermia is caused either by obstructive or secretory dysfunction. Differential diagnosis is determined by physical examination, testis biopsy, and genetic and endocrine testing. Azoospermia in conjunction with a pH of less than 7 and a volume of 1 mL or less is associated with congenital, bilateral absence of the vas deferens.

The finding of elevated sperm count (between 250 and 350 X 10^6 /mL) is associated with diminished reproductive ability and miscarriage. Abnormal morphology and motility are more common in men with sperm counts above 350 X 10^6 mL.

Evaluation of sperm vitality is of limited diagnostic value, as this parameter can be adversely affected by abnormalities of any genital organ.

Normal laboratory findings
Patients with normal semen analysis results likely have fertility-compatible sperm.

Timing of Monitoring
Two semen analyses should be performed as part of an initial screening after a male has been unsuccessful at reproducing for 1 year.

COLLECTION/STORAGE INFORMATION
- Sample should be produced by masturbation without artificial lubrication into a wide-mouth sterile glass or plastic specimen cup. The entire ejaculate must be collected for accurate interpretation; partial ejaculate samples should be identified as 'incomplete'.
- Two samples are required. The first sample should be collected between 48 hours and 7 days after the initiation of abstinence. Collect the second sample 7 days to 3 weeks after the first sample, after 48 hours to 7 days of abstinence. Results between samples can vary considerably; if substantial differences are observed the collection of additional samples may be indicated.
- Keep samples warm between 20°C and 40°C during transportation to the laboratory. Spermatozoa must be separated from seminal plasma within 1 hour of collection. Analyze immediately in cases of suspected low motility.

Serologic test for Aspergillus

TEST DEFINITION
Detection or measurement of *Aspergillus* antigens and antibodies in serum

SYNONYMS
- Aspergillus antibody assay

REFERENCE RANGE
- Adults and children: negative
  Please refer to your institution's reference ranges as lab normals may vary.

INDICATIONS
Suspected allergic bronchopulmonary aspergillosis (ABPA)
    Strength of Recommendation: Class I
    Strength of Evidence: Category B
    Results Interpretation:
    Serology positive
    Diagnostic criteria for allergic bronchopulmonary aspergillosis (ABPA) include: elevated levels (compared with non-ABPA asthmatics) of serum IgE and IgG anti-*Aspergillus fumigatus* antibodies, total serum IgE concentration greater than 1000 ng/mL, and the presence of precipitating antibodies against *Aspergillus fumigatus*, in an asthmatic patient with proximal bronchiectasis and immediate cutaneous reactivity to *A fumigatus*.

    Patients who have a positive serology test finding, but no roentgenographic changes, are designated as being 'ABPA-Seropositive'.

Suspected invasive pulmonary aspergillosis in immunocompromised patients
    Strength of Recommendation: Class IIa
    Strength of Evidence: Category B
    Results Interpretation:
    Serology positive

A positive serology test for *Aspergillus* suggests the possibility of invasive aspergillosis in immunocompromised patients.

Direct antigen testing can be used to screen for *Aspergillus* invasive infections in at-risk (neutropenic) patients, but antibody screening is not useful in such patients.

A positive serology finding for *Aspergillus* in at-risk patients is an indication that a full workup should be done.

If the patient is started on antifungal therapy, *Aspergillus* antigen titers may be used to monitor patient response, however, high assay variability may occur.

The *Aspergillus* galactomannan antigen can be detected in serum and other body fluids (eg, urine, bronchoalveolar lavage (BAL), cerebrospinal fluid).

The detection rates for *Aspergillus* galactomannan antigen are lower in serum compared to body fluids such as BAL, as the antigen quickly forms immunocomplexes and is rapidly removed from the bloodstream.

Combining *Aspergillus* antigen testing with polymerase chain reaction (PCR) testing may yield higher sensitivity than using only a single method to detect *Aspergillus*.

Definitive diagnosis of invasive pulmonary aspergillosis requires a finding of *Aspergillus* hyphae in tissue sections, or a positive mycology culture.

Negative laboratory findings
- A negative serology finding for *Aspergillus* does not rule out invasive aspergillosis, as current tests may have a high false negative rate.

CLINICAL NOTES

The *Aspergillus* antigen test detects galactomannan, an *Aspergillus* cell-wall component released by growing hyphae.

COLLECTION/STORAGE INFORMATION
- Collect venous specimen in a red-top or serum separator tube (SST).

LOINC CODES
- Code: 9492-0 (*Short Name* - Aspergillus IgM Ser-aCnc)
- Code: 7808-9 (*Short Name* - Aspergillus Ab Ser Ql)
- Code: 7105-0 (*Short Name* - A nidulans IgE Qn)
- Code: 16414-5 (*Short Name* - A amstelodami Ab Qn)
- Code: 7106-8 (*Short Name* - Aspergillus IgE Qn)
- Code: 23953-3 (*Short Name* - Aspergillus Ab Titr CSF CF)
- Code: 31233-0 (*Short Name* - Aspergillus Ab CSF-aCnc)
- Code: 7807-1 (*Short Name* - Aspergillus Ab Ser-aCnc)
- Code: 18426-7 (*Short Name* - Aspergillus Ab CSF Ql)
- Code: 31228-0 (*Short Name* - A clavatus Ab Ser Ql)
- Code: 23660-4 (*Short Name* - Aspergillus Ab Titr Ser EIA)
- Code: 18416-8 (*Short Name* - A nidulans IgG Qn)
- Code: 6026-9 (*Short Name* - A terreus IgE Qn)
- Code: 31231-4 (*Short Name* - A nidulans Ab Ser Ql)
- Code: 7107-6 (*Short Name* - Aspergillus IgG Qn)
- Code: 5053-4 (*Short Name* - Aspergillus Ab Titr Ser CF)
- Code: 6027-7 (*Short Name* - A versicolor IgE Qn)
- Code: 5052-6 (*Short Name* - Aspergillus Ab Ser Ql ID)
- Code: 23956-6 (*Short Name* - Aspergillus Ab Titr CSF)
- Code: 31234-8 (*Short Name* - A terreus Ab Ser Ql)
- Code: 9491-2 (*Short Name* - Aspergillus IgA Ser-aCnc)
- Code: 22087-1 (*Short Name* - Aspergillus Ab Titr Ser)

Serologic test for Blastomyces

TEST DEFINITION
The detection and titer measurement of *Blastomyces* antibodies in serum for evaluation of blastomycosis fungal infection

SYNONYMS
- Blastomyces antibody assay

REFERENCE RANGE
Negative
Please refer to your institution's reference ranges as lab normals may vary.

INDICATIONS
Suspected blastomycosis
> **Strength of Recommendation:** Class IIb
> **Strength of Evidence:** Category C
> **Results Interpretation:**
> **Fungal antibody titer - finding**
> A 4-fold increase in *Blastomyces* serology titers between disease onset and 3 to 4 weeks later indicates probable blastomycosis infection. A titer of 1:8 to 1:16 by enzyme immunoassay is suggestive of infection.
> A positive immunodiffusion test in the appropriate clinical setting tentatively diagnoses blastomycosis, however, a negative test does not exclude it.
> A complement fixation titer of 1:8 or greater against the yeast-form homogenate-supernatant antigen indicates probable infection.
> Cross-reactions can occur in histoplasmosis or coccidioidomycosis infection.
> Culture and microscopic exam remain the diagnostic methods of choice.
> **Timing of Monitoring**
> Serology testing should be done at onset of disease and 3 to 4 weeks later.

CLINICAL NOTES
Identification of the fungus *Blastomyces* by stain or culture remains the primary method of diagnosis.

COLLECTION/STORAGE INFORMATION
Draw serum at onset of disease and 3 to 4 weeks later.

LOINC CODES
- Code: 18197-4 (*Short Name* - Blastomyces Ab CSF QI)
- Code: 27386-2 (*Short Name* - Blastomyces Ab Fld QI ID)
- Code: 23670-3 (*Short Name* - Blastomyces Ab Ser QI)
- Code: 18200-6 (*Short Name* - Blastomyces IgM Ser QI)

Serologic test for Candida

TEST DEFINITION
Serologic test for detection of antibody against *Candida*

SYNONYMS
- Candida antibody assay

REFERENCE RANGE
- Negative
  Please refer to your institution's reference ranges as lab normals may vary.

INDICATIONS

Suspected systemic candidiasis
    Strength of Recommendation: Class IIb
    Strength of Evidence: Category B
Results Interpretation:
Serology positive
- Findings:
  - Production of ≥1 band is positive
  - Latex agglutination and immunodiffusion titers ≥1:8 suggest invasive candidiasis
  - Latex agglutination titers of 1:4 and positive immunodiffusion are evidence of early stages of colonization or early invasion of *Candida* species
  - Four-fold rise in titer between acute and convalescent sera is presumptive of systemic candidiasis. Four-fold decrease in titer may indicate successful chemotherapy or eradication of colonization
  - ≥2 ng of serum mannan antigen by enzyme immunoassay is suggestive of invasive candidiasis

  False Results
  A negative result does not rule out disease, especially in immunocompromised patients in whom antibodies are not reliably produced.
  A positive result may occur with colonization of *Candida* species or *Torulopsis glabrata*.
  Severe vaginitis or mucocutaneous candidiasis can produce positive serologic results.
Frequency of Monitoring
Draw blood serum at onset of disease and two to three weeks later, if required.

CLINICAL NOTES

Antigens or metabolites helpful in the diagnosis of invasive candidiasis include cell wall mannoprotein (mannan), heat labile antigen, D-arabinitol, and enolase. The enolase antigen is highly specific for the*Candida* species. Mannan rapidly clears from the blood and occurs in low levels, requiring frequent sampling. A positive mannan test confirms diagnosis of invasive candidiasis and also correlates with disseminated non-albicans candidiasis.

COLLECTION/STORAGE INFORMATION

- Collect serum sample at disease onset and 2 to 3 weeks later if clinically indicated:

LOINC CODES

- Code: 26636-1 (*Short Name* - Candida Ab Ser Ql)
- Code: 35270-8 (*Short Name* - Candida Ab Ser Ql ID)

Serologic test for Coxiella burnetii

TEST DEFINITION

Measurement of antibodies to *Coxiella burnetii* in blood for the evaluation and management of acute and chronic Q fever and related diseases

SYNONYMS

- Coxiella burnetii antibody assay

REFERENCE RANGE

- Adults and Children: Negative
  Please refer to your institution's reference ranges as lab normals may vary.

INDICATIONS

Suspected Q fever
    Strength of Recommendation: Class IIa
    Strength of Evidence: Category C

Results Interpretation:
Abnormal laboratory findings
- Cut-off titers using microimmunofluorescence are as follows:
  - Acute infection, anti-phase II IgG: Antibody titer >1:200
  - Acute infection, anti-phase II IgM: Antibody titer >1:50
  - Chronic infection, anti-phase I IgG: Antibody titer >1:800
  - Chronic infection, anti-phase I IgA: Antibody titer >1:100

  Using the microimmunofluorescence technique (IFA), seroconversion can be detected within one to two weeks of symptom onset with 90% of cases detected by the third week. Antibody titers peak 4 to 8 weeks after the onset of acute Q fever, then gradually subside over the subsequent 12 months. Due to its low cross-reactivity, seroconversion or a fourfold rise in antibody titers can be considered diagnostic for Q fever, using the IFA technique.

  A reoccurrence of high titers or the persistence of high levels of anti-phase I antibodies may be indicative of the onset of chronic Q fever infection.

  Antibody titers are useful to monitor response to treatment, particularly in Q fever endocarditis.

  IgM titers may not be beneficial in diagnosing Q fever, due to their potential variability.

  Active Q fever is highly unlikely if phase II IgG antibody titers are less than or equal to 1:100 in a single serum sample. If the sample was collected at least 1.5 months after the onset of symptoms the diagnosis of Q fever can be definitively ruled out.

  The presence of both an anti-phase II IgG antibody titer greater than or equal to 200, and a IgM antibody titer greater than or equal to 50, is 100% predictive of acute Q fever infection. Titers gradually increase following the onset of symptoms, and are often not found early in the disease process. These titer findings are observed in only 10% of patients during the second week, 50% of patients during the third week, and 70% of patients during the fourth week, following symptom onset.. Anti-phase I antibodies are indicative of chronic Q fever; anti-phase I IgG antibody titers greater than or equal to 800 are considered highly predictive of Q fever endocarditis.

  Using the complement fixation test (CF), anti-phase II antibodies of greater than or equal to 40, and anti-phase I antibodies of greater than 200, are indicative of acute and chronic Q fever, respectively. Seroconversion using this method takes 2 to 3 weeks, and is not as commonly used as IFA and enzyme-linked immunosorbent assay (ELISA).

  Using the ELISA test, proposed cut-off values of greater than or equal to 1,024 for anti-phase II IgG and greater than or equal to 512 for anti-phase II IgM for acute Q fever, and greater than or equal to 128 for anti-phase I IgG and IgM antibody for chronic Q fever, have been proposed.

  Results are increased in recent Q fever vaccination.

Frequency of Monitoring
  Obtain serial serologic tests monthly for at least 6 months following acute Q fever diagnosis.

COLLECTION/STORAGE INFORMATION
- Collect blood sample in a marbled top tube.
- Because of its highly infectious nature, *Coxiella burnetii* specimens should be handled by experienced personnel wearing mask and gloves, in a biosafety level 3 laboratory.

LOINC CODES
- Code: 16677-7 (*Short Name* - C burnet IgG Ser-aCnc)
- Code: 23018-5 (*Short Name* - C burnet Ab Ser QI IF)
- Code: 16678-5 (*Short Name* - C burnet IgM Ser-aCnc)
- Code: 23020-1 (*Short Name* - C burnet Ab Ser QI)
- Code: 25335-1 (*Short Name* - C burnet IgG Titr Ser)
- Code: 7828-7 (*Short Name* - C burnet Ab Ser-aCnc)
- Code: 23017-7 (*Short Name* - C burnet Ab Ser QI CF)
- Code: 30213-3 (*Short Name* - C burnet IgM Ser QI)
- Code: 5100-3 (*Short Name* - C burnet Ab Titr Ser CF)
- Code: 25336-9 (*Short Name* - C burnet IgM Titr Ser)
- Code: 32566-2 (*Short Name* - C burnet Ab Titr CSF)
- Code: 30212-5 (*Short Name* - C burnet IgG Ser QI)
- Code: 22211-7 (*Short Name* - C burnet Ab Titr Ser)

Serum 5-nucleotidase measurement

TEST DEFINITION
Measurement of 5'-nucleotidase in serum for the evaluation and management of hepatobiliary disease, including liver metastases

SYNONYMS
- Serum 5-nucleotidase
- Serum 5-nucleotidase level

REFERENCE RANGE
- Adults: 0-11 units/L (0.02-0.18 microkat/L)
  Please refer to your institution's reference ranges as lab normals may vary.

INDICATIONS
Suspected liver disease
> **Strength of Recommendation:** Class IIb
> **Strength of Evidence:** Category B
> **Results Interpretation:**
> **Increased level (laboratory finding)**
> Increased serum 5'-nucleotidase (5'NT) activity predominately occurs in hepatobiliary disease and is common in patients with intrahepatic obstruction. In contrast to serum alkaline phosphatase (AP), elevated 5'NT levels are rarely seen in osteoblastic disease, childhood, or pregnancy.
> In hepatobiliary disease, serum 5'NT activity typically parallels increases in serum AP activity; however, if the origin of an elevated serum AP level is unclear, a normal 5'NT value does not necessarily rule out hepatic disease. There are rare cases of liver dysfunction in which only one of the enzymes is elevated, and 5'NT activity may not increase proportionately in individual patients.
> In general, serum 5'NT levels are markedly increased in patients with cholestatic disease, and parallel those of gamma-glutamyl transferase (GGT) and AP.
> Detection of hepatobiliary disease by serum enzyme activity is improved when both 5'NT and serum AP are measured.

Suspected metastasis to the liver
> **Strength of Recommendation:** Class IIb
> **Strength of Evidence:** Category C
> **Results Interpretation:**
> **Increased level (laboratory finding)**
> Elevated serum 5'-nucleotidase (5'NT) in cancer patients may suggest the presence of liver metastases; however, elevated levels may be found in some cases of primary tumor alone or extrahepatic metastasis.

CLINICAL NOTES
Serum 5'-nucleotidase levels are generally low during childhood, increase during adolescence, and reach a plateau after age 50.

COLLECTION/STORAGE INFORMATION
- Specimen Collection and Handling:
  - Collect serum or plasma (heparin) specimen.
  - Specimen is stable for 4 days at 4°C.
  - Specimen is stable for 4 months if frozen.

LOINC CODES
- Code: 1690-7 (*Short Name* - 5NT Ser-cCnc)

Serum C reactive protein level

TEST DEFINITION
Measures serum C-reactive protein (CRP), an acute phase reactant that is a biomarker of inflammation

REFERENCE RANGE
- Adults: 0.08-3.1 mg/L
- Adults (high sensitivity): 0.02-8 mg/L
  Please refer to your institution's reference ranges as lab normals may vary.

INDICATIONS
Suspected meningococcemia in children with associated septic shock and purpura
  Results Interpretation:
  Increased C-reactive protein level
    C-reactive protein measurements have moderate diagnostic but not prognostic value for meningococcal disease..

Bacterial meningitis
  Results Interpretation:
  Increased C-reactive protein level
    C-reactive protein (CRP) levels maybe increased up to 100-fold or more with a bacterial infection.
    CRP measurement is most useful for monitoring patient response to therapy after primary diagnosis of invasive infectious or inflammatory disease.

Community-acquired pneumonia
  Results Interpretation:
  Increased C-reactive protein level
    C-reactive protein (CRP) is elevated in about 25% of patients with pneumonia, but it is not helpful in discriminating between viral and bacterial pneumonia in children.
    One retrospective study did demonstrate that CRP levels in patients with lower respiratory tract infections were higher in patients requiring hospitalization.
    Antibiotic treatment failure or the evolvement of infective complications may be demonstrated by unremittingly elevated or increasing c-reactive protein levels.
    CRP may be a useful adjunct for diagnosing Legionella pneumonia. In 1 study, the odds of having a CRP level greater than 25 mg/dL were almost 7 times higher in patients with Legionella infection than in those with pneumonia due to other causes. A different study found similar CRP levels in patients with Legionella and pneumococcal pneumonia.
  Decreased level (laboratory finding)
    CRP levels fall rapidly in accordance with clinical recovery.

Coronary artery disease
    Strength of Recommendation: Class IIa
    Strength of Evidence: Category A
  Results Interpretation:
  Increased C-reactive protein level
    C-reactive protein (CRP) levels greater than 10 mg/L increase risk of death 4-fold compared with CRP levels less than 3 mg/L.
    A serum CRP concentration above 3 mg/L correlates with a poorer prognosis in patients with unstable angina.
    Increased levels of high-sensitivity CRP (hs-CRP) has been shown to be associated with the risk of subsequent fatality in patients with acute coronary syndrome.
    CRP may be an important general marker of increased risk for cardiovascular events, including death, however, AHA/CDC guidelines recommend against basing management of coronary disease on CRP screening.

Rheumatoid arthritis
    Strength of Recommendation: Class IIa
    Strength of Evidence: Category C

Results Interpretation:
Increased C-reactive protein level

C- reactive protein (CRP) greater than 1 mg/dL indicates an inflammatory process but it is nonspecific. Levels may be useful in monitoring therapy.

Single measurements of CRP may remain within range of normal while reflecting elevation for an individual patient. Serial measurements are more helpful in assessing disease activity.

CRP is helpful in the management of rheumatoid arthritis since its levels will fall as inflammation subsides.

Serum marker to assess the severity of acute pancreatitis
Results Interpretation:
Increased C-reactive protein level

C-reactive protein levels greater than 150 mg/L at 48 hours predict disease severity.

Suspected and known Kawasaki disease
Results Interpretation:
Increased level (laboratory finding)

A C-reactive protein (CRP) level of 3 mg/dL or greater is found in nearly all cases of Kawasaki disease (KD) during the acute febrile stage.

CRP concentrations greater than 10 mg/dL have been associated with a poor response to intravenous immunoglobulin.

Elevated CRP has been used as part of some scoring systems to identify KD patients at high risk of developing coronary artery lesions.

Suspected and known malaria
Results Interpretation:
Increased C-reactive protein level

C-reactive protein levels correlates well with the severity of P falciparum malaria and is useful in following the response to therapy.

Suspected and known osteomyelitis
Results Interpretation:
Increased C-reactive protein level

The serum C-reactive protein is elevated in 90% of children with osteomyelitis overall and in almost all patients with vertebral osteomyelitis.

Suspected appendicitis
Strength of Recommendation: Class IIb
Strength of Evidence: Category B
Results Interpretation:
Increased C-reactive protein level

C-reactive protein (CRP) is elevated in relation to severity of appendiceal inflammation, such as with appendiceal perforation or abscess formation.

When CRP and leucocyte count are both normal, acute appendicitis is unlikely.

Suspected pelvic inflammatory disease (PID)
Strength of Recommendation: Class IIb
Strength of Evidence: Category B
Results Interpretation:
Increased C-reactive protein level

An elevated C-reactive protein (CRP) level supports the diagnosis of pelvic inflammatory disease (PID).

A CRP level reflects the extent and severity of PID more closely than erythrocyte sedimentation rate or WBC count determinations.

Suspected sepsis
Strength of Recommendation: Class IIb
Strength of Evidence: Category C
Results Interpretation:
Increased C-reactive protein level

Studies show elevated C-reactive protein (CRP) levels in patients with systemic inflammatory response syndrome.

A CRP level greater than 2 standard deviations above normal is an indicator of inflammation.

C-reactive protein (CRP) is elevated at the onset of infection (greater than 20 mg/L) and will increase during the initial course, then decrease as the patient recovers. In patients who do not recover, levels remain high. Behavior of CRP is not affected by the patient's immunologic status.

Timing of Monitoring

An acute phase serum protein can be measured as a serial index of severity of infection.

COMMON PANELS
- Arthritis panel
- Collagen/Lupus panel

ABNORMAL RESULTS
- Results increased in:
  - Trauma
  - Following surgical procedures
  - Cigarette smoking
  - Diabetes mellitus

COLLECTION/STORAGE INFORMATION
- Specimen Collection and Handling:
  - Collect serum sample
  - Avoid hemolytic and lipemic specimens
  - Analyze fresh specimen or store at 4°C or less than 72 hours
  - Specimen is stable frozen at -20°C for 6 months or indefinitely at -70°C

LOINC CODES
- Code: 30522-7 (*Short Name* - CRP Ser High Sens-mCnc)
- Code: 11039-5 (*Short Name* - CRP Ser QI)
- Code: 1988-5 (*Short Name* - CRP Ser-mCnc)
- Code: 14634-0 (*Short Name* - CRP Titr Ser)

Serum alkaline phosphatase measurement

TEST DEFINITION
Measurement of alkaline phosphatase in serum for the evaluation of bone and liver disease

SYNONYMS
- Serum alkaline phosphatase level

REFERENCE RANGE
- Adults: 30 units/L-120 units/L (0.5 nkat/L to 2 nkat/L)
- Children: < 350 units/L
- Adolescent (male): < 500 units/L
- Adolescent (female > 15 years): 25 units/L-100 units/L
  Please refer to your institution's reference ranges as lab normals may vary.

INDICATIONS
Suspected bone metastasis
   Results Interpretation:
   Alkaline phosphatase raised

In the presence of known malignancy, an elevated alkaline phosphatase is suggestive of metastatic disease. Further evaluation is required before the metastatic site can be determined and metastasis confirmed.

   False Results

Because alkaline phosphatase is not specific to one tissue or one disease, elevated levels may reflect other, unrelated pathology. Further analysis is required to assess the etiology of an increased ALP level.

Suspected cholecystitis
Strength of Recommendation: Class IIa
Strength of Evidence: Category B
Results Interpretation:
Alkaline phosphatase raised
In patients with hepatobiliary obstruction, an elevated alkaline phosphatase is observed in 30% to 40% of patients. In one study, the combination of a bilirubin level greater than 3 mg/dL with an alkaline phosphatase level greater than 250 IU/L had a 76% probability of an associated common duct stone.

Alkaline phosphatase values typically return to normal within one week after symptoms resolve unless suppuration ensues.

False Results
Elevated alkaline phosphatase can only be interpreted in conjunction with other clinical findings and diagnostic tests since it is not is not tissue or disease specific.

Suspected drug-induced liver disease
Strength of Recommendation: Class I
Strength of Evidence: Category C
Results Interpretation:
Alkaline phosphatase raised
Cholestatic liver injury may be characterized by a predominant initial elevation of serum alkaline phosphatase levels relatively more prominent than increases in the ALT or AST levels.

Suspected inflammatory liver disease, including hepatitis
Strength of Recommendation: Class IIa
Strength of Evidence: Category C
Results Interpretation:
Alkaline phosphatase level - finding
Mildly elevated levels of alkaline phosphatase may occur in hepatitis.

Markedly increased levels of alkaline phosphatase indicate cholestasis. Isolated elevation of alkaline phosphatase, confirmed by gamma glutamyl transpeptidase (GGTP) to be hepatic in origin, is strongly suggestive of an infiltrative process, either localized or a systemic granulomatous disorder.

Alkaline phosphatase is also present in bone and will be elevated in growing children and in people with fractured bones and certain diseases of the bone.

COMMON PANELS
• Hepatic function panel

CLINICAL NOTES
Alkaline phosphatase (ALP) is derived from bone, hepatic, intestinal, and placental tissues. Additional diagnostic specificity can be obtained through the analysis of tissue specific ALP isoenyzmes.

COLLECTION/STORAGE INFORMATION
Specimen Collection and Handling:
• Note the age and gender of the patient on test requisition
• Obtain a 5 mL fasting venous blood sample
• Avoid use of an anticoagulant containing tube
• Analyze or refrigerate immediately

LOINC CODES
• Code: 6768-6 (*Short Name* - ALP SerPl-cCnc)

Serum alpha-2 macroglobulin level

TEST DEFINITION
Measurement of alpha$_2$ macroglobulin in serum for the evaluation and management of certain gastrointestinal and renal disorders

REFERENCE RANGE

- Adult males (radial immunodiffusion): 150-350 mg/dL (1.5-3.5 g/L)
- Adult females (radial immunodiffusion): 175-420 mg/dL (1.75-4.2 g/L)
  Please refer to your institution's reference ranges as lab normals may vary.

INDICATIONS

Nephrotic syndrome
> **Strength of Recommendation:** Class IIb
> **Strength of Evidence:** Category B
> **Results Interpretation:**
> **Increased level (laboratory finding)**
> Alpha$_2$ macroglobulin levels are higher in patients with active nephrotic syndrome and to decrease following treatment in patients with nephrotic syndrome.

Suspected hepatic fibrosis in patients with hepatitis C
> **Strength of Recommendation:** Class IIb
> **Strength of Evidence:** Category B
> **Results Interpretation:**
> **Increased level (laboratory finding)**
> Elevated levels of alpha$_2$ macroglobulin appear to correlate with increased severity of fibrosis in patients with hepatitis C. In combination with 5 other markers (alpha$_2$ globulin, total bilirubin, gamma globulin, apolipoprotein A$_1$, and gamma-glutamyltransferase [GGT]), alpha$_2$ macroglobulin may be predictive of severe fibrosis or cirrhosis in these patients.

ABNORMAL RESULTS

- Results increased in:
  - Female adults
  - Male children
  - Newborns
  - Exercise
  - Pregnancy

COLLECTION/STORAGE INFORMATION

- Specimen Collection and Handling:
  - Collect in lavender-top (EDTA) or red-top (serum) tube.
  - May be stored for 2 days at 4°C and for 7 days at -20°C

LOINC CODES

- Code: 1835-8 (*Short Name* - A2 Macroglob Ser-mCnc)

Serum amikacin measurement

TEST DEFINITION

Measurement of serum amikacin levels

SYNONYMS

- Serum amikacin level

REFERENCE RANGE

- Adult, therapeutic level:
- Peak: 25-35 microgram/mL (43-60 micromole/L)
- Trough: 4-8 microgram/mL (6.8-13.7 micromole/L)
  Please refer to your institution's reference ranges as lab normals may vary.

INDICATIONS

Suspected amikacin toxicity

Strength of Recommendation: Class IIa

Strength of Evidence: Category C

Results Interpretation:

Toxicity of drug

Trough levels, as a direct measure of amikacin tissue concentration, are a more accurate predictor of toxicity than peak levels. Peak levels are more predictive of therapeutic response.

In specific patient populations (ie, those on prolonged amikacin therapy, with renal dysfunction, or with life-threatening infections), frequent testing of peak and trough levels minimizes the risk of ototoxicity. Nephrotoxicity with amikacin is uncommon, but is more highly correlated with trough levels as opposed to peak levels..

- Adult, toxic level:
  - Peak: >35 micrograms/mL (>60 micromole/L)
  - Trough: >10 micrograms/mL (>17 micromole/L)
  Trough levels greater than 10 micrograms/mL have sometimes been associated with ototoxicity.

Therapeutic drug level monitoring during amikacin therapy

Strength of Recommendation: Class IIa

Strength of Evidence: Category C

Results Interpretation:

Therapeutic drug level - finding

Testing of peak and trough amikacin levels helps ensure appropriate and individualized therapeutic dosing adjustments, optimization of treatment, and prevention of bacterial adaptive resistance. Peak levels are monitored primarily to predict therapeutic effect, while trough levels are most useful in predicting toxicity.

Timing of Monitoring

Timing of peak and trough sampling is crucial. The specimen for a peak serum amikacin concentration should be obtained at the end of a 1-hour continuous infusion, 30 minutes after the end of a 30-minute continuous infusion, or 1 hour after an intramuscular injection. A trough concentration should be drawn within 30 minutes of the subsequent dose.

CLINICAL NOTES

Immunoassay results may be falsely elevated when amikacin is given concomitantly with kanamycin or tobramycin.

LOINC CODES

- Code: 31097-9 (*Short Name* - Amikacin Peak EID SerPl-mCnc)
- Code: 15098-7 (*Short Name* - Amikacin Ran SerPl-sCnc)
- Code: 31099-5 (*Short Name* - Amikacin Random EID SerPl-mCnc)
- Code: 31098-7 (*Short Name* - Amikacin Trough EID SerPl-mCnc)
- Code: 3319-1 (*Short Name* - Amikacin Peak SerPl-mCnc)

Serum amiodarone measurement

TEST DEFINITION

Measurement of amiodarone in serum to assess therapeutic concentrations for the treatment of cardiac dysrhythmias and to evaluate suspected amiodarone toxicity

SYNONYMS

- Serum amiodarone level

REFERENCE RANGE

- Adults: Therapeutic Concentration, 0.5-2.5 mcg/mL (0.8-3.9 micromol/L)
  Please refer to your institution's reference ranges as lab normals may vary.

INDICATIONS

Amiodarone measurement to monitor drug levels during therapy
> **Strength of Recommendation:** Class III
> **Strength of Evidence:** Category B

Results Interpretation:

Drug level - finding
> The relationship between plasma concentrations and therapeutic effect is not well established.
>
> One study reported good to excellent clinical response in patients with sustained paroxysmal ventricular tachycardia with serum concentrations of 0.8 to 2.8 mcg/mL after at least 10 days of therapy with 200 mg orally three times daily.
>
> Plasma concentrations above 0.5 mcg/mL may be necessary to achieve therapeutic efficacy; however, limited data are available correlating plasma levels with clinical effects.

Suspected amiodarone poisoning or exposure
> **Strength of Recommendation:** Class IIb
> **Strength of Evidence:** Category C

Results Interpretation:

Increased level (laboratory finding)
> Serum amiodarone levels may confirm the diagnosis of acute exposure but are not clinically useful. ECG monitoring may be necessary for several days following an overdose.
>
> Toxic effects have been observed with plasma levels of 2.5 to 6.7 mcg/mL for amiodarone and 102 to 149 ng/dL for desethylamiodarone (active metabolite).
>
> Although plasma levels of either the parent compound or the active metabolite may not accurately predict toxicity, serum levels will decline as toxicity symptoms improve.

CLINICAL NOTES

Routine monitoring of amiodarone levels is not recommended because of limited clinical efficacy both in guiding long-term therapy and in the prevention of toxicity.

COLLECTION/STORAGE INFORMATION

- Specimen Collection and Handling:
  - Collect serum or plasma in EDTA tube.
  - Specimens can be stored at -20°C for at least 6 months.

LOINC CODES

- Code: 15099-5 (*Short Name* - Amiodarone SerPl-sCnc)
- Code: 3330-8 (*Short Name* - Amiodarone SerPl-mCnc)
- Code: 29207-8 (*Short Name* - Amiodarone Fld-mCnc)

Serum androstenedione measurement

TEST DEFINITION

Measurement of serum androstenedione for evaluation of suspected virilizing syndromes or anabolic steroid abuse

SYNONYMS

- Serum androstenedione level

REFERENCE RANGE

- Female, 1 to 10 years: 8-50 ng/dL (0.3-1.7 nmol/L)
- Female, 10 to 17 years: 8-240 ng/dL (0.3-8.4 nmol/L)
- Adult female: 85-275 ng/dL (3-9.6 nmol/L)
- Adult male: 75-205 ng/dL (2.6-7.2 nmol/L)

Please refer to your institution's reference ranges as lab normals may vary.

INDICATIONS

Suspected anabolic steroid abuse
> **Strength of Recommendation:** Class IIb
> **Strength of Evidence:** Category C
Results Interpretation:
Serum androstenedione abnormal
> Elevated androstenedione levels are consistent with suspected exogenous anabolic steroid use. Additional analysis is necessary for confirmation.

Suspected virilizing syndromes
> **Strength of Recommendation:** Class IIb
> **Strength of Evidence:** Category B
Results Interpretation:
Serum androstenedione abnormal
> There is a correlation between increased androstenedione levels and hyperandrogenism. Further evaluation is necessary for diagnosis and to differentiate between ovarian and adrenal sources for the elevated serum androstenedione.

CLINICAL NOTES

In healthy women conversion of androstenedione to testosterone accounts for approximately half the circulating level of testosterone; the adrenals and ovaries contribute approximately equally to the remaining amount.

COLLECTION/STORAGE INFORMATION

- Specimen collection and handling:
  - Place specimen on ice and perform assay within one hour of collection.
  - If unable to perform assay within one hour of collection, store at -20°C.
  - Collect specimen at least 1 week before or after menstrual period.

LOINC CODES

- Code: 1854-9 (*Short Name* - Androst SerPl-mCnc)
- Code: 32587-8 (*Short Name* - Androst 2H p chal SerPl-sCnc)
- Code: 32299-0 (*Short Name* - Androst BS SerPl-sCnc)
- Code: 32588-6 (*Short Name* - Androst 1H p chal SerPl-sCnc)
- Code: 24407-9 (*Short Name* - Androst BS SerPl-mCnc)

Serum angiotensin-converting enzyme measurement

TEST DEFINITION

Measurement of angiotensin-converting enzyme in serum for the evaluation of granulomatous diseases and vascular pathologies involving endothelial abnormalities

SYNONYMS

- Serum angiotensin-converting enzyme level

REFERENCE RANGE

- <40 units/L (<670 nkat/L)
  Please refer to your institution's reference ranges as lab normals may vary.

INDICATIONS

Suspected and known sarcoidosis
> **Strength of Recommendation:** Class IIa
> **Strength of Evidence:** Category B

Results Interpretation:
Positive laboratory findings
   Serum angiotensin-converting enzyme (ACE) may be of value in diagnosing sarcoidosis; however, due to low specificity, a negative result does not rule out the disease. In known sarcoidosis, ACE levels correlate with clinical symptoms, making serial testing a useful adjunct in following disease progression, and for predicting relapse.

Suspected Gaucher's disease
   Strength of Recommendation: Class IIa
   Strength of Evidence: Category B
   Results Interpretation:
   Increased level (laboratory finding)
   Elevated levels of angiotensin-converting enzyme (ACE) may aid in the diagnosis of Gaucher's disease; ACE levels may correlate with disease severity.

Suspected leprosy
   Strength of Recommendation: Class IIb
   Strength of Evidence: Category B
   Results Interpretation:
   Increased level (laboratory finding)
   While elevated angiotensin-converting enzyme (ACE) levels are often present in various forms of leprosy, testing for ACE is not helpful in differentiating sarcoidosis from leprosy, or differentiating lepromatous from tuberculoid leprosy.

CLINICAL NOTES
   Because of the numerous assay methods used to measure angiotensin-converting enzyme (ACE) and lack of standardization in reference ranges, it is important to use the same method and same lab during serial testing.
   Normal values in children are higher than in adults, and higher levels have been observed in boys as compared to girls at puberty. Circulating ACE levels in healthy individuals when measured over time tend to be stable, while inter-individual variability can range by as much as six-fold in healthy persons.

COLLECTION/STORAGE INFORMATION
• Specimen is stable at 4°C for 1 week and may be stored for 6 months at −20°C.

LOINC CODES
• Code: 22675-3 (*Short Name* - ACE SerPl-cCnc)

Serum apolipoprotein A-I measurement

TEST DEFINITION
   Measurement of apolipoprotein A-1 in serum or plasma for evaluating risk of coronary artery disease and for diagnosis of familial Mediterranean fever with amyloidosis

SYNONYMS
• Serum apolipoprotein A-I level

REFERENCE RANGE
• Adults: 119-240 mg/dL (1.2-2.4 g/L)
   Please refer to your institution's reference ranges as lab normals may vary.

INDICATIONS
Hyperlipidemia and/or family history of coronary artery disease
   Strength of Recommendation: Class IIb
   Strength of Evidence: Category B

Results Interpretation:
Decreased level (laboratory finding)
   Low levels of serum apolipoprotein A-1 (apoA-1), correlating with decreased high density lipoprotein levels, may be predictive of an increased risk of coronary artery disease. Increased levels of ApoA-1 may have a cardioprotective effect.

Suspected familial Mediterranean fever with amyloidosis
   Strength of Recommendation: Class IIb
   Strength of Evidence: Category B
Results Interpretation:
Decreased level (laboratory finding)
   In patients with familial Mediterranean fever, lower levels of apolipoprotein A-1 may correlate with an increased likelihood of developing systemic amyloidosis.

ABNORMAL RESULTS
- Results increased in:
  - Pregnancy
  - Exercise
  - Weight reduction
- Results decreased in:
  - Chronic renal failure
  - Smoking
  - Diabetes

COLLECTION/STORAGE INFORMATION
- Specimen Collection and Handling:
  - Obtain fasting specimen (serum or plasma) in EDTA-containing tube
  - Store at 4° C up to 4 days and -20° C up to 6 months
  - Store with preservative (thimerosal) at -20° C up to 3 years and at -70° C for longer than 3 years

LOINC CODES
- Code: 1869-7 (*Short Name* - Apo A-I SerPl-mCnc)

Serum apolipoprotein B measurement

TEST DEFINITION
   The measurement of apolipoprotein B in serum to evaluate the risk for the development of coronary artery disease, hyperlipidemia, and related disorders

SYNONYMS
- Serum apolipoprotein B level

REFERENCE RANGE
- 52 - 163 mg/dL (0.52 - 1.63 g/L)
   Please refer to your institution's reference ranges as lab normals may vary.

INDICATIONS
Risk screening for coronary artery disease
   Strength of Recommendation: Class IIb
   Strength of Evidence: Category A
Results Interpretation:
Increased level (laboratory finding)
   Elevated apolipoprotein B (apoB) level is a predictor of potential coronary artery disease. However, given its historical lack of measurement standardization and lack of sensitivity compared to other CHD risk factors, as well as cost-effectiveness issues, apoB is not recommended for general clinical use, and has limited value in CHD risk assessment. The high correlation between non-HDL cholesterol and apoB level makes non-HDL an acceptable surrogate marker for total apoB.

COLLECTION/STORAGE INFORMATION
- Have patient fast for 12 hours prior to sample collection.
- Collect serum sample in a lavender (EDTA) top tube.
- Serum sample is stable for one week at 4°C, or up to 1 year at −70°C.

LOINC CODES
- Code: 1873-9 (*Short Name* - Apo B48 SerPl-mCnc)
- Code: 1884-6 (*Short Name* - Apo B SerPl-mCnc)

Serum calcium measurement

TEST DEFINITION
Measurement of total calcium concentration in serum for the evaluation and management of disorders affecting calcium metabolism

SYNONYMS
- Serum calcium level

REFERENCE RANGE
- Adults: 9-10.5 mg/dL (2.2-2.6 mmol/L)
- Premature infants: 6.2-11 mg/dL (1.55-2.75 mmol/L)
- Neonates, cord blood: 8.2-11.2 mg/dL (2.05-2.8 mmol/L)
- Neonates, 0 to 10 days: 7.6-10.4 mg/dL (1.9-2.6 mmol/L)
- Children, 10 days to 24 months: 9-11 mg/dL (2.25-2.75 mmol/L)
- Children, 2 to 12 years: 8.8-10.8 mg/dL (2.2-2.7 mmol/L)
- Children, 12 to 18 years: 8.4-10.2 mg/dL (2.1-2.55 mmol/L)

Please refer to your institution's reference ranges as lab normals may vary.

INDICATIONS
Hypomagnesemia and suspected hypercalcemia
   Results Interpretation:
   Hypocalcemia
   Hypocalcemia frequently develops as a result of magnesium deficiency, possibly because of suppression of parathyroid hormone (PTH) secretion and end-organ resistance to PTH or as a direct effect of magnesium depletion on bone, independent of the effects of PTH.
   Hypocalcemia is not a result of hypercalciuria and generally corrects spontaneously once the primary magnesium deficiency is corrected.
   The degree of hypocalcemia is usually related to the severity of magnesium deficiency; however, hypocalcemia refractory to replacement therapy may develop in the presence of only small deficiencies of magnesium.

Suspected and known meningococcal disease in pediatric patients
   Results Interpretation:
   Hypocalcemia
   Hypocalcemia is a common finding in meningococcal disease.

Electrical trauma
   Results Interpretation:
   Hypocalcemia
   Concentrations of serum calcium less than 6.3 mg/dL have been noted in patients who have sustained electrical trauma.
   Although hypocalcemia may be associated with acute renal failure (usually within 3 days), hypocalcemia associated with electrical trauma is much more severe because of metastatic calcification in necrotic muscle, which occurs independently of renal failure.
   Tetany usually is not a feature, even with these low calcium levels, as long as the patient remains acidotic.

Known and suspected renal failure
    Strength of Recommendation: Class I
    Strength of Evidence: Category C
    Results Interpretation:
    Hypocalcemia

In acute renal failure (ARF), hypocalcemia (usually ranging from 6.3 to 8.3 mg/dL) is common and develops rapidly after disease onset. Hypocalcemia typically begins early during the oliguric phase and lasts through the diuretic phase of ARF.

In chronic renal failure (CRF), hypocalcemia appears to be a risk factor for mortality and for the development of bone disease and secondary hyperparathyroidism. A finding of hypocalcemia suggests moderate to severe CRF.

In patients with a GFR of 15 to 59 mL/minute (chronic kidney disease stages 3 and 4), serum levels of total corrected calcium should be maintained within the normal range. In patients with a GFR of less than 15 mL/minute or in patients on dialysis (chronic kidney disease stage 5), the serum total corrected calcium should be maintained at the lower end of normal (8.4 mg/dL to 9.5 mg/dL). If the serum total corrected calcium rises above 10.2 mg/dL in stage 5 patients, any medications or dialysate content that may be contributory should be adjusted.

In patients with chronic kidney disease stages 3 through 5, hypocalcemia should be treated if the serum total corrected calcium is below the lower end of normal (less than 8.4 mg/dL) and the patient is symptomatic or the parathyroid hormone (PTH) level is above the target range.

    Frequency of Monitoring

Serum calcium levels should be obtained every 12 months in Stage 3 chronic kidney disease (CKD) patients (GFR 30 to 59 mL/minute/1.73 m^2), every 3 months in Stage 4 patients (GFR 15 to 29 mL/minute/1.73 m^2), and every month in Stage 5 patients (GFR less than 15 mL/minute/1.73 m^2, or dialysis-dependent). More frequent serum calcium measurements are indicated in patients being treated for abnormal calcium levels.

Pancreatitis
    Results Interpretation:
    Hypocalcemia

Hypocalcemia occurs in 30% to 60% of patients with pancreatitis, although the exact pathogenesis is not well understood.

Hypocalcemia likely reflects imbalances in various hormones (including glucagon, calcitonin, and parathyroid hormone), the ability of free fatty acid-albumin complexes to bind calcium, and the concomitant presence of hypoalbuminemia.

A calcium level of less than 8 mg/dL is associated with a poor outcome.

Rhabdomyolysis
    Results Interpretation:

Hypercalcemia may occur in patients with rhabdomyolysis following skeletal muscle trauma and follows initial decreased calcium levels in 20% of patients with rhabdomyolysis and renal failure. It occurs in the diuretic phase of renal failure and is accompanied by hypercalciuria, hypophosphatemia, and phosphaturia. The rise in calcium levels is due to liberation of calcium salts previously precipitated by necrotic skeletal muscle.

    Hypocalcemia

Concentrations of serum calcium less than 6.3 mg/dL have been noted in rhabdomyolysis. Hypocalcemia has been found early in the course of the condition in more than 60% of patients. Tetany is usually not a feature as long as the patient remains acidotic.

Hypocalcemia in the setting of rhabdomyolysis is associated with acute renal failure (usually within 3 days) and metastatic calcification in necrotic muscle, which occurs independently of renal failure.

Suspected and known primary hyperparathyroidism
    Strength of Recommendation: Class I
    Strength of Evidence: Category C
    Results Interpretation:

Elevated levels of serum calcium and parathyroid hormone (PTH) are essentially diagnostic of primary hyperparathyroidism, although this pattern also may be seen in cases of familial hypocalciuric hypercalcemia or when the patient is taking lithium or thiazide diuretics.

The majority of patients with primary hyperparathyroidism have both elevated serum PTH and serum calcium levels. In most patients, the serum calcium level is elevated to the level of 10.2 to 12 mg/dL, although the value may fluctuate from high-normal to high in some cases.

Occasionally, patients may present with calcium levels elevated to the life-threatening range, a state known as parathyroid crisis or acute primary hyperparathyroidism. This may occur in 6% to 14% of cases, with a serum calcium level above 15 mg/dL and accompanying symptoms of central nervous system (CNS) dysfunction (confusion, disorientation, coma), anorexia, nausea, weight loss, weakness, fatigue, and dehydration.

Particularly in the USA, most patients present with asymptomatic mild hypercalcemia with levels elevated less than 1 mg/dL above the upper limit of normal, often discovered on routine screening. In other parts of the world, however, such as parts of Western Europe and Asia, patients may present with more severe and/or symptomatic hypercalcemia.

According to the 2002 National Institutes of Health (NIH) Workshop guidelines, surgery is recommended when the serum calcium level is elevated more than 1 mg/dL above the upper limit of normal.

Normal serum calcium level

Primary hyperparathyroidism may occur in the setting of normal calcium and elevated PTH levels; this condition is usually diagnosed in the process of working up osteoporosis or osteopenia.

Some patients with primary hyperparathyroidism who have mildly elevated calcium levels (less than 0.5 mg/dL above the upper limit of normal) may have a normal serum calcium concentration on some measurements.

Frequency of Monitoring

According to the 2002 National Institutes of Health (NIH) Workshop guidelines, serum calcium should be monitored every 6 months in patients with primary hyperparathyroidism not undergoing surgery.

Suspected heat stroke
Results Interpretation:
Hypocalcemia

Hypocalcemia may be present due to sequestration of calcium in damaged muscle of heat stroke patients. However, it has also been seen in patients without evidence of muscle damage.

In one series, hypocalcemia was present in about 55% of patients with exertional heat stroke.

Hypercalcemia is sometimes seen in the acute phase, but only with accompanying severe muscle or soft tissue damage and acute oliguric renal failure

Hypercalcemia is commonly seen in the second week of recovery. It is postulated that this is due to excessive parathormone production secondary to initial hypocalcemia.

Suspected hemorrhagic shock
Results Interpretation:
Abnormal laboratory findings

With shock, cytoplasmic calcium increases, presumably secondary to cellular membrane leakage. A persistent increase in cellular calcium directly correlates with cell death.

Suspected hypercalcemia
Strength of Recommendation: Class I
Strength of Evidence: Category C
Results Interpretation:

Hypercalcemia is defined as a serum calcium level greater than 10.5 mg/dL.

Mild hypercalcemia (less than 12 mg/dL), which is often episodic, is the usual pattern seen in hyperparathyroidism. Repeat determinations of the serum calcium level may be necessary in these patients.

Severe hypercalcemia (greater than 14 mg/dL) usually occurs in malignant disease or other nonparathyroid disease states. Rarely, patients with hyperparathyroidism or parathyroid carcinoma will present in acute hypercalcemic crisis.

A calcium level greater than 13.5 mg/dL should be treated aggressively, regardless of symptoms.

Suspected hypocalcemia
Strength of Recommendation: Class I
Strength of Evidence: Category C
Results Interpretation:
Hypocalcemia

A decreased serum calcium concentration (less than 8.5 mg/dL) is critical in the diagnosis of hypocalcemia; however, the measured value must be interpreted carefully because the ionized fraction determines the likelihood of the patient being symptomatic.

Symptoms of hypocalcemia are correlated principally with the rate and degree of decline in calcium serum concentration. Calcium should be repleted, usually parenterally, in patients who are symptomatic.

In acidosis, there is increased dissociation of calcium from albumin.

Normal serum calcium level

In the presence of alkalosis, there is enhanced binding of calcium to albumin, although the total calcium level will be unchanged. For this reason, tetany may occur in the presence of a normal total serum calcium concentration. If hypocalcemic tetany is suspected, arterial pH and serum ionized calcium level should be measured.

Suspected necrotizing fasciitis
Results Interpretation:
Lowered laboratory findings

A moderate decrease in the serum calcium level may be noted in patients with necrotizing fasciitis, presumably due to the binding of calcium with fatty acids formed in the gut by bacterial lipase.

Suspected or known measles
Results Interpretation:
Hypocalcemia

Transitory, asymptomatic hypocalcemia associated with a decrease in the parathyroid hormone level has been reported during epidemics of measles in nonvaccinated young adults.

In one series, serum calcium less than 2 mmol/L was present in 54% of hospitalized adults with measles.

Hypocalcemia has also been reported in children and may be severe. One series found serum calcium levels less than 1.87 mmol/L in 11 of 15 children with severe measles. Phosphorus levels were normal to low, suggesting decreased absorption or malnutrition rather than hypoparathyroidism.

Suspected pheochromocytoma
Results Interpretation:

Hypercalcemia may be present in persons with pheochromocytoma in the absence of parathyroid disease. It resolves after tumor resection. Hypercalcemia is present in patients who have multiple endocrine neoplasia type II A with their hyperparathyroidism being a result of parathyroid hyperplasia or a parathyroid adenoma.

Suspected toxic shock syndrome
Results Interpretation:
Hypocalcemia

Hypocalcemia, which can be severe, occurs in over 50% of patients with toxic shock syndrome (TSS) and usually resolves in 1 to 2 weeks. The degree of hypocalcemia observed in TSS is greater than that expected with the decrease in plasma proteins associated with TSS. Hypocalcemia is thought to be due to a direct effect of toxin on the calcium-parathyroid hormone mechanism or may be due to hypercalcitoninemia.

Serum albumin concentration directly effects total serum calcium; for every 1 g/dL decrease in serum albumin there is a corresponding 0.8 mg/dL decrease in total serum calcium.

Ionized calcium levels are inversely related to serum albumin concentration; total calcium may be low in hypoalbuminemia while ionized calcium is normal. Symptoms usually develop when ionized calcium is below 2.5 mg/dL.

Tumor lysis syndrome
Strength of Recommendation: Class I
Strength of Evidence: Category C
Results Interpretation:
Hypocalcemia

In tumor lysis syndrome, hypocalcemia may be caused by the precipitation of calcium phosphate, which can occur when the solubility product of calcium and phosphate is exceeded. Hypocalcemia may lead to muscle cramps, tetany, cardiac dysrhythmias, or seizures. Because of the risk of calcium phosphate precipitation, asymptomatic hypocalcemia should not be treated.

Frequency of Monitoring

In patients at risk for tumor lysis syndrome, serum chemistries should be obtained every 12 hours.

COMMON PANELS

- Basic metabolic panel
- Bone and joint panel
- Comprehensive metabolic panel
- Diabetic management panel
- Electrolyte panel
- Enteral/Parenteral nutritional management panel
- General health panel

- Hypertension panel
- Pancreatic panel
- Parathyroid panel
- Renal panel
- Transplant panel

ABNORMAL RESULTS
- Results increased in:
    - Dehydration
    - Polycythemia vera
- Results decreased in:
    - Hepatic cirrhosis

CLINICAL NOTES
To correct for hypoalbuminemia, add 0.8 mg/dL (2 mmol/L) to the total calcium serum concentration for each 1-g/dL decrease in serum albumin, although some data suggest that this adjustment may not provide an accurate prediction of the ionized calcium concentration.

COLLECTION/STORAGE INFORMATION
- Patient Preparation:
    - Have patient avoid exercise prior to specimen collection.
    - If possible, collect specimen while patient is fasting.
- Specimen Collection and Handling:
    - Collect specimen in marbled-top tube.
    - Avoid prolonged venous stasis, which may cause a false elevation in the serum calcium level.

LOINC CODES
- Code: 2000-8 (*Short Name* - Calcium SerPl-sCnc)
- Code: 17861-6 (*Short Name* - Calcium SerPl-mCnc)

Serum ceruloplasmin measurement

TEST DEFINITION
Measurement of ceruloplasmin in serum for the evaluation and management of copper-related disorders

SYNONYMS
- Serum caeruloplasmin level
- Serum caeruloplasmin measurement
- Serum ceruloplasmin level

REFERENCE RANGE
- Adults: 27-37 mg/dL (270-370 mg/L)
- Infants, 1 day to 3 months: 5-18 mg/dL (50-180 mg/L)
- Infants, 6 to 12 months: 33-43 mg/dL (330-430 mg/L)
- Children, 13 to 36 months: 26-55 mg/dL (260-550 mg/L)
- Children, 4 to 5 years: 27-56 mg/dL (270-560 mg/L)
- Children, 6 to 7 years: 24-48 mg/dL (240-480 mg/L)
- Children, older than 7 years: 20-54 mg/dL (200-540 mg/L)
    Please refer to your institution's reference ranges as lab normals may vary.

INDICATIONS
Suspected copper deficiency
        Strength of Recommendation: Class IIa
        Strength of Evidence: Category C

Results Interpretation:
Decreased level (laboratory finding)
In Menkes' disease, there is decreased copper absorption from the intestine, causing systemic copper and ceruloplasmin deficiencies.

Suspected Wilson's disease
Strength of Recommendation: Class IIa
Strength of Evidence: Category C
Results Interpretation:
Decreased level (laboratory finding)
Although a serum ceruloplasmin level is generally considered the most useful screening test for Wilson's disease, a low ceruloplasmin level cannot by itself establish the diagnosis. In symptomatic Wilson's disease, urinary copper levels are usually elevated, and liver biopsy may confirm the diagnosis.

ABNORMAL RESULTS
- Results increased in:
  - Pregnancy
  - Inflammation
  - Tissue necrosis
  - Trauma

CLINICAL NOTES
Serum ceruloplasmin levels measured immunochemically are almost always higher than levels measured enzymatically because immunologic methods measure the non-copper-bound apoprotein, which has no enzymatic activity, in addition to the copper-bound form. The oxidase assay has a lower detection limit than the nephelometric assay.

COLLECTION/STORAGE INFORMATION
- Specimen Collection and Handling:
  - Collect serum in red top tube.
  - May store at 4°C for 3 days or at -20°C for up to 4 weeks

LOINC CODES
- Code: 2064-4 (*Short Name* - Ceruloplasmin Ser-mCnc)

Serum chloride measurement

TEST DEFINITION
Measurement of serum chloride concentrations for the assessment of certain disorders manifesting with electrolyte abnormalities

SYNONYMS
- Serum chloride level

REFERENCE RANGE
- Adults: 98-106 mEq/L (98-106 mmol/L)
- Premature neonates: 95-110 mEq/L (95-110 mmol/L)
- Neonates, cord blood: 96-104 mEq/L (96-104 mmol/L)
- Neonates, 0 to 30 days: 98-113 mEq/L (98-113 mmol/L)
- Children, older than 30 days: 98-107 mEq/L (98-107 mmol/L)
Please refer to your institution's reference ranges as lab normals may vary.

INDICATIONS

Hypokalemia
Results Interpretation:
Increased level (laboratory finding)
High serum chloride levels with hypokalemia are usually associated with low serum bicarbonate levels and may reflect either metabolic acidosis (eg, diarrhea, renal tubular acidosis) or respiratory alkalosis (eg, cirrhosis, sepsis, salicylate poisoning).
Decreased level (laboratory finding)
Low serum chloride levels with hypokalemia are usually associated with increased serum bicarbonate and metabolic alkalosis, suggesting diuretic use, vomiting, hyperaldosteronism, or abuse of licorice or laxatives as the etiology of hypokalemia.

Initial evaluation and monitoring of diabetic ketoacidosis
Strength of Recommendation: Class I
Strength of Evidence: Category C
Results Interpretation:
Hyperchloremia
Chloride measurement is used to calculate plasma anion gap.

Hyperchloremic normal anion gap metabolic acidosis is present on admission in about 10% of patients with diabetic ketoacidosis (DKA) and is present in nearly all patients after resolution of ketonemia. During treatment, severity of hyperchloremia can be exacerbated by excessive chloride administration of 0.9% sodium chloride for hydration. In general, hyperchloremic metabolic acidosis is self-limiting with reduction in chloride load and judicious use of hydrating solution.
Frequency of Monitoring
Serum chloride should be monitored every 2 to 4 hours during treatment.

Metabolic acidosis
Results Interpretation:
Increased level (laboratory finding)
An elevated serum chloride level occurs in hyperchloremic acidosis, a metabolic acidosis in which the anion gap is normal. Hyperchloremia secondary to dehydration or a chronic respiratory alkalosis must be distinguished from hyperchloremic acidosis. Evaluation of the patient's history and arterial blood gases will distinguish normal anion gap metabolic acidosis from respiratory alkalosis.

Evaluation of the serum sodium level may aid in distinguishing hyperchloremia primarily due to dehydration from that due to metabolic acidosis. Hypernatremia suggests the presence of dehydration. If the serum chloride level remains high after a correction is made for the degree of dehydration, then an acid-base disturbance is also present.

Suspected acid-base balance disorder
Strength of Recommendation: Class IIa
Strength of Evidence: Category B
Results Interpretation:
Chloride level - finding
In critically ill patients, changes in chloride concentration appear to have the greatest impact upon base excess and, therefore, the overall metabolic acid-base state.
Hyperchloremia
In normal anion gap metabolic acidosis, an elevated serum chloride level occurs when the serum sodium level is normal.
Hypochloremia
In metabolic alkalosis, the serum electrolyte pattern is characterized by an elevated total CO2 content, hypochloremia, and hypokalemia.

Suspected pyloric stenosis
Strength of Recommendation: Class IIa
Strength of Evidence: Category B
Results Interpretation:
Hypochloremia
In infants with recurrent vomiting, a serum chloride concentration less than or equal to 98 mmol/L may be predictive of pyloric stenosis; however, given the test's low sensitivity, a higher serum chloride level would not be helpful in ruling out pyloric stenosis.

Hypochloremic, hypokalemic metabolic alkalosis is the classic electrolyte and acid-base imbalance that is pathognomonic of pyloric stenosis. In one series, hypochloremia was present on admission in approximately

25% of cases. The 'classic' metabolic derangements associated with pyloric stenosis are seen much less frequently than in past years, however. One study showed no electrolyte abnormalities at presentation in 88% of infants with pyloric stenosis treated since 1975.

Persistent vomiting leads to hypochloremia, with a serum chloride concentration in the range of 60 to 75 mEq/L; this implies a longer duration of illness with the consequent clinical changes.

Plasma chloride level may be a reliable and valid parameter for assessing and correcting hypochloremic alkalemia during fluid resuscitation, using a target level of 106 mmol/L.

COMMON PANELS
- Basic metabolic panel
- Comprehensive metabolic panel
- Diabetic management panel
- Electrolyte panel
- Enteral/Parenteral nutritional management panel
- General health panel
- Hypertension panel
- Renal panel

ABNORMAL RESULTS
- Results increased in:
    - Hypertriglyceridemia (colorimetric assay)
- Results decreased in:
    - Acute intermittent porphyria
    - Postprandial state

CLINICAL NOTES
Changes in chloride concentration typically reflect changes in sodium concentration. When this is not the case, an acid-base disorder is usually present.

COLLECTION/STORAGE INFORMATION
- Collect specimen while patient is fasting.
- Collect specimen in red marbled-top tube.
- Avoid hemolysis.

LOINC CODES
- Code: 2075-0 (*Short Name* - Chloride SerPl-sCnc)

Serum cholesterol measurement

TEST DEFINITION
Measurement of total cholesterol from serum to evaluate cardiovascular risk profile

SYNONYMS
- Serum cholesterol level

REFERENCE RANGE
- Adults: <200 mg/dL (<5.17 mmol/L)
- Pediatrics: <170 mg/dL (< 4.40 mmol/L)
  Please refer to your institution's reference ranges as lab normals may vary.

INDICATIONS
HIV with suspected lipodystrophy secondary to protease inhibitors
    Results Interpretation:
    Hypercholesterolemia
        Elevated cholesterol and triglyceride levels (greater than 5.5 mmol/L and greater than 2 mmol/L, respectively) can be seen within a syndrome (ie, lipodystrophy) of hyperlipidemia, fat wasting, central adiposity, and insulin resistance in HIV-infected patients on protease-inhibitor therapy.

Suspected hypercholesterolemia
>> **Strength of Recommendation:** Class I
>> **Strength of Evidence:** Category A
> **Results Interpretation:**
> **Hypercholesterolemia**
>> A total cholesterol of less than 200 mg/dL is desirable. A total cholesterol of 200 mg/dL to 239 mg/dL is considered borderline high, and a level of 240 mg/dL is considered high. Cholesterol goals may be lower in patients at high risk for coronary heart disease..

COMMON PANELS
- Lipid profile

ABNORMAL RESULTS
- Results increased in:
  - Age
  - Diet high in saturated fat
  - Male gender
  - Winter
- Results decreased in:
  - Malaria
  - Spring and summer

COLLECTION/STORAGE INFORMATION
- Specimen Collection and Handling
  - Use heparinized or EDTA containing tube
  - Separate serum from cells within 2 hours
  - Store at 4°C up to 7 days
  - Store at -20°C up to 3 months
  - Store at -70°C for longer than 3 months to several years
  - Avoid repeated freezing and thawing

LOINC CODES
- Code: 14647-2 (*Short Name* - Cholest SerPl-sCnc)
- Code: 9342-7 (*Short Name* - Cholest SerPl Qn)
- Code: 2093-3 (*Short Name* - Cholest SerPl-mCnc)

Serum cortisol measurement

TEST DEFINITION
Measurement of cortisol in serum for evaluation of adrenal dysfunction.

SYNONYMS
- Serum cortisol level

REFERENCE RANGE
- Adults:
- 8 AM to noon: 5-25 mcg/dL (138-690 nmol/L)
- 8 PM to 8 AM: 0-10 mcg/dL (0-276 nmol/L)
  Please refer to your institution's reference ranges as lab normals may vary.

INDICATIONS
Suspected adrenal insufficiency, eg, Addison's Disease
>> **Strength of Recommendation:** Class IIa
>> **Strength of Evidence:** Category B

Results Interpretation:
Decreased cortisol level

An unstimulated serum cortisol value less than 80 nmol/L, in the absence of corticosteroid-binding globulin deficiency, soundly implies adrenal insufficiency.

Decreased morning cortisol levels are consistent with a diagnosis of adrenal insufficiency.

Timing of Monitoring

An unstimulated cortisol level should be obtained between 6 AM and 9 AM.

Suspected Cushing's syndrome

Strength of Recommendation: Class IIa
Strength of Evidence: Category B
Results Interpretation:
Increased cortisol level

An elevated midnight cortisol level is consistent with a diagnosis of Cushing's syndrome.

Timing of Monitoring

Midnight is the optimal time for obtaining a cortisol level in patients with suspected hypercortisolism. This time period correlates with lowest diurnal cortisol levels.

ABNORMAL RESULTS

- Results increased in:
  - Depression
  - Hyperthyroidism
  - Hypoglycemia
  - Obesity
  - Pregnancy
  - Stress
- Results decreased in:
  - Cirrhosis
  - Hepatitis
  - Hypothyroidism

CLINICAL NOTES

Because tests for serum cortisol measure both free (bioactive) and protein-bound (non active) cortisol, additional testing for only free cortisol in urine may be useful.

COLLECTION/STORAGE INFORMATION

- Specimen Collection and Handling:
  - Obtain sample in a heparinized tube.
  - Store at 4° C for up to two days.
  - Freeze sample for storage beyond two days.

LOINC CODES

- Code: 32315-4 (*Short Name* - Cortis BS SerPl-sCnc)
- Code: 9813-7 (*Short Name* - Cortis AM SerPl-mCnc)
- Code: 9812-9 (*Short Name* - Cortis PM SerPl-mCnc)
- Code: 14679-5 (*Short Name* - Cortis AM SerPl-sCnc)
- Code: 2143-6 (*Short Name* - Cortis SerPl-mCnc)
- Code: 14678-7 (*Short Name* - Cortis PM SerPl-sCnc)

Serum creatine kinase measurement

TEST DEFINITION

Measurement of creatine kinase in serum for the evaluation of tissue damage, particularly muscle

SYNONYMS

- Serum CK measurement

REFERENCE RANGE
- Adult females: 40-150 units/L (0.67-2.5 microkat/L)
- Adult males: 60-400 units/L (1-6.67 microkat/L)
  Please refer to your institution's reference ranges as lab normals may vary.

INDICATIONS
Neuroleptic malignant syndrome
Results Interpretation:
Increased creatine kinase level

Serum creatine kinase (CK) levels may be more than 3 times the upper limit of normal. The majority of patients have levels of 2,000 to 15,000 units/L, although levels may range from less than 2,000 to 100,000 units/L. Extremely high CK levels may indicate the development of rhabdomyolysis, which can lead to renal failure.

Increased CK levels result from sustained muscle rigidity and myonecrosis in the setting of hyperpyrexia and are probably not directly linked to the underlying pathogenesis of neuroleptic malignant syndrome.

Suspected heat stroke
Results Interpretation:
Increased creatine kinase level

Serum creatine kinase level is elevated in most cases of heat stroke, indicating tissue disruption.

Peak serum creatine kinase levels greater than 10,000 units/L may be seen in patients with hypocalcemic exertional heat stroke, and may be useful in predicting acute renal failure.

Suspected HIV myopathy
Results Interpretation:
Increased creatine kinase level

Increased creatine kinase levels are seen in patients with HIV polymyositis, the most common myopathy associated with HIV infection. It may be difficult to differentiate HIV-related myopathy from myopathy associated with antiretroviral therapy.

Suspected muscle necrosis in patients with electrical or lightning trauma
Results Interpretation:
Increased creatine kinase level

Creatine kinase levels will rise in proportion to the amount of generalized muscle necrosis following electrical or lightning trauma. Acute myocardial infarction following electrical injury is rare.

Suspected Reye syndrome
Results Interpretation:
Increased creatine kinase level

Creatine kinase levels may be elevated in Reye syndrome.

Suspected rhabdomyolysis
Strength of Recommendation: Class IIa
Strength of Evidence: Category C
Results Interpretation:
Increased creatine kinase level

The hallmark of the diagnosis of rhabdomyolysis is an increase of creatine kinase to greater than 5 times normal without evidence of brain or cardiac injury.

Creatine kinase elevations tend to peak 24 to 48 hours after the initial insult, then gradually decrease in 5 to 7 days.

In tight fascial compartment injury, creatine kinase levels may again rise after 3 days to 5 days, secondary to the increased edema and further muscle necrosis.

In rhabdomyolysis, creatine kinase levels are markedly elevated, usually greater than 10 times the upper limit of normal and are associated with myalgia.

Suspected severe acute respiratory syndrome
Results Interpretation:
Increased creatine kinase level

Early in the respiratory phase of severe acute respiratory syndrome, elevated creatine kinase levels (as high as 3000 International Units/L) have been reported.

Suspected statin-induced myopathy
    Results Interpretation:
    Increased creatine kinase level
        Statin-induced rhabdomyolysis is defined as a creatine kinase (CK) level greater than 10 times upper limit of normal, and elevated creatinine levels. Markedly increased creatine kinase (CK) levels (greater than 10 times upper limit of normal [ULN]) have been reported in less than 0.08% of patients receiving statin therapy., most commonly seen in patients with major comorbidities and in patients receiving combination therapy.
        Statin-induced myositis is defined as muscle complaints with CK elevations. Some patients receiving statin therapy may have elevations in CK levels without any muscle complaints. The incidence of CK level elevations of less than 10 times ULN in patients treated with statin therapy is not known.

COMMON PANELS
- Cardiac injury panel

ABNORMAL RESULTS
- Results increased in:
  - Trauma
  - Surgery
  - Generalized convulsions
  - Malignant hyperpyrexia
  - Prolonged hypothermia
  - Delirium tremens
  - Acute psychotic reactions
  - Intramuscular injection
  - Chronic obstructive lung disease
  - Short-term strenuous exercise
- Results decreased in:
  - Small muscle mass
  - Sedentary lifestyle
  - Bedrest

COLLECTION/STORAGE INFORMATION
- Specimen Collection and Handling:
  - Collect 5 mL blood sample in a red top tube.
  - Avoid hemolysis.

LOINC CODES
- Code: 24335-2 (*Short Name* - CK Pan SerPl)
- Code: 2157-6 (*Short Name* - CK SerPl-cCnc)

Serum dehydroepiandrosterone measurement

TEST DEFINITION
Measurement of dehydroepiandrosterone (DHEA) in serum for the evaluation of adrenal dysfunction

SYNONYMS
- Serum dehydroepiandrosterone level
- Serum DHEA level

REFERENCE RANGE
- Adult males: 180-1,250 ng/dL (6.24-41.6 nmol/L)
- Adult females: 130-980 ng/dL (4.5-34 nmol/L)
- Premature infants: 80-3,150 ng/dL (2.8-109.3 nmol/L)
- Cord: 200-1,590 ng/dL (6.9-55.1 nmol/L)

- Newborn, 1 to 30 days: 50-760 ng/dL (1.7-26.3 nmol/L)
- Infants, 1 to 6 months: 26-385 ng/dL (0.9-13.4 nmol/L)
- Infants, 6 to 12 months: 18-95 ng/dL (0.6-3.3 nmol/L)
- Children, 1 to 6 years: <20-130 ng/dL (<0.7-4.5 nmol/L)
- Children, 6 to 8 years: <20-275 ng/dL (<0.7-9.5 nmol/L)
- Children, 8 to 10 years: 31-345 ng/dL (1.1-12 nmol/L)
- Male Tanner stages:
- Tanner stage 1: 31-345 ng/dL (1.1-12 nmol/L)
- Tanner stage 2: 110-495 ng/dL (3.8-17.2 nmol/L)
- Tanner stage 3: 170-585 ng/dL (5.9-20.3 nmol/L)
- Tanner stage 4: 160-640 ng/dL (5.5-22.2 nmol/L)
- Tanner stage 5: 250-900 ng/dL (8.7-31.2 nmol/L)
- Female Tanner stages:
- Tanner stage 1: 31-345 ng/dL (1.1-12 nmol/L)
- Tanner stage 2: 150-570 ng/dL (5.2-19.8 nmol/L)
- Tanner stage 3: 200-600 ng/dL (6.9-20.8 nmol/L)
- Tanner stage 4: 200-780 ng/dL (6.9-27 nmol/L)
- Tanner stage 5: 215-850 ng/dL (7.5-29.5 nmol/L)
  Please refer to your institution's reference ranges as lab normals may vary.

INDICATIONS
Suspected androgen decline in aging men (ADAM)
> **Strength of Recommendation:** Class IIb
> **Strength of Evidence:** Category C
> **Results Interpretation:**
> **Male climacteric**
> Dehydroepiandrosterone (DHEA) concentrations peak in males between the ages of 20 and 30 years, then decline. By age 70 to 80 years, concentrations are 20% of what they were at 20 to 30 years, with the greatest decline occurring by age 50 to 60 years. Although DHEA concentrations exhibit diurnal variation, this effect is less prominent in the elderly.

ABNORMAL RESULTS
- Results increased in:
  - Exercise
  - Noontime food intake
  - Smoking
- Results decreased in:
  - Anorexia nervosa
  - Depression (AM levels)
  - End-stage renal disease
  - Non-insulin dependent diabetes mellitus
  - Schizophrenia
  - Systemic lupus erythematosus

CLINICAL NOTES
DHEA levels are highest in the morning.

COLLECTION/STORAGE INFORMATION
- Collect serum in red top tube
- Refrigerate for up to 2 days or freeze at -20° C for up to 2 months

LOINC CODES
- Code: 16735-3 (*Short Name* - DHEA p chal SerPl-mCnc)
- Code: 12591-4 (*Short Name* - DHEA sp3 p chal SerPl-mCnc)
- Code: 15054-0 (*Short Name* - DHEA SerPl-sCnc)
- Code: 12592-2 (*Short Name* - DHEA sp4 p chal SerPl-mCnc)
- Code: 12593-0 (*Short Name* - DHEA sp5 p chal SerPl-mCnc)
- Code: 12594-8 (*Short Name* - DHEA sp6 p chal SerPl-mCnc)
- Code: 2193-1 (*Short Name* - DHEA SerPl-mCnc)
- Code: 16734-6 (*Short Name* - DHEA BS SerPl-mCnc)

- Code: 16733-8 (*Short Name* - DHEA sp9 p chal SerPl-mCnc)
- Code: 12590-6 (*Short Name* - DHEA sp2 p chal SerPl-mCnc)

Serum dibucaine number

TEST DEFINITION
A calculated number providing a functional assessment of pseudocholinesterase (butyrylcholinesterase, plasma cholinesterase, serum cholinesterase, non specific cholinesterase) activity

REFERENCE RANGE
- The clinically accepted normal range for dibucaine number is ≥ 70
- Dibucaine Number (DN) = {1 - (pseudocholinesterase activity in presence of inhibitor/pseudocholinesterase activity in absence of inhibitor)} x 100

Please refer to your institution's reference ranges as lab normals may vary.

INDICATIONS
Screen for pseudocholinesterase deficiency in patients with a family history of prolonged neuromuscular blockade during surgical procedures

Strength of Recommendation: Class IIa
Strength of Evidence: Category B
Results Interpretation:
Abnormal decrease in number

A low dibucaine number reflects a degree of functional impairment of the pseudocholinesterase enzyme, leading to prolongation of neuromuscular blockade following succinylcholine or mivacurium administration.

The most common genetic polymorphism for pseudocholinesterase associated with an abnormal dibucaine number is the A variant. In this variant, the amino acid aspartate is replaced with a glycine at amino acid 70 (G70D).

Heterozygotes, representing approximately 3 in 100 persons, typically have a dibucaine number of approximately 62. Heterozygotes have recovery from neuromuscular blockade from succinylcholine (suxamethonium) or mivacurium that is 3 to 8 times that of normal patients.

Approximately one person in 4,000 is a homozygote. These patients typically have a dibucaine number of about 20, which results in prolongation of neuromuscular blockade of up to 60 times that of normal.

Suspected pseudocholinesterase deficiency in patients with known prolonged muscular block occurring during surgical procedures

Strength of Recommendation: Class IIa
Strength of Evidence: Category B
Results Interpretation:
Abnormal decrease in number

A low dibucaine number reflects a degree of functional impairment of the pseudocholinesterase enzyme, leading to prolongation of neuromuscular blockade following administration of succinylcholine or mivacurium.

The most common genetic polymorphism for pseudocholinesterase associated with an abnormal dibucaine number is the A variant. In this variant, the amino acid aspartate is replaced with a glycine at amino acid 70 (G70D).

Heterozygotes, representing approximately 3 in 100 persons, typically have a dibucaine number of approximately 62. Heterozygotes have recovery from neuromuscular blockade from succinylcholine (suxamethonium) or mivacurium that is 3 to 8 times that of normal patients.

Approximately one person in 4,000 is a homozygote. These patients typically have a dibucaine number of about 20, which results in prolongation of neuromuscular blockade of up to 60 times that of normal.

CLINICAL NOTES
Genetic analysis has identified numerous variants of the gene that codes for pseudocholinesterase. Abnormal variants have been identified that, when tested, will have normal dibucaine numbers. Though unusual, some of the resulting protein variants (like the normal phenotype) are significantly inhibited by dibucaine. Still, these variants do not hydrolyze succinylcholine or related compounds normally and can only be identified by additional testing.

COLLECTION/STORAGE INFORMATION
- Collect venous blood in a heparinized (green-top) tube; separate plasma.
- Sample is stable at room temperature for 6 hours, at 4°C for 1 week, and at -70°C for 6 months.
- Prevent repeated thawing, freezing or hemolysis of sample.

LOINC CODES
- Code: 22754-6 (*Short Name* - Dibucaine Number Ser-aCnc)
- Code: 3554-3 (*Short Name* - Dibucaine Number Ser-mCnc)

Serum erythropoietin measurement

TEST DEFINITION
Serum or plasma erythropoietin levels used in the differential diagnosis of certain disorders of erythrocyte production

SYNONYMS
- Serum erythropoetin level
- Serum erythropoetin measurement

REFERENCE RANGE
- Adults: 5-36 international units/L
  Please refer to your institution's reference ranges as lab normals may vary.

INDICATIONS
Anemia in diabetes mellitus with suspected subclinical renal impairment
  Strength of Recommendation: Class IIb
  Strength of Evidence: Category C
  Results Interpretation:
  Decreased protein hormone level
  Impaired erythropoietin production in the presence of declining hemoglobin levels may contribute to anemia in diabetic patients. This impairment may manifest in subclinical kidney disease without reduction in glomerular filtration rate (GFR).

Differential diagnosis of polycythemia
  Strength of Recommendation: Class IIb
  Strength of Evidence: Category B
  Results Interpretation:
  Increased erythropoietin level
  - Increased erythropoietin (EPO) levels are highly correlated with secondary disease.
  - Normal EPO levels suggest relative polycythemia.
  - Decrease EPO levels are consistent with polycythemia vera.

COMMON PANELS
- Renal panel

CLINICAL NOTES
Morning erythropoietin values may be higher than afternoon values because of diurnal secretory patterns.

COLLECTION/STORAGE INFORMATION
Specimen Collection and Handling
- Collect 5 mL of venous blood in EDTA containing (lavender-top) tube

LOINC CODES
- Code: 14714-0 (*Short Name* - EPO Ser-sCnc)
- Code: 15061-5 (*Short Name* - EPO SerPl-aCnc)
- Code: 2237-6 (*Short Name* - EPO Ser-mCnc)

Serum estradiol measurement

TEST DEFINITION
Measurement of estradiol in serum or plasma.

SYNONYMS
- Serum estradiol level
- Serum oestradiol level
- Serum oestradiol measurement

REFERENCE RANGE
- Postmenopausal female: <59 pg/mL (217 pmol/L):
- Menstruating Adult Female
- Follicular phase: <20-145 pg/mL (184-532 pmol/L)
- Midcycle peak: 112-443 pg/mL (411-1,626 pmol/L)
- Luteal phase: <20-241 pg/mL (184-885 pmol/L)
- Adult Male: <20 pg/mL (184 pmol/L)
- Female Tanner Stages
- Tanner stage 1: 5-10 pg/mL (18-37 pmol/L)
- Tanner stage 2: 5-115 pg/mL (18-422 pmol/L)
- Tanner stage 3: 5-180 pg/mL (18-661 pmol/L)
- Tanner stage 4: 25-345 pg/mL (92-1,266 pmol/L)
- Tanner stage 5: 25-410 pg/mL (92-1,505 pmol/L)
- Male Tanner Stages
- Tanner stage 1: 3-15 pg/mL (11-55 pmol/L)
- Tanner stage 2: 3-10 pg/mL (11-37 pmol/L)
- Tanner stage 3: 5-15 pg/mL (18-55 pmol/L)
- Tanner stage 4: 3-40 pg/mL (11-147 pmol/L)
- Tanner stage 5: 15-45 pg/mL (55-165 pmol/L)
- Male and female children, 6 months to 10 years: <15 pg/mL (<55 pmol/L)
- Female infant, 30-60 days: 5-50 pg/mL (18-184 pmol/L)
- Male infant, 30-60 days old: 10-32 pg/mL (37-117 pmol/L)
- Cord blood: 3,000-29,000 pg/mL (11,010-106,430 pmol/L)
  Please refer to your institution's reference ranges as lab normals may vary.

INDICATIONS
Hypothalamic amenorrhea secondary to suspected anorexia nervosa
>   **Strength of Recommendation:** Class IIb
>   **Strength of Evidence:** Category C
> **Results Interpretation:**
> **Decreased estradiol level**
>   In anorexia nervosa, amenorrhea is a reflection of hypothalamic dysfunction caused by severe restriction of dietary fat, weight loss, and exercise. When gonadotropin releasing hormone (GnRH) is completely suppressed, hypogonadatropic hypogonadism results, with accompanying severely decreased estrogen levels.
>   When GnRH is incompletely suppressed, some follicular growth and estradiol secretion can continue, but the level of estradiol produced may be inadequate to stimulate the development of a dominant follicle and the resulting corpus luteum.

Suspected estrogen-secreting tumor
>   **Strength of Recommendation:** Class IIa
>   **Strength of Evidence:** Category C
> **Results Interpretation:**
> **Increased estradiol level**
>   Serum estradiol and other estrogens may be elevated secondary to estrogen-secreting tumors. Estradiol measurement may assist in making the diagnosis of estrogen-secreting neoplasm.

Suspected hypogonadism
>   **Strength of Recommendation:** Class IIa
>   **Strength of Evidence:** Category C

Results Interpretation:
Increased estradiol level

In males with primary hypogonadism (testicular failure) and secondary hypogonadism (pituitary or hypothalamic failure), estradiol level is increased.

In males at puberty, serum estrogens are increased due to conversion of testosterone to estradiol.

Decreased estradiol level

In females with primary or secondary hypogonadism, serum estradiol is consistently low and in the postmenopausal range (ie, less than 59 pg/mL [217 pmol/L]).

Suspected ovulation

Strength of Recommendation: Class IIa
Strength of Evidence: Category C
Results Interpretation:
Finding of ovulation

Serial estradiol measurements are used to monitor follicular growth and predict ovulation in females with spontaneous menstrual cycles. Serum estradiol rises steadily during the second half of the follicular phase, reaching a peak 1 to 2 days before ovulation when the average concentration is approximately 1,000 pmol/L.

Suspected polycystic ovary syndrome (PCOS)

Strength of Recommendation: Class IIb
Strength of Evidence: Category C
Results Interpretation:
Irregular periods

Abnormally secreted estrogen results in chronic anovulation in polycystic ovary syndrome (PCOS). Serum concentrations of estradiol (both total and free) are within the normal range for the early follicular and mid-follicular phases of the menstrual cycle.

The pattern of estrogen secretion in PCOS differs from a normal menstrual cycle due to a lack of preovulatory or midluteal increase in estradiol concentrations.

Frequency of Monitoring

Serial estradiol measurement during the menstrual cycle may be useful in combination with ultrasonography to investigate ovulatory dysfunction.

Timing of Monitoring

Blood can be collected at any time of the day.

Suspected precocious puberty

Strength of Recommendation: Class IIa
Strength of Evidence: Category C
Results Interpretation:
Increased estradiol level

In precocious puberty, estradiol level is typically increased. In rare cases, estradiol level is undetectable.

In pseudoprecocious puberty, serum estradiol levels are increased as a result of estrogen secretion, usually by ovarian or adrenal tumors, or by stimulation of the ovaries by hCG from an hCG-secreting tumor.

ABNORMAL RESULTS

- Results increased in:
  - Obesity
  - Hyperthyroidism
  - Liver disease
  - Gynecomastia
  - Precocious puberty Results decreased in:
  - Vegetarians
  - Turner's Syndrome
  - Menopause

CLINICAL NOTES

- Estradiol is the most potent estrogen.
- Primary sites of estradiol synthesis include ovaries, testes, adrenal cortex, peripheral tissues, and placenta.
- Estradiol is eliminated in the liver.
- Pre-ovulatory ovarian follicle is main source of estrogen during reproductive years.

- Estradiol secretion can vary as much as 50% in a 30-minute time frame in the pre-ovulatory period in females, requiring serial measurements to assess follicular growth or to monitor estradiol levels during spontaneous and stimulated cycles.
- Considerable variation exists with all current and new methods of estradiol testing. Interpret results within the context of other clinical parameters.

COLLECTION/STORAGE INFORMATION
- Specimen Collection and Handling:
  - Collect serum in red top tube
  - May be stored in glass tube at 2°C to 8°C for 2 days, otherwise freeze and store at -20°C
  - Note the time of sampling and menstrual cycle day for nonpregnant women

LOINC CODES
- Code: 14960-9 (*Short Name* - Estradiol Free % SerPl)
- Code: 13883-4 (*Short Name* - Estradiol Bioavail % SerPl)
- Code: 24414-5 (*Short Name* - Estradiol BS SerPl-mCnc)
- Code: 17844-2 (*Short Name* - Estradiol Alb Bnd SerPl-mCnc)
- Code: 2243-4 (*Short Name* - Estradiol SerPl-mCnc)
- Code: 12596-3 (*Short Name* - Estradiol 3H p chal SerPl-mCnc)
- Code: 13884-2 (*Short Name* - Estradiol Bioavail SerPl-mCnc)
- Code: 14715-7 (*Short Name* - Estradiol SerPl-sCnc)

Serum ferritin measurement

TEST DEFINITION
Measurement of the body's major iron storage protein to evaluate the body's total iron stores, in uncomplicated iron deficiency states, iron overload states (ie, hemochromatosis), and to monitor response to iron therapy

SYNONYMS
- Serum ferritin level

REFERENCE RANGE
- Adult males: 30-300 ng/mL (30-300 mcg/L)
- Adult females: 10-200 ng/mL (10-200 mcg/L)
- Newborns: 25-200 ng/mL (25-200 mcg/L)
- Children, 1 month: 200-600 ng/mL (200-600 mcg/L)
- Children, 2-5 months: 50-200 ng/mL (50-200 mcg/L)
- Children, 6 months-15 years: 7-140 ng/mL (7-140 mcg/L)
  Please refer to your institution's reference ranges as lab normals may vary.

INDICATIONS
Suspected acute respiratory distress syndrome (ARDS)
　　Results Interpretation:
　　Serum ferritin high
　　　　Serum ferritin levels are significantly increased in patients at risk of acute respiratory distress syndrome (ARDS) and in established cases, as compared with healthy controls.

Suspected adult-onset Still's disease
　　Strength of Recommendation: Class IIb
　　Strength of Evidence: Category B
　　Results Interpretation:
　　Increased level (laboratory finding)
　　　　An increase in serum ferritin level may be suggestive of adult-onset Still's disease (AOSD). Ferritin levels greater than 1,000 mcg/L in women and 1,500 mcg/L in men (five times the upper limit of normal) have been associated with AOSD. In patients with inactive disease, ferritin may have limited clinical utility.
　　　　In one retrospective multicenter study of 169 patients, the combined use of serum ferritin (five times the upper limit of normal) and glycosylated ferritin (less than or equal to 20%) was useful in the differential diagnosis of AOSD.

Suspected hemochromatosis
> **Strength of Recommendation:** Class IIa
> **Strength of Evidence:** Category C

Results Interpretation:

Increased level (laboratory finding)

Serum ferritin concentrations vary with age and sex; however values more than 2 standard deviations above the appropriate mean are considered abnormal. The combination of an elevated ferritin value that is twice normal, and an elevated transferrin saturation (60% for men and 50% for women) is suggestive of iron overload.

The diagnosis of hemochromatosis is based on several parameters: an elevated serum ferritin level (greater than or equal to 200 mcg/L in premenopausal women and greater than or equal to 300 mcg/L in men or postmenopausal women), a transferrin saturation of 55% or more, or evidence of liver disease.

Normal laboratory findings

Normal ferritin levels do not exclude the diagnosis of hemochromatosis, but do suggest that substantial hepatic overload has not yet occurred. Elevated transferrin saturation is the earliest evidence of hemochromatosis and may be seen before elevation in ferritin levels

Frequency of Monitoring

In patients with transferrin saturation of 45% to 55%, repeat ferritin levels in 2 years if initial results are normal. In patients with transferrin saturation greater than 55%, reevaluate ferritin levels annually or biennially.

Suspected iron deficiency anemia
> **Strength of Recommendation:** Class IIa
> **Strength of Evidence:** Category C

Results Interpretation:

Ferritin level low

A ferritin level of 15 mcg/L or less is a marker of depleted or absent iron stores, and confirms iron deficiency anemia in the presence of low Hgb or HCT.

As ferritin levels may be normal or increased in anemia of chronic disease, using a cutoff level of 30 mcg/L or less may be more accurate in detecting concomitant iron deficiency anemia.

A low serum ferritin concentration is an early finding in iron deficiency, and may detect declining body iron stores before overt anemia develops.

A low serum ferritin concentration develops earlier than the drop in hemoglobin concentration, hematocrit, erythrocyte count, and MCV or the increase in red-cell distribution width and free erythrocyte protoporphyrin.

The cutoff value for serum ferritin for the diagnosis of iron deficiency is 8 to 12 mcg/L (8 to 12 ng/mL) in children aged 1 to 5 years.

Serum ferritin normal

A small proportion of iron-deficient patients may have a normal serum ferritin level, because serum ferritin is also an acute-phase reactant.

Serum ferritin high

The serum ferritin concentration does not reflect iron stores in persons with chronic disorders such as rheumatoid arthritis, chronic infections, or malignancies. With liver injury, as in hepatitis, the serum ferritin concentration is increased, often markedly so. In each of these disorders, the serum ferritin concentration is elevated, and this elevation may mask concomitant iron deficiency.

Some rheumatologists have adopted the rule that if the serum ferritin concentration is over 90 mcg/L in a patient with rheumatoid arthritis, concurrent iron deficiency is unlikely.

Suspected preterm labor

Results Interpretation:

Serum ferritin high

High third trimester maternal serum markers of ferritin are associated with preterm delivery and markers of maternal infection. Statistically significant elevations are seen in serum ferritin levels of women who will develop preterm labor and delivery.

High plasma ferritin levels, especially at 26 weeks, were strongly associated with subsequent preterm delivery and low birth weight in a study of black women.

COMMON PANELS

• Iron panel

COLLECTION/STORAGE INFORMATION
- Specimen Collection and Handling:
  - Collect sample in a marbled top tube.
  - Avoid violent mixing which may denature ferritin.
  - Store sample for up to 7 days at 2°C to 8°C or for 6 months at -20°C
- Patient Preparation:
  - Have patient fast prior to blood draw.

LOINC CODES
- Code: 2276-4 (*Short Name* - Ferritin Ser-mCnc)
- Code: 20567-4 (*Short Name* - Ferritin Ser EIA-mCnc)
- Code: 14723-1 (*Short Name* - Ferritin Ser-sCnc)

Serum flecainide level

TEST DEFINITION
Measuring of flecainide levels in serum or plasma for therapeutic monitoring and assessment of toxicity.

REFERENCE RANGE
- Adults: 0.2-1 mg/L (0.5-2.4 micromol/L)
  Please refer to your institution's reference ranges as lab normals may vary.

INDICATIONS
Flecainide therapeutic drug monitoring
> **Strength of Recommendation:** Class IIb
> **Strength of Evidence:** Category B
> **Results Interpretation:**
> **Therapeutic drug level - finding**
> The therapeutic range for flecainide is 0.2 to 1 mg/L (0.5 micromol/L to 2.4 micromol/L). Levels below 0.2 mg/L (0.5 micromol/L) are sub-therapeutic and levels greater than 1 mg/L (2.4 micromol/L) predispose to toxicity.
> **Frequency of Monitoring**
> Flecainide reaches steady state in 3 to 5 days following treatment initiation. During this period, monitoring of serum levels is indicated.
> Levels should also be closely monitored in patients with conditions that may impair drug clearance and/or metabolism. More frequent monitoring and dosing adjustments may be necessary in these patients to avoid toxicity.
> **Timing of Monitoring**
> Flecainide levels should be assayed one hour prior to next dosing (trough).

ABNORMAL RESULTS
- Results increased by:
  - Decreased cardiac output
  - Renal disease
  - Urinary alkalinization
  - Liver disease
  - Interference with cytochrome P450 2D6 enzymes
- Results decreased by:
  - Induction of cytochrome P450 2D6 enzymes
  - Urinary acidification

COLLECTION/STORAGE INFORMATION
- Specimen Collection and Handling:
  - Collect blood for flecainide measurement one hour prior to the next dose (trough)
  - Obtain sample in a heparinized or EDTA containing tube

LOINC CODES
- Code: 15105-0 (*Short Name* - Flecainide SerPl-sCnc)
- Code: 3638-4 (*Short Name* - Flecainide SerPl-mCnc)

Serum follicle stimulating hormone measurement

TEST DEFINITION
Measurement of follicle stimulating hormone (FSH) level in serum for the evaluation and management of endocrine disorders

SYNONYMS
- Serum follicle stimulating hormone level

REFERENCE RANGE
- Female, menstruating:
- Follicular phase: 3-20 milli-International Units/mL (3-20 International Units/L)
- Ovulatory phase: 9-26 milli-International Units/mL (9-26 International Units/L)
- Luteal phase: 1-12 milli-International Units/mL (1-12 International Units/L)
- Postmenopausal: 18-153 milli-International Units/mL (18-153 International Units/L)
- Male: 1-12 milli-International Units/mL (1-12 International Units/L).
- Female 2-11 months: 0.10-11.3 milli-International Units/mL (0.19-11.3 International Units/L)
- Male 2-11 months: 0.19-11.3 milli-International Units/mL (0.19-11.3 International Units/L)
- Female 1-10 years: 0.68-6.7 milli-International Units/mL (0.68-6.7 International Units/L)
- Male 1-10 years: 0.3-4.6 milli-International Units/mL (0.3-4.6 International Units/L)
- Puberty, Tanner stages (TS):
- TS 1-2 Female: 0.68-6.7 milli-International Units/mL (0.68-6.7 International Units/L)
- TS 3-4 Female: 1-7.4 milli-International Units/mL (1-7.4 International Units/L)
- TS 5 Female: 1-9.2 milli-International Units/mL (1-9.2 International Units/L)
- Puberty, Tanner stages (TS):
- TS 1-2 Male: 0.3-4.6 milli-International Units/mL (0.3-4.6 International Units/L)
- TS 3-4 Male: 1.24-15.4 milli-International Units/mL (1.24-15.4 International Units/L)
- TS 5 Male: 1.53-6.8 milli-International Units/mL (1.53-6.8 International Units/L)
  Please refer to your institution's reference ranges as lab normals may vary.

INDICATIONS
Primary or secondary amenorrhea
> **Strength of Recommendation:** Class IIa
> **Strength of Evidence:** Category C
> **Results Interpretation:**
> **Decreased pituitary follicle stimulating hormone**
> Low follicle-stimulating hormone (FSH) levels indicate hypogonadotropic hypogonadism or hypothalamic dysfunction. In these disorders, gonadotropin-releasing hormone secretion is very low, which results in low levels of FSH, luteinizing hormone, and estradiol. Most patients have hypothalamic dysfunction without apparent organic (hypothalamic or anterior pituitary) disease.
> **Increased pituitary follicle stimulating hormone level**
> A follicle-stimulating hormone level in the castrate range (greater than 30 International Units/L) in combination with a low estradiol level (less than 60 pmol/L) is diagnostic of ovarian failure or, rarely, resistant ovary syndrome.
> **Normal hormone production**
> About 30% of women with secondary amenorrhea have normal levels of gonadotropins (ie, follicle-stimulating hormone and luteinizing hormone). Women with normogonadotropic anovulation usually have polycystic ovaries.

Suspected hypogonadism
> **Strength of Recommendation:** Class IIa
> **Strength of Evidence:** Category C

Results Interpretation:
Increased pituitary follicle stimulating hormone level
- Men:
  - Increased levels of serum follicle-stimulating hormone (FSH) and luteinizing hormone (LH) suggest primary testicular failure in men.
  - In men, the diagnosis of hypogonadism is first suggested by a decrease in sperm count or testosterone, and is confirmed by elevated gonadotropin levels.
  - After puberty onset, men with Klinefelter syndrome have uniformly elevated FSH and LH levels, regardless of the serum testosterone level. Before puberty onset, the FSH, LH, and testosterone levels are normal.
  - In men, an isolated increase in FSH levels with normal LH and testosterone levels suggests failure of the testicular germ cell compartment.
- Women: If obtained during the early follicular phase, follicle-stimulating hormone (FSH) levels greater than 10 International Units/L indicate reduced ovarian reserve, and levels greater than 40 International Units/L indicate ovarian failure.

Decreased pituitary follicle stimulating hormone
- Men:
  - Patients with low or normal FSH and LH levels and low testosterone levels, are categorized as having hypogonadotropic hypogonadism. Men with a selective decrease of LH and FSH without any apparent cause, and with normal function of the other pituitary hormones, are categorized as having isolated gonadotropin deficiency or idiopathic hypogonadotropic hypogonadism.
  - In Kallman syndrome (classic hypogonadotropic hypogonadism) FSH, testosterone and LH levels will be low.
- Women:
  - In the early follicular phase, FSH levels less than 5 International Units/L suggest hypothalamic or pituitary dysfunction.
  - FSH, LH and estradiol levels in women with hypogonadotrophic hypogonadism will be low, regardless of the cause.

Normal laboratory findings
- Men with azoospermia and normal follicle-stimulating hormone (FSH), luteinizing hormone (LH) and testosterone levels may have an obstructive lesion requiring further evaluation.

Suspected menopause
Strength of Recommendation: Class IIb
Strength of Evidence: Category B
Results Interpretation:
Increased pituitary follicle stimulating hormone level
The cutoff value of 40 International Units/L is not independently useful for clinical determination of postmenopausal status.

High levels of follicle-stimulating hormone (FSH) alone should not be used to diagnose menopause in menstruating women.

In women aged 45 to 55 years without a uterus or hot flashes, follicle stimulating hormone (FSH) levels greater than 30 International Units/L suggest menopause.

During the perimenopause, follicle stimulating hormone (FSH) levels may rise to postmenopausal levels during some cycles, but return to premenopausal levels in subsequent cycles; in addition, pulsatile secretory patterns complicate results interpretation.

Suspected premature ovarian failure
Results Interpretation:
Increased pituitary follicle stimulating hormone level
Premature ovarian failure is characterized by elevated follicle stimulating hormone (FSH) levels before the age of 40, and it is the result of premature depletion of the oocyte-follicle complex.

To predict ongoing pregnancy rates for assisted reproductive procedures
Strength of Recommendation: Class III
Strength of Evidence: Category B
Results Interpretation:
Increased pituitary follicle stimulating hormone level
Cutoff values, used to test ovarian reserve, range from 10 to 25 milli-International Units/mL; variations are due to laboratory factors, such as laboratory technique and, reference standards.

A high basal follicle-stimulating hormone (FSH) level identifies women who are very unlikely to have an ongoing pregnancy after in vitro fertilization. However, a definitive basal FSH level requires such a high cutoff level that the proportion of patients with a positive test is small.

Frequency of Monitoring

Once an elevated basal (day 3) follicle-stimulating hormone (FSH) level is attained, repeated testing during subsequent cycles, even if FSH values are normal, has no apparent utility (eg, does not improve the prognostic value).

Timing of Monitoring

Blood sampling for follicle-stimulating hormone (FSH) levels is recommended on menstrual cycle day 3, because FSH levels are reported to be at or near maximum at that time. Measurements of basal FSH levels on cycle days 2 to 5 do not vary significantly, but blood should be drawn before cycle day 4 if an estradiol measurement is included.

ABNORMAL RESULTS

- Results increased in:
    - Alcoholism
    - Post-castration
- Results decreased in:
    - Hemochromatosis
    - Anorexia nervosa
    - Pregnancy
    - Severe illness
    - Hyperprolactinemia
    - Sickle cell disease

CLINICAL NOTES

Because follicle stimulating hormone levels vary throughout the day and during different phases of the menstrual cycle, clinical assessment may require pooled or multiple serial blood specimens. However, a single specimen is often sufficient in persons with high gonadotropin levels (eg, anorchism or postmenopausal women).

COLLECTION/STORAGE INFORMATION

- Collection and Handling Information:
    - Collect 7 mL of venous blood in a red top tube
    - Store refrigerated or frozen. Stable for 8 days at room temperature and for 14 days at 4°C

LOINC CODES

- Code: 2288-9 (*Short Name* - A-FSH SerPl-sCnc)
- Code: 20433-9 (*Short Name* - FSH SerPl 2nd IRP-aCnc)
- Code: 27942-2 (*Short Name* - FSH SerPl-mCnc)
- Code: 27140-3 (*Short Name* - A-FSH SerPl-mCnc)
- Code: 2289-7 (*Short Name* - B-FSH SerPl-sCnc)
- Code: 15067-2 (*Short Name* - FSH SerPl-aCnc)

Serum free triiodothyronine measurement

TEST DEFINITION

Measurement of free triiodothyronine (fT_3) levels in serum for the evaluation and management of thyroid disorders

SYNONYMS

- Serum free T3 level
- Serum free triiodothyronine level

REFERENCE RANGE

- Adults: 1.4-4.4 pg/mL (0.22-6.78 pmol/L)
- Neonates older than 37 weeks (cord blood): 15-391 pg/dL (0.2-6 pmol/L)
- Pregnancy, 1st trimester: 211-383 pg/dL (3.2-5.9 pmol/L)

- Pregnancy, 2nd trimester: 196-338 pg/dL (3-5.2 pmol/L)
- Pregnancy, 3rd trimester: 196-338 pg/dL (3-5.2 pmol/L)
  Please refer to your institution's reference ranges as lab normals may vary.

INDICATIONS

Suspected hyperthyroidism
> **Strength of Recommendation:** Class IIa
> **Strength of Evidence:** Category C

Results Interpretation:
Increased triiodothyronine level
> An elevated free triiodothyronine (fT_3) level in conjunction with a low thyroid stimulating hormone (TSH) and elevated free thyroxine (fT_4) is diagnostic for primary hyperthyroidism.

Normal laboratory findings
> A normal fT_3 level may occur in conjunction with a low TSH and normal fT_4 in subclinical primary hyperthyroidism, which is most often seen in the elderly.

Suspected triiodothyronine (T_3) thyrotoxicosis
> **Strength of Recommendation:** Class IIa
> **Strength of Evidence:** Category C

Results Interpretation:
Increased triiodothyronine level
> In triiodothyronine (T_3) toxicosis, there is an increase in serum free T_3 with normal free thyroxine (fT_4) and low thyroid stimulating hormone (TSH) levels. This entity occurs in less than 5% of thyrotoxicosis patients in North America.

COMMON PANELS

- Transplant panel

ABNORMAL RESULTS

- Results increased in high altitude.
- Results decreased in acute illness.

CLINICAL NOTES

Peak serum values of free triiodothyronine (fT_3) occur from 2 to 4 hours post-administration of thyroid preparations containing T_3. Stable levels of serum T_3 will be reached after weeks of treatment. Measuring free instead of total triiodothyronine levels will largely bypass having to account for changes in thyroid-binding protein concentration, although extreme changes in these protein concentrations may still affect free-hormone assays.

COLLECTION/STORAGE INFORMATION

- Collect serum sample.
- Although sample is stable for 7 days at room temperature, storage at 4°C or in freezer is preferred.

LOINC CODES

- Code: 25807-9 (*Short Name* - T3Free sp5 p chal SerPl-sCnc)
- Code: 25808-7 (*Short Name* - T3Free sp6 p chal SerPl-sCnc)
- Code: 25809-5 (*Short Name* - T3Free sp7 p chal SerPl-sCnc)
- Code: 25811-1 (*Short Name* - T3Free sp9 p chal SerPl-sCnc)
- Code: 25805-3 (*Short Name* - T3Free sp3 p chal SerPl-sCnc)
- Code: 25806-1 (*Short Name* - T3Free sp4 p chal SerPl-sCnc)

Serum fructosamine measurement

TEST DEFINITION

Measurement of fructosamines for the evaluation of intermediate-term (2 to 3 weeks) blood sugar concentration (control)

Synonyms
- Serum fructosamine level

Reference Range
- Adults (NBT): 1.61-2.68 mmol/L
- Adults (colorimetry, affinity chromatography): 1%-2% of total protein (0.01-0.02 fraction of total protein)
- Children: 5% below adult levels
  Please refer to your institution's reference ranges as lab normals may vary.

Indications
Diabetes mellitus monitoring
> **Strength of Recommendation:** Class IIb
> **Strength of Evidence:** Category B
> **Results Interpretation:**
> **Increased level (laboratory finding)**
> Regardless of technique used, the fructosamine assay appears to be useful for monitoring diabetes, with moderate correlation with glucose and Hgb A1$_c$. Fructosamine reflects the mean glucose concentration over 2 to 3 weeks in contrast with Hgb A1$_c$, which reflects the mean glucose concentration over 6 to 8 weeks because albumin and other proteins have a half-life of 2.5 to 23 days compared with 60 days for Hgb.

Abnormal Results
- High uric acid
- High bilirubin level

Clinical Notes
Fructosamine levels may be particularly useful when hemoglobin A1$_c$ cannot be measured accurately (eg, hemoglobinopathies, hemolytic anemias).

Contraindications
The fructosamine assay should not be performed when serum albumin is less than or equal to 3 mg/dL.

Collection/Storage Information
- Collect in marble-top (serum separator) tube

LOINC Codes
- Code: 2294-7 (*Short Name* - Fructosamine Ser-cCnc)
- Code: 15069-8 (*Short Name* - Fructosamine Ser-sCnc)

Serum gamma-glutamyl transferase measurement

Test Definition
Measurement of gamma-glutamyltransferase (gamma-glutamyltranspeptidase) in serum for the evaluation and management of hepatobiliary dysfunction

Synonyms
- Serum gamma-glutamyl transferase level

Reference Range
- Adults: 1-94 units/L
- Neonates, cord blood: 11-194 units/L (0.19-3.3 microkatal/L)
- Neonates, 0 to 1 month: 0-151 units/L (0-2.57 microkatal/L)
- Infants, 1 to 2 months: 0-114 units/L (0-1.94 microkatal/L)
- Infants, 2 to 4 months: 0-81 units/L (0-1.38 microkatal/L)
- Infants, 4 to 7 months: 0-34 units/L (0-0.58 microkatal/L)

- Children, 7 months to 15 years: 0-25 units/L (0-0.43 microkatal/L)
Please refer to your institution's reference ranges as lab normals may vary.

INDICATIONS
Suspected alcohol abuse
    Strength of Recommendation: Class IIb
    Strength of Evidence: Category B
    Results Interpretation:
    Gamma-glutamyl transferase raised
        From 35% to 85% of heavy drinkers have increased gamma-glutamyltransferase (GGT) levels after episodes of acute drinking; GGT is believed to be the most sensitive indicator of recent heavy drinking.
        An elevated GGT appears to have moderate sensitivity and high specificity for identifying active drinkers.

COMMON PANELS
- General health panel
- Hepatic function panel

ABNORMAL RESULTS
- Results increased in:
  - Infectious mononucleosis
  - Renal transplant
  - Hyperthyroidism
  - Myotonic dystrophy
  - Diabetes mellitus
  - African ancestry
  - Obesity
  - Moderate to heavy smoking
  - Acute renal failure
  - Stroke
  - Myocardial infarction
- Results decreased in :
  - Women
  - Hypothyroidism
  - Pregnancy

COLLECTION/STORAGE INFORMATION
- Collect serum in red top tube.
- May store specimen for 1 month at 4°C or 1 year at -20°C

LOINC CODES
- Code: 2324-2 (*Short Name* - GGT SerPl-cCnc)

Serum glomerular basement membrane antibody level

TEST DEFINITION
    Detection of anti-glomerular basement membrane (anti-GBM) antibodies in serum for the evaluation of anti-GBM related pulmonary and renal disorders

REFERENCE RANGE
- Adults, qualitative: Negative
- Adults, quantitative: <5 units/mL (<5 kunits/L)
Please refer to your institution's reference ranges as lab normals may vary.

INDICATIONS

Suspected antiglomerular basement membrane antibody-mediated glomerulonephritis
  Strength of Recommendation: Class IIa
  Strength of Evidence: Category C
  Results Interpretation:
  Glomerular basement membrane antibodies present
    Borderline values can be seen in latent and active antiglomerular basement membrane (anti-GBM) disease, while levels greater than 100 units may reflect active disease.
    A positive enzyme immunoassay result may require confirmation by the indirect fluorescent antibody method using human kidney tissue.

Suspected Goodpasture syndrome
  Strength of Recommendation: Class IIa
  Strength of Evidence: Category C
  Results Interpretation:
  Glomerular basement membrane antibodies present
    Borderline values can be seen in latent and active antiglomerular basement membrane (anti-GBM) disease, whereas levels greater than 100 units may reflect active disease.
    Because Goodpasture disease is most often monophasic, recurrence of autoantibody production is uncommon, although continued autoantibody production has been reported in rare cases of clinical relapse.
    A positive enzyme immunoassay result may require confirmation by the indirect fluorescent antibody method using human kidney tissue.

COLLECTION/STORAGE INFORMATION
- Store sample at -20°C.

LOINC CODES
- Code: 29994-1 (*Short Name* - GBM IgG Ser QI IF)
- Code: 29997-4 (*Short Name* - GBM IgG Ser EIA-aCnc)
- Code: 21093-0 (*Short Name* - GBM IgG Ser IF-Imp)
- Code: 31254-6 (*Short Name* - GBM IgG Ser-aCnc)
- Code: 16433-5 (*Short Name* - GBM Ab Ser QI)
- Code: 5056-7 (*Short Name* - GBM Ab Ser QI IF)
- Code: 29995-8 (*Short Name* - GBM IgA Ser QI IF)
- Code: 10862-1 (*Short Name* - GBM Ab Titr Ser)
- Code: 31255-3 (*Short Name* - GBM IgG Ser QI)
- Code: 31252-0 (*Short Name* - GBM Ab Ser-aCnc)
- Code: 31253-8 (*Short Name* - GBM IgA Ser QI)
- Code: 9329-4 (*Short Name* - GBM Ab Ser EIA-aCnc)
- Code: 16434-3 (*Short Name* - GBM Ab Ser IF-aCnc)

Serum haptoglobin measurement

TEST DEFINITION
   Measurement of haptoglobin serum concentrations for diagnosis and clinical management of hemolytic disorders

SYNONYMS
- Serum haptoglobin level

REFERENCE RANGE
- Adults: 16-199 mg/dL (0.16-1.99 g/L)
- Newborns: 5-48 mg/dL (50-480 mg/L)
- Ahaptoglobinemia is not uncommon in the neonate, and may persist up to the age of 3 months in up to 90% of infants.
- Children, 6 months to 16 years: 25-138 mg/dL (250-1380 mg/L)
  Please refer to your institution's reference ranges as lab normals may vary.

INDICATIONS

Dissolution of hematoma
>**Strength of Recommendation:** Class IIb
>**Strength of Evidence:** Category C

Results Interpretation:
Lowered hematology findings
Reduced serum haptoglobin concentrations are associated with the dissolution of organized hematomas and other hemorrhagic debris.

Infectious disease management
>**Strength of Recommendation:** Class IIb
>**Strength of Evidence:** Category C

Results Interpretation:
Raised hematology findings
Haptoglobin is an acute phase reactant protein; increased serum concentrations are routinely seen in acute and chronic infection.

Haptoglobin serum concentrations may rise 3 to 8-fold in response to acute or chronic bacterial or parasitic infection (including localized infections).

Severe liver disease
>**Strength of Recommendation:** Class IIb
>**Strength of Evidence:** Category C

Results Interpretation:
Lowered hematology findings
Reduced serum haptoglobin concentrations, in severe hepatocellular pathology, represent a primary deficiency state due either to failed hepatic haptoglobin biosynthesis or to depressed hepatocyte secretion of haptoglobin.

Suspected blood transfusion reaction
>**Strength of Recommendation:** Class IIa
>**Strength of Evidence:** Category C

Results Interpretation:
Lowered hematology findings
Low serum haptoglobin concentrations occur in association with hemolytic blood transfusion reactions.

Suspected hemolytic anemia
>**Strength of Recommendation:** Class IIa
>**Strength of Evidence:** Category C

Results Interpretation:
Lowered hematology findings
Low serum concentrations of haptoglobin occur in both intravascular and extravascular hemolysis, in erythroblastosis fetalis, and in hemoglobinopathies represented by sickle cell anemia and the thalassemias.

A complete absence of free serum haptoglobin may be seen with intravascular hemolysis.

A serum haptoglobin cut-off level of 0.2 g/L is considered useful in differentiating between primary and secondary hemolytic anemia.

Haptoglobin is an acute phase reactant. If hemolysis occurs concomitantly with an acute inflammatory state, the hemolysis-induced decline in haptoglobin serum concentration will occur substantially faster compared with the acute-phase induction of haptoglobin synthesis.

COMMON PANELS
- Hemolysis panel

ABNORMAL RESULTS
- Results increased in:
  - Biliary obstruction
  - Major depression, unipolar
- Results decreased in:
  - Pregnancy
  - Subacute bacterial endocarditis

Clinical Notes

As an acute-phase reactant, serum haptoglobin concentrations display bidirectional changes during inflammation. Since inflammatory states often coexist with hemolytic conditions, serum haptoglobin concentrations should be interpreted concurrently with the serology findings of at least one other acute phase reactant not affected by hemolysis.

Collection/Storage Information
- Specimen Collection and Handling:
  - Avoid specimen hemolysis
  - May store at -20°C for 2 weeks

LOINC Codes
- Code: 4542-7 (*Short Name* - Haptoglob Ser-mCnc)

Serum iron measurement

Test Definition
Measurement of iron in serum for the evaluation and management of iron status and imbalances

Synonyms
- Serum iron level

Reference Range
- Adults: 50-150 mcg/dL (9-27 micromols/L)
  Please refer to your institution's reference ranges as lab normals may vary.

Indications
Suspected and known iron toxicity
> **Strength of Recommendation:** Class IIb
> **Strength of Evidence:** Category B
> **Results Interpretation:**
> **Increased level (laboratory finding)**
> Serum levels greater than 350 mcg/dL may be potentially toxic, and deferoxamine therapy may be indicated if clinical symptoms or acidosis are also present. Levels greater than 500 mcg/dL have been suggested as an indication for chelation therapy.
> Serum iron levels after acute iron ingestion may vary widely and are inconsistent predictors of iron toxicity, whether considered alone or when combined with total iron binding capacity.

Suspected hemochromatosis
> **Strength of Recommendation:** Class IIb
> **Strength of Evidence:** Category B
> **Results Interpretation:**
> **Abnormal laboratory findings**
> Although serum iron may be higher in homozygous patients with clinical hemochromatosis, it is not an accurate predictor of the disease.

Suspected iron deficiency
> **Strength of Recommendation:** Class IIb
> **Strength of Evidence:** Category B
> **Results Interpretation:**
> **Lowered laboratory findings**
> Low serum iron in the presence of elevated total iron-binding capacity and low serum ferritin is considered diagnostic for iron deficiency. Because of the wide variety of factors that affect serum iron levels, serum iron alone is of limited clinical utility.

Suspected neuroleptic malignant syndrome
Results Interpretation:
Serum iron low
Serum iron levels less than 10 micromol/L have been noted in 95% of patients. Serum iron has been shown to decrease from a mean of 15 micromol/L before neuroleptic malignant syndrome (NMS) to 6 micromol/L after onset (mean drop of 60%) and to return to normal upon resolution of NMS. Such findings suggest that the extremely low serum iron levels that occur during NMS do not merely precede the episode but are specific to the disorder itself.

COMMON PANELS
- Anemia panel
- Iron panel

CLINICAL NOTES
Many factors can cause fluctuations in serum iron levels, including diurnal variations, fasting, dietary intake of iron-rich foods and supplements, alcohol ingestion, recent transfusion and some medications. Low serum levels are associated with inflammation, infection, stress and injury.
Adult serum iron levels are approximately 10 to 15% higher in males than in females.

COLLECTION/STORAGE INFORMATION
Specimens should be drawn after an overnight fast and before other specimens that require anticoagulated tubes. Hemolysis will render results indeterminate.

LOINC CODES
- Code: 14797-5 (*Short Name* - Iron SerPl-Imp)
- Code: 14801-5 (*Short Name* - Iron Satn Ser-sRto)
- Code: 2498-4 (*Short Name* - Iron SerPl-mCnc)
- Code: 14798-3 (*Short Name* - Iron SerPl-sCnc)

Serum ketone level

TEST DEFINITION
Measurement of serum or plasma ketones, specifically acetoacetate, for analysis of ketone-producing glyco-genolytic disorders

REFERENCE RANGE
- Negative: < 1 mg/dL (< 0.1 mmol/L)
  Please refer to your institution's reference ranges as lab normals may vary.

INDICATIONS
Initial evaluation of suspected hyperglycemic hyperosmolar state
Strength of Recommendation: Class I
Strength of Evidence: Category C
Results Interpretation:
Ketonemia
Serum ketones are small in hyperglycemic hyperosmolar state.

Suspected alcoholic ketoacidosis (AKA)
Strength of Recommendation: Class IIb
Strength of Evidence: Category C
Results Interpretation:
Increased level (laboratory finding)
Elevated serum ketones, in conjunction with patient history, is consistent with alcoholic ketoacidosis. However, the predominant ketone, beta-hydroxybutyrate (BOHB), is not detected by the nitroprusside reaction. Because acetoacetate (AcAc) levels are not always markedly elevated in ketoacidosis, this test may inaccurately report a weakly positive or even negative serum ketone finding.

The ratio of BOHB to AcAc is approximately 6:1 in alcoholic ketoacidosis (AKA). Since the nitroprusside reaction does not detect BOHB, some patients with AKA will have negative, or only weakly positive, test results for serum ketone bodies.

Suspected and known diabetic ketoacidosis (DKA)
    Strength of Recommendation: Class IIa
    Strength of Evidence: Category C
    Results Interpretation:
    Ketonemia
        Positive serum ketones are part of the diagnostic criteria for mild, moderate, and severe diabetic ketoacidosis (DKA). Because the predominant ketone, beta-hydroxybutyrate, is not detected by the nitroprusside reaction method, serum ketone levels (acetoacetate and acetone) may plateau with appropriate insulin therapy despite a net reduction in ketone levels, giving the false impression that the DKA is not improving. Ketonemia usually takes longer to clear than hyperglycemia does.

CLINICAL NOTES
    The nitroprusside reaction is a semi-quantitative test that detects only acetoacetate and acetone. The predominant ketone formed by ketogenesis is beta-hydroxybutyrate. Test results must be interpreted with caution as acetoacetate levels, alone, may not accurately reflect serum ketone levels at diagnosis or during the treatment of ketoacidosis.

COLLECTION/STORAGE INFORMATION
- Collect plasma or serum specimen after overnight fast
- Cover specimen and transport immediately to laboratory.
- Avoid hemolysis.
- If analysis is not performed immediately, freeze specimen at -80°C to avoid significant acetoacetate degradation.

LOINC CODES
- Code: 33058-9 (*Short Name* - Ketones SerPl-mCnc)
- Code: 2513-0 (*Short Name* - Ketones SerPl Ql)

Serum lipase measurement

TEST DEFINITION
    Measurement of lipase in serum for evaluation of pancreatic dysfunction

SYNONYMS
- Serum lipase level

REFERENCE RANGE
- Adults: 0-160 units/L (0-2.66 microkatal/L)
    Please refer to your institution's reference ranges as lab normals may vary.

INDICATIONS
Hemolytic uremic syndrome (HUS)
    Results Interpretation:
    Increased serum lipase level
        Elevated levels of serum lipase may aid in the diagnosis of pancreatitis in hemolytic uremic syndrome. Pancreatitis is not considered to be present unless elevations are greater than 4 times the normal value or other evidence of pancreatitis is present.

Hyperlipasemia in multiple organ failure
    Strength of Recommendation: Class IIb
    Strength of Evidence: Category B

Results Interpretation:
Increased serum lipase level
In comparison with intensive care unit (ICU) patients without serum lipase levels elevated above the upper limit of normal, ICU patients with serum lipase levels elevated above the upper limit of normal may have longer lengths of stay in the ICU, increased duration of mechanical ventilation, significantly higher multiple-organ dysfunction scores, and similar mortality.

Suspected acute pancreatitis
Strength of Recommendation: Class IIa
Strength of Evidence: Category B
Results Interpretation:
Increased serum lipase level
Lipase specificity is maximized by increasing the upper limit of the normal reference values. A diagnostic threshold 2 to 3 times normal provides the best achievable specificity without compromising sensitivity.
Lipase levels increase within 4 to 8 hours after the onset of acute pancreatitis, peak at 24 hours, and decrease within 8 to 14 days. Lipase elevation rarely persists beyond 14 days; prolonged increases typically signal poor prognosis or the presence of a pancreatic cyst.

COMMON PANELS
• Pancreatic panel

ABNORMAL RESULTS
• Results increased in mumps and extrapancreatic injury

CLINICAL NOTES
Assays are highly dependent on substrate used. Assays that contain colipase and bile salts are more specific for pancreatic lipase.

COLLECTION/STORAGE INFORMATION
• Store refrigerated or frozen

Serum lithium measurement

TEST DEFINITION
Measurement of lithium levels in serum to facilitate therapeutic or toxicity monitoring

SYNONYMS
• Serum lithium level

REFERENCE RANGE
• Therapeutic range: 0.6 mEq/L-1.2 mEq/L (0.6 mmols/L-1.2 mmols/L)
Please refer to your institution's reference ranges as lab normals may vary.

INDICATIONS
Drug level monitoring during lithium therapy
Strength of Recommendation: Class I
Strength of Evidence: Category B
Results Interpretation:
Lithium: blood level - finding
Lithium levels above 0.8 mmol/L increase the likelihood of a therapeutic response; levels up to 1 mmol/L are usually adequate for prophylaxis and maintenance. Some patients may exhibit a therapeutic response at levels below 0.8 mmol/L. Individual patient response can be quite variable.
Some patients may experience poor response or toxicity despite lithium levels within the therapeutic range. Fluctuating lithium levels may be indicative of a patient's poor compliance.
Rapid changes in lithium levels may lead to greater symptom recurrence.
A blood concentration of at least 0.4 mmol/L is necessary for antidepressant augmentation.

Frequency of Monitoring
Lithium levels should be monitored at least every 6 months after a patient has become stable.
Timing of Monitoring
Lithium levels should be obtained 12 hours after the patient's last dose.

Suspected lithium toxicity
Strength of Recommendation: Class I
Strength of Evidence: Category B
Results Interpretation:
Lithium level high - toxic
The toxic level for lithium is greater than 2 mEq/L (2 mmol/L).

Symptoms of mild to moderate intoxication may occur at concentrations up to 2 mEq/L to 3 mEq/L, and include lethargy, drowsiness, photophobia, coarse hand tremor, muscle weakness and myoclonic twitches, nausea, vomiting, diarrhea, ataxia, nystagmus, confusion, choreoathetosis, agitation, and ECG changes.

Symptoms of severe intoxication may occur at concentrations above 2.5 mEq/L to 3.5 mEq/L, and include grossly impaired consciousness, increased deep tendon reflexes, seizures, syncope, renal insufficiency, coma, cardiovascular instability, and death.

A lithium level above 1.5 mEq/L may be indicative of lithium toxicity in patients with chronic intoxication from long-term lithium therapy. Patients with acute intoxication have less of a correlation between lithium levels and toxic symptoms.

Toxicity may be predicted in some patients when lithium levels are above 1.43 mmol/L, although some patients may experience toxicity at levels within the normal therapeutic range.

A lithium level greater than 1.5 mEq/L may lead to subacute renal impairment.

Lithium levels above 4 mEq/L in chronic intoxication patients may require hemodialysis; lithium levels above 6 mEq/L likely require hemodialysis in all patients.

Neurotoxicity and other symptoms of lithium intoxication may be noted in patients with only moderately elevated lithium blood levels, particularly in older patient populations.
Timing of Monitoring
Lithium levels for patients suspected or known to have chronic poisoning should be obtained 12 hours after the patient's last dose.

COLLECTION/STORAGE INFORMATION
- Specimen Collection and Handling:
  - Draw serum (or plasma in heparin or EDTA tube) 12 hours after last dose.
  - Separate cells from plasma/serum if test not performed in 4 hours.
  - Store up to 24 hours at room temperature or at -20°C indefinitely.

LOINC CODES
- Code: 3720-0 (*Short Name* - Lithium SerPl Ql)
- Code: 14334-7 (*Short Name* - Lithium SerPl-sCnc)
- Code: 3719-2 (*Short Name* - Lithium SerPl-mCnc)

Serum methylmalonic acid level

TEST DEFINITION
Measurement of serum methylmalonic acid (MMA) level to assess vitamin B_{12} (cobalamin) deficiency

SYNONYMS
- Serum methylmalonic acid measurement

REFERENCE RANGE
- Adults: <4.72 mcg/dL (0.4 micromol/L)
- Neonates: 0.36 ± 0.26 micromol/L
Please refer to your institution's reference ranges as lab normals may vary.

INDICATIONS

Suspected vitamin B$_{12}$ (cobalamin) deficiency

    Strength of Recommendation: Class IIa

    Strength of Evidence: Category B

    Results Interpretation:

    Methylmalonic acidemia

    Serum methylmalonic acid (MMA) levels, elevated more than 0.4 micromol/L, are an early indicator of cobalamin (Cbl) deficiency because normal metabolism of MMA is dependent upon Cbl.

    A deficiency can indicate problems with intestinal absorption, digestion, or an inadequate diet.

    With an elevated MMA, patients may exhibit symptoms of Cbl deficiency, such as changes in behavior, mental status, or neuropathy, prior to hematologic changes like anemia.

    Healthy infants, less than one year old, may have increased serum or urinary MMA levels due to undeveloped organ or enzyme systems or defective Cbl function.

    Though useful for screening purposes particularly in the elderly, serial monitoring is not recommended as results are variable and do not correspond reliably with treatment of Cbl deficiency.

ABNORMAL RESULTS

- Results increased in:
  - Renal insufficiency
  - Hereditary inability to metabolize MMA (rare)

CLINICAL NOTES

    Methylmalonic acid (MMA) in serum, plasma, or urine is a unique indicator of cobalamine (Cbl) deficiency, though urine MMA levels are more specific due to urinary MMA being normalized to urine creatinine.

COLLECTION/STORAGE INFORMATION

- Specimen Collection and Handling:
  - Draw fasting specimen.
  - Analyze serum fresh or store at -70°C.

LOINC CODES

- Code: 13964-2 (*Short Name* - MMA SerPl-sCnc)
- Code: 2629-4 (*Short Name* - MMA SerPl-mCnc)

Serum molybdenum level

TEST DEFINITION

    Measurement of molybdenum in serum for evaluation and management of deficiency or toxicity or biomonitoring.

REFERENCE RANGE

    Adults and Children: 0.1-3 mcg/L (1-31.3 mmol/L)

    Please refer to your institution's reference ranges as lab normals may vary.

INDICATIONS

Suspected molybdenum deficiency

    Strength of Recommendation: Class IIb

    Strength of Evidence: Category C

    Results Interpretation:

    Decreased level (laboratory finding)

    Molybdenum deficiency in adults is a benign condition and is relatively asymptomatic.

    Decreased serum molybdenum reflects low dietary intake.

    Molybdenum deficiency induced by long-term total parenteral nutrition may result in conditions caused by reduced activity of sulfite and xanthine oxidase.

COLLECTION/STORAGE INFORMATION

- Collect specimen in a metal-free container

LOINC CODES
- Code: 25481-3 (*Short Name* - Molybdenum SerPl-sCnc)
- Code: 5698-6 (*Short Name* - Molybdenum SerPl-mCnc)

Serum potassium measurement

TEST DEFINITION
Measurement of potassium in serum for the evaluation and management of disorders (most commonly renal) affecting potassium balance

SYNONYMS
- Serum potassium level

REFERENCE RANGE
- Adults: 3.5-5 mEq/L (3.5-5 mmol/L)
- Premature neonates, cord blood: 5-10.2 mEq/L (5-10.2 mmol/L)
- Premature neonates, 48 hours: 3-6 mEq/L (3-6 mmol/L)
- Neonates, cord blood: 5.6-12 mEq/L (5.6-12 mmol/L)
- Neonates: 3.7-5.9 mEq/L (3.7-5.9 mmol/L)
- Infants: 4.1-5.3 mEq/L (4.1-5.3 mmol/L)
- Children: 3.4-4.7 mEq/L (3.4-4.7 mmol/L)
  Please refer to your institution's reference ranges as lab normals may vary.

INDICATIONS
Peripheral vascular disease with arterial embolism and severe muscle ischemia
  Results Interpretation:
  Hyperkalemia
    Muscle necrosis secondary to prolonged hypoxia will lead to the release of intracellular potassium and subsequent elevation of the serum potassium level. If not recognized and treated, elevated potassium could lead to cardiac arrhythmias and death.

Ascites in the setting of liver cirrhosis
  Results Interpretation:
  Hyperkalemia
    Hyperkalemia is almost always secondary to potassium-sparing diuretics, such as spironolactone, in combination with a high potassium diet consisting of fruits and salt substitutes.
  Hypokalemia
    Loop diuretics cause potassium loss and can lead to hypokalemia, sometimes manifesting as worsening encephalopathy.

Hypomagnesemia and suspected hypokalemia
  Results Interpretation:
  Hypokalemia
    Patients with hypomagnesemia are twice as likely to have decreased serum potassium levels than are normomagnesemic patients. Conversely, hypomagnesemia is present in approximately 40% of patients with hypokalemia.
    Hypokalemia results from a shift of potassium into the extracellular fluid, which, in turn increases urinary potassium losses. In this setting, magnesium repletion will usually correct the hypokalemia.

Suspected and known meningococcal septic shock in pediatric patients
  Results Interpretation:
  Potassium level - finding
    Potassium levels appear to correlate with mortality in children with meningococcal septic shock.

CABG
  Strength of Recommendation: Class IIb
  Strength of Evidence: Category B

Results Interpretation:
Abnormal biochemistry findings
In patients undergoing CABG, serum potassium levels less than 3.5 mmol/L predispose to perioperative arrhythmia. Potassium levels over 5.5 mmol/L may predispose to postoperative atrial fibrillation/flutter. Potassium levels at either extreme may increase the risk of death or need for cardiopulmonary resuscitation.

Heart failure
Strength of Recommendation: Class I
Strength of Evidence: Category B
Results Interpretation:
Potassium level - finding
It is particularly important to monitor serum potassium levels in patients with heart failure because the medications used for treatment may influence or be affected by the potassium level.
Some experts recommend that the target level of potassium for heart failure patients should be between 4.5 and 5.5 mmol/L. The serum potassium level appears to be inversely correlated with prognosis.
Hyperkalemia
Higher potassium levels appear to decrease the risk of ventricular dysrhythmias.
Hyperkalemia may occur in patients taking a combination of angiotensin converting enzyme (ACE) inhibitors and spironolactone.
A significant rise in serum potassium levels can occur abruptly, especially during an exacerbation of heart failure (HF), in patients with severe HF who receive oral potassium supplementation, even when the supplemental potassium dose remains constant and potassium-sparing diuretics are not used. The mechanism is probably due to further deterioration of the already severely compromised cardiac function, which results in tissue hypoperfusion and metabolic acidosis. Hypoperfusion leads to a decrease in GFR that, when combined with metabolic acidosis, results in decreased potassium excretion.
Hypokalemia
Hypokalemia appears to increase the risk of ventricular dysrhythmia. Survivors of sudden cardiac death often have low potassium levels, and mortality is higher in heart failure patients receiving non-potassium sparing diuretics. A serum potassium level of 4.1 mmol/L appears to confer an increased risk of death in class I, II, and III heart failure patients compared with a potassium level of 4.4 mmol/L.
Hypokalemia often occurs in those patients being treated with diuretics. Hypokalemia may also increase the risk of digoxin toxicity.

Hypercalcemia
Results Interpretation:
Hyperkalemia
Hyperkalemia may occur with hypercalcemia, especially when the elevated calcium level has caused renal failure.
Hypokalemia
Hypokalemia is the most common electrolyte disturbance of acute hypercalcemia, particularly that associated with diuretic use, malignancy, milk-alkali syndrome, granulomatous disease, hypervitaminosis D, and, less frequently, hyperparathyroidism.

Hypothermic patients in cardiac arrest
Strength of Recommendation: Class I
Strength of Evidence: Category C
Results Interpretation:
Hyperkalemia
Decision to pursue treatment of hypothermic cardiac arrest patients should not be based on laboratory values or presenting core temperature. A pH of 6.51, core temperature of 14°C, and potassium level of 11.8 mEq/L have been reported in neurologically intact survivors.

Initial evaluation and monitoring of diabetic ketoacidosis
Strength of Recommendation: Class I
Strength of Evidence: Category C
Results Interpretation:
Hyperkalemia
Insulin deficiency, hypertonicity, and acidemia may cause an extracellular shift of potassium and increased serum potassium concentration.

Low serum potassium level - finding

Low-normal or low serum potassium on presentation indicates severe total-body potassium deficiency. Because treatment may further deplete potassium and provoke cardiac dysrhythmia, conscientious cardiac monitoring and more vigorous potassium replacement is required.

Normal serum potassium level

Potassium replacement should be initiated for levels below 5.5 mEq/L in patients with adequate urine output.

Frequency of Monitoring

Monitor potassium level every 2 to 4 hours until patient is stable.

Initial evaluation and monitoring of hyperosmolar hyperglycemic state

Strength of Recommendation: Class I
Strength of Evidence: Category C
Results Interpretation:

Hyperkalemia

Insulin deficiency, hypertonicity, and acidemia may cause an extracellular shift of potassium and increased serum potassium concentration.

Low serum potassium level - finding

Low-normal or low serum potassium on presentation indicates severe total-body potassium deficiency. Because treatment may further deplete potassium and provoke cardiac dysrhythmias, conscientious cardiac monitoring and more vigorous potassium replacement is required.

Normal serum potassium level

Potassium replacement should be initiated for levels below 5.5 mEq/L in patients with adequate urine output.

Frequency of Monitoring

Monitor potassium level every 2 to 4 hours until patient is stable.

Metabolic acidosis

Strength of Recommendation: Class I
Strength of Evidence: Category C
Results Interpretation:

Potassium level - finding

The effects of metabolic acidosis on the plasma potassium level depend on the cause and duration of the acidosis. The complex pathophysiologic interactions occurring in various types of metabolic acidosis may raise, lower, or have no effect on the serum potassium level.

Uncomplicated acute organic acidosis (eg, alcoholic ketoacidosis, lactic acidosis, or methanol, ethylene glycol, salicylate, or paraldehyde ingestion) is not usually associated with a significant change in potassium concentrations. This may reflect the fact that the hydrogen ion and associated anion move into cells together, not requiring the movement of potassium out of the cell.

Acute acidemias (eg, HCl, NH_4 Cl, uremia) are more likely to be associated with elevations in serum potassium. Generally, a decrease of 0.1 units in pH gives rise to a serum potassium increase of 0.6 mmol/L in these conditions.

Hypokalemia

Several causes of nonanion gap acidosis are associated with hypokalemia, including diarrhea, renal tubular acidosis (RTA) types 1 and 2, laxative abuse, and urinary diversions.

Hyperkalemia

In acidosis associated with mineral acids (end stage uremic acidosis, ammonium chloride-induced acidosis), increases in serum potassium occur through a shift from the intracellular to the extracellular compartment to maintain electrical neutrality as hydrogen ions enter cells.

In chronic nonanion gap metabolic acidosis, associated hyperkalemia suggests the existence of tissue necrosis, low aldosterone hormonal levels, or failure of the kidney to respond to aldosterone.

Metabolic alkalosis

Results Interpretation:

Hypokalemia

Hypokalemia is almost invariably a characteristic of the serum electrolyte pattern seen in metabolic alkalosis (along with an elevated total CO_2 content and hypochloremia); however, the exact nature of the relationship between serum potassium and blood pH may not be as straightforward.

The decreased potassium level is primarily related to renal excretion at the distal tubule, as well as to aldosterone production in the face of extracellular fluid (ECF) volume depletion with subsequent potassium loss. It is also secondary to the shift of potassium into the cells in exchange for hydrogen.

Although potassium depletion contributes to the maintenance of an elevated plasma HCO_3 in metabolic alkalosis, the alkalosis can be corrected without provision of potassium despite potassium deficits as high as 350 to 450 mEq/L.

Rhabdomyolysis
Strength of Recommendation: Class I
Strength of Evidence: Category C
Results Interpretation:
Hyperkalemia

In rhabdomyolysis, rupture of muscle cell membranes causes the release of large amounts of intracellular potassium into the extracellular fluid.

The absence of hyperkalemia should not rule out the diagnosis of rhabdomyolysis, especially in patients with normally functioning kidneys.

In rhabdomyolysis, the rate of rise in the potassium level is 2 to 3 times that of other causes of renal failure.

In the presence of oliguria and acidosis, the potassium released can cause fulminant hyperkalemia.

Hypokalemia

Subclinical rhabdomyolysis may be common in hypokalemic patients. In the presence of moderately severe potassium deficiency, a fundamental defect in muscle membrane integrity occurs, characterized by a subnormal resting membrane potential and elevation of serum creatine kinase levels. Associated with this is the inability of the muscle to maintain normal levels of glycogen. If the muscle is subjected to intense exercise, the utilization of energy is impaired and vasodilatation is prevented, leading to ischemia and necrosis.

Severe adrenal insufficiency (adrenal crisis)
Results Interpretation:
Hyperkalemia

Hyperkalemia is a common finding in patients with primary adrenal insufficiency.

The potassium level in adrenal crisis is usually moderately increased (6 mEq/L), but a level exceeding 7 mEq/L is uncommon.

Because aldosterone's action on the renal distal tubules increases the secretion of potassium, aldosterone deficiency will result in potassium retention, usually manifesting as hyperkalemic metabolic acidosis.

Normal serum potassium level

The initial potassium level may be normal in adrenal crisis if protracted vomiting has occurred.

Hypokalemia

The initial potassium level may be low in adrenal crisis if protracted vomiting has occurred.

Suspected acute coronary syndrome
Strength of Recommendation: Class I
Strength of Evidence: Category C
Results Interpretation:
Hypokalemia

Hypokalemia in acute myocardial infarction patients is associated with an increased risk of developing ventricular fibrillation.

Timing of Monitoring

Serum potassium should be measured in all patients who present with suspected acute coronary syndrome.

Suspected and known asthma
Results Interpretation:
Hypokalemia

- Signs and symptoms associated with hypokalemia:
  - Mild hypokalemia (3 to 3.5 mEq/L): Usually asymptomatic
  - Moderate hypokalemia (2.5 to 3 mEq/L): Weakness, constipation, fatigue, malaise, rhabdomyolysis, polyuria, nausea, vomiting, irritability, somnolence, depression
  - Severe hypokalemia (<2.5 mEq/L): Paralysis, respiratory failure, metabolic alkalosis, psychosis, ileus, and arrhythmias, including asystole

Suspected and known atrial fibrillation
Strength of Recommendation: Class I
Strength of Evidence: Category C

Results Interpretation:
Hypokalemia
Low potassium levels can contribute to the development of atrial fibrillation. Additionally, all patients, especially those on digoxin, should have potassium levels corrected prior to cardioversion.
Timing of Monitoring
Potassium and other electrolyte levels should be obtained prior to cardioversion, especially in patients who receive digoxin.

Suspected and known ovarian hyperstimulation syndrome
Results Interpretation:
Hyperkalemia
Serum potassium may be increased in patients with ovarian hyperstimulation syndrome (OHSS) due to vascular hyperpermeability, which can result in rapid dynamic changes in potassium levels. A potassium level greater than 5 mEq/L indicates grade 5 OHSS and is an indication for hospital admission.

Suspected and known renal failure
Strength of Recommendation: Class I
Strength of Evidence: Category C
Results Interpretation:
Hyperkalemia
In acute renal failure life-threatening levels of serum potassium greater than 7 mmol/L are commonly seen. In patients with chronic renal failure, moderate hyperkalemia ranging from 6.1 mmol/L to 6.9 mmol/L is usually well tolerated.
Hyperkalemia is commonly observed in the oliguric phase of acute renal failure. In chronic renal insufficiency, however, hyperkalemia is usually not encountered until the GFR is less than 25% of normal.

Suspected heat stroke
Results Interpretation:
Hypokalemia
Hypokalemia may be present in the early stages of heat stroke.
A low potassium level secondary to sweating may be seen in mild to moderate cases of exertional heat stroke. Potassium concentration in sweat averages 9 mEq/L.
Hypokalemia may occasionally be seen in elderly patients with nonexertional heat stroke, possibly due to preexisting drug-induced losses or loss due to sweating.
Hypokalemia may be secondary to respiratory alkalosis.
Hyperkalemia
Hyperkalemia may occur in severe cases of exertional heat stroke and may develop later as a result of tissue destruction, renal failure, or metabolic acidosis.

Suspected hemorrhagic shock
Results Interpretation:
Potassium level - finding
Hyperkalemia is an expected finding in severe shock and trauma but occurs only occasionally.

Suspected hyperkalemia
Strength of Recommendation: Class I
Strength of Evidence: Category C
Results Interpretation:
Hyperkalemia
- Hyperkalemia is often defined as a potassium concentration above 5 mEq/L. The severity is dependent on the rapidity of the rise of potassium.
- Classification of hyperkalemia:
  - Mild hyperkalemia: Serum potassium level 5 to 6 mEq/L
  - Moderate hyperkalemia: Serum potassium level >6 mEq/L to 7 mEq/L
  - Severe hyperkalemia: Serum potassium level >7 mEq/L
- Potassium levels and effects on ECG:
  - 5.5 mEq/L to 6 mEq/L: Tall, peaked T waves in precordial leads
  - >6 mEq/L to 7 mEq/L: Prolonged PR interval and QRS duration, prolonged terminal conduction waves (S waves in leads I, V_5, V_6), diffuse QRS conduction abnormality not classic for right or left bundle branch block
  - >7 mEq/L to 8 mEq/L: Progressive flattening of P wave
  - >8 mEq/L to 10 mEq/L: Sine wave appearance (merging of QRS with T wave)

- >10 mEq/L to 12 mEq/L: Ventricular fibrillation, asystole
- Although progressive levels of hyperkalemia may be roughly correlated with ECG findings, the rate of the rise of serum potassium concentration is more important than the absolute level.
- Although the presence of ECG findings rules out pseudohyperkalemia, the absence of ECG findings does not rule out true hyperkalemia.
- The rate of development of hyperkalemia is an important factor in determining the cardiac effects. If the disorder develops slowly, as in chronic renal failure, ECG manifestations may be minimal or absent with potassium levels of 7 to 7.5 mEq/L.
- Ventricular fibrillation usually results from rapidly progressive hyperkalemia, while asystole is most often seen in patients with the slow development of severe hyperkalemia.

Suspected hyperventilation
Results Interpretation:
Abnormal laboratory findings
Potassium level rises about 1.2 mEq/L but then decreases in response to the induced alkalosis of hyperventilation syndrome (HVS).

Suspected hypokalemia
Strength of Recommendation: Class I
Strength of Evidence: Category C
Results Interpretation:
Hypokalemia
- Signs and symptoms associated with hypokalemia:
  - Mild hypokalemia (3 to 3.5 mEq/L): Usually asymptomatic
  - Moderate hypokalemia (2.5 to 3 mEq/L): Weakness, constipation, fatigue, malaise, rhabdomyolysis, polyuria, nausea, vomiting, irritability, somnolence, depression
  - Severe hypokalemia (<2.5 mEq/L): Paralysis, respiratory failure, metabolic alkalosis, ileus, and arrhythmias, including asystole
  Hypokalemia may lead to asystole, especially in patients with underlying heart disease. Prompt recognition and treatment may rapidly reverse asystole.
- Serum potassium level and total body potassium deficit (assuming hypokalemia was not caused by intracellular shifting of potassium):
  - Serum level 3 to 3.5 mEq/L: Total body deficit 150 to 300 mEq/1.73 m^2
  - Serum level 2.5 to 3 mEq/L: Total body deficit 300 mEq/1.73 m^2 to 500 mEq/1.73 m^2
  - Serum level <2.5 mEq/L: Total body deficit greater than 500 mEq/1.73 m^2

Suspected Kawaski disease
Results Interpretation:
Decreased level (laboratory finding)
In one study lower levels of serum potassium were an independent risk factor of giant aneurysms.

Suspected pyloric stenosis
Results Interpretation:
Hypokalemia
A hypochloremic, hypokalemic metabolic alkalosis is the classic electrolyte and acid-base imbalance that is pathognomonic of pyloric stenosis. In 1 series, hypokalemia was present on admission in about 10% of cases. However, the 'classic' metabolic derangements associated with pyloric stenosis are seen much less frequently than in past years. One study showed no electrolyte abnormalities at presentation in 88% of infants with pyloric stenosis treated since 1975.

Persistent vomiting leads to the loss of gastric juice containing hydrochloric acid, sodium, potassium, and water. The resulting volume depletion stimulates the release of renin and aldosterone, ultimately resulting in the exchange of sodium for potassium at the distal renal tubules. Bicarbonate anions are reabsorbed avidly in the kidneys to compensate for the loss of chloride ions. These events produce self perpetuating hypokalemia, hypochloremia, and metabolic alkalosis.
Normal serum potassium level
Total body potassium depletion may be assumed even if the serum level is normal.

Thermal burn
   Results Interpretation:
   Hyperkalemia
      During the early resuscitation period, circulating levels of potassium are commonly increased due to a release of potassium from burn-injured cells and may be further elevated by acidosis. Cardiac function may be adversely influenced.
   Hypokalemia
      Hypokalemia is seen during the postresuscitative period (third postburn day) due to fluid diuresis and intracellular potassium shifts. Use of aqueous topical agents may cause transeschar leeching of potassium resulting in hypokalemia.

Ventricular tachycardia
   Results Interpretation:
   Hypokalemia
      Hypokalemia causes myocardium irritability and is a common cause of ventricular tachycardia and Torsade de pointes, especially in patients with underlying heart disease. Hypokalemia-induced cardiac conduction abnormalities are rarely seen in patients without a history of cardiac disease.
      Hypokalemia may affect the action of antiarrhythmic drugs by altering the electrophysiologic properties of the myocardium, potentially negating some of the antiarrhythmic activity of the drug.

COMMON PANELS

- Basic metabolic panel
- Comprehensive metabolic panel
- Diabetic management panel
- Electrolyte panel
- Enteral/Parenteral nutritional management panel
- General health panel
- Hypertension panel
- Renal panel
- Transplant panel

COLLECTION/STORAGE INFORMATION

- Specimen Collection and Handling:
    - Obtain 5 mL of venous blood sample in a serum or heparinized vacutainer tube.
    - To prevent hemolysis (which can cause potassium levels to rise by 10% to 20%), avoid having patient open and close fist during collection, and avoid using tourniquet. If a tourniquet must be used, release after needle is inserted in vein.

LOINC CODES

- Code: 12813-2 (*Short Name* - Potassium #3 SerPl-sCnc)
- Code: 22760-3 (*Short Name* - Potassium SerPl-mCnc)
- Code: 12812-4 (*Short Name* - Potassium sp2 SerPl-sCnc)
- Code: 29349-8 (*Short Name* - Potassium p dial SerPl-sCnc)

Serum prealbumin level

TEST DEFINITION

Measurement of prealbumin in serum for the evaluation and management of nutritional status

REFERENCE RANGE

- Adults: 19.5-35.8 mg/dL (195-358 mg/L)
  Please refer to your institution's reference ranges as lab normals may vary.

INDICATIONS

Known or suspected nutritional deficiency
      Strength of Recommendation: Class IIa
      Strength of Evidence: Category B

Results Interpretation:
Lowered biochemistry findings

A serum prealbumin level of less than 110 mg/L is associated with a substantial metabolic deficit, and the prompt initiation of nutritional support should be considered. Levels between 110 mg/L and 150 mg/L are below normal and indicate heightened risk. A value of less than 50 mg/L is predictive of poorer prognosis. An upward trend in prealbumin levels during refeeding is indicative of sufficient treatment response, while continued low levels despite adequate nutritional support are associated with poorer outcomes.

Prealbumin levels drop quickly in the absence of adequate caloric intake; severe calorie restriction will cause a drop in levels within 3 or 4 days even when protein intake is adequate, and will quickly return to normal once appropriate nutritional support is initiated.

Prealbumin will decrease substantially in the presence of inflammatory responses such as sepsis and trauma, and in a wide variety of liver disorders. Increased levels have been reported in renal disease while other studies have not found a significant association between prealbumin levels and renal function. Because C-reactive protein increases and prealbumin decreases in the acute-phase response, the addition of a C-reactive protein test in patients with low prealbumin who are not responding to treatment, may help to determine to what degree the low prealbumin level is caused by acuity, versus poor nutritional state. An increased prealbumin level in the presence of a decreased C-reactive protein suggests a more positive anabolic state.

Due to its short half life of about 2 days, prealbumin is a better predictor of visceral protein status than albumin. Prealbumin is not directly affected by albumin levels or fluid status.

Frequency of Monitoring

Prealbumin levels are recommended twice weekly in recuperating patients, and may be required more frequently in critically ill patients with rapid losses.

Timing of Monitoring

A surgical patient with a level less than 110 mg/L will require immediate postoperative nutritional support and possible feeding tube placement intraoperatively. A prealbumin level should be obtained by the third to fifth postoperative day, since prealbumin drops to its lowest level at that time.

COLLECTION/STORAGE INFORMATION
- Stable at 4°C for up to 72 hours, -20°C for 6 months, or -70°C indefinitely

LOINC CODES
- Code: 14338-8 (*Short Name* - Prealb SerPl-mCnc)
- Code: 6793-4 (*Short Name* - Prealb SerPl EIA-mCnc)
- Code: 3037-9 (*Short Name* - Prealb SerPl-cCnc)
- Code: 2877-9 (*Short Name* - Prealb SerPl Elph-mCnc)

Serum prolactin measurement

TEST DEFINITION
Measurement of prolactin levels in serum for evaluation and management of disease

SYNONYMS
- Serum prolactin level

REFERENCE RANGE
- Adult females: 0-20 ng/mL (0-20 mcg/L).
- Pregnancy, third trimester: 95-473 ng/mL (95-473 mcg/L)
- Adult males: 0-15 ng/mL (0-15 mcg/L).
- Cord blood: 45-539 ng/mL (45-539 mcg/L)
- Newborn, 1 to 7 days: 30-495 ng/mL (30-495 mcg/L)
- Females in puberty:
- Tanner stage 1:
- 3.6-12 ng/mL (3.6-12 mcg/L)
- Tanner stage 2-3:
- 2.6-18 ng/mL (2.6-18 mcg/L)
- Tanner stage 4-5:
- 3.2-20 ng/mL (3.2-20 mcg/L)

- Males in puberty:
- Tanner stage 1
- <10 ng/mL (<10 mcg/L)
- Tanner stage 2-3
- <6.1 ng/mL <6.1 mcg/L)
- Tanner stage 4-5
- 2.8-11 ng/mL (2.8-11 mcg/L)
  Please refer to your institution's reference ranges as lab normals may vary.

INDICATIONS
Erectile dysfunction with suspected hyperprolactinemia
Strength of Recommendation: Class IIa
Strength of Evidence: Category C
Results Interpretation:
Prolactin level raised
About 80% of men with significant hyperprolactinemia (eg, serum prolactin level greater than 50 ng/mL) complain of diminished libido and erectile dysfunction.

Hyperprolactinemia has many potential causes, including medications (eg, psychotropics, spirono-lactone), hypothyroidism with increased thyrotropin, chest wall injuries, and compression of the pituitary stalk.

Generally, a cranial MRI is indicated to rule out a pituitary adenoma.
Timing of Monitoring
Prolactin measurement is not a primary screening tool for erectile dysfunction, but it should be evaluated if serum testosterone is abnormally low.

Suspected hyperprolactinemia with amenorrhea
Results Interpretation:
Increased prolactin level
Elevated serum prolactin indicates hyperprolactinemia, which is the most common pituitary cause of secondary amenorrhea. Elevated prolactin levels inhibit pulsatile gonadotropin-releasing hormone (GnRH) by the hypothalamus; GnRH is needed for the secretion of pituitary gonadotropin, which will in turn promote follicular development and ovulation.

Hyperprolactinemia can be caused by drugs that inhibit dopamine action such as antipsychotics; risper-idone treatment results in persistent hyperprolactinemia to the same or greater degree as seen with older neuroleptics. Hyperprolactinemia also occurs as a result of prolactin-secreting adenomas, idiopathic hyper-prolactinemia, and primary hypothyroidism.

Suspected prolactin-secreting pituitary adenoma (prolactinoma)
Strength of Recommendation: Class IIa
Strength of Evidence: Category B
Results Interpretation:
Increased prolactin level
Elevated prolactin levels in the range of 25 to 200 mcg/L is suggestive of pituitary adenoma.

Serum prolactin levels parallel tumor size; macroadenomas (greater than or equal to 10 mm diameter) are associated with prolactin levels over 250 mcg/L and may exceed 1000 mcg/L
Frequency of Monitoring
Due to the influence of stress and the pulsative secretion of prolactin, any test level of 25 to 40 mcg/L should be repeated to confirm hyperprolactinemia.

Suspected seizure disorder
Strength of Recommendation: Class IIa
Strength of Evidence: Category B
Results Interpretation:
Increased prolactin level
Serum prolactin is released at the onset of a generalized tonic-clonic seizure, reaching a peak increase at 15 to 25 minutes after the event.
Prolactin level normal
A normal prolactin level in and of itself is insufficient to diagnose psychogenic nonepileptic seizure or to rule out the possibility of generalized tonic-clonic, complex partial, or other epileptic seizure.

Neonatal serum prolactin levels can vary substantially based on gestational and postnatal age, and may be affected by encephalopathy.

Timing of Monitoring

Ideally, serum prolactin should be measured 10 to 20 minutes after an event, although levels will remain elevated for up to an hour. Serum prolactin drawn more than 6 hours after an epileptic seizure is most likely reflective of the patient's baseline level.

DRUG/LAB INTERACTIONS

- Veralipride - an increase in serum prolactin levels

ABNORMAL RESULTS

- Results increased in:
  - Chest wall stimulation
  - Granulomatous infiltration of the hypothalamus
  - Head trauma, severe
  - Hypothyroidism, primary
  - Renal failure, chronic
  - Stress, physical and psychological

CLINICAL NOTES

Due to nocturnal circadian fluctuations, prolactin levels may rise by 50% to 100% before awakening, while levels are stable while awake (CHEN2005)

COLLECTION/STORAGE INFORMATION

- Specimen Collection and Handling:
  - Collect sample in a red top or serum separator tube.
  - Store specimen at 4°C for up to 24 hours or freeze for long term storage.

LOINC CODES

- Code: 20434-7 (*Short Name* - Prolactin SerPl 3rd IS-aCnc)
- Code: 20568-2 (*Short Name* - Prolactin SerPl EIA-mCnc)
- Code: 2842-3 (*Short Name* - Prolactin SerPl-mCnc)
- Code: 15081-3 (*Short Name* - Prolactin SerPl-aCnc)

Serum protein electrophoresis

TEST DEFINITION

Differentiation of serum proteins in the evaluation and management of inflammatory and neoplastic conditions and hepatic, renal, and bone disease.

SYNONYMS

- SPEP

REFERENCE RANGE

- Adults:
- Albumin fraction: 3.5-5.5 g/dL (35-55 g/L)
- Alpha$_1$ globulin fraction: 0.2-0.4 g/dL (2-4 g/L)
- Alpha$_2$ globulin fraction: 0.5-0.9 g/dL (5-9 g/L)
- Beta globulin fraction: 0.6-1.1 g/dL (6-11 g/L)
- Gamma globulin fraction: 0.7-1.7 g/dL (7-17 g/L)
- Globulin fraction: 2-3.5 g/dL (20-35 g/L)
- Neonates 0 to 15 days:
- 'Albumin fraction: 3.0-3.9 g/dL (30-39 g/L)
- Alpha$_1$ globulin fraction: 0.1-0.3 g/dL (1-3 g/L)
- Alpha$_2$ globulin fraction: 0.3-0.6 g/dL (3-6 g/L)
- Beta globulin fraction: 0.4-0.6 g/dL (4-6 g/L)
- Gamma globulin fraction: 0.7-1.4 g/dL (7-14 g/L)
- Infants 15 days to 1 year:
- Albumin fraction: 2.2-4.8 g/dL (22-48 g/L)

- Alpha$_1$ globulin fraction: 0.1-0.3 g/dL (1-3 g/L)
- Alpha$_2$ globulin fraction: 0.5-0.9 g/dL (5-9 g/L)
- Beta globulin fraction: 0.5-0.9 g/dL (5-9 g/L)
- Gamma globulin fraction: 0.5-1.3 g/dL (5-13 g/L)
- Children 1 to 16 years:
- Albumin fraction: 3.6-5.2 g/dL (36-52 g/L)
- Alpha$_1$ globulin fraction: 0.1-0.4 g/dL (1-4 g/L)
- Alpha$_2$ globulin fraction: 0.5-1.2 g/dL (5-12 g/L)
- Beta globulin fraction: 0.5-1.1 g/dL (5-11 g/L)
- Gamma globulin fraction; 0.5-1.7 g/dL (5-17 g/L)
- Adolescents 16 to 18 years:
- Albumin fraction: 3.9-5.1 g/mL (39-51 g/L)
- Alpha$_1$ globulin fraction: 0.2-0.4 g/dL (2-4 g/L)
- Alpha$_2$ globulin fraction: 0.4-0.8 g/dL (4-8 g/L)
- Beta globulin fraction; 0.5-1.0 g/dL (5-10 g/L)
- Gamma globulin fraction: 0.6-1.2 g/dL (6-12 g/L)
- Monoclonal and polyclonal spikes are absent in normal SPEP
  Please refer to your institution's reference ranges as lab normals may vary.

INDICATIONS
Suspected amyloidosis
> **Strength of Recommendation:** Class IIa
> **Strength of Evidence:** Category C
Results Interpretation:
Increased immunoglobulin
> A localized peak in the gamma-globulin area, a monoclonal protein (M-protein), suggests the presence of amyloidosis or other monoclonal gammopathy. If amyloidosis is strongly suspected despite a normal SPEP, further testing should be done.
Decreased immunoglobulin
> Up to 20% of primary amyloidosis cases may show hypogammaglobulinemia in the SPEP.

Suspected monoclonal gammopathy
> **Strength of Recommendation:** Class IIa
> **Strength of Evidence:** Category C
Results Interpretation:
Increased immunoglobulin
- A localized peak in the gamma-globulin area, a monoclonal protein (M-protein), is associated with a variety of monoclonal gammopathies, which can be defined more specifically with further testing. These include:
  - Multiple Myeloma:
    - Over 95% of symptomatic patients have a monoclonal protein in serum, urine, or both
    - M protein appears as a spike in the alpha$_2$, beta, or gamma regions and is usually >3 g/dL
    - Hyperviscosity syndrome, though uncommon, may occur with M-protein in excess of 6 g/dL
  - Asymptomatic Multiple Myeloma:
    - Monoclonal peaks are >2.5 g/dL in 85% of patients
    - Bence Jones protein levels >50 mg/dL are associated with accelerated disease progression
  - POEMS Syndrome
    - POEMS = peripheral neuropathy, organomegaly, endocrine deficiency, monoclonal gammopathy, skin pigmentation
    - 75% of patients have IgAL or IgGL monoclonal protein
  - Waldenstr|f-m's Macroglobulinemia
    - IgM monoclonal protein ≥3 g/dL
    - Cryoglobulinemia or hyperviscosity syndrome may be found
  - Amyloidosis
    - Small monoclonal immunoglobulin on SPEP, most often IgM
  - Monoclonal Gammopathy of Undetermined Significance (MGUS)
    - Low monoclonal IgG, IgA, or IgM peak ≤2.5 g/dL in asymptomatic older patients
    - 1.5% of MGUS patients progress to multiple myeloma, amyloidosis, or Waldenstr|f-m's disease annually
  - Solitary Plasmacytoma
    - A monoclonal protein of <2.5 g/dL is found in 50% of patients with a single destructive bone lesion
  - Heavy Chain Disease

- Monoclonal immunoglobulins without any light chains, found in lymphoma-like diseases
- IgG heavy chain disease looks like Hodgkin's lymphoma
- IgA heavy chain disease causes a small bowel lymphocytic infiltrate with malabsorption
- IgM heavy chain disease resembles chronic lymphocytic leukemia

False Results

Up to 8% of healthy elderly patients have a monoclonal gammopathy.

Suspected multiple myeloma

Strength of Recommendation: Class IIa
Strength of Evidence: Category C
Results Interpretation:
Increased immunoglobulin

A localized peak in the gamma-globulin area, a monoclonal protein (M-protein), suggests multiple myeloma or other monoclonal gammopathy. The M-protein level is usually greater than 3 g/dL in multiple myeloma. If the SPEP is normal but suspicion for multiple myeloma remains high, immunofixation is helpful.

Decreased immunoglobulin

About 10% of multiple myeloma patients may show hypogammaglobulinemia on SPEP.

Suspected Waldenstr|f-m's macroglobulinemia

Strength of Recommendation: Class IIa
Strength of Evidence: Category C
Results Interpretation:
Increased immunoglobulin

A localized peak in the gamma-globulin area, a monoclonal protein (M-protein) suggests the presence of Waldenstr|f-m's macroglobulinemia or other monoclonal gammopathy. More specific tests can further define the gammopathy. Waldenstr|f-m's macroglobulinemia usually produces a monoclonal IgM at levels greater than or equal to 1 g/dL.

COMMON PANELS

- Bone and joint panel
- Comprehensive metabolic panel
- Hepatic function panel
- Parathyroid panel
- Renal panel
- Transplant panel

COLLECTION/STORAGE INFORMATION

- Specimen Collection and Handling
  - Obtain 7 mL of blood in a marbled topped tube
  - If not analyzed fresh, store specimen at 4° C for up to 72 hours, stable for six months frozen at -20° C, and indefinitely at -70° C

LOINC CODES

- Code: 20577-3 (*Short Name* - Prot SerPl Elph-mCnc)
- Code: 13980-8 (*Short Name* - Alb % SerPl Elph)
- Code: 24351-9 (*Short Name* - Prot Elph Pan Ser)

Serum quantitative HCG measurement

TEST DEFINITION

Quantitative measurement of human chorionic gonadotropin (hCG) levels in serum for evaluation and management of pregnancy complications and trophoblastic disease

SYNONYMS

- Serum total HCG level
- Serum total HCG measurement

REFERENCE RANGE

- Males: <5 milliInternational Units/mL (<5 International Units/L)
- Females, nonpregnant:: <5 milliInternational Units/mL (<5 International Units/L)
- Normal ranges during 1st trimester:
- ≤1 week: 5-50 milliInternational Units/mL (5-50 International Units/L)
- 2 weeks: 50-500 milliInternational Units/mL (50-500 International Units/L)
- 3 weeks: 100-10,000 milliInternational Units/mL (100-10,000 International Units/L)
- 4 weeks: 1,000-30,000 milliInternational Units/mL (1,000-30,000 International Units/L)
- 5 weeks: 3,500-115,000 milliInternational Units/mL (3,500-115,000 International Units/L)
- 6-8 weeks: 12,000-270,000 milliInternational Units/mL (12,000-270,000 International Units/L)
- 12 weeks: 15,000-220,000 milliInternational Units/mL (15,000-220,000 International Units/L)

Please refer to your institution's reference ranges as lab normals may vary.

INDICATIONS

Suspected ectopic pregnancy

    Strength of Recommendation: Class I

    Strength of Evidence: Category B

Results Interpretation:

Decreased human chorionic gonadotropin level

- Levels:
  - The mean plasma concentration of human chorionic gonadotropin (hCG) is significantly lower for ectopic pregnancy than for a viable intrauterine pregnancy, but there is no definitive laboratory test permitting distinction between them. A consistently declining hCG level indicates a nonviable pregnancy.
  - Serum hCG levels are more useful in distinguishing abnormal from normal pregnancies than in distinguishing ectopic from intrauterine pregnancies.
- Doubling:
  - In a normal intrauterine pregnancy, hCG levels double roughly every 2 days. The rate decreases from about every 1.5 days in early pregnancy to about every 3 days at 6 to 7 weeks' gestation, at which point the reliability of serial testing may be diminished.
  - In an abnormal intrauterine pregnancy or ectopic pregnancy, beta hCG production is impaired, with longer doubling times (about 7 days in an ectopic pregnancy).
- Discriminatory zone:
  - The range of serum hCG concentration above which a normal intrauterine pregnancy can be visualized consistently is called the discriminatory zone. That zone varies with the hCG assay used, the reference standard with which it is calibrated, and the available ultrasound resolution; findings also may be compromised by obesity, fibroids, and the axis of the uterus.
  - An intrauterine gestational sac in a normal uterus usually can be seen with transvaginal ultrasound when the hCG level is between 1,000 and 1,200 milliInternational Units/mL. When the hCG level exceeds the discriminatory zone, the absence of an intrauterine gestational sac on ultrasound is suggestive of ectopic pregnancy (but also can occur with a multiple-gestation or failed intrauterine pregnancy).
  - Patients with a nondiagnostic transvaginal ultrasound and a serum hCG level greater than 2,000 milliInternational Units/mL have an increased likelihood of ectopic pregnancy and should be referred for follow-up.
  - Patients with abdominal pain or vaginal bleeding and a serum hCG level less than 1,500 milliInternational Units/mL have a substantially increased risk of ectopic pregnancy, while the likelihood of normal pregnancy is low. The American College of Emergency Physicians recommends that transvaginal ultrasound be considered in patients with serum hCG levels of less than 1,000 milliInternational Units/mL because ultrasound may detect an intrauterine or ectopic pregnancy.
  - When the beta hCG is greater than 1,500 milliInternational Units/mL (5 to 6 weeks' gestation), transvaginal ultrasound reliably detects intrauterine pregnancies as early as 1 week after missed menses.
  - In patients with symptoms suggestive of an ectopic pregnancy who have indeterminate transvaginal ultrasound findings, the rate of change of serial beta hCG levels is predictive of an ectopic pregnancy. Patients with increasing hCG values and an empty endometrial cavity on ultrasound are at greatest risk of an ectopic pregnancy; almost two thirds of such patients subsequently have an ectopic pregnancy confirmed.
- Complicating factors:
  - Quantitation of serum beta hCG is complicated by the existence of 3 different reference standards for hCG assays, the existence of multiple antibodies in commercial assays, and confusing nomenclature. These factors can cause varying and inconsistent results and can affect the interpretation of results and clinical management.
- Post-treatment:

- The elimination of hCG after treatment of ectopic pregnancy follows a 2-phase distribution: the major elimination has a half-life of 5 to 9 hours, and a second, longer phase has a half-life of 22 to 32 hours. Beta hCG levels may increase during the first 4 days after methotrexate treatment.
- Limitations of serial testing:
  - There is an inability to distinguish a failing intrauterine pregnancy from an ectopic pregnancy.
  - There is an inherent 48-hour delay.

Frequency of Monitoring

Serial quantitative beta human chorionic gonadotropin (hCG) levels should be drawn every 48 hours in patients with an indeterminate ultrasound suspected to have an ectopic pregnancy.

Suspected pregnancy
Strength of Recommendation: Class IIa
Strength of Evidence: Category C
Results Interpretation:
Increased human chorionic gonadotropin level

A positive serum human chorionic gonadotropin (hCG) confirms pregnancy. Quantitative levels of serum hCG increase with advancing gestational age. A single hCG value cannot, however, be used to determine viability or gestational age due to the variable range of results. Levels that double every two days are consistent with a viable intrauterine pregnancy.

Suspected spontaneous abortion
Strength of Recommendation: Class IIa
Strength of Evidence: Category B
Results Interpretation:
Decreased human chorionic gonadotropin level

A single human chorionic gonadotropin (hCG) level does not aid in the diagnosis of spontaneous abortion. Levels normally rise rapidly during the first 12 to 24 weeks of pregnancy, doubling approximately every three days in the presence of an intact pregnancy. Serial hCG levels that fail to double are strongly suggestive of a nonviable pregnancy. A spontaneous decline of serial hCG levels to under 5 milli-International Units/mL without medical or surgical intervention defines a spontaneous abortion.

Frequency of Monitoring

Quantitative human chorionic gonadotropin levels should be measured every 2 to 3 days when monitoring for suspected spontaneous abortion.

Suspected testicular cancer
Results Interpretation:
Increased human chorionic gonadotropin level

Elevated levels of serum human chorionic gonadotropin (hCG) are found in 15% to 20% of seminomatous and 40% to 50% of nonseminomatous germ cell testicular tumors. Testicular tumors with elevated hCG (greater than 300 to 1,000 International Units/L) almost always indicate nonseminomatous tumors.

Only the beta-subunit of hCG is present in many testicular tumors. Separate tests for total hCG and beta-hCG may detect relapses earlier.

Persistent elevations of hCG suggest a lack of response to therapy.

Frequency of Monitoring

Patient monitoring includes tumor marker assessments every 2 to 4 weeks for the first year post-initial therapy and less frequently for up to 5 years.

Suspected trophoblastic disease
Strength of Recommendation: Class I
Strength of Evidence: Category C
Results Interpretation:
Increased human chorionic gonadotropin level

- Persistently elevated levels of human chorionic gonadotropin (hCG) in the absence of pregnancy may indicate trophoblastic disease.
- Trophoblastic disease such as molar pregnancy may progress to neoplasia. HCG levels can be used to make the diagnosis of neoplasia with these criteria:
  - hCG plateaus over a 3-week or longer period, measuring levels on days 1, 7, 14, and 21
  - hCG rises in 3 weekly consecutive measurements over 2 or more weeks, measuring levels on days 1, 7, and 14
  - hCG remains elevated for 6 months or longer
- Elevated levels of the variant beta-hCG (greater than 3% of total hCG) suggest trophoblastic neoplasia such as choriocarcinoma.

- Hyperglycosylated hCG, an hCG variant also known as invasive trophoblast antigen, may differentiate between invasive and noninvasive trophoblastic disease.
- Measurement of hCG variants nicked hCG and nicked free beta-hCG is critical in monitoring trophoblastic disease when total hCG has decreased to under 100 milliInternational Units/mL, as these may be the only immunoreactive forms left after treatment.

False Results

False-positive serum human chorionic gonadotropin (hCG) results are not uncommon, depending on the assay used, and could lead to unnecessary treatment. Positive results should be confirmed by other means before treatment is undertaken.

CLINICAL NOTES

Several variants of human chorionic gonadotropin exist. Available assays use different antibodies and measure different combinations of variants. Matching the clinical data with the appropriate assay becomes significant when monitoring other than normal pregnancies.

COLLECTION/STORAGE INFORMATION

- Specimen Collection and Handling:
  - Store specimen at 2°C to 8°C for up to 24 hours.
  - After 24 hours, freeze specimen at −20°C. :

LOINC CODES

- Code: 2119-6 (*Short Name* - HCG Ser-sCnc)
- Code: 19080-1 (*Short Name* - HCG Ser-aCnc)

Serum theophylline level

TEST DEFINITION

Measurement of theophylline levels in serum for therapeutic monitoring and suspected toxicity

REFERENCE RANGE

- Adults: 8-20 micrograms/mL (44-111 micromols/L)
- Neonatal apnea: 6-11 mg/L
  Please refer to your institution's reference ranges as lab normals may vary.

INDICATIONS

Suspected theophylline toxicity
    Strength of Recommendation: Class I
    Strength of Evidence: Category C
    Results Interpretation:
    Theophylline level high
        Although toxicity has been observed at levels as low as 15 mg/L (15 microgram/mL), toxicity is most commonly observed at levels greater than 20 mg/L (20 microgram/mL).
        The risk of toxicity is greater in patients with levels above 25 microgram/mL or with significant risk factors including ICU admission, prior seizures, or arrhythmias. Critically ill patients may manifest signs of toxicity with only mildly elevated serum concentrations.
        Patients with acute theophylline intoxication have a 50% probability of major toxicity at peak serum theophylline concentration of 611 micromole/L (110 mg/L).
    Frequency of Monitoring
        Frequency of monitoring in the overdosed patient depends on the clinical severity and the nature of the intervention. If therapeutic interventions (eg, hemodialysis) are used, more frequent monitoring is done. Conversely, if drug withdrawal is the only intervention, levels are measured after several half-lives. Monitoring usually continues until values are less than 20 mg/L (less than 20 microgram/mL).

Theophylline monitoring
    Strength of Recommendation: Class I
    Strength of Evidence: Category C

Results Interpretation:
Theophylline level therapeutic
- The established therapeutic range should be used as a guide only, due to theophylline's narrow therapeutic index and daily variations in plasma theophylline clearance.
- Although large variability in theophylline elimination occurs, individual patient variability is usually relatively small in the absence of confounding factors such as drug interactions.
- In otherwise healthy patients, levels below 25 microgram/mL are usually not associated with a substantial risk of major theophylline toxicity.
- Bronchodilatory, antiinflammatory, and immunomodulatory effects of theophylline may be adequate for some patients at serum levels lower than 10 microgram/mL.
- Time to steady state is as follows:
  - Adults: 2 to 3 days
  - Children: 1 to 2 days
  - Infants: 1 to 5 days
  - Neonates/Premature infants: About 6 days
  - Healthy newborns: About 5 days

Frequency of Monitoring
Following intravenous administration, monitoring is performed until a stable steady-state is reached, and again when therapy changes from intravenous to oral formulation.

One or two measurements of serum concentration may be all that is needed to determine the appropriate oral dosage of theophylline therapy.

Theophylline should be measured after 1 to 2 half-lives after initiation of treatment, and again at 5 half-lives, to ensure steady-state concentration. Additionally, after the patient has switched to oral medication, a theophylline level should be obtained after 5 half-lives. Half-life varies from 4 hours (healthy adult smokers) to 25 hours in cirrhotic patients.

Timing of Monitoring
During administration of intravenous theophylline, a serum theophylline level should be obtained 4 to 6 hours after the start of the infusion; the infusion should be stopped for 15 minutes before the sample is taken.

If a loading dose is administered in the acute care setting, obtain a theophylline measurement prior to - and again about 1 hour after - the loading dose is administered to allow for calculation of the infusion dose and to verify the concentration.

Patients on oral theophylline should have peak and trough levels drawn. Peak sample should be drawn 15 minutes following elixir dose, 2 hours after regular-release dose, and 4 to 6 hours after a modified-release dose. Slow-release formulas create a 'steady-state' condition, and thus do not require peak and trough measurements.

Due to circadian rhythms of theophylline metabolism, repeat samples for measurement of trough concentration should be taken at the same time of day to allow direct result comparison.

ABNORMAL RESULTS
- Serum concentration increased in:
  - Obesity
  - High carbohydrate, low protein diet
  - Premature babies and neonates
  - Elderly patients
  - Prolonged fever has been shown to slow the elimination of theophylline
- Serum concentration reduced in:
  - Low carbohydrate, high protein diet
    - Physical activity
  - Cigarette or marijuana smoking increases the elimination of theophylline 1.5 to 2 times

CLINICAL NOTES
In an epidemiologic investigation of 36,000 ambulatory patients, the overall risk for serious toxic reactions to theophylline was rare; however, risk was five times greater among elderly patients and those taking cimetidine.

COLLECTION/STORAGE INFORMATION
- Specimen Collection and Handling:
  - Collect heel puncture specimen for neonates
  - Collect serum or plasma specimen in serum separator (red marble) tube
  - Screen the patient for cigarette use

LOINC CODES
- Code: 32116-6 (*Short Name* - Theophylline Trough SerPl-sCnc)
- Code: 14915-3 (*Short Name* - Theophylline SerPl-sCnc)
- Code: 32115-8 (*Short Name* - Theophylline Peak SerPl-sCnc)
- Code: 4049-3 (*Short Name* - Theophylline SerPl-mCnc)

Serum total T4 measurement

TEST DEFINITION
Measurement of total thyroxine (T_4) that is bound to plasma protein in serum for evaluation of thyroid function

SYNONYMS
- Serum total T4 level
- Serum total thyroxine level

REFERENCE RANGE
- Adults: 4.5-10.9 microg/dL (58-140 nmol/L)
  Please refer to your institution's reference ranges as lab normals may vary.

INDICATIONS
Suspected subacute thyroiditis
>   **Strength of Recommendation:** Class I
>   **Strength of Evidence:** Category C
>   **Results Interpretation:**
>   **Increased thyroxine level**
>   In subacute thyroiditis, thyroxine levels are usually elevated at presentation, then fall to normal as symptoms resolve.
>   Increased thyroxine (T_4) levels are found at presentation in 76% to 88% of patients with subacute thyroiditis.
>   **Decreased thyroxine level**
>   In the late phase of subacute thyroiditis, the thyroxine (T_4) level falls and may be low if colloid reserves are depleted.

COMMON PANELS
- Thyroid panel
- Transplant panel

ABNORMAL RESULTS
- Conditions that affect thyroxine-binding globulin levels may cause misleading results in total thyroxine measurement:

CLINICAL NOTES
The combination of thyroxine (T_4) and other thyroid function test results plus clinical findings is vital in the management of the patient with thyroid disease.

COLLECTION/STORAGE INFORMATION
- Specimen Collection and Handling:
  - Collect serum sample in a red top tube.
  - Refrigerate specimen immediately.

Serum total protein measurement

TEST DEFINITION
Measurement of total protein in serum to evaluate disorders affecting albumin or immunoglobulin levels

SYNONYMS
- Serum total protein level

REFERENCE RANGE
- Adults: 5.5-8 g/dL (55-80 g/L)
  Please refer to your institution's reference ranges as lab normals may vary.

INDICATIONS
Henoch-Schonlein purpura
  Results Interpretation:
  Decreased serum protein level
    A decrease in total serum protein and albumin are suggestive of renal involvement.

Suspected hyponatremia
  Results Interpretation:
  Hyperproteinemia
    Proteinemia may cause pseudohyponatremia. With severe proteinemia, the plasma appears viscous. This occurs in multiple myeloma.
    The degree of sodium depression can be estimated by multiplying any serum protein concentration greater than 8 g/dL by 0.25.

Suspected monoclonal gammopathy
    Strength of Recommendation: Class IIb
    Strength of Evidence: Category C
  Results Interpretation:
  Increased serum protein level
    Multiple myeloma or other monoclonal gammopathies may be incidentally discovered by an elevated serum total protein, which should trigger a serum protein electrophoresis (SPEP).

COMMON PANELS
- Bone and joint panel
- Comprehensive metabolic panel
- Enteral/Parenteral nutritional management panel
- Hepatic function panel
- Parathyroid panel
- Renal panel
- Transplant panel

ABNORMAL RESULTS
- Results increased in:
  - Upright position for several hours after rising (highest level at mid-morning)
  - Venous stasis
  - Short-term high-protein diet
  - Strenuous exercise
  - Male sex
  - Hyperglycemia
  - Severe hyperlipidemia
  - Marked dehydration
- Results decreased in:
  - Overnight recumbent position
  - Elderly during summer months
  - Advanced age in nonsmokers (0.5-1 g/L per decade)
  - Prolonged bed rest

CLINICAL NOTES
While an abnormal total serum protein reflects underlying disease, it does not by itself identify a specific disorder.

Serum albumin (and immunoglobulin, when indicated) should be measured in conjunction with total serum protein.

- Specimen Collection and Handling:
  - Collect serum in red top tube.
  - Avoid prolonged application of tourniquet (increases protein concentration in sample).
  - Obtain sample distal to intravenous infusion site (local hemodilution can result in erroneously low values).
  - Store at 4° C for <72 hours, or freeze at -20° C for 6 months or at -70° C indefinitely.

Serum unconjugated bilirubin measurement

TEST DEFINITION
Measurement of unconjugated bilirubin levels in blood for the evaluation and management of hematologic, hepatic or biliary dysfunction

SYNONYMS
- Serum indirect bilirubin measurement
- Serum unconjugated bilirubin level

REFERENCE RANGE
- Adults: 0.2-0.7 mg/dL (3.4-12 micromol/L)
  Please refer to your institution's reference ranges as lab normals may vary.

INDICATIONS
Sickle cell disease
  Results Interpretation:
  Unconjugated hyperbilirubinemia
  Baseline elevations of indirect (unconjugated) serum bilirubin levels occur secondary to chronic hemolysis in sickle cell disease. Steady state levels are typically 2.3 ± 1.9 mg/dL.
  A relative increase in the baseline hyperbilirubinemia without change in direct (conjugated) bilirubin levels suggests increased red cell destruction, as found in hyperhemolytic sickle cell crisis.
  A relative decrease in baseline hyperbilirubinemia can occur in painful sickle crises, suggesting other causes of anemia than hemolysis such as aplastic or sequestration crisis.
  Conditions associated with increased indirect bilirubin in sickle cell disease include transfusion hepatitis and acute hepatic crisis.

Suspected biliary obstruction
  Results Interpretation:
  Unconjugated hyperbilirubinemia
  Elevated bilirubin and alkaline phosphatase are consistent with biliary obstruction or cholangitis.
  Serum bilirubin levels are elevated in 8% to 37% of cases of cholecystitis, usually to less than 5 mg/dL (less than 85.5 micromol/L), and the higher the bilirubin level, the more likely that stones will be present in the common duct.

Suspected Crigler-Najjar syndrome type I or II
  Strength of Recommendation: Class IIa
  Strength of Evidence: Category C
  Results Interpretation:
  Unconjugated hyperbilirubinemia
  Unconjugated hyperbilirubinemia due to a severe deficiency of uridine diphosphate glucuronosyltransferase is seen in Crigler-Najjar syndrome. In type II Crigler-Najjar syndrome, serum bilirubin levels are rarely in excess of 20 mg/dL, while type I Crigler-Najjar syndrome is more severe and is often accompanied by kernicterus shortly after birth.

Suspected Gilbert's syndrome
  Strength of Recommendation: Class IIa
  Strength of Evidence: Category C

Results Interpretation:
Unconjugated hyperbilirubinemia

Unconjugated hyperbilirubinemia, in the absence of liver disease and hemolysis, that increases 2 to 3 times when an individual is placed on a 400 kcal diet for 3 days is consistent with Gilbert's syndrome.

Suspected neonatal physiologic jaundice
   Strength of Recommendation: Class IIa
   Strength of Evidence: Category C
Results Interpretation:
Unconjugated hyperbilirubinemia

Indirect bilirubin levels peaking in the first days of life at approximately 5 to 6 mg/dL in full-term neonates (up to the first week of life for preterm and some Asian neonates), then declining over several weeks, are consistent with physiologic jaundice. Indirect bilirubin levels exceeding 17 mg/dL in full-term infants may indicate a cause other than physiologic jaundice.

Physiologic jaundice appears in full-term infants after the first 24 hours of life, peaking on day 4 or 5 of life, while physiologic jaundice in preterm infants does not appear until 48 hours after birth, lasting up to 2 weeks.

Suspected pyloric stenosis
   Strength of Recommendation: Class IIb
   Strength of Evidence: Category C
Results Interpretation:
Unconjugated hyperbilirubinemia

Indirect bilirubin levels are elevated in 2% to 3% of infants with pyloric stenosis. Levels may reach 5 to 10 mg/dL but rarely exceed 20 mg/dL.

Enhanced enterohepatic circulation of indirect bilirubin, reduced hepatic glucuronyl transferase activity, and reduction in hepatic perfusion have been postulated as causes of the indirect hyperbilirubinemia.

COMMON PANELS

- Comprehensive metabolic panel
- Hemolysis panel
- Hepatic function panel
- Transfusion reaction workup
- Transplant panel

ABNORMAL RESULTS

- Results increased in:
  - Prolonged fasting

CLINICAL NOTES

Unconjugated bilirubin, also called indirect bilirubin, is protein-bound. Routine exams generally measure total bilirubin, which may then be broken down into unconjugated (indirect) and conjugated (direct) forms. Unconjugated results may not be reported by all laboratories.

COLLECTION/STORAGE INFORMATION

- Specimen Collection and Handling:
  - Collect 5 mL of non-hemolyzed venous blood from fasting patient.
  - Protect from sample from ultraviolet light (sunlight).
  - Refrigerate sample.

LOINC CODES

- Code: 1971-1 (*Short Name* - Bilirubin Indirect SerPl-mCnc)
- Code: 14630-8 (*Short Name* - Bilirub Indirect SerPl-sCnc)

Serum uric acid measurement

TEST DEFINITION

Measurement of uric acid in serum for the evaluation of nucleoprotein metabolism or kidney disease

Synonyms
- Serum uric acid

Reference Range
- Adult males: 2.5-8 mg/dL (150-480 micromol/L)
- Adult females: 1.5-6 mg/dL (90-360 micromol/L)
  Please refer to your institution's reference ranges as lab normals may vary.

Indications
Tumor lysis syndrome
Results Interpretation:
Increased uric acid level
Cell breakdown is the major source of increased uric acid levels. Increased uric acid levels may also result from increased production or decreased excretion of uric acid, or both.

Diagnosis and monitoring of tumor lysis syndrome
Results Interpretation:
Hyperuricemia
Hyperuricemia results from the release of purine nucleic acids that metabolize into uric acid after spontaneous or cytotoxic therapy-induced lysis. This causes rapid increases in plasma and renal tubular concentrations. Uric acid nephropathy should be suspected when the uric acid: creatinine ratio is greater than 1.

In TLS, a uric acid level greater than 9 mg/dL is treated with hydration, allopurinol and alkalinization of the urine. Dialysis should be considered for a uric acid level greater than 10 mg/dL.

Timing of Monitoring
In tumor lysis syndrome, hyperuricemia develops 48 to 72 hours after cytotoxic therapy is begun.

Gout related to suspected hyperuricemia
Strength of Recommendation: Class IIb
Strength of Evidence: Category C
Results Interpretation:
Hyperuricemia
Hyperuricemia does not establish the diagnosis of gout; however, as uric acid levels rise above 600 micromol/L, the risk for developing gout also rises.

Approximately 80% to 90% of persons with a serum uric acid level greater than 9 mg/dL (uricase method) develop gout, although the degree of elevation does not necessarily correlate with disease severity. Hyperuricemia in gout patients increases the risk of kidney stones.

Although a single low serum uric acid level does not exclude gout, a series of low values makes the diagnosis less likely.

In patients with hyperuricemia, a 24-hour uric acid excretion of more than 800 mg indicates overproduction; a 24-hour uric acid excretion of less than 600 mg indicates hypoexcretion, possibly due to renal tubular defect. In the presence of hyperuricemia, even normal uric acid excretion is evidence of hypoexcretion of the increased urate load, which is filtered at the glomerulus.

Kidney stone related to suspected hyperuricemia
Strength of Recommendation: Class I
Strength of Evidence: Category B
Results Interpretation:
Increased uric acid level
Most patients with increased serum uric acid levels are asymptomatic and do not have renal calculi; however, hyperuricemia increases the risk of developing kidney stones, often in association with gouty arthritis.

Normal or high plasma uric acid levels may be seen in patients with pure uric acid stones. Patients may have either normal or high urinary uric acid excretion.

Increased serum uric acid levels are seen in some patients with nephrolithiasis.

Increased serum uric acid levels can be caused by increased dietary intake of purines, increase in uric acid production, or decrease in excretion.

Leukemia
Results Interpretation:
Increased uric acid level
Aggressive hematologic malignancies, including leukemia, may be associated with increased uric acid production resulting in hyperuricemia (values greater than 7 mg/dL).

Suspected heat stroke
Results Interpretation:
Increased uric acid level
Hyperuricemia is common in heat stroke and may contribute to renal dysfunction.

Suspected hyponatremia
Results Interpretation:
Increased uric acid level
Uric acid levels may be useful in the differential diagnosis of hyponatremia. An increased serum uric acid level (greater than 0.3 mmol/L) may be suggestive of hypovolemic hyponatremia.
Decreased uric acid level
Decreased uric acid levels (less than 0.24 mmol/L) are commonly seen in patients with SIADH.

Suspected or known hypertensive disorder
Results Interpretation:
Hyperuricemia
- Hyperuricemia is typically defined as serum uric acid (SUA) levels >6.5 mg/dL or >7 mg/dL in men and >6 mg/dL in women.
- Although SUA levels are an independent predictor of hypertension incidence and longitudinal blood pressure progression in various patient populations, SUA levels are unlikely to be a good screening tool for risk stratification of specific individuals at risk for developing hypertension.
- An SUA level >5.5 mg/dL in an adolescent with otherwise unexplained hypertension and normal renal function strongly suggests primary hypertension and tends to rule out white-coat hypertension or secondary hypertension.
- Although the SUA level is likely to increase, gout is uncommon in patients receiving ≤50 mg/day of hydrochlorothiazide or ≤25 mg/day of chlorthalidone.
- Methods to reduce high SUA levels include decreasing or eliminating the diuretic dose, or adding losartan (an angiotensin receptor blocker) because it attenuates the diuretic-induced increase in SUA levels compared with a beta blocker.

Suspected pregnancy-induced hypertension
Strength of Recommendation: Class IIa
Strength of Evidence: Category B
Results Interpretation:
Increased uric acid level
In women with chronic hypertension, increased uric acid levels may be helpful in identifying those with increased likelihood of developing superimposed preeclampsia, and may precede the signs and symptoms of the disease.
Uric acid clearance is decreased in preeclamptic women and serum uric acid concentration is increased. Preeclampsia is characterized by shallow implantation, hypoxic maternal-fetal exchange and higher trophoblast tissue turnover resulting in higher levels of xanthine, hypoxanthine, and cytokines. This may lead to hyperuricemia and increased oxidative stress that is seen in preeclampsia.
Increased uric acid level precedes the onset of heavy proteinuria (greater than 5 g/24 hours) in pregnancies complicated by preeclampsia.
Hyperuricemia reflects renal retention of urate and correlates with renal histologic changes; however, this finding in itself does not constitute an indication for delivery.

Suspected rhabdomyolysis
Strength of Recommendation: Class IIb
Strength of Evidence: Category C
Results Interpretation:
Increased uric acid level
Skeletal muscle injury leads to an overproduction of uric acid with subsequent hyperuricemia, especially in the patient with exertional rhabdomyolysis.

COMMON PANELS
- Arthritis panel
- Bone and joint panel
- General health panel
- Prenatal screening panel

ABNORMAL RESULTS
- Results increased in:
  - Purine-rich diet
  - Vigorous exercise

COLLECTION/STORAGE INFORMATION
- Collect sample in a red top tube.
- Store specimen at 4°C for 3 to 5 days, and at -20°C for 6 months.

LOINC CODES
- Code: 35232-8 (*Short Name* - Urate SerPl-msCnc)
- Code: 14933-6 (*Short Name* - Urate SerPl-sCnc)
- Code: 3084-1 (*Short Name* - Urate SerPl-mCnc)

Serum vitamin B12 measurement

TEST DEFINITION
Measurement of vitamin B_{12} in serum for evaluation of deficiencies as a result of inadequate dietary intake or malabsorption

SYNONYMS
- Serum vitamin B12 level

REFERENCE RANGE
- Adults: >250 pg/mL (>185 pmol/L)
- Newborns: 160-1300 pg/mL (118-959 pmol/L)
  Please refer to your institution's reference ranges as lab normals may vary.

INDICATIONS
Suspected vitamin B12 (cobalamin) deficiency secondary to pernicous anemia
>   **Strength of Recommendation:** Class I
>   **Strength of Evidence:** Category B
> **Results Interpretation:**
> **Decreased vitamin B12**
>   Serum cobalamin levels less than 74 pmol/L indicate a probable cobalamin deficiency. Patients with borderline or slightly lower than normal levels (74 pmol/L to 221 pmol/L) may have a cobalamin deficiency, but further testing is needed. Serum methylmalonic acid and total homocysteine are usually elevated in most patients with cobalamin deficiency. When serum cobalamin levels are greater than 221 pmol/L, cobalamin deficiency is unlikely.
>   Pernicious anemia associated with chronic atrophic gastritis is the most common cause of vitamin B_{12} deficiency. Determination of serum cobalamin deficiency with a normal serum folate may be useful in diagnosing pernicious anemia when serum parameters are set below 150 pmol/L and a malabsorption etiology is determined by Schilling test with intrinsic factor or intrinsic factor antibody screening.

Dementia related to vitamin B_{12} deficiency
>   **Strength of Recommendation:** Class IIa
>   **Strength of Evidence:** Category B
> **Results Interpretation:**
> **Decreased vitamin B12**
>   Serum vitamin B_{12} levels less than or equal to 150 pmol/L may be related to the development of Alzheimer's disease and dementia in the elderly.

CLINICAL NOTES

In cases where a likely diagnosis of vitamin B_{12} deficiency can not be reached with serum vitamin B_{12} measurements, determination of serum methylmalonic acid and homocysteine may provide additional discriminative information.

COLLECTION/STORAGE INFORMATION

- Patient Preparation:
    - Instruct patient to fast overnight
    - Instruct patient to abstain from heparin, ascorbic acid, or fluoride prior to draw
- Specimen Collection and Handling:
    - Protect specimen from light
    - Specimens are stable overnight at 8°C and for 8 weeks at -20°C
    - Avoid repeated freezing and thawing of specimen
    - When ruling out malabsorption as the cause of vitamin B_{12} deficiency, draw sample prior to performing Schilling test

LOINC CODES

- Code: 15039-1 (*Short Name* - Cobalamin Ser-sCnc)

Serum vitamin E measurement

TEST DEFINITION

Measurement of vitamin E (alpha tocopherol) in serum to evaluate nutritional status

SYNONYMS

- Serum vitamin E level

REFERENCE RANGE

- Adults: 5-18 mcg/mL (12-42 micromol/L)
- Children, 0 to 12 years: 0.3 -0.9 mg/dL (7-21 micromol/L)
- Adolescents, >12 to 18 years: 0.6-1 mg/dL (14-23 micromol/L)
  Please refer to your institution's reference ranges as lab normals may vary.

INDICATIONS

Suspected vitamin E deficiency due to intestinal malabsorption of lipophilic vitamins.
      Strength of Recommendation: Class IIa
      Strength of Evidence: Category C
Results Interpretation:
Vitamin E deficiency
- Vitamin E Deficiency:
    - Adults: <5 mcg/mL (<12 micromol/L)
    - Adolescents: <0.6 mg/dL (<14 micromol/L)
    - Children: <0.3 mg/dL (<7 micromol/L)

Insufficient dietary intake rarely results in vitamin E deficiency; however, vitamin E deficiency and low tocopherol levels are associated with intestinal lipid malabsorption disorders.

Intestinal malabsorption of fat is characterized by the development of steatorrhea, and an associated loss of tocopherols. Studies of children with cystic fibrosis have found that the severity of prolonged fat malabsorption and steatorrhea positively correlated with severe vitamin E deficiency and low serum tocopherol levels.

Vitamin E deficiency and low serum tocopherol concentration are common in premature infants due to poor tissue storage at birth and intestinal malabsorption for the first 2 to 3 months of life.

Serum tocopherol levels vary with total serum lipids and beta-lipoprotein levels. Low lipid levels can result in low serum tocopherol levels in the absence of vitamin E deficiency; hyperlipemia can result in normal tocopherol serum levels when tissue deficiencies actually exist.

CLINICAL NOTES

Vitamin E serum levels are influenced by the serum total lipid level.

COLLECTION/STORAGE INFORMATION

- Patient Preparation:
  - Instruct patient to fast prior to test.
- Specimen Collection and Handling:
  - Collect serum specimen in a red top tube.
  - Protect specimen from light.
  - Serum is stable for 4 weeks at 4° C and for 1 year at -20° C.

LOINC CODES

- Code: 1823-4 (*Short Name* - A-Tocopherol Vit E Ser-mCnc)
- Code: 14590-4 (*Short Name* - A-Tocopherol Vit E Ser-sCnc)

Serum vitamin K measurement

TEST DEFINITION

Measurement of vitamin K in serum to assess vitamin K status.

SYNONYMS

- Serum vitamin K level

REFERENCE RANGE

- Adults: 0.13-1.19 ng/mL (0.29-2.64 nmol/L)
  Please refer to your institution's reference ranges as lab normals may vary.

INDICATIONS

Suspected Vitamin K deficiency
  Strength of Recommendation: Class IIb
  Strength of Evidence: Category B
Results Interpretation:
Vitamin K deficiency
  Decreased vitamin K levels are observed after malabsorptive bariatric surgery.
  Plasma vitamin K does not reflect liver reserve.
  Fasting phylloquinone levels are highest in patients with the apolipoprotein E2 variant.
  Phylloquinone levels are higher after meals, lower in debilitated patients and decrease with dietary vitamin K restrictions. Menaquinone is present in smaller amounts than phylloquinone in plasma.
  Timing of Monitoring
  Serum vitamin K should be measured at more than one time point due to temporal variations.

COLLECTION/STORAGE INFORMATION

- Specimen Collection and Handling:
  - Obtain a fasting blood sample.
  - Do not freeze and thaw repeatedly.
  - Do not expose the sample to ultraviolet light.
  - Sample is stable at -20°C for 2 to 3 months.

LOINC CODES

- Code: 9622-2 (*Short Name* - Phytonadione Plas-mCnc)

Sickle cell identification, solubility method

TEST DEFINITION

A qualitative screening test to detect presence of hemoglobin S or other sickling hemoglobins

SYNONYMS
- Sickle solubility test
- Sickling, turbidometric method

REFERENCE RANGE
- Adults and Children: Negative
  Please refer to your institution's reference ranges as lab normals may vary.

INDICATIONS
Suspected carrier state for hemoglobinopathy trait in pregnant women
> **Strength of Recommendation:** Class IIa
> **Strength of Evidence:** Category C
> **Results Interpretation:**
> **Positive laboratory findings**
> A positive solubility test identifies possible carriers of a hemoglobinopathy trait or disease. Results should be confirmed with hemoglobin electrophoresis to determine the abnormal hemoglobin.

Suspected sickle cell trait or disease
> **Strength of Recommendation:** Class IIa
> **Strength of Evidence:** Category B
> **Results Interpretation:**
> **Positive laboratory findings**
> Sickle cell screening can help to determine the prevalence of sickle cell trait and disease in a community and identify the at-risk population. A positive solubility test result, however, does not distinguish between sickle cell trait and sickle cell anemia, nor does it provide data regarding other hemoglobinopathies. All positive tests should be confirmed by Hgb electrophoresis or HPLC.

> **False Results**
> If severe anemia (Hgb <8 g/dL) or polycythemia is present, the solubility test is inaccurate unless steps are made to use washed erythrocytes, or use hemolysates with a standard Hgb concentration.
> In a prospective population study of 3,246 individuals from India, the solubility test had a false-positive and false-negative result of 2% and 3%, respectively.

CLINICAL NOTES
Any positive solubility test should be confirmed by high-performance liquid chromatography (HPLC) or hemoglobin electrophoresis.

COLLECTION/STORAGE INFORMATION
- Specimen Collection and Handling:
  - Collect specimen in EDTA, heparin, or citrate tube
  - Serum sample can be stored for up to 20 days at 4° C

Sickling test

TEST DEFINITION
Detection of sickling in a low-oxygen environment as a screen for the presence of Hgb S or other rare sickling hemoglobins

SYNONYMS
- Sickle test

REFERENCE RANGE
- Adults and Children: Negative
  Please refer to your institution's reference ranges as lab normals may vary.

INDICATIONS

Suspected sickle cell disease
Results Interpretation:
Positive hematology findings
The sickling test will be positive when Hgb S is present in concentrations above 25%.

Because the sickling test cannot differentiate between heterozygotes and homozygotes for Hgb S, a positive result should be followed by hemoglobin electrophoresis.

ABNORMAL RESULTS

- Results decreased in:
  - Recent blood transfusion (within the last 3 to 4 months)
  - Polycythemia
  - Infants younger than 3 months

CLINICAL NOTES

The sickling test has essentially been replaced by the solubility test.

COLLECTION/STORAGE INFORMATION

- Specimen Collection and Handling:
  - Collect whole blood (in EDTA, heparin, or oxalate tube) or capillary blood.
  - Stable up to 20 days at 4°C

Smooth muscle antibody measurement

TEST DEFINITION

Measurement of antibodies to cytoskeletal proteins in serum for the evaluation of certain autoimmune liver diseases

SYNONYMS

- Anti-smooth muscle antibody measurement
- Anti-smooth muscle autoantibody level

REFERENCE RANGE

- Adults: Negative at 1:20 dilution
Please refer to your institution's reference ranges as lab normals may vary.

INDICATIONS

Suspected autoimmune hepatitis (AIH)
Strength of Recommendation: Class IIa
Strength of Evidence: Category B
Results Interpretation:
Smooth muscle antibodies positive
Smooth muscle antibody (SMA) titers greater than or equal to 1:80 are suggestive of the diagnosis of autoimmune hepatitis (AIH). In adult patients, titers of less than or equal to 1:40 are not indicative of AIH.

Increased SMA titers often accompany increased ANA titers. In pediatric AIH type 1 patients, SMA may be the only autoantibody marker and may be as low as 1:40 in very young patients.

Detection of anti-F-actin antibody is considered indicative of autoimmune hepatitis, since the F-actin specific antibody has high sensitivity.

Detection of smooth muscle antibody peritubular (SMA-T) pattern is highly specific for he diagnosis of type 1 autoimmune hepatitis.

ABNORMAL RESULTS

- Results increased in:
  - Rheumatic disorders
  - Certain infectious diseases, including infectious mononucleosis
  - Cancer

CLINICAL NOTES
Low smooth muscle antibody titers may be detected in normal adults.

COLLECTION/STORAGE INFORMATION
- Collect 7 mL of blood in red or marbled-top tube
- Store at -20°C

LOINC CODES
- Code: 30557-3 (*Short Name* - Sm Mus IgG Ser QI)
- Code: 8095-2 (*Short Name* - Sm Mus Ab Titr Ser)
- Code: 14252-1 (*Short Name* - Sm Mus Ab Ser QI)
- Code: 26971-2 (*Short Name* - Sm Mus Ab Ser QI IF)
- Code: 17593-5 (*Short Name* - Sm Mus Ab Swt QI)
- Code: 31629-9 (*Short Name* - Sm Mus Ab Ser-aCnc)

Sodium measurement, serum

TEST DEFINITION
The measurement of serum or plasma sodium levels for diagnosis and management of water and electrolyte disorders

SYNONYMS
- Serum sodium
- Serum sodium level

REFERENCE RANGE
- Adults: 136-145 mEq/L (136-145 mmol/L)
- Adults >90 years: 132-146 mEq/L (132-146 mmol/L)
- Premature infants, cord blood: 116-140 mEq/L (116-140 mmol/L)
- Premature infants at 48 hours: 128-148 mEq/L (128-148 mmol/L)
- Full term neonates, cord blood: 126-166 mEq/L (126-166 mmol/L)
- Full term neonates: 133-146 mEq/L (133-146 mmol/L)
- Children: 138-146 mEq/L (138-146 mmol/L)

Please refer to your institution's reference ranges as lab normals may vary.

INDICATIONS
Patients hospitalized for community-acquired pneumonia
Strength of Recommendation: Class IIa
Strength of Evidence: Category C
Results Interpretation:
Hyponatremia
A sodium level less than 130 mmol/L is a marker of disease severity in the Patient Outcomes Research Team (PORT) Pneumonia Severity Index.
Hyponatremia (sodium value 134 mmol/L or less) was present in 45% of children with pneumonia in 1 study.

Ascites in the setting of liver cirrhosis
Results Interpretation:
Hyponatremia
Hyponatremia is present in one third of patients with ascites secondary to liver cirrhosis and is frequently a stable, although undesirable, condition. It is thought to be due to reduced free water loss. Treatment with diuretics contributes to hyponatremia.
Hypernatremia
Hypernatremia may be encountered in patients with ascites secondary to liver cirrhosis. Patients treated with lactulose may develop profound diarrhea and free water loss leading to increased serum sodium levels.

Dehydration
Results Interpretation:
Hypernatremia
Hypernatremia may be present in patients with dehydration.

The loss of hypotonic fluids secondary to diarrhea in patients with gastroenteritis, especially infants, may lead to the development of hypernatremia.

Diarrhea associated with gastroenteritis
Results Interpretation:
Hypernatremia
Increased sodium levels may occur with excessive water loss in excess of sodium excretion, or abnormal replacement of fluid losses with fluids having a high sodium content, eg, boiled skim milk.

Hypernatremic dehydration associated with rotavirus enteritis may be more common than previously thought.
Hyponatremia
Decreased sodium levels may be produced by abnormally large sodium losses via the gastrointestinal tract or by excessive water intake as treatment for the diarrhea.

Decreased sodium levels are most commonly associated with *Salmonella* infections.

Initial evaluation and monitoring of hyperosmolar hyperglycemic state
Strength of Recommendation: Class I
Strength of Evidence: Category C
Results Interpretation:
Hyponatremia
Serum sodium measurement should be obtained in all patients with suspected hyperosmolar hyperglycemic state (HHS) as significant derangements in sodium are common. Measured sodium also is used to calculate serum osmolality and anion gap.

In HHS, hyperglycemia causes water to be drawn from intracellular to extracellular space, causing hyponatremia without hypotonicity. Serum sodium level typically decreases 1.6 mEq/dL for every 100 mg/dL increase in serum glucose level above normal. Correct serum sodium by adding 1.6 mEq to the measured sodium serum sodium for each 100 mg/dL of glucose over 100 mg/dL. The corrected serum sodium level should be calculated to adjust for the dilutional effect of hyperglycemia. It is important to consider that mild hyponatremia in the presence of an extremely high serum glucose level may represent a corrected hypernatremic value.

False Results
In laboratories using volumetric testing or dilution of samples with ion-specific electrodes, severe hyperlipidemia may reduce serum sodium level, factiously leading to pseudohyponatremia. Rectify by clearing lipemic blood prior to sodium measurement or by using undiluted samples with ion-specific electrodes.
Hypernatremia
Hypernatremia occurs gradually in hyperosmolar hyperglycemic state (HHS) as fluid loss and dehydration become severe. Typical total body sodium deficit in HHS is 5 to 13 mEq/kg, and the mean sodium level is 143 mEq/L.

False Results
In laboratories using volumetric testing or dilution of samples with ion-specific electrodes, severe hyperlipidemia may reduce serum sodium level, factiously leading to pseudohyponatremia. Rectify by clearing lipemic blood prior to sodium measurement or by using undiluted samples with ion-specific electrodes.
Frequency of Monitoring
During therapy, check the sodium level every 2 to 4 hours until the patient is stable.

Suspected and known diabetic ketoacidosis
Strength of Recommendation: Class I
Strength of Evidence: Category C
Results Interpretation:
Hyponatremia
An increased plasma glucose concentration will increase plasma osmolality and produce dilutional hyponatremia secondary to the movement of water along the osmotic gradient.

Sodium is also lost in the urine secondary to osmotic diuresis. Total body sodium stores may be normal despite a reduced plasma sodium concentration.

Typical total body sodium deficit in diabetic ketoacidosis (DKA) is 7 to 10 mEq/kg, mean sodium level is 134 mEq/L. Plasma sodium will decrease by approximately 1.6 mEq/L with every elevation of 100 mg/dL in plasma glucose above normal.

Hyponatremia may be seen in patients with metabolic acidosis secondary to chronic renal failure.

False Results
Severe hyperlipidemia or hyperproteinemia may reduce serum sodium level, factiously leading to pseudohyponatremia.

Hypernatremia
Serum sodium level may be elevated with large free water losses.

False Results
Severe hyperlipidemia or hyperproteinemia may reduce serum sodium level, factiously leading to pseudohyponatremia.

Frequency of Monitoring
Obtain serum sodium level as part of the initial laboratory evaluation in suspected diabetic ketoacidosis (DKA).

Assess sodium level every 1 to 4 hours during treatment, depending on clinical response.

Suspected and known ovarian hyperstimulation syndrome
Results Interpretation:
Hyponatremia
Decreased sodium is a common finding in patients with ovarian hyperstimulation syndrome (OHSS) who have developed ascites. Vascular hyperpermeability in OHSS can result in rapid dynamic changes of sodium levels. A sodium level less than 135 mEq/L indicates possible grade 5 OHSS and is an indication for hospital admission.

Suspected and known Rocky Mountain spotted fever
Results Interpretation:
Hyponatremia
A serum sodium level less than 130 mEq/L, secondary to an increase in vascular permeability that results in a decrease in plasma volume and a subsequent increase in antidiuretic hormone (ADH) secretion, is present in about 50% of patients with Rocky Mountain spotted fever.

Suspected child abuse
Results Interpretation:
Hypernatremia
Hypernatremia may be indicative of water deprivation related to toilet training or punishment.
Hyponatremia
Hyponatremia without underlying disease may be evidence of chronic child abuse due to intentional water intoxication.

Suspected heat illness
Results Interpretation:
Hyponatremia
Hyponatremia is the most common cause of serious illness related to prolonged exercise in heat and may be associated with overhydration.

Hyponatremia is suggested by altered mental status or by seizures without hyperpyrexia or hypogly-cemia, and the development or progression of these symptoms after exercise has ceased. Nausea, vomiting, headache, and dizziness are common symptoms but do not predict serum sodium level.

In heat cramps, hyponatremia is common in patients with isolated cramps.

In heat exhaustion, hyponatremia is common in cases due to salt depletion.

In heat stroke, the serum sodium level may be high, normal, or low based on the relative balance between sodium and water loss, although hyponatremia has been reported in up to 60% of patients.
Hypernatremia
In heat stroke, the serum sodium level may be high, normal, or low based on the relative balance between sodium and water loss.

Sodium levels may be greater than 180 mEq.

Suspected hemorrhagic shock
    Results Interpretation:
    Serum sodium level abnormal
        Hyponatremia occurs with hypo-osmolar fluid resuscitation and renal water retention in response to an increased antidiuretic hormone secretion secondary to hypovolemia. Hypernatremia frequently occurs following the use of hypertonic sodium solutions for resuscitation.

Suspected hypernatremia
    Strength of Recommendation: Class I
    Strength of Evidence: Category C
    Results Interpretation:
    Hypernatremia
        A serum or plasma sodium (Na) level higher than 145 mEq/L (145 mmol/L) defines hypernatremia in an adult.
- The correlation between absolute serum/plasma Na levels and symptoms and signs (primarily CNS) is modest, largely because a slow increase in Na levels (chronic hypernatremia) is better tolerated than a rapid increase (acute hypernatremia, defined as documented development in less than 48 hours). Nonetheless, reported correlations include:
  - With Na levels of 148 to 154 mEq/L, intense thirst is the only common symptom.
  - With Na levels less than 160 mEq/L, elderly patients typically have few symptoms, but there is a 20% mortality in symptomatic patients.
  - With Na levels greater than 160 mEq/L, there is a 60% to 75% mortality rate. Symptomatic infants with diarrheal dehydration often have severe acidosis and prerenal azotemia.

Suspected hyponatremia
    Strength of Recommendation: Class I
    Strength of Evidence: Category C
    Results Interpretation:
    Hyponatremia
        Hyponatremia is a sodium plasma or serum concentration less than 136 mEq/L (ratio of sodium to volume of plasma). It is not a reflection of the amount of total body sodium. Severe hyponatremia is apparent when the plasma sodium concentration is less than 120 mEq/L.
        The severity of presentation correlates with both rapidity with which hyponatremia develops and the degree of decrease in sodium levels. Acute hyponatremia (ie, a rapid drop or a level less than 120 mEq/L) may be associated with severe symptoms; chronic hyponatremia (ie, a gradual drop in sodium level) may present with minimal to severe symptoms.
        Clinical effects are secondary to shift of water into cells, with neurologic manifestations primarily due to cerebral edema.
- Manifestations associated with a decreasing sodium level:
  - Na 131-136 mEq/L: Usually asymptomatic
  - Na 125-130 mEq/L: Asymptomatic or gastrointestinal symptoms predominate
  - Na <125 mEq/L: CNS findings predominate (eg, weakness, lethargy, confusion
  - Na <115 mEq/L: Severe CNS findings (eg, coma, seizures, hypoactive reflexes)

    False Results
        Pseudohyponatremia in the setting of severe hypertriglyceridemia or paraproteinemia may be seen when sodium concentration is measured by means of flame photometry. Direct measurement of serum sodium with an ion-specific electrode has all but eliminated this laboratory artifact.

Suspected malaria
    Results Interpretation:
    Hyponatremia
        Hyponatremia is common in patients with malaria and is associated with the severity of parasitemia in adults, but not in children.
        It may be the result of intravascular volume expansion occurring as a compensatory response to vasodilation caused by the malarial endotoxins. The fluid and electrolyte balance may be further altered by the marked diaphoresis, vomiting, and decreased fluid intake that accompany the malarial paroxysms.
        In children with severe malaria, hyponatremic sodium depletion that exceeds water depletion is much more likely that is SIADH. If hypotonic or isotonic solutions are used when restricting fluids, they may exacerbate hyponatremia in children who have an appropriate antidiuretic hormone response. This may contribute to increase intracranial pressure and predispose to seizures.

Suspected necrotizing fasciitis
Results Interpretation:
Serum sodium level abnormal
Serum sodium levels of less than 135 mmol/L may help distinguish necrotizing fasciitis from non-necrotizing fascial infections. This is supported when classic 'hard' signs of necrotizing fasciitis such as, hypotension, crepitance, skin necrosis, bullae, or gas on x-ray are absent.

Suspected or known hemolytic uremic syndrome (HUS)
Results Interpretation:
Hyponatremia
Decreased sodium levels are a common feature (70% to 75% of patients) of hemolytic uremic syndrome (HUS) and reflect enteric electrolyte losses and renal impairment.

Hyponatremia may result in seizures, which occur within 24 hours of the lowest recorded serum sodium concentration in two thirds of cases.

Hyponatremia may result from rehydration with hypotonic saline. The state of hydration does not correlate with hyponatremia.

Suspected or known seizures, including status epilepticus
Results Interpretation:
Serum sodium level abnormal
Status epilepticus can occur with any cause of hyponatremia if the level is low enough. The serum level that produces seizures is unknown but is usually in the range of 110 to 115 mEq/L; the seizure activity may be more related to the rapidity of the drop rather than to the absolute sodium level.

In one study, neurologic signs were found in more than 50% of the study patients with a serum sodium level of 151 to 188; seizures occurred most commonly during rehydration.

Suspected or known viral encephalitis
Results Interpretation:
Hyponatremia
As SIADH is a common complication of viral encephalitis, serum sodium should be closely monitored.

Hyponatremia is reported in 30% to 40% of patients with West Nile virus infection, especially those with encephalitis.

Hyponatremia may occur in any type of encephalitis due to SIADH, usually becoming clinically apparent only at serum sodium levels less than 115 milliequivalents/L, at which point seizures occur.

Suspected porphyria
Results Interpretation:
Decreased level (laboratory finding)
A decrease in sodium is a classic feature of acute porphyria, which may be profound. Syndrome of inappropriate antidiuretic hormone secretion (SIADH) is generally considered an important etiologic factor, reflecting damage of the hypothalamic supraoptic nuclei by the activity of porphyria.

A proposed explanation is that sodium-losing nephropathy occurs secondary to the toxic effect of aminolevulinic acid on the renal tubules.

Suspected subarachnoid hemorrhage
Results Interpretation:
Hypernatremia
Hypernatremia is the most severe electrolyte imbalance occurring after subarachnoid hemorrhage (SAH). It develops in about 20% of patients during acute SAH, most commonly within a few days. It is associated with poor outcome, independent of other predictors of outcome, including age and initial Glasgow Coma Score, but does not increase the risk of symptomatic vasospasm.

Treatment is difficult because attempts to treat the hypernatremia and hyperosmolarity with hypotonic solutions generally lead to an exacerbation of intracranial hypertension.

Hyponatremia
Hyponatremia is a common consequence of SAH, occurring in about 30% of cases. It is more frequently associated with anterior or middle cerebral artery aneurysms.

Brain natriuretic peptide, probably promoted by noradrenaline release in SAH, is believed to cause hyponatremia.

Subsequent passive diuresis may lead to hypovolemia, which may impair cerebral blood flow, resulting in cerebral ischemia.

Typically, the sodium level starts decreasing about the fourth day post-SAH and, if uncorrected, severe hyponatremia will develop by the end of the first week.

The incidence of delayed cerebral ischemia after aneurysmal SAH is increased in patients with hyponatremia, whether or not they were treated with fluid restriction.

Hyponatremia in SAH is not associated with either symptomatic vasospasm or poor outcome.

Thermal burn
Results Interpretation:
Serum sodium level abnormal

Hypernatremia frequently occurs in burn patients who do not receive adequate amounts of free water since large amounts of water are lost from burn wounds.

Sodium rich albumin solutions may also contribute to the development of hypernatremia.
Frequency of Monitoring

Serum sodium measurements should be obtained upon admission and every 4 to 6 hours during fluid resuscitation.

COMMON PANELS

- Basic metabolic panel
- Comprehensive metabolic panel
- Electrolyte panel

CLINICAL NOTES

To calculate the 'corrected' sodium for the dilutional effects of marked hyperglycemia, increase the serum sodium value by 1.3 to 1.6 mEq/L for every 100 mg/dL (5.56 mmol/L) increase in serum glucose.

Marked hyperlipemia or hyperproteinemia can cause pseudohyponatremia (ie, falsely low sodium levels), if the laboratory uses indirect reading (diluted plasma), ion-selective electrodes, or flame photometry. Pseudohyponatremia does not occur with direct reading (undiluted plasma) ion-selective electrodes.

COLLECTION/STORAGE INFORMATION

- Specimen Collection and Handling:
  - Collect venous blood specimen in a serum (red- or marbled-top) tube or plasma (eg, lithium [not sodium] heparin]) tube
  - Avoid hemolysis, and centrifuge blood as soon as possible

LOINC CODES

- Code: 2951-2 (*Short Name* - Sodium SerPl-sCnc)

Soluble transferrin receptor test

TEST DEFINITION

Measurement of serum concentration of soluble transferrin receptor for the evaluation of anemia

REFERENCE RANGE

- Adults: 9.6-29.6 nmol/L
- Blacks: 9% increase in normal values
- Residence at high altitude: 9% increase in normal values
  Please refer to your institution's reference ranges as lab normals may vary.

INDICATIONS

Suspected iron deficiency anemia
   Strength of Recommendation: Class IIa
   Strength of Evidence: Category B
   Results Interpretation:
   Increased level (laboratory finding)

An increased level of sTfR indicates iron deficiency. The most clinically useful aspect of the assay is in determining the etiology of iron-deficient erythropoiesis and in discriminating iron deficiency anemia from anemia of chronic disease.

CLINICAL NOTES

The normal range for soluble transferrin receptor varies with different assay methods; however, the relative changes in soluble transferrin receptor concentration in different disease states are remarkably similar regardless of the assay used.

COLLECTION/STORAGE INFORMATION

• Collect specimen in a red top tube

LOINC CODES

• Code: 30248-9 (*Short Name* - sTfR SerPl-mCnc)

Sporothrix schenckii antibody assay

TEST DEFINITION

Measurement of antibodies to *Sporothrix schenckii* in serum or cerebrospinal fluid (CSF) for the diagnosis of sporotrichosis

REFERENCE RANGE

• Negative (titer <1:8)
  Please refer to your institution's reference ranges as lab normals may vary.

INDICATIONS

Suspected sporotrichosis
    Strength of Recommendation: Class IIa
    Strength of Evidence: Category B
Results Interpretation:
Serology positive
• Positive titers (serum and cerebrospinal fluid [CSF]): ≥1:8
  Both the tube and slide latex agglutination assays appear to have high sensitivity and specificity for sporotrichosis.
  Serology may turn positive before and therefore be more helpful than culture in making the diagnosis of sporotrichosis meningitis.

COLLECTION/STORAGE INFORMATION

• Specimen Collection and Handling:
  • Use red top tube to collect serum.
  • Use sterile tube to collect cerebrospinal fluid (CSF).

LOINC CODES

• Code: 13241-5 (*Short Name* - S schenckii IgG Ser-aCnc)
• Code: 13243-1 (*Short Name* - S schenckii IgA Ser-aCnc)
• Code: 27937-2 (*Short Name* - S schenckii Ab Titr Ser)
• Code: 13242-3 (*Short Name* - S schenckii IgM Ser-aCnc)
• Code: 26864-9 (*Short Name* - S schenckii Ab Ser LA-aCnc)

St. Louis encephalitis virus antibody assay

TEST DEFINITION

Detection of antibodies to St. Louis encephalitis in serum to aid in the diagnosis and management of St. Louis encephalitis

SYNONYMS

• Serologic test for St. Louis encephalitis virus

REFERENCE RANGE
- Hemagglutination inhibition (HI) titer <1:10
  Please refer to your institution's reference ranges as lab normals may vary.

INDICATIONS
Suspected or known St. Louis encephalitis
> **Strength of Recommendation:** Class IIb
> **Strength of Evidence:** Category C
> **Results Interpretation:**
> **Positive immunology findings**

A single positive SLE-specific IgM antibody level with IgM antibody-capture enzyme-linked immunosorbent assay (MAC-ELISA) found in cerebrospinal fluid (CSF) is sufficient to confirm an SLE infection as IgM does not cross the blood-brain barrier.

The presence of SLE-specific IgM identified by enzyme-linked immunoassay (EIA)/MAC-ELISA testing plus an SLE-positive IgG antibody in the same or a later specimen by another serologic assay (eg, neutralization or hemagglutination) is diagnostic for SLE disease.

A 4-fold or greater change in a plaque-reduction neutralizing test antibody titer in paired sera specimens is diagnostic for SLE disease.

Due to cross-reactivity with other flaviviruses, including West Nile virus, and the lingering presence of IgG antibody, a positive IgG is not diagnostic of past or present infection. Conversely, the presence of IgM antibody can be considered provisional evidence of infection. Patient age, clinical presentation, season, location of exposure, occurrence of similar cases in the same geographic area and other epidemiological factors must be considered when evaluating serologic results.

An algorithm has been developed to help differentiate SLE from WNV encephalitis.

Because cross-reactivity of flaviviruses does not permit precise viral identification, a second assay is routinely performed to verify the causative organism.

Timing of Monitoring

Blood samples should be obtained at disease onset and 2 to 4 weeks later for acute and convalescent specimen analysis.

In a public health laboratory study of serum specimens collected from 69 SLE-confirmed patients using IgM antibody capture enzyme immunoassay (MAC-ELISA), 71% of specimens were positive for IgM antibodies when collected 0 to 3 days after symptom onset, 99% were positive when collected 4 to 21 days after onset, 91% were positive when collected 22 to 67 days after onset, and 29% remained positive at 115 to 251 days after illness onset.

CLINICAL NOTES

For a presumptive diagnosis of recent acute infection by serological testing a 4-fold increase in IgG between the acute and the convalescent sera must occur, however definitive diagnosis requires virus isolation. In general, viral-specific IgM appears during the first week of primary infection with levels becoming undetectable within 6 to 8 weeks, although it can remain detectable for extended periods of time. IgM specificity and sensitivity can be improved by removing rheumatoid factor and IgG to reduce competition with IgM for viral antigen. Viral-specific IgG appears 1 to 2 weeks after primary infection and reaches peak levels at 4 to 8 weeks, but remains detectable indefinitely. During reinfection IgM may reappear ephemerally in low levels while IgG will increase rapidly and peak at higher levels than are seen in primary infection. Factors such as infection site and immune status can alter these findings and specific viruses may produce different patterns.

COLLECTION/STORAGE INFORMATION
- Transport immediately to lab
- Freeze specimen if not immediately processed

LOINC CODES
- Code: 22513-6 (*Short Name* - SLEV IgM Titr CSF)
- Code: 24201-6 (*Short Name* - SLEV Ab sp1 Titr Ser IF)
- Code: 20806-6 (*Short Name* - SLEV Ab Ser QI)
- Code: 29822-4 (*Short Name* - SLEV Ab Titr XXX)
- Code: 21510-3 (*Short Name* - SLEV IgM Titr CSF IF)
- Code: 29796-0 (*Short Name* - SLEV Ab Titr CSF Nt)
- Code: 8023-4 (*Short Name* - SLEV Ab Ser QI EIA)
- Code: 8022-6 (*Short Name* - SLEV Ab Ser CF-aCnc)
- Code: 29783-8 (*Short Name* - SLEV Ab Titr XXX Nt)

- Code: 5365-2 (*Short Name* - SLEV Ab Ser-aCnc)
- Code: 21509-5 (*Short Name* - SLEV IgG Titr CSF IF)
- Code: 10906-6 (*Short Name* - SLEV IgG Titr Ser IF)
- Code: 13231-6 (*Short Name* - SLEV IgM CSF-aCnc)
- Code: 9634-7 (*Short Name* - SLEV IgG Titr XXX)
- Code: 22509-4 (*Short Name* - SLEV Ab Titr CSF)
- Code: 9577-8 (*Short Name* - SLEV Ab Titr CSF IF)
- Code: 8016-8 (*Short Name* - SLEV IgG Ser-aCnc)
- Code: 22510-2 (*Short Name* - SLEV Ab Titr Ser)
- Code: 24275-0 (*Short Name* - SLEV Ab sp1 Titr Ser)
- Code: 8024-2 (*Short Name* - SLEV Ab Ser QI IF)
- Code: 10907-4 (*Short Name* - SLEV IgM Titr Ser IF)
- Code: 8021-8 (*Short Name* - SLEV Ab CSF QI EIA)
- Code: 29809-1 (*Short Name* - SLEV Ab Titr Ser Nt)
- Code: 22514-4 (*Short Name* - SLEV IgM Titr Ser)
- Code: 24202-4 (*Short Name* - SLEV Ab sp2 Titr Ser IF)
- Code: 9635-4 (*Short Name* - SLEV IgM Titr XXX)
- Code: 24276-8 (*Short Name* - SLEV Ab #2 Titr Ser)
- Code: 8017-6 (*Short Name* - SLEV IgM Ser-aCnc)
- Code: 22507-8 (*Short Name* - SLEV Ab CSF QI)
- Code: 17558-8 (*Short Name* - SLEV Ab CSF-aCnc)
- Code: 13230-8 (*Short Name* - SLEV IgG CSF-aCnc)
- Code: 22511-0 (*Short Name* - SLEV IgG Titr CSF)
- Code: 31617-4 (*Short Name* - SLEV Ab XXX-aCnc)
- Code: 9578-6 (*Short Name* - SLEV Ab Titr Ser IF)
- Code: 22512-8 (*Short Name* - SLEV IgG Titr Ser)

Stool culture

TEST DEFINITION
Detection and screening of stool for enteric pathogens (eg, *Salmonella* spp., *Shigella* spp., and *Campylobacter* spp.)

SYNONYMS
- Faeces culture
- Feces culture
- Microbial stool culture

REFERENCE RANGE
- Adults and Children: Negative
  Please refer to your institution's reference ranges as lab normals may vary.

INDICATIONS
Suspected infectious gastroenteritis
    Strength of Recommendation: Class IIa
    Strength of Evidence: Category B
Results Interpretation:
Stool culture positive
    Results are usually available within 2 or 3 days when the suspected causative organisms are one or more of the following: *Salmonella*, *Shigella*, *Campylobacter*, enterohemorrhagic E *Coli*, *Vibrio*, or B *Cerus*. Cultures for enterotoxigenic and enteropathogenic E *Coli* are available from research laboratories.

    The best clinical predictor of a positive stool culture for inflammatory diarrhea is the combination of diarrhea persisting for greater than 24 hours, fever (greater than 37.7°C), and either blood in the stool or abdominal pain with nausea or vomiting.

    In laboratories where routine culture for Campylobacter has been instituted, C *jejuni* is the most common isolate and, combined with *Salmonella* spp, comprises approximately 90% of the stool pathogens.

    FREQUENCY: A single specimen collection can recover up to 96.9% of pathogens (excluding heavy growth of yeast and S *aureus*) found in a stool sample; subsequent analysis of two or more specimens produces a cumulative yield of 99% or more.

Suspected or known diarrheal disorder
Results Interpretation:
Positive microbiology findings

Traveler's diarrhea is often due to enterotoxigenic *E. coli*.

In laboratories where routine culture for *Campylobacter* has been instituted, *C jejuni* is the most common isolate and, combined with salmonella species, comprises approximately 90% of the stool pathogens.

Results usually are available within 2 or 3 days when the suspected causative organisms are *Salmonella*, *Shigella, Campylobacter,* enterohemorrhagic *E coli, Vibrio,* or *B cereus.* Cultures for enterotoxigenic and enteropathogenic *E coli* are available only from research laboratories.

Timing of Monitoring

Patients returning from a developing country or a primitive area with acute diarrhea that does not resolve and becomes chronic should be evaluated for chronic bacterial enteric pathogens and protozoal and parasitic infections, and if no etiology is identified, endoscopy is recommended for visualization and histologic assessment.

Patients with acute diarrheal illness (eg, bloody diarrhea, persistent or recurrent diarrhea, or dehydration from diarrhea) should be investigated. When epidemiologic factors and health safety are critical factors (ie, bloody diarrhea in someone with presumptive community-acquired salmonella or shigella infection), patients should be evaluated.

Suspected or known hemolytic uremic syndrome (HUS)
Results Interpretation:
Stool sample culture negative

If routine stool cultures are negative, cultures for *Escherichia coli* O157:H7 should be performed, particularly in geographic areas where this serotype is prevalent (eg, the Pacific Northwest and Canada).

Stool culture positive

Numerous bacterial, rickettsial, and viral organisms have been cultured from stool specimens of hemolytic uremic syndrome (HUS) patients.

Timing of Monitoring

Recovery of *Escherichia coli* O157:H7 is highly dependent on obtaining stool cultures within 6 days of the onset of diarrhea.

CLINICAL NOTES

A selective approach to diagnosis patients with diarrheal disease is advised, due to the high cost of routine stool cultures and low yield (less than 10%).

Routine cultures identify the most common of pathogens: *Shigella, Salmonella, Campylobacter, Aeromonas,* and *Yersinia.*

Additional cultures should be requested, based on clinical and historical features, (eg, patient's symptoms, time to onset, age, travel history, food/water exposure, homosexual exposure, recent antibiotic use). Other pathogens that may produce illness (eg, *Vibrio* spp., *Yersinia* spp., or *Clostridium difficile*) can be included with a routine stool culture.

COLLECTION/STORAGE INFORMATION

- Specimen Collection and Handling:
  - Collect freshly passed stool in a closed container; rectal swabs can be used but often yield less enteric pathogens.
  - Transport specimen immediately to lab; do not refrigerate.
  - Place specimens in a transport medium (eg, glycerol-buffered saline for *Salmonella* or *Shigella* or alkaline peptone water for *Vibrio* spp.) if there is a delay of several hours in transport to the lab.

LOINC CODES

- Code: 17968-9 (*Short Name* - Stl Cult org #6)
- Code: 625-4 (*Short Name* - Stl Cult)
- Code: 17964-8 (*Short Name* - Stl Cult org #2)
- Code: 17967-1 (*Short Name* - Stl Cult org #5)
- Code: 17965-5 (*Short Name* - Stl Cult org #3)
- Code: 17966-3 (*Short Name* - Stl Cult org #4)

Surfactant albumin ratio, amniotic fluid

TEST DEFINITION
Quantitative measurement of the surfactant to albumin ratio in amniotic fluid or vaginal pool specimens for the evaluation of fetal lung maturity.

SYNONYMS
• Fetal lung maturity test by fluorescence polarization

REFERENCE RANGE
• TDx FLM II assay (Abbott Laboratories, Abbott Park, IL):
• Mature: ≥55 mg surfactant/g albumin
• Immature: ≤39 mg surfactant/g albumin :
  Please refer to your institution's reference ranges as lab normals may vary.

INDICATIONS
At risk for respiratory distress syndrome in the newborn
> **Strength of Recommendation:** Class IIa
> **Strength of Evidence:** Category B
> **Results Interpretation:**
> **Abnormal laboratory findings**
> Fetal lung maturity test by fluorescence polarization (FPOL) values >55 mg/g are suggestive of mature lung development in the fetus. FPOL values <40 mg/g are indicative of immature fetal lungs and are associated with a higher incidence of respiratory distress syndrome.

> **False Results**
> Specimens contaminated with blood may produce false results; mature results may produce less mature (lower) values, and immature results may produce more mature (higher) values as a result of contamination.
> **Timing of Monitoring**
> Testing for fetal lung maturity is recommended prior to elective delivery at less than 39 weeks gestation unless fetal maturity can be reasonably determined by an alternative method such as fetal ultrasound measurement, documented continuous fetal heart tones for 20 to 30 weeks by nonelectronic fetoscope or Doppler, respectively, or the absence of a positive human chorionic gonadotropin pregnancy test for at least 36 weeks previously. Fetal lung maturity testing of amniotic fluid prior to 33 weeks gestation offers limited clinical utility as fetal lung maturity is unlikely at this gestational age.

COLLECTION/STORAGE INFORMATION
Amniotic fluid samples are stable for 24 hours at 4°C and 16 hours at room temperature. Samples stored at -20°C do not provide reliable results.

A minimum of 10 mL of uncontaminated amniotic fluid is recommended. Collection of amniotic fluid in the amber tube commonly included in amniotic trays is not necessary for fetal lung maturity testing; the amber tube is required for bilirubin testing only.

LOINC CODES
• Code: 30562-3 (*Short Name* - Surfactant/Alb Amn-mRto)

Synovial fluid analysis

TEST DEFINITION
Measurement of characteristics and biochemical parameters of synovial fluid for the evaluation and management of joint disease

REFERENCE RANGE
• Characteristics of Normal Synovial Fluid:
• Volume: Up to 3.5 mL

- Color: Pale yellow
- Clarity: Clear
- Viscosity: High (strings 3-6 mm long)
- Spontaneous clot formation: None
- Hyaluronate content: 3-4 g/L, decreases with age
- Cytologic examination:
- Erythrocytes: $<2 \times 10^9$ /L
- Leukocytes: $<0.2 \times 10^9$ /L
- Cytological sediment:
- Monocytes/macrophages: Approximately 60%
- Lymphocytes: Approximately 30%
- Neutrophilic granulocytes: Approximately 10% (<25%)
- Biochemical parameters:
- Glucose: Approximately same as plasma concentration (3.3-5.3 mmol/L)
- Uric acid: Identical to plasma concentration
- Total protein: 10-30 g/L
- Lactate: 1-1.8 mmol/L
- Lactate dehydrogenase: <4.8 microkatal/L
- Acid phosphatase: Negative
- Immunoglobulins: Approximately half of plasma concentration
- Rheumatoid factor: Negative
- Bacteria: Negative
- Crystals: Negative
- Fibrinogen: Negative
  Please refer to your institution's reference ranges as lab normals may vary.

INDICATIONS
Suspected brucella arthritis
Results Interpretation:
Abnormal laboratory findings
In brucella arthritis, synovial fluid is exudative with WBC counts between 180 and 10,250/mm^3.

Suspected gout or pseudogout
Strength of Recommendation: Class IIa
Strength of Evidence: Category B
Results Interpretation:
Synovial fluid: crystals
Identification of crystals in synovial fluid is specific for the diagnoses of gout and pseudogout. Sodium urate crystals appear on polarized light microscopy in the form of small needles and are found both inside and outside of leukocytes, sometimes piercing through the leukocyte during acute episodes. Crystals appear yellow when they are parallel to the gamma plane of the compensator and blue when they are perpendicular. Urate crystals may also occur as spherulites with negative birefringence and may require special staining to distinguish them from fat particles, although they are not typically present without the more typical needle-like crystals.
Calcium pyrophosphate crystals are found in cells, are rhomboid, and appear flatter; they do not penetrate the cell membrane. These crystals appear blue when they are parallel to the axis of the compensator.
Crystals with negative birefringence may correlate with acute gout; those with positive birefringence may correlate with pseudogout. The presence of crystals can help to differentiate gout and pseudogout from other causes of inflammatory arthritis.
Crystal arthropathy can exist along with bacterial arthritis.
White blood cell finding
In gout, the synovial fluid WBC count is usually 10,000 to 75,000/mm^3. High counts may indicate coexisting septic arthritis.
Negative microbiology findings
In gout, culture and Gram stain of synovial fluid is negative for organisms.

Suspected inflammatory or noninflammatory arthritis
Strength of Recommendation: Class IIa
Strength of Evidence: Category C

Results Interpretation:
Synovial fluid finding
- Inflammatory effusion suggestive of arthritis includes:
  - Volume: >3.5 mL
  - Color: Yellow-greyish
  - Clarity: Turbid
  - Viscosity: Low
  - Spontaneous clot formation: Yes
  - Leukocytes: 3 to 50 x 10^9 /L
  - Polymorphonuclear cells: >75%
  - Crystals: May or may not be present
  - Bacteria: Negative
  - Glucose: Normal to low
  - Total protein: >40 g/L
  - Uric acid: Normal to increased
  - Lactate: 4.2 to 6.9 mmol/L
  - Lactate dehydrogenase: Increased
  - Acid phosphatase: >100 nkat/L (rheumatoid arthritis)
  - Immunoglobulins: Increased
  - Rheumatoid factor: Positive or negative
- Non-inflammatory effusion suggestive of arthritis includes:
  - Volume: >3.5 mL
  - Color: Yellow
  - Clarity: Slightly turbid
  - Viscosity: High
  - Spontaneous clot formation: No
  - Leukocytes: <3 x 10^9 /L
  - Bacteria: Negative
  - Glucose: Normal
  - Total protein: Normal
  - Uric acid: Normal
  - Lactate: <4.2 mmol/L
  - Lactate dehydrogenase: Normal
  - Acid phosphatase: Up to 40 nkat/L
  - Immunoglobulins: Normal
  - Rheumatoid factor: Negative

White blood cell finding

The synovial fluid WBC count in rheumatoid arthritis (RA) is usually in the range of 3000 to 30,000 mm^3 (mean is usually 15,500 mm^3); although ranges of 300 to 75,000 mm^3 have been noted. The percentage of polymorphonuclear leukocytes is usually 60% to 70%. While a low WBC count does not rule out RA, it does make the diagnosis less likely.

In rheumatic fever, synovial fluid from affected joints contain 10,000 to 100,000 WBC/mm^3 ; mostly neutrophils.

In Lyme disease arthritis, the mean WBC count is 24,500/mm^3, with a range of 2100 to 72,250/mm^3. The differential count consists primarily of granulocytes and ranges from 16% to 88% (median 80%).

In early-onset arthritis associated with Kawasaki disease, synovial fluid examination reveals grossly purulent fluid with intense inflammatory reactions. The mean WBC count is 135,000/mm^3, but counts as high as 350,000/mm$_3$ have been reported. There is a predominance of polymorphonuclear cells. Late-onset arthritis has a lesser inflammatory reaction with a typical type II reaction and a WBC count ranging from 20,000 to 60,000/mm^3 (mean 40,000/mm^3). Cultures are negative.

Synovial fluid analysis may be useful to identify viral arthritis infections (eg, Ross River virus, rubella), but does not distinguish between them. Early cellular pattern suggests viral infection; paucity of neutrophils in early and late stages help rule out other arthropathies. Cell count ranges from 1.1 to 60 x 10^9 /L and are entirely or predominantly mononuclear.

Suspected osteoarthritis
Results Interpretation:
White blood cell finding

Typically, in osteoarthritic joint fluid, the cell count is below 1,000 cells/mm^3, no crystals are seen, the glucose level is normal, and the fluid viscosity is normal.

Suspected septic arthritis
Strength of Recommendation: Class I
Strength of Evidence: Category C
Results Interpretation:
Synovial fluid finding
- Characteristics of synovial fluid from a suspected septic effusion:
  - Volume: >3.5 mL
  - Color: Green-greyish
  - Clarity: Turbid, purulent
  - Viscosity: Low
  - Spontaneous clot formation: Yes
  - Leukocytes: >50 x 10^9 /L
  - PMN: >85%
  - Crystals: Negative
  - Bacteria: Positive
  - Glucose: Decreased
  - Total protein: 30 to 60 g/L
  - Uric acid: Normal
  - Lactate: >9 mmol/L
  - Lactate dehydrogenase: Increased
  - Acid phosphatase: Increased
  - Immunoglobulins: Increased
  - Rheumatoid factor: Negative

Leukocytosis
A synovial WBC count greater than 50,000/mm^3 and greater than 90% neutrophils strongly suggests infection; however, lower counts do not rule out septic arthritis.
In patients with disseminated gonococcal infections, the synovial fluid WBC count is increased (mean counts of 50,000 to 100,000/mm^3), with greater than 90% neutrophils; however, counts as low as 7000/mm^3 have been associated with positive cultures. Lower leukocyte counts are more common early in the course of bacterial arthritis in patients with disseminated gonococcal infection, and in partially-treated patients.

White blood cell finding
Response to therapy can be guided by reductions in WBC counts after 1 week. If there is no reduction in the WBC count, the likelihood of complete recovery is reduced.

Decreased glucose level
Measurement of glucose in synovial fluid rarely contributes significant information and is not recommended as part of the initial diagnostic evaluation. A low level is suggestive of an infected joint, but is present in only about 50% of patients with septic arthritis. A low level can also occur in rheumatoid arthritis.

Protein level - finding
The synovial fluid protein level is elevated (mean 5.7 g/dL) in patients with disseminated gonococcal infection.

Increased C-reactive protein level
Elevated C-reactive protein is strongly supportive of septic arthritis in children with monoarthritis and is especially helpful in diagnosing septic hip. C-reactive protein was found to be elevated in 98% of cases of adult-onset septic arthritis.

CLINICAL NOTES

It is recommended that synovial fluid samples with high viscosity be treated with hyaluronidase enzyme to reduce viscosity and allow easier and more accurate diagnosis.

COLLECTION/STORAGE INFORMATION

- Specimen Collection and Handling:
  - The following tubes are used for the components of synovial fluid analysis:
    - Cell count, differential: lavender top
    - Protein, glucose: red top
    - Gram stain, culture: sterile syringe
    - Microscopic crystal examination: green top
    - Cytology: sterile syringe or container
  - Send first sample of fluid for microbiological testing in a sterile container; second sample of fluid is usually sent for biochemical and cytology testing.
  - Examine sample within one hour; cell lysis is likely if examination is delayed for longer than one hour.

LOINC CODES

- Code: 13357-9 (*Short Name* - Synovial Cells Fld-aCnc)
- Code: 14363-6 (*Short Name* - Gram Stn Snv)
- Code: 621-3 (*Short Name* - Snv BFld Cult)

T4 newborn screen

TEST DEFINITION

Measurement of thyroxine (T4) from dried capillary blood spots for congenital hypothyroid screening in newborns

SYNONYMS

- T4 neonatal screen
- Thyroid screen for newborn

REFERENCE RANGE

- Serum: 58-160 nmol/L (4.5-12.6 mcg/dL). Reference values are method dependent, and age and laboratory specific.
- Normal ranges and percentile cutoffs are often independently determined by each screening program. A cutoff of less than 10% is frequently utilized.
  Please refer to your institution's reference ranges as lab normals may vary.

INDICATIONS

Newborn screening for congenital hypothyroidism
    Strength of Recommendation: Class IIa
    Strength of Evidence: Category B
    Results Interpretation:
    Thyroid function tests abnormal

During the first 2 weeks of life, newborns presenting with a low thyroxine (T4) level and a thyroid stimulating hormone (TSH) level greater than 40 mU/L by filter paper specimen are considered to have a presumptive diagnosis of primary congenital hypothyroidism; confirmatory testing of serum and immediate clinical evaluation are required to confirm the diagnosis. This presentation may also be due to maternal antibodies or maternal medications such as iodine. Substantially elevated TSH levels require immediate evaluation, regardless of T4 results. However, no treatment is required in nearly all cases of transient newborn hypothyroidism in which the mother is taking antithyroid medication, as both T4 and TSH levels return to normal within 1 to 3 weeks without intervention.

Normal TSH and low T4 levels can be caused by pituitary or hypothalmic disorders, thyroid-binding globulin (TBG) deficiency, or secondary hypothyroidism; these findings may also be seen in premature infants. An elevated TSH level in the presence of a normal T4 level can be due to hypothyroidism or TSH surge. In both instances, rescreening and possible diagnostic workup are recommended, to include T4, triiodothyronine (T3) uptake, either free T4 or T4 index, and TSH testing. Additional supplemental tests and procedures such as serum TBG and ultrasound imaging of the thyroid may also be appropriate.

Preterm infants younger than 34 weeks gestation are typically born with substantially lower T4 levels than full-term infants, and levels continue to fall during the first few weeks of life. These infants also experience a small first-day TSH surge, complicating the evaluation of laboratory results. Reference values specific for premature infants should be utilized when evaluating these test results. Preterm infants born before 32 weeks are particularly prone to transient hypothyroidism and should therefore have repeat thyroid testing at 32 week gestation. Some premature infants with primary hypothyroidism may not present with a TSH elevation immediately, necessitating serial thyroid testing.

    False Results

While hemolysis, lipemia and hyperbilirubinemia do not substantially alter immunoassay results, free fatty acids can interfere with the ability of thyroxine (T4) to bind to serum binding proteins, leading to low T4 levels in patients with non-thyroid conditions.

Timing of Monitoring

Thyroid screening specimens should not be collected until at least 24 hours after birth, since postnatal thyroid stimulating hormone (TSH) surge occurs during this time period. Some screening programs include the collection of a second specimen 1 to 2 weeks after birth, a method which can identify up to 10% of patients whose initial test was negative.

CLINICAL NOTES

Dried whole blood spots are stable for months or years when stored with a drying agent.

COLLECTION/STORAGE INFORMATION

Do not touch the filter paper during specimen collection. Apply the second largest blood drop to the filter paper circle from one side of the filter paper only; avoid using the first drop of blood. Use additional drops of blood as needed to completely fill all required circles one at a time. Let the filter paper dry on a flat surface at room temperature for 3 to 4 hours. Keep specimens out of direct sunlight. Specimens should be packed in low gas-permeable, zip-closure bags with a drying agent and humidity indicator cards, and forwarded to the screening laboratory within 24 hours of collection. Filter paper must meet National Committee for Clinical Laboratory Standards (NCCLS) standards.

LOINC CODES

• Code: 20451-1 (*Short Name* - T4 Bld Ql)

TGF-Beta assay

TEST DEFINITION

Measurement of the cytokine transforming growth factor (TGF)-beta levels in serum or plasma; may be useful as a marker in certain disease states, primarily cancer

INDICATIONS

Colorectal cancer

> **Strength of Recommendation:** Class IIb
> **Strength of Evidence:** Category B
> **Results Interpretation:**
> **Increased level (laboratory finding)**
>
> Transforming growth factor-beta $_1$ (TGF-beta$_1$) levels are significantly increased in colorectal cancer patients and may be reflective of disease severity.

Hepatocellular carcinoma (HCC)

> **Strength of Recommendation:** Class IIb
> **Strength of Evidence:** Category B
> **Results Interpretation:**
> **Increased level (laboratory finding)**
>
> Levels of transforming growth factor-beta$_1$ (TGF-beta$_1$) appear to be higher in patients with hepatocellular carcinoma, and in patients with metastasis compared to those without metastasis.

Invasive breast cancer

> **Strength of Recommendation:** Class IIb
> **Strength of Evidence:** Category B
> **Results Interpretation:**
> **Increased level (laboratory finding)**
>
> Transforming growth factor-beta$_1$ (TGF-beta$_1$) levels are significantly increased in breast cancer patients with advanced lymph node status, advanced TNM stage, and more advanced histologic grade, based upon data from 1 small cohort study.

Myelofibrosis
Results Interpretation:
Increased level (laboratory finding)
Elevated levels of transforming growth factor-beta (TGF-beta) have been found in patients with idiopathic and secondary myelofibrosis, suggesting that TGF-beta may become useful as a prognostic indicator of this disease.

Prostate cancer
Strength of Recommendation: Class IIb
Strength of Evidence: Category C
Results Interpretation:
Increased level (laboratory finding)
Elevated levels of transforming growth factor-beta$_1$ (TGF-beta$_1$) appear to be predictive of higher grade pathologic stage and worsened disease progression in men with prostate cancer.

CLINICAL NOTES
TGF-beta is a cytokine that modulates cell-cell interactions by binding to cell surface receptors and initiating an intracellular cascade. It is known to influence apoptosis, strengthen the extracellular matrix, and increase angiogenesis, among other functions.

COLLECTION/STORAGE INFORMATION
- Collect blood in a heparinized (green) tube.
- Store sample at -20°C or at -70° C until ready for assay.

Testosterone measurement, total

TEST DEFINITION
Measurement of total testosterone in serum for the evaluation of gonadal hormone function

REFERENCE RANGE
- Adult males (morning): 270-1070 ng/dL (9.36-37.1 nmol/L)
- Adult females (morning): 6-86 ng/dL (0.21-2.98 nmol/L)
- Pregnant women: 3 to 4 times normal
- Postmenopausal women: 8-35 ng/dL (0.28-1.22 nmol/L)
- Premature neonates, male: 37-198 ng/dL (1.28-6.87 nmol/L)
- Premature neonates, female: 5-22 ng/dL (0.17-0.76 nmol/L)
- Neonates, male: 75-400 ng/dL (2.6-13.9 nmol/L)
- Neonates, female: 20-64 ng/dL (0.69-2.22 nmol/L)
- Children, male, 1 to 5 months: 1-177 ng/dL (0.03-6.14 nmol/L)
- Children, female, 1 to 5 months: 1-5 ng/dL (0.03-0.17 nmol/L)
- Children, males, 6-11 months: 2-7 ng/dL (0.07-0.24 nmol/L)
- Children, females, 6 to 11 months: 2-5 ng/dL (0.07-0.24 nmol/L)
- Children, males, 1 to 5 years: 2-25 ng/dL (0.07-0.87 nmol/L)
- Children, females, 1 to 5 years: 2-10 ng/dL (0.07-0.35 nmol/L)
- Children, males, 6 to 9 years: 3-30 ng/dL (0.10-1.04 nmol/L)
- Children, females, 6 to 9 years: 2-20 ng/dL (0.07-0.69 nmol/L)
- Male Tanner stages:
- Tanner stage 1: 2-23 ng/dL (0.07-0.8 nmol/L)
- Tanner stage 2: 5-70 ng/dL (0.17-2.43 nmol/L)
- Tanner stage 3: 15-280 ng/dL (0.52-9.72 nmol/L)
- Tanner stage 4: 105-545 ng/dL (3.64-18.91 nmol/L)
- Tanner stage 5: 265-800 ng/dL (9.19-27.76 nmol/L)
- Female Tanner stages:
- Tanner stage 1: 2-10 ng/dL (0.07-0.35 nmol/L)
- Tanner stage 2: 5-30 ng/dL (0.17-1.04 nmol/L)
- Tanner stage 3: 10-30 ng/dL (0.35-1.04 nmol/L)
- Tanner stage 4: 15-40 ng/dL (0.52-1.39 nmol/L)
- Tanner stage 5: 10-40 ng/dL (0.35-1.39 nmol/L)
- **Please refer to your institution's reference ranges as lab normals may vary.**

INDICATIONS

Men at risk for hip fracture
  Strength of Recommendation: Class IIb
  Strength of Evidence: Category B
Results Interpretation:
Decreased testosterone level
  Below normal levels of testosterone may be a risk factor for hip fracture in men.

Suspected adrenocortical tumor
  Strength of Recommendation: Class IIa
  Strength of Evidence: Category C
Results Interpretation:
Increased testosterone level
  Total testosterone levels may be elevated in adults with adrenocortical carcinoma and virilization syndrome..
  Testosterone levels are typically elevated in children with adrenocortical carcinoma and virilizing features and are generally higher in children with pure virilizing symptoms compared to children with mixed Cushing virilizing syndrome.

Suspected congenital adrenal hyperplasia
  Strength of Recommendation: Class IIb
  Strength of Evidence: Category C
Results Interpretation:
Increased testosterone level
  Serum testosterone levels may be increased in congenital adrenal hyperplasia.

Suspected hypogonadism in men
  Strength of Recommendation: Class I
  Strength of Evidence: Category C
Results Interpretation:
Decreased testosterone level
  Low total testosterone levels in men should be interpreted in conjunction with a free testosterone level or sex hormone-binding globulin level. Total testosterone levels may be decreased due aging or various disorders of hypergonadotropic hypogonadism or hypogonadotropic hypogonadism..
  There is hourly variation in testosterone levels, and normal men may have periodic decline below the normal range. In young men, highest values occur at 8 AM and lowest in the late afternoon.
  Although there are no specific recommendations regarding therapy for older men with symptomatic hypogonadism, men with a total testosterone level of less than 200 ng/mL may be potential candidates for therapy. A level of 2.5 standard deviations below the mean testosterone value for young normal males (approximately 319 ng/dL) has been used in some studies.
Timing of Monitoring
  Blood sample for total testosterone should preferably be drawn in the morning because of diurnal variation. Morning sampling may not be mandatory as diurnal pattern is lost with aging.
  Testosterone levels should be repeated in patients with subnormal levels, especially patients with no definite signs or symptoms of hypogonadism.

Suspected polycystic ovary syndrome
  Strength of Recommendation: Class IIa
  Strength of Evidence: Category C
Results Interpretation:
Increased testosterone level
  Total testosterone is at the upper range of normal or modestly elevated in women with polycystic ovary syndrome.
  Patients with testosterone levels greater than 2 ng/mL should be evaluated for ovarian or adrenal androgen-producing tumors; however, this cut-off level has poor sensitivity and specificity.

COLLECTION/STORAGE INFORMATION

- Specimen Collection and Handling:
  - Collect 5 mL of venous blood sample at 7 AM in a marbled red top tube.
  - Take pooled samples at different times throughout the day to nullify diurnal variation.
  - Specify age and gender on laboratory request.

Tetanus antibody assay

TEST DEFINITION
Measurement of antibodies to tetanus antitoxin in serum for the evaluation of immunity status.

SYNONYMS
- Serologic test for Tetanus

REFERENCE RANGE
While studies on anti-tetanus toxin responses to vaccine define seroprotection as ≥0.1 International Units/mL, other researchers have suggested that a level of ≥0.15 International Units/mL is more reliably predictive of immunity regardless of vaccination history.
Please refer to your institution's reference ranges as lab normals may vary.

INDICATIONS
Evaluation of immunity status to tetanus.
> **Strength of Recommendation:** Class IIa
> **Strength of Evidence:** Category B
> **Results Interpretation:**
> **Abnormal immunology findings**
>> Antibody levels below the recommended threshold suggest incomplete protection. While a 3-dose primary series of tetanus vaccine generally provides seroprotection for 10 years or longer, antibody levels can be expected to drop as the length of time since the last tetanus vaccination increases.
>> Health care providers should evaluate tetanus immunity status at every opportunity, and vaccinate as necessary. Those at higher risk include diabetics, older adults, intravenous drug users, persons of Hispanic ethnicity, pregnant women and those who have not received a primary vaccination series.

LOINC CODES
- Code: 5093-0 (*Short Name* - C tetani Ab Ser Ql)
- Code: 16627-2 (*Short Name* - C tetani Ab sp2 Ser-aCnc)
- Code: 25536-4 (*Short Name* - C tetani Toxoid IgE RAST Ql)
- Code: 26643-7 (*Short Name* - C tetani Tox Ab Ser Ql)
- Code: 16626-4 (*Short Name* - C tetani Ab sp1 Ser-aCnc)
- Code: 6367-7 (*Short Name* - C tetani IgG Ser EIA-aCnc)
- Code: 19760-8 (*Short Name* - C tetani Toxoid IgE Qn)
- Code: 32775-9 (*Short Name* - C tetani Toxoid Ab Qn)
- Code: 33469-8 (*Short Name* - C tetani IgG Ser Ql)
- Code: 22203-4 (*Short Name* - C tetani IgG Ser-aCnc)
- Code: 5092-2 (*Short Name* - C tetani Ab Ser-aCnc)

Thallium measurement, blood

TEST DEFINITION
Measurement of thallium in whole blood for diagnosis of thallium toxicity/poisoning

REFERENCE RANGE
- Adults and children: <0.5 mcg/dL (<24.5 nmol/L)
Please refer to your institution's reference ranges as lab normals may vary.

INDICATIONS
Suspected thallium poisoning
> **Strength of Recommendation:** Class IIa
> **Strength of Evidence:** Category C

Results Interpretation:
Thallium toxicity
Whole blood thallium levels of greater than or equal to 10 mcg/dL (0.5 micromol/L) indicate thallium tox-
icity.

COLLECTION/STORAGE INFORMATION
- Specimen Collection and Handling:
    - Collect whole blood (sodium heparin tube) in a metal-free container
    - Do not allow specimen to contact metal or dusts with metal
    - Use of EDTA may affect results

LOINC CODES
- Code: 32114-1 (*Short Name* - Thallium Bld QI)
- Code: 25173-6 (*Short Name* - Thallium Bld-sCnc)

Thallium measurement, urine

TEST DEFINITION
Measurement of thallium in urine for diagnosis and monitoring of thallium toxicity/poisoning

REFERENCE RANGE
- Adults and children: <2 mcg/L (<9.8 nmol/L)
Please refer to your institution's reference ranges as lab normals may vary.

INDICATIONS
Monitoring response to treatment for thallium poisoning
    Strength of Recommendation: Class IIa
    Strength of Evidence: Category C
Results Interpretation:
Thallium toxicity
Treatment may be discontinued when urine values are less than 0.5 mg/24 hours.

Suspected thallium poisoning
    Strength of Recommendation: Class IIa
    Strength of Evidence: Category C
Results Interpretation:
Thallium toxicity
Clinical toxicity is indicated with 24-hour urine thallium levels of greater than or equal to 1 mg/L (4.9
micromol/L).

COMMON PANELS
- Heavy metal screen, urine

COLLECTION/STORAGE INFORMATION
- Specimen Collection and Handling:
    - Collect all urine over a 24-hour period in a metal-free container
    - The specimen remains stable for 7 days at room temperature

LOINC CODES
- Code: 29938-8 (*Short Name* - Thallium/creat 24H Ur-mRto)
- Code: 13469-2 (*Short Name* - Thallium/creat Ur-mRto)
- Code: 30929-4 (*Short Name* - Thallium ?Tm Ur-mCnc)
- Code: 21558-2 (*Short Name* - Thallium 24H Ur-mCnc)

Throat culture

TEST DEFINITION

Detection of bacteria by routine throat culture most commonly collected for screening and management of Group A beta-hemolytic streptococci infection

REFERENCE RANGE

- Adults and Children: Negative
  Please refer to your institution's reference ranges as lab normals may vary.

INDICATIONS

Confirmation of suspected streptococcal pharyngitis in children and adolescents with a negative antigen-detection (rapid strep) test
      Strength of Recommendation: Class I
      Strength of Evidence: Category B
      Results Interpretation:
      Throat swab culture positive
      Definitive results may take between 24 and 48 hours. Antibiotics should not routinely be initiated while awaiting throat culture results unless rapid streptococcal antigen screening is positive.

Suspected streptococcal pharyngitis in adults
      Strength of Recommendation: Class IIb
      Strength of Evidence: Category B
      Results Interpretation:
      Throat swab culture positive
      Definitive results may take between 24 and 48 hours. Antibiotics should not routinely be initiated while awaiting throat culture results unless rapid streptococcal antigen screen is positive.

Obtain in patients with epiglottitis after the airway is secured
      Results Interpretation:
      Positive microbiology findings
      In adults, throat and blood cultures may yield different pathogens.
      No definable pathogen is isolated in the majority of patients with mild epiglottitis. The inability to isolate any organism may be partially due to the presence of anaerobes.

CLINICAL NOTES

Perform throat cultures routinely for patients with a history of rheumatic fever. Consider throat cultures for patients who develop even mild acute pharyngitis during outbreaks of either acute rheumatic fever or post-streptococcal acute glomerulonephritis.

Throat cultures are indicated to confirm a negative rapid antigen-detection (RAD; rapid strep) test result in children and adolescents, but this remains controversial. It has been suggested that throat culture confirmation of a negative RAD may only be necessary in individuals with a history of rheumatic fever or family members of patients with rheumatic fever. It is also not recommended for routine primary evaluation of adults with pharyngitis or for confirmation of negative antigen-detection tests when test sensitivity exceeds 80%.

COLLECTION/STORAGE INFORMATION

- Specimen Collection and Handling:
  - Depress tongue with tongue blade and swab back and forth across the pharynx to collect specimen.
  - Collect specimen in a sterile tube or transport medium.
  - Transport to lab as soon as possible or refrigerate for a short time if delay in transport to lab.
  - Transport to another lab requires placing the specimen onto a filter paper strip.

LOINC CODES

- Code: 17902-8 (*Short Name* - Thrt Aerobe Cult org #5)
- Code: 17901-0 (*Short Name* - Thrt Aerobe Cult org #4)
- Code: 17900-2 (*Short Name* - Thrt Aerobe Cult org #3)
- Code: 626-2 (*Short Name* - Thrt Cult)

Thrombin time

TEST DEFINITION
Measurement of the late phase of coagulation to assess conversion of fibrinogen to fibrin

SYNONYMS
- Fibrin time
- Thrombin time - observation
- TT - Thrombin time

REFERENCE RANGE
- Adults: 16-24 seconds
  Please refer to your institution's reference ranges as lab normals may vary.

INDICATIONS
Screening for suspected congenital or acquired dysfibrinogenemia
 Strength of Recommendation: Class IIa
 Strength of Evidence: Category C
Results Interpretation:
Increased level (laboratory finding)
 Prolonged thrombin time suggests the presence of dysfibrinogenemia.
Decreased level (laboratory finding)
 A decreased thrombin time is found with only one dysfibrinogen.

Suspected clotting abnormality in amyloidosis
 Strength of Recommendation: Class IIb
 Strength of Evidence: Category C
Results Interpretation:
Increased level (laboratory finding)
 Although prolonged thrombin time and reptilase time are associated with amyloidosis, they do not appear to cause bleeding manifestations. A prolonged thrombin time in a patient without evidence of a bleeding disorder might suggest that amyloidosis should be included in the differential diagnosis.

Suspected DIC
 Strength of Recommendation: Class IIa
 Strength of Evidence: Category C
Results Interpretation:
Thrombin time abnormal
 Thrombin time is prolonged in DIC because of fibrinogen consumption.

COMMON PANELS
- Disseminated intravascular coagulopathy panel
- Hypercoagulation panel
- Transplant panel

COLLECTION/STORAGE INFORMATION
- Specimen Collection and Handling:
  - Collect sample in buffered citrate (blue-top) tube.
  - Sample is stable for 7 days at room temperature or 23 days at 4°C.

Thyroglobulin antibody measurement

TEST DEFINITION
Measurement of thyroglobulin autoimmune antibody (TgAb) in serum for evaluation of suspected or known thyroid disorders

Synonyms

- Anti-thyroglobulin antibody measurement

Reference Range

- Adults:
- Enzyme-linked immunosorbent assay: <5 International Units/mL (<0.3 kiloInternational Units/L)
- Radioimmunoassay: <20 International Units/mL (<20 kiloInternational Units/L)
- Tanned RBC agglutination: ≤ 1:10
- Indirect immunofluorescence microscopy: Negative
  Please refer to your institution's reference ranges as lab normals may vary.

Indications

Suspected chronic autoimmune thyroiditis due to Hashimoto's disease or atrophic thyroiditis
    Strength of Recommendation: Class IIb
    Strength of Evidence: Category C
Results Interpretation:
Autoantibody titer positive
    Testing for thyroid antibodies, along with determination of serum thyrotropin, may confirm a diagnosis of chronic autoimmune thyroiditis. Titers of thyroglobulin antibodies (TgAb) are often higher in patients with the atrophic thyroiditis form of chronic autoimmune thyroiditis versus the Hashimoto's goiter form. Ten percent of the normal population have measurable levels of the thyroglobulin antibody (TgAb). Up to 20% of female patients, without having any clinical signs of Hashimoto's disease, have measurable levels of TgAb.
Timing of Monitoring
    The presence of anti-thyroid antibodies has been associated with a doubling of the normal rate for spontaneous abortions, thus women with recurrent spontaneous abortions should be checked for these antibodies prior to attempting to becoming pregnant again.

Suspected Graves' disease
    Strength of Recommendation: Class IIa
    Strength of Evidence: Category B
Results Interpretation:
Antibody studies abnormal
    High levels of thyroglobulin antibody (TgAb) are consistent with autoimmune thyroid disease, which includes Graves' disease, as well as Hashimoto's. Graves' disease patients with positive titers of TgAb prior to drug treatment may have decreased rates of hyperthyroidism relapse after treatment.

Suspected thyroid cancer
    Strength of Recommendation: Class I
    Strength of Evidence: Category B
Results Interpretation:
Postoperative state
    The prevalence of thyroglobulin antibody (TgAb) in the general population is 10.1%. Of patients with differentiated thyroid carcinoma (DTC), 25% have detectable levels of thyroglobulin antibody (TgAb) with rates higher for women. Continued positive results for TgAb postoperatively may indicate persistent tumor tissue; negative results may reflect disease-free status. Testing for TgAb should be done with the more sensitive immunoassay technique. TgAb monitoring alone (without thyroglobulin testing) may be sufficient for tracking thyroid tumor activity.
Frequency of Monitoring
    Thyroglobulin antibody (TgAb) testing should be ordered each time a thyroglobulin level is checked in TgAb-positive patients.
Timing of Monitoring
    Thyroglobulin antibody testing is performed after thyroid tumor removal surgery as an adjunctive check for the persistence of tumor.

Clinical Notes

    Serial testing (done for monitoring purposes) should be performed by the same laboratory, using the same test method to insure uniformity of results.

COLLECTION/STORAGE INFORMATION
- Specimen Collection and Handling:
    - Collect venous blood specimen in a marbled serum separator tube (SST)
    - Store specimen at -20°C

LOINC CODES
- Code: 15210-8 (*Short Name* - Thyroglob Ab Ser Ql)
- Code: 5381-9 (*Short Name* - Thyroglob Ab Titr Ser LA)
- Code: 8098-6 (*Short Name* - Thyroglob Ab Ser-aCnc)
- Code: 5380-1 (*Short Name* - Thyroglob Ab Ser RIA-aCnc)

Thyroid stimulating hormone measurement

TEST DEFINITION
Measurement of thyroid stimulating hormone (TSH) in serum for the evaluation and management of thyroid dysfunction

SYNONYMS
- Thyroid stimulating hormone level
- Thyrotropin measurement
- Thyrotropin stimulating hormone measurement
- TSH level
- TSH measurement
- TSH - Thyroid stimulating hormone level

REFERENCE RANGE
- Adults: 0.5-4.7 microunits/mL (0.5-4.7 milliunits/L)
- Pregnancy (1st trimester): 0.3-4.5 microunits/mL (0.3-4.5 milliunits/L)
- Pregnancy (2nd trimester): 0.5-4.6 microunits/mL (0.5-4.6 milliunits/L)
- Pregnancy (3rd trimester): 0.8-5.2 microunits/mL (0.8-5.2 milliunits/L)

Please refer to your institution's reference ranges as lab normals may vary.

INDICATIONS
Gout
   Results Interpretation:
   Abnormal laboratory findings
   In patients with urate crystals present in synovial fluid indicating gout, a thyroid stimulating hormone (TSH) level aids in assessing thyroid function. Hypothyroidism may be associated with gout.

Suspected and known atrial fibrillation.
   Strength of Recommendation: Class I
   Strength of Evidence: Category C
   Results Interpretation:
   Decreased thyroid stimulating hormone level
   Subnormal thyroid stimulating hormone (TSH) is consistent with hyperthyroidism. Subclinical hyperthyroidism is a reversible cause of atrial fibrillation (AF) in elderly patients and is relatively common. The Framingham Study found an association of low serum TSH with a 3-fold increase in developing AF over the next 10 years.
   Timing of Monitoring
   Tests for thyroid function are indicated for first episodes of atrial fibrillation (AF), episodes where ventricular rate is difficult to control, in elderly individuals presenting with AF, and when AF recurs unexpectedly after cardioversion.

Suspected and known hypothyroidism
   Strength of Recommendation: Class IIa
   Strength of Evidence: Category C

Results Interpretation:
Increased thyroid stimulating hormone level

A thyroid stimulating hormone level greater that 20 milliInternational Units/L in association with a low free thyroxine (T_4) confirms the diagnosis of hypothyroidism. In some cases, levels may be as high as 200 milliInternational Units/L. Lower elevations (less than 20 milliInternational Units/L), in conjunction with a normal thyroid hormone level, may indicate subclinical hypothyroidism.

In secondary hypothyroidism, TSH levels may be normal, low, or high.

Drug monitoring done

In thyroid replacement therapy for hypothyroidism, the therapeutic goal is to achieve a TSH level in the midnormal range (1 to 2 milliInternational Units/L).

In thyroid replacement for subclinical hypothyroidism, the target TSH level is 0.03 to 3 milliInternational Units/mL.

Timing of Monitoring

It may take 6 to 8 weeks or longer for the thyroid stimulating hormone level to equilibrate after the initiation of thyroid hormone replacement in hypothyroid patients.

In hypothyroidism, once the TSH level is in the normal range, a follow-up visit in 6 months and then annually is the common schedule.

Subclinical hypothyroidism with thyroid hormone replacement may be evaluated annually once a stable TSH level has been reached.

Suspected hyperthyroidism

Strength of Recommendation: Class IIa
Strength of Evidence: Category C
Results Interpretation:
Decreased thyroid stimulating hormone level

A thyroid stimulating hormone (TSH) level less than 0.1 milliInternationalUnits/L strongly suggests the diagnosis of hyperthyroidism, particularly when accompanied by a high free T_4 or high free T_3 level.

If a 3rd generation assay is not available, T_4 and T_3 levels should be measured in addition to TSH to arrive at an accurate diagnosis.

In patients with subclinical hyperthyroidism, the TSH level may be slightly higher ranging from less than 0.1 milliInternationalUnits/L to the lower limit of the normal range.

In hyperthyroid patients who undergo treatment with radioactive iodine, an elevated TSH in conjunction with a normal T_4 indicates a 5% to 15% risk of progression to hypothyroidism at 1 year.

COMMON PANELS

- Anemia panel
- General health panel
- Thyroid panel
- Transplant panel

ABNORMAL RESULTS

- Results increased in:
  - Hospitalized patients
  - Acute psychiatric illness
  - Adrenal insufficiency
- Results decreased in:
  - Hospitalized patients
  - Blacks
  - First trimester pregnancy

CLINICAL NOTES

Thyroid stimulating hormone is the single most reliable test for detecting thyroid disorders. Third-generation tests have a lower detection limit of 0.01 to 0.02 milliInternationalUnits/L, in contrast to the first-generation tests, which had a detection limit of 1 to 2 milliInternationalUnits/L.

COLLECTION/STORAGE INFORMATION

- Draw blood in red marbled tube
- Store at 4° C for up to 7 days or freeze for up to 1 month

LOINC CODES
- Code: 26998-5 (*Short Name* - TSH Sal-aCnc)
- Code: 20452-9 (*Short Name* - TSH Bld Ql)

Total iron binding capacity measurement

TEST DEFINITION
Indirect measurement of transferrin in serum to evaluate iron availability to tissues

REFERENCE RANGE
- Adults: 250-370 mcg/dL (45-66 micromol/L)
  Please refer to your institution's reference ranges as lab normals may vary.

INDICATIONS
Abnormal liver function tests
    Strength of Recommendation: Class IIa
    Strength of Evidence: Category C
    Results Interpretation:
    Decreased level (laboratory finding)
        Total iron binding capacity (TIBC) is decreased in iron overload conditions that can occur with liver disease, eg, cirrhosis, chronic liver disease, and hemachromatosis.
        A decreased TIBC together with unexplained abnormal liver function tests (LFTs) is suggestive of hemochromatosis.
        Liver damage can affect transferrin levels. Decreased levels of transferrin are reflected in decreased TIBC related to liver damage.

Suspected hemochromatosis
    Strength of Recommendation: Class IIa
    Strength of Evidence: Category C
    Results Interpretation:
    Decreased level (laboratory finding)
        A decreased total iron binding capacity (TIBC), together with an increased transferrin saturation and an elevated serum iron level, is highly suggestive of hemochromatosis.
        A fasting transferrin saturation greater than 45% is highly sensitive in detecting individuals with hereditary hemochromatosis.

Suspected iron-deficiency anemia
    Strength of Recommendation: Class IIa
    Strength of Evidence: Category C
    Results Interpretation:
    Increased level (laboratory finding)
        An elevated total iron binding capacity (TIBC), together with a decreased serum iron level and a decreased transferrin saturation level, indicates iron deficiency anemia. However, there may be no elevation of TIBC in iron-deficient patients with chronic blood loss plus chronic infection.

COMMON PANELS
- Iron panel

ABNORMAL RESULTS
- Results decreased in protein-deficient diets (eg, Kwashiorkor).

CLINICAL NOTES
    Total iron binding capacity (TIBC) is a measurement of transferrin, the primary iron-transport protein. TIBC is a calculated value, based on serum or plasma iron levels. TIBC reflects the amount of iron needed to fully bind the transferrin receptor sites in serum. Thus factors that affect iron measurements may also affect TIBC determination. Transferrin can be directly measured by immunologic techniques. TIBC normal levels depend on the method used for the iron measurement.

The plasma iron level plus TIBC together reflect iron availability status, not iron stores. Transferrin saturation (amount of plasma iron divided by TIBC) is a more useful test than TIBC for determining iron availability.

COLLECTION/STORAGE INFORMATION
- Specimen Collection and Handling:
  - Collect venous blood specimen in a marbled serum separator tube (SST).
  - Draw specimen in the morning (circadian rhythm affects iron levels).
  - Avoid specimen hemolysis.
- Patient Preparation:
  - Have patient fast prior to blood draw.

Total pyridinolines measurement

TEST DEFINITION
The measurement of total pyridinolines (pyridinoline and deoxypyridinoline) in urine for evaluation and management of diseases involving bone resorption

SYNONYMS
- Total pyridinolines

REFERENCE RANGE
- Adult males ≥ 18 years:
- Pyridinoline: 20-61 nmol/mmol creatinine
- Deoxypyridinoline: 4-19 nmol/mmol creatinine .
- Premenopausal females ≥18 years:
- Pyridinoline: 22-89 nmol/mmol creatinine
- Deoxypyridinoline: 4-21 nmol/mmol creatinine .
  Please refer to your institution's reference ranges as lab normals may vary.

INDICATIONS
Management of metastatic bone disease in prostate cancer
> **Strength of Recommendation:** Class IIb
> **Strength of Evidence:** Category B
> **Results Interpretation:**
> **Increased level (laboratory finding)**
> Elevated urinary levels of pyridinoline and deoxypyridinoline appear to correlate with increased pain in patients with metastatic bone disease secondary to prostate cancer. Elevated deoxypyridinoline levels may be predictive of skeletal complications.

Suspected osteoporosis.
> **Strength of Recommendation:** Class IIb
> **Strength of Evidence:** Category B
> **Results Interpretation:**
> **Increased level (laboratory finding)**
> Elevated free levels of urine deoxypyridinoline may indicate an increased risk of hip fracture secondary to osteoporosis.

ABNORMAL RESULTS
- Results Increased in:
  - Nighttime
  - Luteal phase of menstrual cycle
  - Puberty
  - Winter
  - Bone fracture
  - Non-weightbearing
  - Prolonged bedrest

CLINICAL NOTES

Because of diurnal, menstrual phase, and seasonal variations, total urine pyridinolines can be difficult to interpret on specimens taken at different times from the same individual. Deoxypyridinoline is more specific for bone, while pyridinoline is more specific for cartilage, ligaments, and tendons.

COLLECTION/STORAGE INFORMATION

- Specimen Collection and Handling:
  - Obtain 24-hour urine collection
  - Preserve specimen with 25 mL of HCL (6 mol/L)
  - Refrigerate or store in freezer

Transferrin saturation index

TEST DEFINITION

Calculation of the saturated fraction of iron in serum for the evaluation of iron status

SYNONYMS

- Percent iron saturation

REFERENCE RANGE

- Adult, males: 20-50%
- Adult, females: 15-50%
  Please refer to your institution's reference ranges as lab normals may vary.

INDICATIONS

Suspected hemochromatosis
　　Strength of Recommendation: Class IIa
　　Strength of Evidence: Category B
　　Results Interpretation:
　　Abnormal laboratory findings
　　　　A serum transferrin saturation greater than 60% in men and 50% in premenopausal women suggests hemochromatosis. Adolescents with hemochromatosis will usually have increased percent iron saturation, but will not likely express complications until adulthood.
　　　　Following phlebotomy therapy, a substantial decrease in percent iron saturation to less than 15% is considered confirmation of successful iron depletion. Serum ferritin will usually return to normal before transferrin saturation.

Suspected or known iron deficiency
　　Strength of Recommendation: Class IIa
　　Strength of Evidence: Category C
　　Results Interpretation:
　　Lowered laboratory findings
　　　　An iron saturation less than 16% indicates a depletion of iron stores or inflammation. An iron saturation less than 16% in the presence of an increased transferrin concentration differentiates iron deficiency from inflammation. Hemoglobin impairment may occur once transferrin saturation levels fall below 15%.

Suspected or known iron overload
　　Strength of Recommendation: Class IIa
　　Strength of Evidence: Category C
　　Results Interpretation:
　　Increased level (laboratory finding)
　　　　An iron saturation greater than 80% in males and greater than 70% in females is suggestive of iron overload.

COMMON PANELS

- Anemia panel
- Iron panel

CLINICAL NOTES

Because of the impact of estrogen on transferrin levels, women taking contraceptive medication, and pregnant and premenstrual women will have increased transferrin saturation levels, while levels will drop in women during menses. Increased levels can also be caused by sample contamination, liver disease and erythrocyte disorders. Sleep deprivation, alcohol ingestion and stress can lower levels. Overnight fasting will increase transferrin saturation levels in the morning and decrease levels in the afternoon due to the diurnal variations in serum iron, and the effect of fasting, dietary intake and absorption on serum iron concentrations. Males have 15% to 20% higher transferrin saturation levels than females.

COLLECTION/STORAGE INFORMATION

- Avoid hemolysis after drawing serum sample.
- To obtain the highest, most stable serum iron levels, samples should be drawn after an overnight fast.

LOINC CODES

- Code: 2505-6 (*Short Name* - Iron/TIBC SerPl-mRto)

Tricyclic antidepressant measurement

TEST DEFINITION

Measurement of the serum level of the tricyclic class of antidepressant drugs

SYNONYMS

- Tricyclic screening

INDICATIONS

Measurement of tricyclic antidepressant drug level in suspected accidental or intentional overdose
   Strength of Recommendation: Class IIb
   Strength of Evidence: Category C
   Results Interpretation:
   Blood drug level high
      Plasma levels of tricyclic antidepressants do not accurately predict clinical complications.. A QRS interval greater than 100 milliseconds presents a more accurate assessment of cardiotoxicity.

Measurement of tricyclic antidepressants in serum for therapeutic drug monitoring
   Strength of Recommendation: Class IIb
   Strength of Evidence: Category B
   Results Interpretation:
   Blood drug levels - finding
      At least 25% of patients do not have an adequate clinical response to tricyclic antidepressants (TCA). However, therapeutic TCA levels are correlated with significantly better outcomes at clinical endpoints. Therefore, blood levels can be useful in monitoring the response by looking at the following: appropriateness of therapy, compliance, potential for toxicity, effects of drug to drug interactions on steady state concentrations, and establishing individual target concentrations.

DRUG/LAB INTERACTIONS

- Quetiapine - a false-positive urine tricyclic antidepressant assay

ABNORMAL RESULTS

- Results increased in:
  - Hypoalbuminemia
  - Acidemia
- Results decreased in:
  - Malignancy
  - Inflammation
  - Hepatorenal disease

CLINICAL NOTES

The relationship between serum tricyclic antidepressant (TCA) levels and clinical response is inconsistent. However, TCA levels may be useful in monitoring treatment, side effects, altered metabolism, and in verifying compliance.

COLLECTION/STORAGE INFORMATION

- Specimen Collection and Handling:
    - Collect specimen 10 to 14 hours after last dose of once-daily therapy or 4 to 6 hours after divided-dose therapy
    - Collect serum or plasma specimen in EDTA tube
    - May keep sample at room temperature for one week, for 4 weeks at 4°C, or for more than one year at −20°C
    - Avoid use of gel separator tubes which may lower blood concentration of tricyclic antidepressants
    - Avoid hemolyzed specimens which may cause variable effects

LOINC CODES

- Code: 15111-8 (*Short Name* - Tricyclics SerPl-sCnc)
- Code: 16181-0 (*Short Name* - Tricyclics Ur Cnfrn-mCnc)
- Code: 6799-1 (*Short Name* - Tricyclics Ur Ql EIA)
- Code: 19318-5 (*Short Name* - Tricyclics CtOff Ur Cnfrn-mCnc)
- Code: 4073-3 (*Short Name* - Tricyclics SerPl Ql)
- Code: 10552-8 (*Short Name* - Tricyclics SerPl-mCnc)
- Code: 11004-9 (*Short Name* - Tricyclics Ur Ql)
- Code: 29228-4 (*Short Name* - Tricyclics Fld-mCnc)
- Code: 19316-9 (*Short Name* - Tricyclics Pos Ur Cfm)
- Code: 19315-1 (*Short Name* - Tricyclics Ur Ql Cfm)

Triglycerides measurement

TEST DEFINITION

Measurement of triglycerides in blood for the evaluation and management of lipid disorders and coronary heart disease risk

SYNONYMS

- TG - Triglyceride level
- Triacylglycerols measurement

REFERENCE RANGE

- Adults: <150 mg/dL
- Female neonates, cord blood: 11-76 mg/dL (0.12-0.86 mmol/L)
- Male neonates, cord blood: 13-95 mg/dL (0.15-1.07 mmol/L)
- Females, 0-9 years: 35-110 mg/dL (0.40-1.24 mmol/L)
- Males, 0-9 years: 30-100 mg/dL (0.34-1.13 mmol/L)
- Females, 10-14 years: 37-131 mg/dL (0.42-1.48 mmol/L)
- Males, 10-14 years: 32-125 mg/dL (0.36-1.41 mmol/L)
- Females, 15-18 years: 39-124 mg/dL (0.44-1.4 mmol/L)
- Males, 15-18 years: 37-148 mg/dL (0.42-1.67 mmol/L)
    Please refer to your institution's reference ranges as lab normals may vary.

INDICATIONS

Suspected hypertriglyceridemia in HIV infection
    Strength of Recommendation: Class IIa
    Strength of Evidence: Category B
    Results Interpretation:
    Hypertriglyceridemia
    Elevated triglycerides, greater than 2 mmol/L, can occur in HIV-infected patients receiving highly active antiretroviral therapy. Triglyceride elevation is compound specific, and is increased more with ritonavir than with indinavir, nelfinavir or saquinavir.

Suspected hypertriglyceridemia
> **Strength of Recommendation:** Class I
> **Strength of Evidence:** Category B
> **Results Interpretation:**
> **Hypertriglyceridemia**
> Blood tests for elevated serum triglycerides are valuable in determining the risk of coronary heart disease. The National Cholesterol Education Program guidelines, in the third Adult Treatment Panel (ATP III), established borderline-high triglycerides at 150 to 199 mg/dL. High triglycerides were defined as 200 to 499 mg/dL, and very high triglycerides were designated as greater than 1,000 mg/dL.

Suspected pancreatitis
> **Results Interpretation:**
> **Serum triglycerides raised**
> Elevated triglyceride levels can cause both acute and chronic pancreatitis. Levels equal to or higher than 500 mg/dL are more likely to occur in the inherited hyperlipidemia syndromes and indicate an elevated risk for acute pancreatitis. Levels higher than 1,000 mg/dL indicate an even greater risk of acute pancreatitis, proportional to the elevation above 1,000 mg/dL. The situation is considered urgent when levels exceed 2,000 mg/dL. When acute pancreatitis occurs at these levels, it is usually a component of chylomicronemia syndrome.

COMMON PANELS
- Lipid profile

ABNORMAL RESULTS
- Results increased in:
  - Chronic alcoholism
  - Viral hepatitis
  - Gout
  - Pregnancy
  - Anorexia nervosa
  - Down syndrome
  - Acute intermittent porphyria
- Results decreased in:
  - Parenchymal liver disease
  - Malnutrition
  - Malabsorption

COLLECTION/STORAGE INFORMATION
- Specimen Collection and Handling:
  - Instruct patient to fast for 12 or more hours
  - Collect specimen into an EDTA or heparin tube
  - Separate serum or plasma from cells within 2 hours
  - May be stored for 5 to 7 days at 4°C, 3 months at −20°C, and indefinitely at −70°C

LOINC CODES
- Code: 12228-3 (*Short Name* - Trigl Fld-mCnc)
- Code: 3043-7 (*Short Name* - Trigl Bld-mCnc)
- Code: 22731-4 (*Short Name* - Trigl XXX-sCnc)
- Code: 14449-3 (*Short Name* - Trigl Snv-mCnc)
- Code: 14448-5 (*Short Name* - Trigl Smn-mCnc)
- Code: 29766-3 (*Short Name* - Trigl Fld-sCnc)

Triiodothyronine measurement

TEST DEFINITION
Measurement of total triiodothyronine (T_3) levels for the evaluation and management of thyroid dysfunction

SYNONYMS
- T3 - Triiodothyronine level
- Triiodothyronine level

REFERENCE RANGE
- Adults: 60-181 ng/dL (0.92-2.78 nmol/L)
- Pregnancy (last 5 months): 116-247 ng/dL (1.79-3.8 nmol/L)

Please refer to your institution's reference ranges as lab normals may vary.

INDICATIONS
Suspected hyperthyroidism in patients with thyroid-stimulating hormone (TSH) levels less than 0.1 milli-International Units/L

Strength of Recommendation: Class I
Strength of Evidence: Category C
Results Interpretation:
Increased triiodothyronine level

In hyperthyroidism, elevated total serum triiodothyronine (T_3) levels are used to help confirm the diagnosis of hyperthyroidism in patients with low TSH levels. T_3 levels are usually increased more than thyroxine (T_4) levels.

Suspected T_3 (triiodothyronine) thyrotoxicosis

Strength of Recommendation: Class IIa
Strength of Evidence: Category C
Results Interpretation:
Increased triiodothyronine level

T_3 thyrotoxicosis is diagnosed when the triiodothyronine (T_3) level is elevated and the free thyroxine (T_4) level is normal. This state is considered a subset of hyperthyroidism

COMMON PANELS
- Transplant panel

ABNORMAL RESULTS
- Results decreased in:
  - Severe systemic illness
- Results increased in:
  - Pregnancy

CLINICAL NOTES
About 80% of circulating T_3 comes from the peripheral conversion of thyroxine (T_4). The metabolic activity of T_3 is 5 to 10 times that of T_4. Total T_3 levels generally correspond with free T_3 levels, except when thyroid hormone-binding protein concentrations are abnormal. To evaluate for those binding proteins, T_3 resin uptake or thyroid-binding globulin should be done at the same time as the total T_3.

COLLECTION/STORAGE INFORMATION
- Specimen Collection and Handling:
  - Collect serum sample
  - Store at room temperature or preferably at 4° C for up to 7 days
  - Store at -20° C for up to 30 days

LOINC CODES
- Code: 26879-7 (*Short Name* - T3 Sal-mCnc)

Triple screening test

TEST DEFINITION
Measurement of alpha-fetoprotein, human chorionic-gonadotrophin, and unconjugated estriol for the screening of fetal genetic malformations and neural tube defects.

REFERENCE RANGE

- Human chorionic-gonadotrophin maternal serum:
- 2 weeks after fertilization: 5 -100 milliInternational Units/mL (5 -100 International Units/L)
- 3 weeks after fertilization: 200-3,000 milliInternational Units/mL (200-3,000 International Units/L)
- 4 weeks after fertilization: 10,000-80,000 milliInternational Units/mL (10,000-80,000 International Units/L)
- 5-12 weeks after fertilization: 90,0000-500,000 milliInternational Units/mL (90,0000-500,000 International Units/L)
- 13-24 weeks after fertilization: 5,000-80,000 milliInternational Units/mL (5,000-80,000 International Units/L)
- 26-28 weeks after fertilization: 3,000-15,000 milliInternational Units/mL (3,000-15,000 International Units/L)
- Free estriol maternal serum:
- 22 weeks gestation: 2.6-8 ng/mL (9-27.8 nmol/L)
- 26 weeks gestation: 2.5-13.5 ng/mL (8.7-46.8 nmol/L)
- 30 weeks gestation: 3.5-19 ng/mL (12.1-65.9 nmol/L)
- 34 weeks gestation: 5.3-18.3 ng/mL (18.4-63.5 nmol/L)
- 35 weeks gestation: 5.2-26.4 ng/mL (18.0-91.6 nmol/L)
- 36 weeks gestation: 8.2-28.1 ng/mL (28.4-97.5 nmol/L)
- 37 weeks gestation: 8.0-30.1 ng/mL (27.8-104.4 nmol/L)
- 38 weeks gestation: 8.6-38 ng/mL (29.8-131.9 nmol/L)
- 39 weeks gestation: 7.2-34.3 ng/mL (25-119 nmol/L)
- 40 weeks gestation: 9.6-28.9 ng/mL (33.3-100.3 nmol/L)
- Alpha-fetoprotein maternal serum:
- 14 weeks gestation: 25.6 ng/mL (25.6 mcg/L)
- 15 weeks gestation: 29.9 ng/mL (29.9 mcg/L)
- 16 weeks gestation: 34.8 ng/mL (34.8 mcg/L)
- 17 weeks gestation: 40.6 ng/mL (40.6 mcg/L)
- 18 weeks gestation: 47.3 ng/mL (47.3 mcg/L)
- 19 weeks gestation: 55.1 ng/mL (55.1 mcg/L)
- 20 weeks gestation: 64.3 ng/mL (64.3 mcg/L)
- 21 weeks gestation: 74.9 ng/mL (74.9 mcg/L)

   Please refer to your institution's reference ranges as lab normals may vary.

INDICATIONS

Fetal screening for neural tube defects in at risk women
   Strength of Recommendation: Class IIa
   Strength of Evidence: Category B
   Results Interpretation:
   Abnormal laboratory findings
   Elevated levels of maternal serum alpha-fetoprotein (AFP) identify women at sufficient risk for fetal neural tube defects (NTD) to warrant further testing - such as amniocentesis and ultrasound - and genetic counseling. Positive maternal serum AFP results are not diagnostic for NTD; definitive diagnosis requires AFP and acetylcholinesterase measurement of amniotic fluid in conjunction with ultrasound..
   Amniotic acetylcholinesterase testing is recommended when AFP levels in amniotic fluid exceed the pre-determined cut-off value, normally 2 multiples of the median (MoM) or 2.5 MoM for singleton pregnancies, and 4 MoM to 4.5 MoM for twin pregnancies. Amniotic acetylcholinesterase testing may also be performed in the presence of a normal amniotic fluid AFP when a prior risk of NTD exists, as evidenced by elevated maternal serum AFP, abnormal ultrasound or positive family history.
   Test results must be reinterpreted if a discrepancy in gestational age of 2 or more weeks is found. If the sample was obtained at less than 15 weeks gestation, a new sample should be sent with the accurate gestational age identified.
   Timing of Monitoring
   The ideal window in which to screen for open neural tube defects is between 16 and 18 weeks gestation, but screening between 15 and 20.9 weeks is acceptable. If screening is performed at less than 14 weeks, test performance results will be substantially poorer. Results performance is unchanged after 18 weeks gestation, but fewer options are available after that time in the event that the results are positive.

Screening for fetal trisomy 21 (Down syndrome) in at risk women
   Strength of Recommendation: Class IIa
   Strength of Evidence: Category B

Results Interpretation:
Abnormal laboratory findings

Elevated levels of human chorionic gonadotrophin (hCG) in the presence of low alpha-fetoprotein (AFP) and low unconjugated estriol (uE3) levels identify women at sufficient risk for Down syndrome to warrant further testing - such as amniocentesis and karotyping - and genetic counseling. Positive triple screen results are not diagnostic for Down syndrome; definitive diagnosis requires karyotyping of fetal cells, either by amniocentesis or chorionic villus sampling.

Maternal serum AFP and uE3 increase by a constant percentage per week in the second trimester; AFP increases by 10% to 15% per week while uE3 increases by 20% to 25%. hCG decreases by 25% from 15 to 17 weeks gestation then decreases at a substantially lower rate from 18 to 20 weeks gestation.

Levels of all three analytes are generally higher in women of lighter weight and lower in heavier women, although weight adjustment for Down syndrome does not provide significant improvement in results interpretation. AFP and possibly hCG are 10% to 15% higher in black women than in caucasian women. Correction for maternal insulin dependent diabetes mellitus should be made for AFP.

In 1 in 1,000 pregnancies uE3 will be below the lower assay sensitivity limit (less than 0.1 ng/mL) for no obvious reason; in many cases these pregnancies are males with steroid sulfatase deficiency or other rare metabolic disorders.

Timing of Monitoring

Specificity and sensitivity are essentially unchanged between 15 and 20 weeks gestation for Down syndrome, but because the test is also used to screen for open neural tube defects, the triple maternal screen is optimally obtained between 16 and 18 weeks gestation. If screening is performed at less than 14 weeks, test performance results will be substantially poorer. Reliable results after 20 weeks gestation are possible but the available options may be limited in the presence of a positive test finding. If multiple specimens are drawn, they should be collected at the same time of day since concentrations of unconjugated estriol are lower in the morning than in the evening.

Screening for trisomy 18 (Edward syndrome) in at risk women

Strength of Recommendation: Class IIa
Strength of Evidence: Category B
Results Interpretation:
Abnormal laboratory findings

Decreased levels of human chorionic gonadotrophin (hCG), alpha-fetoprotein (AFP) and unconjugated estriol (uE3) identify women at sufficient risk for trisomy 18 to warrant further testing - such as amniocentesis and karotyping - and genetic counseling. Positive triple screen results are not diagnostic for trisomy 18.

Because trisomy 18 presents with a unique pattern of markers unlike that of Down syndrome, a separate algorithm for estimating an individual's risk is required, and published algorithms are available for trisomy 18. AFP, uE3 and hCG levels should all be adjusted for maternal weight when screening for trisomy 18. Because, unlike Down syndrome, incorrect gestational dating will not cause the marker pattern associated with trisomy 18, redating the pregnancy does not typically provide additional useful information.

Timing of Monitoring

Specificity and sensitivity are essentially unchanged between 15 and 20 weeks gestation for Down syndrome, but because the test is also used to screen for open neural tube defects, results of the triple maternal screen are optimally obtained between 16 and 18 weeks gestation. If multiple specimens are drawn, they should be collected at the same time of day since concentrations of unconjugated estriol are lower in the morning than in the evening.

COMMON PANELS

· Maternal serum triple screen

COLLECTION/STORAGE INFORMATION

· Alpha-fetoprotein and human chorionic-gonadotrophin:
  · Draw 5 mL blood in a red top or serum separator tube.
  · Serum may be stored at 4°C to 8°C for days or at -20°C for years..
· Unconjugated estriol (uE3):
  · Draw 5 mL blood in a red top or serum separator tube.
  · uE3 is not stable in whole blood; serum may be stored at 4°C to 8°C for days..
· For the most reliable results the laboratory may request the following information:
  · Gestational age
  · Maternal weight
  · Maternal race
  · Presence of maternal insulin dependent diabetes mellitus prior to pregnancy

- Number of fetuses
- Time and date of any previous samples collected
- Family history of Down syndrome
- The results of other related diagnostic tests

LOINC CODES
- Code: 35086-8 (*Short Name* - Triple Marker Screen SerPl)

Troponin T cardiac measurement

TEST DEFINITION
Measurement of troponin T, a protein specific to cardiac cells found in the troponin regulatory complex, in serum for the evaluation of myocardial injury

REFERENCE RANGE
- Adults: 0-0.1 ng/mL (0-0.1 mcg/L)
- Each laboratory should determine reference values using specific assays with appropriate quality control.
  Please refer to your institution's reference ranges as lab normals may vary.

INDICATIONS
Acute thromboembolic stroke.
> **Strength of Recommendation:** Class IIb
> **Strength of Evidence:** Category C
Results Interpretation:
Increased troponin T level
> Cardiac damage, as indicated by increased troponin T levels, may be neurally mediated through abnormal autonomic discharges following stroke.
> In acute ischemic stroke, a 3-fold risk of death is seen in patients with elevated troponin T levels measured within 12 to 72 hours of admission.

Suspected acute coronary syndrome
> **Strength of Recommendation:** Class I
> **Strength of Evidence:** Category A
Results Interpretation:
Increased troponin T level
> Troponin T (TnT) levels typically increase within 3 to 12 hours (mean time to peak elevation 12 hours to 2 days) and return to normal within 5 to 14 days of myocardial injury.
> A myocardial infarction (MI) is suspected if an increased cTnT is detected at least once within 24 hours of the index clinical event. An increased cTnT level is defined as a measurement exceeding the 99th percentile of the mean value measurement in a normal control population. Each laboratory should determine reference values using specific assays with appropriate quality control. The actual value that determines a positive test ('rule-in value') will vary by the assay used; physicians should be familiar with the properties of the assay used at their institution.
> A prospective evaluation of 7,115 patients with non-ST-segment elevation acute coronary syndrome (NSTE ACS) from the Global Utilization of Strategies To open Occluded arteries IV (GUSTO-IV) trial validated the cutoff level of 0.01 mcg/L (third-generation cTnT assay). Patients with cTnT levels less than 0.01 mcg/L had low risk for 30-day adverse outcomes (ie, myocardial infarction, death) with a negative predictive value of 0.98.
> Patients with cTnT levels greater than 0.1 mcg/L had higher 30-day mortality rates (5.5%) than those with levels less than or equal to 0.1 mcg/L (2.2%).
Frequency of Monitoring
> Measure serum troponin T (cTnT) at presentation, then 6 to 12 hours after onset of symptoms.
> Serial measurements may be helpful for early assessment of reperfusion in patients undergoing thrombolytic therapy or PTCA; however, due to the slow return of troponins to baseline, they are not the best of the available biochemical cardiac markers to determine successful reperfusion (nor re-infarction).
Timing of Monitoring
> Cardiac troponin levels should be obtained in all patients with chest pain or anginal equivalent suggestive of acute coronary syndrome.

If myocardial infarction may have occurred more than 24 hours before evaluation and if CK levels are not diagnostic, measurement of troponin T should be ordered in the acute care setting.

Suspected cardiac contusion
　Results Interpretation:
　Increased troponin T level
　　Troponin T is significantly higher in blunt chest trauma (BCT) patients with myocardial contusion compared with BCT patients without myocardial contusion. There is no correlation, however, between elevated troponin T levels and long-term outcome.

Suspected pulmonary embolism
　　Strength of Recommendation: Class IIb
　　Strength of Evidence: Category C
　Results Interpretation:
　Increased troponin T level
　　Patients with normal troponin levels can almost certainly be treated with anticoagulant therapy alone, while those with elevated levels require further testing of right ventricular function with echocardiography. Studies have found that patients with acute PE and elevated troponin T levels are at significant risk of a complicated clinical course and a fatal outcome.

ABNORMAL RESULTS
• Results increased in chronic renal failure

CLINICAL NOTES
　Useful in evaluating for acute myocardial infarction in patients following direct current countershock. Studies have shown troponin T levels remain normal in patients following cardioversion unlike total CK and CK-MB which increase significantly.

COLLECTION/STORAGE INFORMATION
• May store for up to 24 hours at 2°C to 8°C or for 3 months at -20°C

LOINC CODES
• Code: 6598-7 (*Short Name* - Troponin T SerPl-mCnc)
• Code: 6597-9 (*Short Name* - Troponin T BldV-mCnc)

Trypanosoma cruzi antibody assay

TEST DEFINITION
　Detection of *Trypanosoma cruzi* antibodies in serum for the diagnosis of Chagas' disease

REFERENCE RANGE
• Negative
　Please refer to your institution's reference ranges as lab normals may vary.

INDICATIONS
Suspected *Trypanosoma cruzi* infection (Chagas disease)
　　Strength of Recommendation: Class IIa
　　Strength of Evidence: Category B
　Results Interpretation:
　Serology positive
　　A positive result on a *Trypanosoma cruzi* antibody assay is essential for the diagnosis of Chagas disease.

　False Results
• False positives may be seen in:
• Leishmaniasis
• Toxoplasmosis
• Schistosomiasis
• Sleeping sickness

CLINICAL NOTES

This test is more useful during the chronic stage of *Trypanosoma cruzi* infection than in the acute phase.

COLLECTION/STORAGE INFORMATION

- Specimen Collection and Handling:
  - Collect serum in red marbled (separation) tube.
  - Freeze specimen if not immediately tested.

LOINC CODES

- Code: 30104-4 (*Short Name* - T cruzi IgG Titr XXX)
- Code: 26989-4 (*Short Name* - T cruzi IgM Ser Ql IF)
- Code: 13290-2 (*Short Name* - T cruzi IgM Ser-aCnc)
- Code: 31691-9 (*Short Name* - T cruzi IgG XXX-aCnc)
- Code: 5398-3 (*Short Name* - T cruzi Ab Titr Ser CF)
- Code: 14094-7 (*Short Name* - T cruzi IgG Titr Ser)
- Code: 25813-7 (*Short Name* - T cruzi Ab Titr Ser IF)
- Code: 8045-7 (*Short Name* - T cruzi Ab Ser-aCnc)
- Code: 13291-0 (*Short Name* - T cruzi IgG Ser-aCnc)
- Code: 30105-1 (*Short Name* - T cruzi IgM Titr XXX)

Tyrosine measurement

TEST DEFINITION

Measurement of tyrosine in plasma or serum for detection of acquired and hereditary amino acid disorders

REFERENCE RANGE

- Premature (fluorometry): 7-24 mg/dL (386-1325 micromol/L)
- Newborn (fluorometry): 1.6-3.7 mg/dL (88-204 micromol/L)
- Premature, 1 day (ion-exchange chromatography): 2.17 ± 1.81 mg/dL (120 ± 100 micromol/L)
- Neonate, 1 day (ion-exchange chromatography): 0.76-1.79 mg/dL (42-99 micromol/L)
- Infants 1 to 3 months (ion-exchange chromatography): 1.48 ± 0.47 mg/dL (82 ± 26 micromol/L)
- Infants 9 to 24 months (ion-exchange chromatography): 0.2-2.21 mg/dL (11-122 micromol/L)
- Children 3 to 10 years (ion-exchange chromatography): 0.56-1.29 mg/dL (31-71 micromol/L)
- Children 6 to 18 years (ion-exchange chromatography): 0.78-1.59 mg/dL (43-88 micromol/L)
- Adults (fluorometry): 0.8-1.3 mg/dL (44-72 micromol/L)
- Adults (ion-exchange chromatography): 0.4-1.58 mg/dL (22-87 micromol/L)
  Please refer to your institution's reference ranges as lab normals may vary.

INDICATIONS

Suspected inborn error of metabolism
> **Strength of Recommendation:** Class IIa
> **Strength of Evidence:** Category C
> **Results Interpretation:**
> **Increased amino acid**

A tyrosine level greater than 200 micromol/L and the presence of succinylacetone in the urine are findings consistent with a diagnosis of hereditary tyrosinemia, while confirmation requires the presence of deficient fumarylacetoacetase (FAH) activity in cultured fibroblasts or liver biopsy specimens. Transient neonatal tyrosinemia is associated with elevated plasma tyrosine and increased tyrosine metabolites in the urine. Premature infants and those receiving hyperalimentation may also have elevated tyrosine levels.

Inherited amino acid disorders are directly related to the absence of an enzyme involved in the metabolism of one or more amino acids; therefore, an elevated plasma level of a particular amino acid is highly suggestive of an inherited metabolic defect. In the majority of cases amino acid and organic acid analysis together permit diagnostic confirmation in infants. Immediate treatment should be initiated when an inborn error of metabolism is suspected, even if a definitive diagnosis has not yet been determined.

COLLECTION/STORAGE INFORMATION

- Specimen Collection and Handling:
  - Immediately place sample in ice water.

- Isolate plasma sample and freeze it within 1 hour; sample stable for 1 week at -20°C.
- Sample should be deproteinized and stored at -70°C for protracted periods of usage.

LOINC CODES

- Code: 25547-1 (*Short Name* - Tyrosine 24H Ur-sRate)
- Code: 32277-6 (*Short Name* - Tyrosine Fld-sCnc)
- Code: 3081-7 (*Short Name* - Tyrosine 24H Ur-mRate)
- Code: 3080-9 (*Short Name* - Tyrosine Ur-mCnc)
- Code: 22642-3 (*Short Name* - Tyrosine CSF-sCnc)
- Code: 26966-2 (*Short Name* - Tyrosine Ur-sCnc)
- Code: 13381-9 (*Short Name* - Tyrosine CSF-mCnc)
- Code: 13901-4 (*Short Name* - Tyrosine Ur QI)
- Code: 30054-1 (*Short Name* - Tyrosine/creat Ur-Rto)
- Code: 32276-8 (*Short Name* - Tyrosine Vitf-sCnc)
- Code: 22739-7 (*Short Name* - Tyrosine XXX-sCnc)
- Code: 30069-9 (*Short Name* - Tyrosine Amn-sCnc)
- Code: 13818-0 (*Short Name* - Tyrosine/creat Ur-mRto)

Undercarboxylated osteocalcin measurement

TEST DEFINITION
Measurement of undercarboxylated osteocalcin in serum for the prediction of hip fracture risk

REFERENCE RANGE
- Adult female: <1.65 ng/mL (in one study [hydroxyapatite binding assay]), although no reference method is available.
  Please refer to your institution's reference ranges as lab normals may vary.

INDICATIONS
Suspected hip fracture
   Strength of Recommendation: Class IIb
   Strength of Evidence: Category B
   Results Interpretation:
   Increased level (laboratory finding)
   Increased levels of serum undercarboxylated osteocalcin signal an increased risk of hip fracture in elderly women.

Suspected vitamin K deficiency.
   Results Interpretation:
   Increased level (laboratory finding)
   Osteocalcin carboxylation, which is required for healthy bone matrix formation, is vitamin K-dependent. Deficiencies of vitamin K and the associated elevations of undercarboxylated osteocalcin levels correlate with an increased hip fracture risk in elderly women.

CLINICAL NOTES
The ELISA is a direct method of testing undercarboxylated osteocalcin, while the hydroxyapatite binding assay is indirect.

Unsaturated iron binding capacity measurement

TEST DEFINITION
Measurement of the unsaturated fraction of transferrin in serum for the evaluation of iron status

SYNONYMS
- Iron, percent saturation, calculated
- Iron/total iron binding capacity ratio measurement
- Transferrin saturation measurement

REFERENCE RANGE
- 110-370 mcg/dL (19.7-66.2 micromol/L)
  Please refer to your institution's reference ranges as lab normals may vary.

INDICATIONS
Suspected hemochromatosis
> **Strength of Recommendation:** Class IIa
> **Strength of Evidence:** Category B
> **Results Interpretation:**
> **Abnormal laboratory findings**
>> In patients at increased risk of hemochromatosis (family history or clinical suspicion), an abnormal unsaturated iron-binding capacity (UIBC) is highly suggestive of hemochromatosis, while a normal UIBC is highly associated with an absence of disease. In low-risk populations UIBC can reliably rule out hemochromatosis, however it cannot reliably rule in disease, even in the presence of abnormal liver function tests.

Suspected or known iron deficiency
> **Strength of Recommendation:** Class IIb
> **Strength of Evidence:** Category C
> **Results Interpretation:**
> **Increased level (laboratory finding)**
>> An elevated unsaturated iron binding capacity (UIBC) suggests iron deficiency.

Suspected or known iron toxicity
> **Strength of Recommendation:** Class IIa
> **Strength of Evidence:** Category C
> **Results Interpretation:**
> **Abnormal biochemistry findings**
>> The unsaturated iron binding capacity assay is useful in estimating potentially toxic iron levels.
> **Timing of Monitoring**
>> If the patient is to be treated with deferoxamine, serum samples should be drawn before administration since this chelator can produce falsely low iron results. However, interference from deferoxamine may be avoided if iron is measured using atomic absorption spectrometry.

LOINC CODES
- Code: 22753-8 (*Short Name* - UIBC SerPl-sCnc)
- Code: 2501-5 (*Short Name* - UIBC SerPl-mCnc)

Ureaplasma urealyticum culture

TEST DEFINITION
Identification of *Ureaplasma urealyticum* by culture of the genitourinary tract

REFERENCE RANGE
- No growth
  Please refer to your institution's reference ranges as lab normals may vary.

INDICATIONS
Suspected *Ureaplasma urealyticum* infection
> **Strength of Recommendation:** Class IIb
> **Strength of Evidence:** Category B

Results Interpretation:
Positive laboratory findings
    Cultures can detect *Ureaplasma urealyticum* in a significant number of women and can be found in women who are asymptomatic for vaginal, cervical, uterine, or tubal infections. A slightly greater, though not statistically significant, association exists between *U urealyticum* infection and infertility than between *U urealyticum* infection and fertility. The relationship between *U urealyticum* and pelvic inflammatory disease has not been firmly established.

COLLECTION/STORAGE INFORMATION
- Specimen Collection and Handling:
    - Using 2 swabs, collect specimen from urethra or endocervix 2 to 5 cm from os.
    - Press swab against side of transport tube.
    - Gently rotate tube.
    - Transport to lab immediately in special transport, albumin-containing medium, such as 2-SP.

LOINC CODES
- Code: 17852-5 (*Short Name* - U urealyticum XXX QI Cult)

Uric acid measurement, urine

TEST DEFINITION
    Measurement of total uric acid excretion in urine for the evaluation of urate production and excretion

REFERENCE RANGE
- Adults (normal diet): 250-800 mg/24 hours (1.49-4.76 mmol/24 hours)
- Adults (purine-free diet): <420 mg/day (<2.48 mmol/day)
- Adults (low-purine diet):
- Males: <480 mg/day (<2.83 mmol/day)
- Females: <400 mg/day (<2.36 mmol/day)
- Adults (high-purine diet): <1000 mg/day (<5.9 mmol/day)
    Please refer to your institution's reference ranges as lab normals may vary.

INDICATIONS
Hyperuricemia
        Strength of Recommendation: Class IIb
        Strength of Evidence: Category C
    Results Interpretation:
    Increased level (laboratory finding)
        Hyperuricuria is defined as greater than 600 mg/24 hours and may be associated with hyperuricemia (such as in primary gout), or may present as an isolated abnormality associated with diet, medications or other factors.
        Increased urate excretion and formation of kidney stones may be the result of protein metabolism in patients with chronic metabolic acidosis.
    Normal laboratory findings
        In the presence of hyperuricemia, a normal uric acid excretion is evidence of underexcretion of the increased urate load filtered at the glomerulus.
        In patients with hyperuricemia, a 24-hour uric acid excretion of less than 600 mg indicates underexcretion due to a renal tubular defect or as a consequence of precipitation of urates in renal tubules, parenchyma, or ureters.

Measurement of urine uric acid levels over 24 hours to detect gout
        Strength of Recommendation: Class IIb
        Strength of Evidence: Category C
    Results Interpretation:
    Increased level (laboratory finding)
        Urate overproduction is defined as a daily urate excretion of greater than 800 to 1,000 mg/24 hours in the absence of an obvious cause such as renal failure or diuretic use.
        Urate overproduction cannot reliably be assessed if the creatinine clearance is below 60 mL/minute.

False Results
False positive results may be seen in patients not following a strict low-purine diet.
Normal laboratory findings
Urate excretion of less than 600 mg/24 hours indicates underexcretion, possible due to renal tubular defect. About 75% of patients with primary (idiopathic) gout have either low or normal excretion of uric acid.
Some patients with gout and uric acid calculi have decreased uric acid excretion and increased serum uric acid levels secondary to tubular reabsorption of urate.

False Results
False positive results may be seen in patients not following a strict low-purine diet.

ABNORMAL RESULTS
- Ethanol ingestion

COLLECTION/STORAGE INFORMATION
- Specimen Collection and Handling :
    - Obtain 24-hour urine collection
    - Add NaOH to keep urine alkaline
    - Do not refrigerate urine sample
    - Uric acid is generally stable in urine for 3 days at room temperature

LOINC CODES
- Code: 3089-0 (*Short Name* - Urate/creat Ur-mRto)
- Code: 14934-4 (*Short Name* - Urate Ur-sCnc)
- Code: 18379-8 (*Short Name* - Urate 6H Ur-mRate)
- Code: 32555-5 (*Short Name* - Urate ?Tm Ur Qn)

Urinary hemosiderin detection

TEST DEFINITION
Qualitative detection of hemosiderin (a catabolite of free hemoglobin found in casts and/or epithelial cells) in urine for the evaluation and management of hemolytic disorders

SYNONYMS
- Urinary haemosiderin detection

REFERENCE RANGE
- Negative
Please refer to your institution's reference ranges as lab normals may vary.

INDICATIONS
Suspected chronic venous insufficiency
    Strength of Recommendation: Class IIb
    Strength of Evidence: Category B
    Results Interpretation:
    Positive laboratory findings
In patients with suspected chronic venous insufficiency, the presence of hemosiderin in urine may be a marker for severe vascular disease. Increasing severity appears to correspond with a greater number of hemosiderin granules in the urinary sediment.

Suspected hemolytic anemia
    Strength of Recommendation: Class IIb
    Strength of Evidence: Category C
    Results Interpretation:
    Positive laboratory findings
A hemosiderin urine test may become positive 2 to 3 days following the hemolytic episode, once the free hemoglobin has been filtered by the glomeruli and reabsorbed by the proximal tubules.

Although hemosiderinuria is not usually found in extravascular hemolysis, it may be present in microangiopathic hemolytic anemia (MAHA) or in paroxysmal nocturnal hemoglobinuria (PNH). Hemosiderinuria typically occurs in conjunction with hemoglobinemia and hemoglobinuria under conditions of severe and rapid intravascular hemolysis.

ABNORMAL RESULTS
- Results increased in:
  - Hemorrhagic pancreatitis

CLINICAL NOTES
Hemosiderin may not be detectable in an alkaline urine sample.

COLLECTION/STORAGE INFORMATION
- Obtain a fresh random urine sample.

Urine amphetamine measurement

TEST DEFINITION
Detection of amphetamine, methamphetamine and other amphetamine-like substances in urine for the evaluation of suspected drug abuse

SYNONYMS
- Urine amphetamine level

REFERENCE RANGE
- Adults and Children: Negative
  Please refer to your institution's reference ranges as lab normals may vary.

INDICATIONS
Suspected amphetamine abuse
>   **Strength of Recommendation:** Class IIa
>   **Strength of Evidence:** Category B
>   **Results Interpretation:**
>   **Amphetamine in urine**
>   Immunoassays are valuable only in differentiating negative from presumptive positive samples. Positive results must be verified by a second independent method with equal or higher sensitivity. The Guidelines for Federal Workplace Testing have set an initial cutoff detection level of 1,000 ng/mL for amphetamine. An initial positive test requires confirmation by chromatography-mass spectometry at a confirmatory cutoff level of 500 ng/mL for both amphetamine and methamphetamine. For a positive methamphetamine result to be valid, the specimen most also contain amphetamine at a concentration equal to or greater than 200 ng/mL by the confirmatory test. The European cutoff value is set at 500 ng/mL.
>
>   Amphetamines are generally detectable in the urine 1 to 3 days following their ingestion or injection.
>   Immunoassays depend on cross-reactivity to detect methylenedioxyamphetamine (MDA), methylenedioxymethylamphetamine (MDM, ecstasy) and methylenedioxyethylamphetamine (MDEA), the latter not tested for in all amphetamine screening tests. While high cutoff levels limit detection to recent ingestion of high doses only, lowering the detection limit produces more false positives, commonly caused by interfering substances such as ephedrine and ranitidine.
>
>   A negative result may reflect specimen dilution or adulteration, or may have been obtained too late after drug exposure to exceed the cutoff threshold level. Positive urine results do not provide information on exposure time, dose ingested or frequency or pattern of use, nor can results be used to predict blood concentration or to determine functional impairment.
>
>   **False Results**
>   A multitude of drugs may produce false-positive results, eg, ephedrine, ranitidine, lofepramine, phenylpropanolamine and trazodone.

COMMON PANELS
- Drugs of abuse testing, urine

COLLECTION/STORAGE INFORMATION
- Maintain chain of custody as appropriate.

LOINC CODES
- Code: 19346-6 (*Short Name* - Amphet Ur-mCnc)
- Code: 19059-5 (*Short Name* - Amphets CtOff Ur-mCnc)
- Code: 16369-1 (*Short Name* - Amphets Ur Ql Cfm)
- Code: 19265-8 (*Short Name* - Amphets Pos Ur Cfm)
- Code: 19344-1 (*Short Name* - Amphet Ur Ql Cnfrn)
- Code: 19267-4 (*Short Name* - Amphets CtOff Ur Cnfrn-mCnc)
- Code: 3349-8 (*Short Name* - Amphets Ur Ql)
- Code: 16234-7 (*Short Name* - Amphet Ur Cnfrn-mCnc)
- Code: 14309-9 (*Short Name* - Amphets Ur Ql Cfm>200 ng/mL)
- Code: 31016-9 (*Short Name* - L-amphet % Ur)

Urine barbiturate measurement

TEST DEFINITION
Detection of barbiturate levels in urine for suspected abuse or overdose

SYNONYMS
- Urine barbiturate level

REFERENCE RANGE
- Adults and Children: Negative
Please refer to your institution's reference ranges as lab normals may vary.

INDICATIONS
Suspected barbiturate abuse
    Strength of Recommendation: Class IIa
    Strength of Evidence: Category B
    Results Interpretation:
    Urine drug levels - finding

A positive qualitative barbiturate urine test result indicates the presence of barbiturate in urine above the cut-off level. Most barbiturates are detectable in urine for up to 2 days after last use, with the exception of phenobarbital, which can be detected for 1 to 3 weeks.

Toxicity requiring therapeutic intervention does not usually occur until the dose has exceeded 5 to 8 mg/kg in children. The fatal dose in non-addicted adults is estimated at 3 to 6 grams.

Individuals who present with a negative drug screen will not generally need further confirmatory testing. Positive results can direct treatment and the initiation of an appropriate rehabilitation program. Drug rehabilitation programs also use point of care testing to verify compliance.

The rapid screening tests such as EMIT, fluorescence polarization immunoassay and thin-layer chromatography (TLC), are used to detect the presence of short- and ultra-short-acting barbiturates in the urine. Because high levels of phenobarbital in urine cross-react with antibodies against short-acting barbiturates, it is important to confirm a positive immunoassay result with TLC. More sophisticated chromatographic procedures such as high performance liquid chromatography and gas chromatography-mass spectrometry (GC-MS) are rarely used for screening purposes, although GC-MS is considered the gold standard due to its high sensitivity and reliability. Liquid chromatography-mass spectroscopy can be used to confirm a drug-of-abuse-assay and is considered a complimentary method to GC-MS.

By law, any confirmatory method is valid, provided it is a completely different method from the primary one. Forensic testing requires an independent confirmatory method, usually GC-MS, in addition to a screen.

Drugs detected using the semiquantitative and qualitative EMIT™ homogenous enzyme immunoassays include secobarbital, amobarbital, butabarbital, pentobarbital, phenobarbital and talbutal. Assay response for samples containing more than one barbiturate may be cumulative.

- Barbiturate cut-off values are as follows. All confirmatory cut-off values were obtained by EMIT® II mono-clonal immunoassay, and all screening cut-off values were obtained by mass spectrometry, unless specified otherwise (cut-off values may be different for different jurisdictions and methods):
  - Pentobarbital: 200 ng/mL confirmation cut-off value; 1,000 ng/mL screening cut-off
  - Secobarbital: 200 ng/mL confirmation cut-off value by EMIT® and QuickScreen™ ; 200 ng/mL screening cut-off
  - Amobarbital: 200 ng/mL confirmation cut-off value; 2,000 ng/mL screening cut-off
  - Butabarbital: 200 ng/mL confirmation cut-off value; 1,000 ng/mL screening cut-off
  - Butalbital: 200 ng/mL confirmation cut-off value; 3,000 ng/mL screening cut-off
  - Phenobarbital: 200 ng/mL confirmation cut-off value; 3,000 ng/mL screening cut-off

COMMON PANELS
- Drugs of abuse testing, urine

CLINICAL NOTES
Urine is generally used as a first line detection screen before quantification in plasma, because the concentration of drugs and their metabolites are higher in urine than in plasma.

COLLECTION/STORAGE INFORMATION
- Follow chain of custody for urine collection, if indicated.

LOINC CODES
- Code: 16429-3 (*Short Name* - Barbiturates Ur Ql Cnfrn)
- Code: 9426-8 (*Short Name* - Barbiturates Ur-mCnc)
- Code: 3377-9 (*Short Name* - Barbiturates Ur Ql)

Urine cannabinoids screening test

TEST DEFINITION
The measurement of cannabinoid metabolites in urine to screen for marijuana exposure

REFERENCE RANGE
- Negative
Please refer to your institution's reference ranges as lab normals may vary.

INDICATIONS
Suspected or known marijuana use
> **Strength of Recommendation:** Class IIa
> **Strength of Evidence:** Category B
> **Results Interpretation:**
> **Positive laboratory findings**
> A positive laboratory evaluation suggests that the individual has been exposed to marijuana by ingestion, smoking, or by passive absorption.
> Positive results for more than eight consecutive days suggests either continuous use or previous chronic, heavy use in a newly abstinent person

> **False Results**
> Intentionally altered samples may yield a false-negative result.
> **Timing of Monitoring**
> Marijuana metabolites can be detected in the urine one hour or more after exposure.
> An infrequent user may have detectable cannabinoid metabolite levels for two to ten days after exposure. The chronic user can have detectable metabolite levels in urine for up to four weeks after the last use.

COMMON PANELS
- Drugs of abuse testing, urine

COLLECTION/STORAGE INFORMATION

- Specimen Collection and Handling:
    - A 20 mL random urine sample should be collected in a tamper-evident container under direct supervision. Specimen temperature and pH may be monitored when sample is used for medicolegal purposes.

LOINC CODES

- Code: 19288-0 (*Short Name* - Cannabinoids Tested Ur Scn)
- Code: 19287-2 (*Short Name* - Cannabinoids Tested Ur Scn)

Urine codeine measurement

TEST DEFINITION

Measurement of codeine in urine

SYNONYMS

- Urine codeine level

REFERENCE RANGE

Negative
Please refer to your institution's reference ranges as lab normals may vary.

INDICATIONS

Suspected codeine abuse.
    Strength of Recommendation: Class IIa
    Strength of Evidence: Category B
    Results Interpretation:
    Positive laboratory findings
    Codeine is reportedly detectable in the urine for 2 to 4 days after last use. However, the period of detection may vary due to user, laboratory, and individual differences in metabolism and excretion rates.
- Codeine may be detected in urine for 1 to 2 days following use per the following cutoff concentrations issued by the Substance Abuse and Mental Health Services Administration (SAMHSA) (formerly National Institute on Drug Abuse) for laboratories certified to conduct drug testing for federal employees:
    - Concentration to separate positive and negative specimens for opiates: 300 ng/mL (1,002 nanomoles/L) morphine equivalents
    - Gas-liquid chromatography with mass spectrometry confirmation: 300 ng/mL (1,002 nanomoles/L) codeine

    The concentration of codeine or morphine in the urine does not correlate with degree of intoxication. A positive urine screen is evidence of opiate use (or poppy seed ingestion) within the last 2 to 4 days but is not proof of acute intoxication.
    Ingestion of poppy seeds may yield measurable urine levels of codeine up to 22 hours post ingestion.

COMMON PANELS

- Drugs of abuse testing, urine

CLINICAL NOTES

The initial test for opiates must employ an immunoassay that meets Food and Drug Administration (FDA) requirements for commercial distribution. It must be a sensitive, rapid, and inexpensive screen to exclude 'true negative' specimens from further consideration.

Detection of codeine found in initial screening by immunoassay is confirmed by gas chromatography-mass spectrometry per mandate of the Substance Abuse and Mental Health Services Administration (SAMHSA) (formerly National Institute on Drug Abuse).

In a method using a single system with solid phase extraction and gas-liquid chromatography with mass spectrometry, opiates were detected at a concentration of 50 micrograms/L.

COLLECTION/STORAGE INFORMATION

- Specimen Collection and Handling
    - Collect urine specimen following chain of custody.

- Store specimen for up to 9 months at -20°C.

LOINC CODES
- Code: 19414-2 (*Short Name* - Codeine CtO Ur Cfm-mCnc)
- Code: 19413-4 (*Short Name* - Codeine CtOff Ur Scn-mCnc)
- Code: 3507-1 (*Short Name* - Codeine Ur QI)
- Code: 3508-9 (*Short Name* - Codeine Ur-mCnc)
- Code: 13641-6 (*Short Name* - Codeine Ur QI SAMHSA Cfm)
- Code: 16250-3 (*Short Name* - Codeine Ur Cnfrn-mCnc)

Urine cotinine measurement

TEST DEFINITION
Measurement of cotinine in urine as an indicator of nicotine intake

SYNONYMS
- Urine cotinine level

REFERENCE RANGE
- Non-smokers: 1-20 ng/mL (6-114 nmol/L)
- Smokers: 300-1300 ng/mL (1703-7378 nmol/L)
  Please refer to your institution's reference ranges as lab normals may vary.

INDICATIONS
Suspected nicotine exposure
> **Strength of Recommendation:** Class IIa
> **Strength of Evidence:** Category B
> **Results Interpretation:**
> **Positive biochemistry findings**
> ELISA-determined concentrations of urinary cotinine are directly proportional to the quantity of daily cigarette consumption, and therefore may be useful for determining both active and passive exposure to nicotine in tobacco smoke.

CLINICAL NOTES
Cotinine levels are stable in body fluids, and are not influenced by factors such as diet or environment.

COLLECTION/STORAGE INFORMATION
- Immediately freeze and store at -20°C

LOINC CODES
- Code: 10366-3 (*Short Name* - Cotinine Ur-mCnc)
- Code: 33796-4 (*Short Name* - Cotinine Ur-sCnc)
- Code: 12293-7 (*Short Name* - Cotinine Ur QI)

Urine culture

TEST DEFINITION
Identification of bacterial colony-forming units (CFU) in urine for the diagnosis and management of urinary tract infections

SYNONYMS
- Microbial urine culture

REFERENCE RANGE

- Negative culture: ≤1000 colony-forming units (CFU)/mL with mixed bacterial species not detected
- Midvoid clean catch specimen positive for one or more bacterial species, measured at counts ≤1000 CFU/mL, is typically considered contaminated and reported as normal
  Please refer to your institution's reference ranges as lab normals may vary.

INDICATIONS

Suspected epididymitis
Results Interpretation:
Abnormal findings on microbiological examination of urine
Positive urine cultures for coliforms or Pseudomonas have been found in 25% of patients with acute epididymitis. The average age of patients with coliform epididymitis was 54 years; the average age for patients with gonococcal or chlamydial epididymitis was 25 years.

In another study, only 2 of 16 patients under 18 years of age with epididymitis had positive urine cultures.

In patients with urinary tract symptoms, the organism that produces cystitis or urethritis is also implicated in the etiology of epididymitis.

Suspected nongonococcal urethritis
Results Interpretation:
Positive microbiology findings
A first voided urine specimen can be processed for *Ureaplasma urealyticum*, although its role in nongonococcal urethritis is controversial.

Suspected prostatitis
Results Interpretation:
Urine culture: organisms - finding
Acute bacterial prostatitis is caused by the same organisms responsible for urinary tract infections such as *Escherichia coli*, *Proteus*, *Klebsiella*, *Enterobacter*, *Pseudomonas*, *Serratia*, and some other less common gram-negative bacteria. Rarely, the infection may be due to *Neisseria gonorrhoeae*. Mixed infections are fairly common.

Suspected sepsis
Strength of Recommendation: Class I
Strength of Evidence: Category C
Results Interpretation:
Abnormal microbiology findings
Escherichia coli is a common organism responsible for urinary tract infection leading to sepsis.

Suspected urinary tract infection (UTI)
Strength of Recommendation: Class IIa
Strength of Evidence: Category C
Results Interpretation:
Bacteriuria
- General, Clinical Evidence of Urinary Tract Infection (UTI):
  - Bacterial counts of greater than or equal to 50,000 colony-forming units (CFU)/mL should undergo identification and susceptibility testing.
  - Short term catheterization specimens with counts greater than or equal to 10^2 CFU/mL typically persist and increase within 48 hours.
  - Most UTIs are caused by enteric bacteria such as *Escherichia coli*.
  - Cultured clean catch midstream specimen is considered contaminated when three or more bacterial species are detected at counts less than or equal to 1000 CFU/mL.
  - In healthy women, the first 10 mL of voided urine can contain normal urethral or perineal flora with counts of 1,000 to 10,000 CFU/mL, making results interpretation more difficult, and reinforcing the need for a midstream specimen.
- Adults, Clinical Evidence of UTI:
  - Acute uncomplicated UTI in women is diagnosed by counts greater than or equal to 10^3 CFU/mL.
  - Acute uncomplicated pyelonephritis is diagnosed by counts greater than or equal to 10^4 CFU/mL.
  - Asymptomatic bacteriuria is diagnosed by counts greater than or equal to 10^5 CFU/mL in 2 consecutive midstream urine cultures collected at least 24 hours apart.
  - UTI in men is diagnosed by counts greater than or equal to 10^4 CFU/mL.

- Complicated UTI, to include long-term indwelling catheter specimens, is diagnosed by counts greater than or equal to 10^5 CFU/mL.
- Children, Clinical Evidence of UTI:
  - Clean catch or bag urine specimen with isolation of a single bacterial species with a colony count of greater than or equal to 10^5 CFU/mL diagnoses UTI.
  - Catheter specimens with 10^3 to 10^5 CFU/mL diagnoses UTI.
  - Suprapubic aspiration specimens with counts greater than 10^2 CFU/mL diagnoses UTI.
  - Catheter specimens from infants with counts greater than or equal to 50,000 CFU/mL diagnoses UTI.

False Results

Urine specimens obtained from bag collection in infants are at increased risk of contamination from periurethral flora and exhibit false-positive rates as high as 70%.

Urine culture screening for asymptomatic bacteriuria in pregnancy
> **Strength of Recommendation:** Class I
> **Strength of Evidence:** Category A
> **Results Interpretation:**
> **Bacteriuria**
>
> Accurate detection with urine culture and early treatment of asymptomatic bacteriuria significantly reduces the risk of pregnancy complications associated with symptomatic urinary tract infections.
>
> Greater than 10^6 colony-forming units (CFU)/mL of the same organism in urine indicates significant bacteriuria. Asymptomatic bacteriuria is defined as greater than or equal to 10^5 CFU/mL of a single bacterial species in 2 consecutive midstream urine cultures collected at least 24 hours apart.
> **Timing of Monitoring**
>
> Urine culture screening for asymptomatic bacteriuria should be performed between 12 and 16 weeks' gestation.
>
> If the urine culture screen is positive, a repeat culture should be performed 7 days after completion of antimicrobial treatment to confirm cure. Monthly screening cultures are recommended until term if the post-treatment culture is negative.

CLINICAL NOTES

Transurethral bladder catheterization and suprapubic aspiration are the recommended methods for obtaining urine specimens from children under 3 years of age.

COLLECTION/STORAGE INFORMATION

- Collect 4 to 10 mL of urine by one of 3 methods to avoid contamination: midstream clean catch, suprapubic aspiration, or catheterization.
- Process catheter and midvoid specimens within 2 hours and suprapubic aspiration specimens immediately.
- If lab processing is delayed 30 minutes or more, refrigerate specimen up to 6 hours and consider adding a preservative such as boric acid.

Urine cystine measurement, qualitative

TEST DEFINITION

Qualitative measurement of cystine in urine for the detection of urinary calculi disorders

REFERENCE RANGE

- Adults: <38.1 mg/day (<317 micromol/day)
- Infants, 10 days to 7 weeks: 2.16-3.37 mg/day (18-28 micromol/day)
- Children, 3 to 12 years: 4.9-30.9 mg/day (41-257 micromol/day)
  Please refer to your institution's reference ranges as lab normals may vary.

INDICATIONS
Suspected cystinuria
> **Strength of Recommendation:** Class IIa
> **Strength of Evidence:** Category C

Results Interpretation:
Increased cystine
Urinary excretion of cystine in excess of 20 mg/day is abnormal. Excretion of greater than 250 mg per day in a 24-hour urine sample diagnoses cystinuria in adults. In children, cystinuria may be diagnosed with levels as low as 75 mg per day.
Urine cystine levels are high for newborns but decrease after the first few months of life.

ABNORMAL RESULTS
- Results increased in first trimester of pregnancy.
- Results decreased in severe burns.

COLLECTION/STORAGE INFORMATION
- Instruct patient to collect first voided morning urine.

LOINC CODES
- Code: 9644-6 (*Short Name* - Cystine Ur Ql)

Urine cystine measurement, quantitative

TEST DEFINITION
Quantitative measurement of cystine in urine for the management of urinary calculi disorders

REFERENCE RANGE
- Adults: <38.1 mg/day (<317 micromol/day)
- Infants, 10 days to 7 weeks: 2.16-3.37 mg/day (18-28 micromol/day)
- Children, 3 to 12 years: 4.9-30.9 mg/day (41-257 micromol/day)
Please refer to your institution's reference ranges as lab normals may vary.

INDICATIONS
Nephrolithiasis attributable to cystinuria
    Strength of Recommendation: Class IIa
    Strength of Evidence: Category B
Results Interpretation:
Increased cystine
An increase in cystine in urine samples may predict nephrolithiasis attributable to cystinuria.
A patient excreting greater than 400 mg/day of cystine is considered to be calculus producing; a non-calculus producing patient excretes less than 400 mg/day. Therapeutic efficacy is determined by the eradication of urinary calculi; however, some patients may exhibit minimal urinary calculi after effective therapy.
Timing of Monitoring
Collect two samples to determine cystinuria: two 24-hour collections or one 16-hour paired with one 8-hour collection.

Urine cystine monitoring
    Strength of Recommendation: Class IIa
    Strength of Evidence: Category C
Results Interpretation:
Increased cystine
An increase in urine cystine levels may signal an increased risk of stone formation in cystinuric patients.
A patient excreting greater than 400 mg/day of cystine is considered to be calculus producing; a non-calculus producing patient excretes less than 400 mg/day.

ABNORMAL RESULTS
- Results increased in first trimester of pregnancy.
- Results decreased in severe burns.

COLLECTION/STORAGE INFORMATION
- Instruct patient to collect either two 24-hour urine specimens or one 16- and one 8-hour urine specimen.

- When conducting two collections, add 15 to 30 ml of 6M hydrochloride to the first bottle, and add either nothing or 20 to 30 ml of 0.3M sodium azide to the second bottle.
- Add 20 mL of toluene to 24-hour collection container.
- May store frozen at -20°C.

LOINC CODES
- Code: 30065-7 (*Short Name* - Cystine/creat Ur-Rto)
- Code: 16709-8 (*Short Name* - Cystine Ur-aCnc)
- Code: 13725-7 (*Short Name* - Cystine/creat Ur-mRto)
- Code: 2178-2 (*Short Name* - Cystine Ur-mCnc)
- Code: 26962-1 (*Short Name* - Cystine Ur-sCnc)

Urine dipstick for hemoglobin

TEST DEFINITION
Urine dipstick for Hgb for the detection of microhematuria

SYNONYMS
- Urine dipstick for haemoglobin

REFERENCE RANGE
- Adults and children: negative
  Please refer to your institution's reference ranges as lab normals may vary.

INDICATIONS
Screening for urologic malignancy
   Strength of Recommendation: Class IIb
   Strength of Evidence: Category B
   Results Interpretation:
   Urine dipstick testing for Hgb is not appropriately sensitive to serve as a screening test for urologic cancers. A full urologic evaluation is not recommended based upon a single positive urine Hgb dipstick test. The advancement of more sensitive assays may offer valuable diagnostic alternatives for patients at risk of urologic malignancy.

Suspected appendicitis
   Results Interpretation:
   Hematuria suggests a ureteral calculus rather than appendicitis; however, a retroileal appendix may cause ureteral inflammation and microscopic hematuria.
   Hematuria may be present in some patients with a ruptured or inflamed appendix in proximity to the urinary tract.

Suspected microhematuria
   Strength of Recommendation: Class IIb
   Strength of Evidence: Category B
   Results Interpretation:
   Microscopic hematuria
   A positive urine dipstick for Hgb has suboptimal correlation with microscopic urinalysis for red blood cells. Further evaluation of dipstick positive samples by microscopy may provide more accurate quantification of suspected microhematuria. When making further diagnostic testing and treatment decisions, microscopic analysis is preferred over dipstick testing.

Suspected myoglobinuria
   Strength of Recommendation: Class IIb
   Strength of Evidence: Category C

Results Interpretation:
Myoglobinuria

Urine dipstick testing identifies the presence of Hgb and not red blood cells, therefore confirmation by urine microscopic exam is necessary to validate the presence of red blood cells. Myoglobinuria in the presence of a negative microscopic urine exam may be suggestive of free hemoglobin from hemolysis or myoglobinuria due to rhabdomyolysis.

Urine dipstick Hgb testing may have value as a screening tool in patients with suspected myoglobinuria.

Suspected necrotizing soft tissue infection
Results Interpretation:
Hemoglobinuria

Hemoglobinuria, indicated by dark-colored urine, occurs secondary to hemolysis in clostridial myonecrosis and necrotizing fasciitis.

ABNORMAL RESULTS

Ingestion of ascorbic acid (350 mg to 1,000 mg daily) can result in a false negative reading.

LOINC CODES

• Code: 5794-3 (*Short Name* - Hgb Ur Ql Test Str)

Urine dipstick for leukocyte esterase

TEST DEFINITION

An indirect measure using a reagent strip to detect leukocyte esterase in urine to assess for pyuria

SYNONYMS

• Urine dipstick for leucocyte esterase
• Urine dipstick for leucocytes
• Urine dipstick for leukocytes
• Urine dipstick for white cells

REFERENCE RANGE

• Adults and Children: Negative or no color change
Please refer to your institution's reference ranges as lab normals may vary.

INDICATIONS
Suspected gonococcal infection
Results Interpretation:
Positive laboratory findings

A positive leukocyte esterase test indicates the presence of nonspecific inflammatory enzymes and not necessarily *Neisseria gonorrhoeae*.

Suspected pyuria in individuals at risk for urinary tract infection
Strength of Recommendation: Class IIa
Strength of Evidence: Category B
Results Interpretation:
Dipstick test finding

Leukocyte esterase examination is a reasonable screening test for pyuria in patients with suspected UTI, but does not directly measure bacteriuria. A negative test cannot exclude UTI in patients in whom signs and symptoms of UTI are ambiguous.

A color change indicates that the enzyme is present; the intensity of the color is proportional to the amount of enzyme present.

False Results

Vaginal fluids or *Trichomonas* can produce false positive results when present as contaminants in urine samples. Oxidizing agents and formalin can also produce false-positive results. The presence of nitrofurantoin and other chromogenic compounds can make color interpretation of the dipstick difficult.

ABNORMAL RESULTS
- Results decreased in:
  - Elevated urine specific gravity
  - Protein
  - Glucose

CLINICAL NOTES
In children, leukocyte esterase can be used for initial assessment of suspected UTI, but may not be reliable in children less than 2 years of age.

Reliance on single parameters of the combined reagent strip may lead to treatment errors. In high risk groups (pregnancy, hospitalized patients), additional testing, including urine culture, should be considered.

COLLECTION/STORAGE INFORMATION
- Specimen Collection and Handling:
  - Obtain urine sample by a clean-catch midstream voided specimen or catheterization
  - Place sample in sterile containers.
  - Process sample immediately or store at 4°C.
  - Specimens can be initially screened with the dipstick and then cultured (gold standard for detecting bacteriuria), if properly obtained.

LOINC CODES
- Code: 5799-2 (*Short Name* - WBC Est Ur Ql Strip)

Urine dipstick for protein

TEST DEFINITION
A semiquantitative measurement of protein concentration in urine

REFERENCE RANGE
- Negative

Please refer to your institution's reference ranges as lab normals may vary.

INDICATIONS
Suspected pre-eclampsia
  Results Interpretation:
  Proteinuria
- A urine dipstick value of 1+ defines proteinuria.
- A urine dipstick value of 2+ or 3+ increases the diagnostic certainty of pre-eclampsia.
- A urine dipstick value of 3+ or greater in two random samples collected four or more hours apart, in the absence of an alternative explanation, indicates severe pre-eclampsia.

Suspected proteinuria
  Results Interpretation:
  Proteinuria
  The degree of proteinuria is determined by the reaction of the urine to the reagent. The results are graded as negative, trace (15 to 30 mg/dL), 1+ (30-100 mg/dL), 2+ (100-300 mg/dL), 3+ (300-100mg/dl), and 4+ ($\geq$1,000 mg/dL)

COMMON PANELS
- Urinalysis

CLINICAL NOTES
Urine dipstick analysis provides only a crude estimate of urine protein concentration. The results are affected by the degree of dilution and the amount of urine excreted.

COLLECTION/STORAGE INFORMATION
- Collect fresh, midstream urine specimen in clean container, free of preservatives

Urine ethanol measurement

TEST DEFINITION
Quantitative measurement of ethanol in urine for the assessment of recent ethanol intake

SYNONYMS
• Urine ethanol level

REFERENCE RANGE
• Adults and Children: Negative
  Please refer to your institution's reference ranges as lab normals may vary.

INDICATIONS
Suspected alcohol intoxication
   Strength of Recommendation: Class IIb
   Strength of Evidence: Category B
   Results Interpretation:
   Positive laboratory findings
      The level of ethanol in urine equating to intoxication differs by state and country statute. Because of variables including amounts of urine in the bladder, physiologic barriers, and specimen collection and handling variations, translating measured urine alcohol concentration into presumed blood alcohol concentration can give inaccurate results.
      Urine ethanol levels soon after ingestion show a urine/blood ratio less than 1. Later, with no ethanol in the stomach, the average urine/blood ratio is 1.3.

ABNORMAL RESULTS
• Results Increased In:
    • Diabetes, resulting from the conversion of urine glucose to ethanol by microorganisms
    • Urinary tract infection

CLINICAL NOTES
Increases in urine output from drinking water or from diuretics will not significantly affect the concentration of alcohol in the urine.
Gas chromatography can detect ethanol concentrations as low as 10 mg/dL and discriminate ethanol from other alcohols, ketones, and hydrocarbons.
Calculating blood alcohol concentration from urine alcohol concentration is inaccurate and does not reflect a true blood alcohol level because of substantial individual variability and pharmacokinetic issues.
Urine ethanol is not generally used for forensic purposes in the United States.

COLLECTION/STORAGE INFORMATION
• Specimen Collection and Handling:
    • Collect 2 urine specimens, one immediately and another 30 to 60 minutes after initial sample.
    • Place urine in sampling tube with 100 mg sodium fluoride to avoid synthesis of ethanol in the specimen.
    • Refrigerate specimen at 4°C until analysis.

LOINC CODES
• Code: 5644-0 (*Short Name* - Ethanol Ur Ql)
• Code: 5645-7 (*Short Name* - Ethanol Ur-mCnc)
• Code: 22745-4 (*Short Name* - Ethanol Ur-sCnc)

Urine flunitrazepam level

TEST DEFINITION
Measurement of flunitrazepam levels in urine for suspected toxicity

REFERENCE RANGE
• Negative
Please refer to your institution's reference ranges as lab normals may vary.

INDICATIONS
Suspected flunitrazepam toxicity such as in sexual assault ('date rape')
   Strength of Recommendation: Class IIb
   Strength of Evidence: Category C
   Results Interpretation:
   Urine drug levels - finding
      A positive test confirms the presence of flunitrazepam metabolites in the urine. Flunitrazepam can be detected in urine up to 72 hours after ingestion of a 2-mg dose.
      Benzodiazepines can be detected in urine as part of a drugs-of-abuse panel, but some commercial toxicology screens do not detect flunitrazepam; therefore, a negative benzodiazepine test does not rule out flunitrazepam ingestion.
      In sexual assault cases, investigating law enforcement personnel should be advised to have the urine sample analyzed by their forensic toxicology laboratory for the flunitrazepam metabolite, 7-amino-flunitrazepam.

   False Results
      Urine specimens can be adulterated by adding various chemicals to urine, such as Visine®, hand soap, Drano®, and bleach, which cause false-negative test results for benzodiazepines.

COMMON PANELS
• Drugs of abuse testing, urine

CLINICAL NOTES
   If a hospital or forensic laboratory is unable to analyze for flunitrazepam, the drug's manufacturer (Hoffman La Roche, Inc), should be contacted for definitive testing.

COLLECTION/STORAGE INFORMATION
• Specimen Collection and Handling:
   • Follow chain of custody for urine collection, if indicated
   • Refrigerate specimen after collection
   • Deliver specimen to lab within 1 hour of collection

LOINC CODES
• Code: 19467-0 (*Short Name* - Flunitrazepam Ur QI Cnfrn)
• Code: 3641-8 (*Short Name* - Flunitrazepam Ur-mCnc)
• Code: 19469-6 (*Short Name* - Flunitrazepam CtOff Ur Cnfrn-mCnc)
• Code: 20528-6 (*Short Name* - Flunitrazepam Ur Cnfrn-mCnc)

Urine methylenedioxymethamphetamine measurement

TEST DEFINITION
   Measurement of urine 3,4-methylenedioxymethamphetamine (MDMA/ecstasy) for the determination of illicit drug use

SYNONYMS
- Urine Methylenedioxymethamphetamine level

REFERENCE RANGE
- Negative
  Please refer to your institution's reference ranges as lab normals may vary.

INDICATIONS
Suspected 3,4-methylenedioxymethamphetamine (MDMA/ecstasy) ingestion
   Results Interpretation:
   Positive laboratory findings
      A standard urine toxicology screen may detect 3,4-methylenedioxymethamphetamine (MDMA/ecstasy) only if very large doses of MDMA have been ingested. MDMA will show up as amphetamines on this screen. The presence of MDMA may be confirmed by specific urine testing.

LOINC CODES
- Code: 19570-1 (*Short Name* - MDMA Ur-mCnc)
- Code: 19572-7 (*Short Name* - MDMA CtO Ur Cfm-mCnc)
- Code: 18358-2 (*Short Name* - MDMA Ur Cnfrn-mCnc)
- Code: 19568-5 (*Short Name* - MDMA Ur Ql Scn)
- Code: 14267-9 (*Short Name* - MDMA Ur Ql)
- Code: 19571-9 (*Short Name* - MDMA CtOff Ur Scn-mCnc)

Urine methylmalonic acid level

TEST DEFINITION
Measurement of urine methylmalonic acid level to assess vitamin B_{12} (cobalamin) deficiency

SYNONYMS
- Urine 2-Methylpropanedioic acid level
- Urine 2-Methylpropanedioic acid measurement
- Urine methylmalonic acid measurement

REFERENCE RANGE
- Normal ranges are technique specific:
- Colorimetry (24 hour urine): ≤11.2 mg/d (≤95 micromol/d)
- Gas-liquid chromatography (24 hour urine): ≤9.0 mg/d (≤76 micromol/d)
- Gas chromatography-mass spectrometry (random urine): <3.76 mg/g creatinine (<3.6 micromol/mol creatinine)
  Please refer to your institution's reference ranges as lab normals may vary.

INDICATIONS
Vitamin B_{12} (cobalamin) deficiency
      Strength of Recommendation: Class IIb
      Strength of Evidence: Category B
   Results Interpretation:
   Abnormal laboratory findings
      A urine methylmalonic acid (uMMA) level of greater than 3.2 mmol/mol creatinine in adults, and cut-off values of 20 to 30 mmol/mol creatinine in infants, may be indicative of early cobalamine (Cbl) deficiency.
      Urine MMA is a sensitive and specific indicator of Cbl function and is useful as both a diagnostic test and to monitor response to therapy. Serum MMA, conversely, may be less specific in renal failure and in conditions of hemoconcentration.
      Urinary MMA, normalized to urine creatinine is usually 40 times higher than serum MMA concentrations.

CLINICAL NOTES
- Valine test results are invalid in methylmalonic aciduria patients.
- Isoleucine is a substitute for valine, but effects are not as evident.

- Decreased urine output renders colorimetric test unreliable.

COLLECTION/STORAGE INFORMATION
- Specimen Collection and Handling:
    - Random urine:
        - Instruct patient to fast overnight.
        - Collect second voided morning urine specimen.
        - Store frozen.
    - 24 hour urine:
        - L-valine is administered immediately prior to commencement of 24-hour urine collection.
        - Add 10 ml HCL, 6 mol/L to urine specimen.
        - Store frozen for up to 3 months.

LOINC CODES
- Code: 29877-8 (*Short Name* - MMA Ur Ql)
- Code: 13775-2 (*Short Name* - MMA/creat 24H Ur-mRto)
- Code: 32287-5 (*Short Name* - MMA Ur-sCnc)
- Code: 2630-2 (*Short Name* - MMA Ur-mCnc)
- Code: 25115-7 (*Short Name* - MMA/creat 24H Ur-sRto)
- Code: 29342-3 (*Short Name* - MMA 24H Ur-mRate)
- Code: 25116-5 (*Short Name* - MMA/creat Ur-sRto)
- Code: 13776-0 (*Short Name* - MMA/creat Ur-mRto)

Urine morphine measurement

TEST DEFINITION
Measurement of morphine in urine for detection and monitoring of suspected abuse

SYNONYMS
- Urine morphine level

REFERENCE RANGE
Negative
Please refer to your institution's reference ranges as lab normals may vary.

INDICATIONS
Suspected or known opioid abuse
      Strength of Recommendation: Class IIa
      Strength of Evidence: Category B
Results Interpretation:
Abnormal laboratory findings
- The Departments of Defense and Health and Human Services use the following steps in the diagnosis of opioid abuse:
    - An immunoassay morphine level of 2000 ng/mL or greater is considered a positive screen and is sent for confirmatory testing.
    - A gas chromatography-mass spectroscopy (GC-MS) morphine level of 4000 ng/mL or greater confirms the presence of morphine.
    - A GC-MS for 6-acetylmorphine (6-AM) is then performed, a level of 10 ng/mL or greater considered positive for heroin.

Detection of morphine in urine may reflect recent morphine, codeine, or heroin use.

Morphine concentrations vary greatly between subjects and are generally higher in urine than in blood. Levels of morphine after ingestion of heroin vary greatly within the same individual.

Although morphine is detectable at lower levels, the generally accepted screening cutoff concentration is 2,000 ng/mL in order to avoid false positives as a result of poppy seed ingestion.

Since a positive result on a morphine immunoassay may be caused by several drugs, the presence of 6-acetylmorphine is often used to confirm suspected heroin use.

Total morphine in urine peaks between 1.2 to 9.3 hours after a single-dose administration.

False positive results may coincide with ingestion of poppy seeds.

ABNORMAL RESULTS
False positive results may coincide with ingestion of poppy seeds.

COLLECTION/STORAGE INFORMATION
- May store at -20°C for up to 9 months.

LOINC CODES
- Code: 20550-0 (*Short Name* - Morphine Free Ur Cnfrn-mCnc)
- Code: 19599-0 (*Short Name* - Morphine CtOff Ur Scn-mCnc)
- Code: 19600-6 (*Short Name* - Morphine CtO Ur Cfm-mCnc)
- Code: 3832-3 (*Short Name* - Morphine 24H Ur-mRate)
- Code: 3831-5 (*Short Name* - Morphine Ur-mCnc)
- Code: 3829-9 (*Short Name* - Morphine Free Ur-mCnc)
- Code: 16251-1 (*Short Name* - Morphine Ur Cfm-mCnc)

Urine nitrite

TEST DEFINITION
Detection of urine nitrites as a screening test for urinary tract infection

REFERENCE RANGE
- Negative
Please refer to your institution's reference ranges as lab normals may vary.

INDICATIONS
Suspected acute renal transplant rejection
> **Strength of Recommendation:** Class IIa
> **Strength of Evidence:** Category B
> **Results Interpretation:**
> **Urine nitrite positive**
>> Urine nitrites may be present in the early stages after a renal transplant due to either urinary tract infection (UTI) or rejection. A urine nitrite level of 3,000 micromol/L or greater indicates renal transplant rejection, whereas levels less than or equal to 1,000 micromol/L are more consistent with UTI.

Suspected urinary tract infection (UTI)
> **Strength of Recommendation:** Class IIa
> **Strength of Evidence:** Category B
> **Results Interpretation:**
> **Urine nitrite positive**
>> Positive dipstick urinalysis for nitrites may indicate the presence of urinary tract infection (UTI). The most accurate results to screen for asymptomatic UTI are obtained by dipstick testing for combinations of urine nitrite and/or leukocyte esterase.
>> For definitive diagnosis, urine culture is the gold standard for diagnosing UTI.
> **Urine nitrite negative**
>> A negative urine dipstick test for nitrite does not rule out urinary tract infection (UTI) in patients with a high likelihood of having the infection.

COMMON PANELS
- Urinalysis

COLLECTION/STORAGE INFORMATION
- Specimen Collection and Handling:
  - Obtain a first morning void midstream urine specimen.
  - Examine specimen immediately or refrigerate.

Urine opiates screening test

TEST DEFINITION
Detection of opiates in urine for suspected overdose or abuse

REFERENCE RANGE
• Negative
Please refer to your institution's reference ranges as lab normals may vary.

INDICATIONS
Suspected opiate abuse
> **Strength of Recommendation:** Class I
> **Strength of Evidence:** Category C

Results Interpretation:
Urine drug levels - finding
> Some urine opiate screens may test positive only for heroin, morphine, and codeine, and may not detect propoxyphene, meperidine, methadone, pentazocine, or oxycodone.
> Opiates may be detected on a urine drug screen within a window of 2 to 5 days, although this will vary depending on the specific opioid, amount involved, route of exposure, and type of assay used.
> Tampering should be suspected if the color or odor of the sample is abnormal, if the pH is less than 3 or greater than 11, if the specific gravity is less than 1.005, if the temperature is less than 90.5°C within 4 minutes after specimen collection, if the creatinine concentration is less than 5 mg/dL, or if the nitrite level is less than 500 mcg/mL.

Positive laboratory findings
> A positive urine drug screen for opiates should typically be followed with a confirmatory quantitative test, typically gas chromatography-mass spectrometry (GC-MS). Although a positive test suggests recent use, it does not distinguish between one-time versus chronic users, establish a pattern or frequency of use, or measure functional impairment.
> The Substance Abuse and Mental Health Services Administration (SAMHSA) has established a cutoff of 2000 ng/mL for opiates on drug screens in the federal workplace. SAMHSA recommends that a test for the heroin metabolite 6-MAM should be performed if the opiate concentration exceeds this level.

Negative laboratory findings
> Because the results of a urine drug screen for opiates is reported as a simple positive or negative, it is possible that opiates may have been present but in a concentration below the reporting threshold.

Frequency of Monitoring
> In a study of 166 patients in methadone maintenance treatment, twice-weekly urine drug screening identified about 50% more illicit opioid users than once-weekly or monthly testing.

COMMON PANELS
• Drugs of abuse testing, urine

ABNORMAL RESULTS
• Results increased in:
  • Poppy seed ingestion

COLLECTION/STORAGE INFORMATION
• Obtain a random urine sample.
• To decrease the possibility of the patient tampering with the sample, urine collection may be directly observed, access to water or cleaning agents should be restricted, and bluing agent may be added to the toilet.
• If the test results could potentially be used as evidence in a court of law, chain of custody should be maintained.
• Record temperature of urine sample at time of collection, then refrigerate specimen.

LOINC CODES
• Code: 21431-2 (*Short Name* - Opiates Ur Ql Scn>2000 ng/m)
• Code: 8222-2 (*Short Name* - Opiates Ur Ql SAMSHA Scn)
• Code: 19295-5 (*Short Name* - Opiates Ur Ql Scn)

Urine pH test

TEST DEFINITION
Measurement of urine pH for the evaluation and management of disorders that affect urine acidity.

REFERENCE RANGE
- Adults: 5-9
- Newborns: 5-7
  Please refer to your institution's reference ranges as lab normals may vary.

INDICATIONS
Nephrolithiasis
   Results Interpretation:
   Decreased level (laboratory finding)
      Alkaline urine (pH greater than 7.5) may be detected in patients with infection by urea-splitting organisms (eg, Proteus).
      Patients with hyperuricosuria have acid urine (pH less than 5.5), which predisposes to uric acid crystallization.

Urinary tract infection
   Results Interpretation:
   Increased level (laboratory finding)
      An alkaline urine occurs in the presence of urinary tract infection with urea-splitting organisms, eg, *Proteus sp.* Urine pH greater than 7 is a clue to the presence of such organisms.

COMMON PANELS
- Urinalysis

ABNORMAL RESULTS
- Results increased in:
    - Diet high in citrus fruits and vegetables
    - Gastric losses from vomiting or nasogastric suction
    - Prolonged time from sample collection
- Results decreased in:
    - Diet high in meat protein or cranberries
    - Potassium depletion

COLLECTION/STORAGE INFORMATION
- Transport specimen to lab immediately or refrigerate:

LOINC CODES
- Code: 27378-9 (*Short Name* - pH 24H Ur-sCnc)
- Code: 2756-5 (*Short Name* - pH Ur-sCnc)

Urine phencyclidine screening test

TEST DEFINITION
Detection of phencyclidine (PCP) in urine for the evaluation and management of suspected PCP exposure

REFERENCE RANGE
- Adults and Children: Negative (less than 25 mcg/L in urine)
  Please refer to your institution's reference ranges as lab normals may vary.

INDICATIONS
Screening for suspected phencyclidine exposure
    Strength of Recommendation: Class IIa
    Strength of Evidence: Category B
    Results Interpretation:
    Positive laboratory findings
        The federally mandated threshold concentration, established by the Substance Abuse and Mental Health Services Administration (SAMHSA), for a positive urine phencyclidine (PCP) test is 25 mcg/L. The National Institute of Drug Addiction guidelines stipulate a cutoff for PCP in urine of 25 nanograms/mL.
        PCP urine concentrations have been reported to be 10 to 20 times greater than plasma concentrations. Urinary excretion of PCP is pH dependent and the PCP level may be undetectable in patients with alkaline urine.
        Urine PCP levels may be detected up to 7 days after a single dose and up to 21 days with chronic exposure. Urine PCP levels do not correlate with clinical toxicity.
        PCP urine concentration cutoff values (CV) below existing standard SAMSHA assay CV may increase the percentage of positive PCP urine screens identified; however, a lower CV may sacrifice positive predictive value accuracy.
        Gas chromatography with mass spectrometry is the preferred method for detection of PCP in urine; limits of detection in the nanogram/mL range are possible with this test technique.
        Sodium chloride, sodium hypochlorite, sodium bicarbonate, and JOY® dishwashing detergent may produce phencyclidine exposure false negative results if used as adulterants when the urine is being analyzed using an Emit® test.

CLINICAL NOTES
    The phencyclidine (PCP) concentration may decrease at variable rates in urine samples stored at room temperature. In specimens stored at -16°C to -20°C significant decreases in PCP levels have not been observed.
    Urine excretion of PCP is pH dependent and the PCP level may be undetectable in patients with alkaline urine. A urine pH should always be obtained in conjunction with the urine PCP level.

COLLECTION/STORAGE INFORMATION
• Store urine samples at -16°C to -20°C.

LOINC CODES
• Code: 8238-8 (*Short Name* - PCP Ur Ql SAMSHA Scn)
• Code: 14311-5 (*Short Name* - PCP Ur Ql Cfm>20 ng/mL)
• Code: 18392-1 (*Short Name* - PCP Ur Ql Cnfrn)
• Code: 3936-2 (*Short Name* - PCP Ur Ql)
• Code: 19659-2 (*Short Name* - PCP Ur Ql Scn)
• Code: 14310-7 (*Short Name* - PCP Ur Ql Scn>25 ng/mL)
• Code: 8237-0 (*Short Name* - PCP Ur Ql SAMHSA Cfm)

Urine pregnancy test

TEST DEFINITION
    Qualitative measurement of human chorionic gonadotropin in urine for the evaluation of pregnancy status

REFERENCE RANGE
• Negative
    Please refer to your institution's reference ranges as lab normals may vary.

INDICATIONS
Suspected pregnancy
    Strength of Recommendation: Class IIa
    Strength of Evidence: Category B

Results Interpretation:
Urine pregnancy test positive
Urine pregnancy tests may become positive as early as 3 days prior to the first missed period or as late as 7 days following the first missed period. Urine human chorionic gonadotropin (hCG) concentrations can vary widely during early pregnancy.
Urine pregnancy test negative
Over-the-counter urine pregnancy tests may be negative around the time of the first missed period, secondary to low urine human chorionic gonadotropin (hCG) levels. Repeat testing in several days may be appropriate if the initial test result is negative.

COLLECTION/STORAGE INFORMATION
- Specimen collection and handling:
  - Collect fresh first-void morning urine specimen
  - May store at 2° to 8° C for up to 48 hours

LOINC CODES
- Code: 2106-3 (*Short Name* - HCG Ur Ql)
- Code: 2107-1 (*Short Name* - HCG Ur-sCnc)
- Code: 25372-4 (*Short Name* - HCG Ur-aCnc)

Urine propoxyphene screening test

TEST DEFINITION
Measurement of propoxyphene in urine for suspected overdose or drug of abuse assessment.

REFERENCE RANGE
- Negative
Please refer to your institution's reference ranges as lab normals may vary.

INDICATIONS
Screening test for suspected propoxyphene overdose or abuse.
Strength of Recommendation: Class I
Strength of Evidence: Category C
Results Interpretation:
Urine drug levels - finding
Detection limits may vary depending on the method used. Several commercial immunoassays report a urine concentration of 300 ng/mL as a positive result.
If propoxyphene poisoning is clinically suspected, a negative analysis should be repeated.

False Results
Since excretion is markedly decreased in alkaline urine (and increased in acid urine), a false-negative test may result when urine pH is 6 or higher

COMMON PANELS
- Drugs of abuse testing, urine

CLINICAL NOTES
Urine detection limits may vary depending on method used.

COLLECTION/STORAGE INFORMATION
- Collect random urine sample

LOINC CODES
- Code: 19429-0 (*Short Name* - Propoxyph Ur Ql Scn)
- Code: 19141-1 (*Short Name* - Propoxyph Ur Ql)

VDRL titer measurement, Cerebrospinal fluid

TEST DEFINITION

Quantitative or qualitative measurement of antibodies to VDRL in cerebrospinal fluid for the diagnosis and management of neurosyphilis.

SYNONYMS

- VDRL (syphilis) titer
- VDRL (syphilis) titre
- VDRL titre measurement

REFERENCE RANGE

- Adults and children: nonreactive
  Please refer to your institution's reference ranges as lab normals may vary.

INDICATIONS

Suspected neurosyphilis in the presence of a positive serum treponemal test, and known neurosyphilis to monitor therapy response

> **Strength of Recommendation:** Class I
> **Strength of Evidence:** Category C
> **Results Interpretation:**
> **Serology positive**
> A positive VDRL-CSF is considered diagnostic for neurosyphilis if significant contamination of CSF with blood does not occur during sample collection. Results must be interpreted in relation to clinical presentation, other test results, and CSF findings. A nonreactive VDRL-CSF does not exclude the diagnosis.
> After treatment, an initially high CSF titer is expected to decline fourfold within a year; a fourfold increase in the serum or CSF VDRL titer probably indicates reinfection.
> **Frequency of Monitoring**
> Quantitative VDRL titers should be done on cerebrospinal fluid at 6 weeks and 3, 6, 12, and 24 months after treatment to assess therapeutic response.

CLINICAL NOTES

Results should be reported quantitatively. Qualitative VDRL results are reported as reactive if large clumps are seen on visual inspection, weakly reactive if small clumps are observed, or nonreactive if no flocculation is seen.

LOINC CODES

- Code: 11084-1 (*Short Name* - Reagin Ab Titr Ser)
- Code: 31146-4 (*Short Name* - VDRL Titr CSF)

VDRL titer measurement, Serum

TEST DEFINITION

Quantitative or qualitative measurement of antibodies to VDRL in serum for the presumptive diagnosis of syphilis.

SYNONYMS

- VDRL (syphilis) titer
- VDRL (syphilis) titre
- VDRL titre measurement

REFERENCE RANGE

- Adults and children: nonreactive
  Please refer to your institution's reference ranges as lab normals may vary.

INDICATIONS

Screening, diagnosis, and therapy response in patients with known or suspected syphilis

    Strength of Recommendation: Class I

    Strength of Evidence: Category C

Results Interpretation:

Serology positive

    A fourfold or greater rise in antibody titer is clinically significant and is considered presumptive for primary syphilis.. A reactive nontreponemal test should be followed up with a confirmatory treponemal test (eg fluorescent treponemal antibody absorbed (FTA-ABS) or T. pallidum particle agglutination (TP-PA). Darkfield examination and direct fluorescent antibody tests of lesion exudate or tissue are the only definitive diagnostic methods for early syphilis.

    A persistent fall in sera titer following the treatment of early syphilis provides essential evidence of an appropriate response to therapy. After adequate treatment, the VDRL will commonly fall about fourfold by 3 or 4 months, eightfold by 6 to 8 months, and will become seronegative or low-grade seroreactive by 12 months in early syphilis, and 24 months in secondary syphilis. A fourfold rise in sera titer or a positive test after 1 year in a patient treated for primary syphilis, or 2 years in a patient treated for secondary syphilis, suggests persistent infection, reinfection, or a biologic false-positive reaction. A VDRL titer of 1:16 or higher is typical with secondary syphilis. The type of rash determines the height of the reagin serologic titer, which in turn influences the speed of the seroreversal response; sera test results from patients with a macular eruption become seronegative sooner than those of patients with either a maculopapular or papular rash. A nonreactive test virtually excludes secondary syphilis in a patient with otherwise compatible mucocutaneous lesions.

    In the absence of treatment in patients with tertiary syphilis, the VDRL slowly returns to normal in almost 50% of cases.

    False Results

Frequency of Monitoring

    VDRL follow-up at 3, 6, and 12 months is recommended in both primary and secondary syphilis to evaluate the adequacy of treatment. Sequential testing should employ the same methodology (e.g. VDRL or RPR), ideally by the same laboratory.

CLINICAL NOTES

    Results should be reported quantitatively. Qualitative VDRL results are reported as reactive if large clumps are seen on visual inspection, weakly reactive if small clumps are observed, or nonreactive if no flocculation is seen.

LOINC CODES

- Code: 11084-1 (*Short Name* - Reagin Ab Titr Ser)
- Code: 31146-4 (*Short Name* - VDRL Titr CSF)

Valine measurement

TEST DEFINITION

    Measurement of valine in plasma or serum for detection of acquired and hereditary amino acid disorders

REFERENCE RANGE

- Premature, 1 day: 1.52 ± 0.59 mg/dL (130 ± 50 micromol/L)
- Neonate, 1 day: 0.94-2.88 mg/dL (80-246 micromol/L)
- Infants 1 to 3 months: 2.27 ± 0.57 mg/dL (194 ± 49 micromol/L)
- Infants 9 to 24 months: 0.67-3.07 mg/dL (57-262 micromol/L)
- Children 3 to 10 years: 1.5-3.31 mg/dL (128-283 micromol/L)
- Children 6 to 18 years: 1.83-3.37 mg/dL (156-288 micromol/L)
- Adults: 1.65-3.71 mg/dL (141-317 micromol/L)

    Please refer to your institution's reference ranges as lab normals may vary.

INDICATIONS

Suspected inborn error of metabolism

    Strength of Recommendation: Class IIa

    Strength of Evidence: Category C

Results Interpretation:
Increased amino acid

Inherited amino acid disorders are directly related to the absence of an enzyme involved in the metabolism of one or more amino acids; therefore, an elevated plasma level of a particular amino acid is highly suggestive of an inherited metabolic defect. In the majority of cases amino acid and organic acid analysis together permit diagnostic confirmation in infants. Immediate treatment should be initiated when an inborn error of metabolism is suspected, even if a definitive diagnosis has not yet been determined.

During acute attacks, maple syrup urine disease (MSUD) is associated with increased levels of leucine, isoleucine, alloisoleucine, valine and related ketoacids.

COLLECTION/STORAGE INFORMATION

- Specimen Collection and Handling:
    - Immediately place sample in ice water.
    - Isolate plasma sample and freeze it within 1 hour; sample stable for 1 week at -20°C.
    - Sample should be deproteinized and stored at -70°C for protracted periods of usage.

LOINC CODES

- Code: 25553-9 (*Short Name* - Valine 24H Ur-sRate)
- Code: 26002-6 (*Short Name* - Valine/creat 24H Ur-sRto)
- Code: 22729-8 (*Short Name* - Valine XXX-sCnc)
- Code: 30064-0 (*Short Name* - Valine/creat Ur-Rto)
- Code: 3119-5 (*Short Name* - Valine Ur-mCnc)
- Code: 26961-3 (*Short Name* - Valine Ur-sCnc)
- Code: 13419-7 (*Short Name* - Valine Amn-mCnc)
- Code: 13822-2 (*Short Name* - Valine/creat Ur-mRto)
- Code: 3120-3 (*Short Name* - Valine 24H Ur-mRate)
- Code: 3116-1 (*Short Name* - Valine CSF-mCnc)
- Code: 9623-0 (*Short Name* - Valine Ur Ql)
- Code: 22649-8 (*Short Name* - Valine CSF-sCnc)
- Code: 32279-2 (*Short Name* - Valine Fld-sCnc)
- Code: 32278-4 (*Short Name* - Valine Vitf-sCnc)
- Code: 26001-8 (*Short Name* - Valine 24H Ur-sCnc)

Verapamil measurement

TEST DEFINITION

Measurement of verapamil levels in serum or plasma to facilitate therapeutic or toxicity monitoring

REFERENCE RANGE

- Therapeutic concentration: 100 ng/mL-500 ng/mL (220 nmol/L-1100 nmol/L)
  Please refer to your institution's reference ranges as lab normals may vary.

INDICATIONS

Drug level monitoring during verapamil therapy or measurement in suspected toxicity
   Strength of Recommendation: Class IIb
   Strength of Evidence: Category B
Results Interpretation:
Blood drug levels - finding

Verapamil therapy is usually monitored by assessing hemodynamic effects rather than by therapeutic drug monitoring. Blood levels of calcium antagonists are not readily available. Blood levels generally do not predict toxicity or direct management but may be of forensic or pharmacokinetic interest.

Toxic levels associated with recovery range from 367 ng/mL (approximately 1 hour after an unknown amount of verapamil was ingested) to 4000 ng/mL (approximately 5 hours after ingestion of 3200 mg). Lethal drug levels have ranged from 690 ng/mL in a 48-year-old male with preexisting liver failure who ingested 1.4 g over 3 days to 8800 ng/mL in a 40 -year-old female following an unknown ingestion.

COLLECTION/STORAGE INFORMATION
• Collect blood in red top (serum), lavender top (EDTA), or green top (heparin) tube.

LOINC CODES
• Code: 4095-6 (*Short Name* - Verapamil Ur QI)
• Code: 4094-9 (*Short Name* - Verapamil SerPl-mCnc)
• Code: 4093-1 (*Short Name* - Verapamil SerPl QI)
• Code: 17767-5 (*Short Name* - Verapamil Ur-mCnc)

Viral culture, Influenzavirus, type A, avian

TEST DEFINITION
Growth of avian influenza A virus in cell culture for the diagnosis of avian influenza A.

SYNONYMS
• Culture for viruses

REFERENCE RANGE
• Adults and children: no growth
Please refer to your institution's reference ranges as lab normals may vary.

INDICATIONS
Suspected avian influenza A
　　　Strength of Recommendation: Class IIa
　　　Strength of Evidence: Category C
　　Results Interpretation:
　　Positive microbiology findings
　　　Virus isolation can provide specific information regarding influenza subtypes and strains. Identification of a previously unknown strain can be performed either by immunofluorescence assay (IFA) using specific monoclonal antibodies or by demonstration of hemagglutination inhibition (HAI). Any specimen testing positive for avian influenza A when infection is suspected should be forwarded to a World Health Organization (WHO) designated laboratory for verification of diagnosis.
　　Timing of Monitoring
　　　Ideally, specimens should be collected within 3 days of symptom onset.

CLINICAL NOTES
US Department of Health and Human Services guidelines state that laboratories isolating highly virulent avian influenza strains must follow biosafety level 3 (BSL-3) conditions with enhancements during interpandemic and pandemic alert periods, and BSL-2 conditions during pandemic periods. Laboratories lacking these capabilities should forward specimens to the Centers for Disease Control. The Centers for Disease Control state that all specimens cultured from patients with suspected H5N1 must be conducted under BSL-3 conditions with enhancements. Clinical specimens from humans and swine should never be processed in the same laboratory.

COLLECTION/STORAGE INFORMATION
Appropriate specimens for culture of avian influenza include nasal and bronchial washes, nasopharyngeal aspirates, nasopharyngeal and throat swabs, tracheal aspirates, and bronchoalveolar lavage. Oropharyngeal swab specimens and lower respiratory tract specimens, such as bronchoalveolar lavage and tracheal aspirates, are preferred because they appear to contain more virus; nasal and nasopharyngeal swab specimens are less optimal because they may contain a lower viral count
　Meticulous collection, handling, and shipping of specimens is imperative to prevent false-negative results.
　Serial specimen collection over several days is optimal; specimens collected within the first 3 days of illness onset are more likely to detect the virus.

To obtain a nasopharyngeal aspirate/wash, instill 1 ml to 1.5 ml nonbacteriostatic saline (pH) into one nostril. Flush a plastic catheter or tubing with 2 ml to 3 ml of saline. Insert tubing into nostril parallel to the palate and aspirate nasopharyngeal secretions. Repeat procedure with second nostril.

To obtain a nasopharyngeal or oropharyngeal swab, insert a swab into the nostril parallel to the palate. Leave the swab in place for a few seconds to absorb secretions. Repeat with second nostril. All swabs used for specimen collection should have an aluminum or plastic shaft and a Dacron tip. Calcium alginate swabs, cotton-tipped swabs, or swabs with wooden shafts should not be used for specimen collection. Place specimen at 4°C immediately after collection.

To collect sputum, have patient rinse mouth with water then expectorate deep cough sputum directly into a sterile screw-cap sputum collection cup or sterile dry container. Use cold packs to keep sample at 4°C for domestic shipping. For international shipping pack in dry ice.

During bronchoalveolar lavage or tracheal aspirate, use a double-tube system to maximize shielding from oropharyngeal secretions; bronchoalveolar lavage is a high-risk, aerosol generating procedure. Centrifuge half of the specimen and fix the cell pellet in formalin. Place the remaining unspun fluid in sterile vials with external caps and internal O-rings. If no O-rings are available, seal tightly with available cap and secure with Parafilm®. Label each specimen with patient's ID and collection date. For domestic shipping use cold packs to keep sample at 4°C. For international shipping, ship fixed cells at room temperature and unfixed cells frozen.

LOINC CODES

- Code: 14455-0 (*Short Name* - Virus Plr Cult)
- Code: 14459-2 (*Short Name* - Virus Pen Cult)
- Code: 5885-9 (*Short Name* - Virus Skn Cult)
- Code: 14460-0 (*Short Name* - Virus Urth Cult)
- Code: 14458-4 (*Short Name* - Virus Spt Cult)
- Code: 5883-4 (*Short Name* - Virus Bld Cult)
- Code: 14454-3 (*Short Name* - Virus Nose Cult)
- Code: 14453-5 (*Short Name* - Virus GenV Cult)
- Code: 6584-7 (*Short Name* - Virus XXX Cult)
- Code: 6608-4 (*Short Name* - Virus Islt Cult)
- Code: 6583-9 (*Short Name* - Virus Smn Cult)
- Code: 5887-5 (*Short Name* - Virus Thrt Cult)
- Code: 5886-7 (*Short Name* - Virus Stl Cult)
- Code: 5884-2 (*Short Name* - Virus CSF Cult)
- Code: 11484-3 (*Short Name* - Virus Amn Cult)
- Code: 14456-8 (*Short Name* - Virus Prt Cult)

Viral culture, eye

TEST DEFINITION

Isolation of a virus from culture obtained by conjunctival swab or scrapings for the evaluation of ocular infections

REFERENCE RANGE

- No growth
  Please refer to your institution's reference ranges as lab normals may vary.

INDICATIONS

Suspected Herpes simplex keratitis
> **Strength of Recommendation:** Class IIa
> **Strength of Evidence:** Category B
> **Results Interpretation:**
> **Positive microbiology findings**
>> The isolation of HSV-1 in culture is diagnostic of Herpes simplex keratitis.

CLINICAL NOTES

Cultures should be obtained within the first week of illness, if possible, because viral yield decreases rapidly beginning 4 days after symptom onset.

COLLECTION/STORAGE INFORMATION
* Specimen Collection and Handling:
    * Place specimen in a viral transport media and transport, maintaining temperature at 4°C.
    * Set up culture within 36 hours of collection for best yield.
    * Freeze specimen at -70°C if no alternative exists.

Viral culture, urine

TEST DEFINITION
Detection of virus by culture of urine for the evaluation and management of viremic infection

REFERENCE RANGE
* Adults and Children: No growth
  Please refer to your institution's reference ranges as lab normals may vary.

INDICATIONS
Suspected adenovirus-associated hemorrhagic cystitis
     Strength of Recommendation: Class IIa
     Strength of Evidence: Category B
     Results Interpretation:
     Positive microbiology findings
         The detection of adenovirus (AdV) by urine viral culture is indicative of an AdV infection.
         It is more probable that transplant patients who develop hemorrhagic cystitis from AdV have reactivation of a latent infection versus a primary infection.

Suspected congenital cytomegalovirus (CMV) infection in newborn infants
     Strength of Recommendation: Class IIa
     Strength of Evidence: Category C
     Results Interpretation:
     Positive microbiology findings
         Detection of cytomegalovirus (CMV) in a patient's urine during the first 2 weeks of life confirms a diagnosis of congenital CMV infection.
         Either standard tissue cell culture or centrifuge-enhanced shell vial culture of urine may be performed to identify CMV; the shell vial method can yield results within 24 to 36 hours while the standard culture can take 2 to 4 weeks.
         Cytomegalovirus is the most common cause of congenital infection, but up to 90% of infants with it may be asymptomatic at birth. Infection with CMV should be suspected in small-for-gestational-age infants, infants with microcephaly, and infants with other signs of congenital infection, eg, prematurity, jaundice, hepatosplenomegaly, petechiae, lethargy.
         Congenital infection can occur either from maternal primary infection or from recurrence of a latent maternal infection. Up to 60% of congenital CMV infections occur as a result of maternal primary infection with transplacental viral transmission to the fetus.
         Congenitally-infected children may continue to shed CMV for many years. Children in daycare who are CMV-positive can easily infect other children and adult caregivers.
     Timing of Monitoring
         Testing to detect congenital cytomegalovirus should be done within the first 2 weeks of life in order to distinguish congenital infection from postnatally acquired infection.

Suspected cytomegalovirus (CMV) disease
     Strength of Recommendation: Class IIb
     Strength of Evidence: Category B
     Results Interpretation:
     Positive microbiology findings
         A positive urine viral culture may indicate an increased risk for developing cytomegalovirus (CMV) disease in immunocompromised patients.
         Urine standard cell culture takes several weeks, limiting its usefulness in making timely treatment decisions for CMV retinitis in AIDS patients. Better tests for treatment purposes include quantitative measurement of CMV DNA by means of plasma or leukocyte PCR.

Negative microbiology findings
Patients who are HIV-positive with consistently negative CMV tests are unlikely to develop CMV disease.
Timing of Monitoring
Culture techniques require the collection of viable virus; specimens should be collected during acute phase illness when active virus is being shed.

Suspected mumps infection
Strength of Recommendation: Class IIa
Strength of Evidence: Category B
Results Interpretation:
Positive microbiology findings
A positive urine shell vial culture can confirm a clinical diagnosis of mumps infection, but takes 2 to 3 days to complete.
Mumps virus present in urine reflects renal involvement, where the mumps virus may be present in urine for up to 2 weeks following initial symptoms.

CLINICAL NOTES

Culture techniques require the collection of viable virus; specimens should be collected during acute phase illness when active virus is being shed. The turnaround time for shell vial technique is shorter than for standard tissue cell technique, which may take up to 3 weeks. Shell vial culture technique uses centrifuge-amplification to promote viral replication; it can improve detection when virus levels are low so that viral antigen can be detected more quickly than by conventional culture.

Viral cultures can become contaminated with other viruses, eg cytomegalovirus standard cell cultures can be contaminated with adenovirus.

COLLECTION/STORAGE INFORMATION
* Specimen Collection and Handling:
  * Obtain appropriate viral transport medium from the laboratory.
  * Collect clean catch or catheterization specimen in a sterile container.
  * Add the specimen to the transport medium, place specimen on ice to maintain temperature at 4°C and transport it to the laboratory immediately.

LOINC CODES
* Code: 14457-6 (*Short Name* - Virus Ur Cult)

Vitamin B6 measurement

TEST DEFINITION
Measurement of pyridoxal-5'-phosphate (PLP), the primary form of vitamin B_6 in plasma, to assess vitamin B_6 status

SYNONYMS
* Pyridoxal phosphate measurement
* Pyridoxine measurement

REFERENCE RANGE
* Adults: 5-30 ng/mL (20-121 nmol/L)
* EGOT index: <1.5
  Please refer to your institution's reference ranges as lab normals may vary.

INDICATIONS
Suspected vitamin B_6 deficiency in chronic alcoholism
Strength of Recommendation: Class IIa
Strength of Evidence: Category B
Results Interpretation:
Vitamin B6 deficiency
A plasma pyridoxal-5'-phosphate (PLP) level less than 5 ng/mL indicates vitamin B_6 deficiency.

A low level of PLP in alcoholics is indicative of pyridoxine (vitamin B$_6$) deficiency. The cause may be ethanol metabolism in the liver, whereby acetaldehyde displaces PLP from albumin and the unbound vitamin is then excreted through the kidneys.

Suspected vitamin B$_6$ deficiency in diabetes mellitus
Strength of Recommendation: Class IIa
Strength of Evidence: Category C
Results Interpretation:
Vitamin B6 deficiency
A plasma pyridoxal-5'-phosphate (PLP) level less than 5 ng/mL indicates vitamin B$_6$ deficiency. Vitamin B$_6$ deficiency has been frequently reported in diabetics.

Low plasma levels of pyridoxine may be seen in diabetics, especially those on insulin therapy and those with poor control of blood glucose.

Suspected vitamin B$_6$ deficiency in patients with carpal tunnel syndrome
Strength of Recommendation: Class IIb
Strength of Evidence: Category C
Results Interpretation:
Vitamin B6 deficiency
Although the reason is unclear, some patients with carpal tunnel syndrome have experienced pain relief from treatment with vitamin B$_6$. Therefore, determining vitamin B$_6$ status may be helpful in patients with carpal tunnel syndrome before surgical treatment, suggesting that those patients without vitamin B$_6$ deficiency are less likely to benefit from pyridoxine treatment and may be better candidates for surgery.

ABNORMAL RESULTS
- Results increased in:
  - Increased dietary vitamin B$_6$ intake
- Results decreased in:
  - Increased dietary protein intake

COLLECTION/STORAGE INFORMATION
- Specimen Collection and Handling:
  - Collect a fasting blood sample.
  - Store plasma at -80°C for up to 10 days.
  - Protect the specimen from exposure to light.
  - Avoid repeated freezing and thawing of sample.

LOINC CODES
- Code: 26915-9 (*Short Name* - Vit B6 Bld Ql)

Vitamin D, 1,25-dihydroxy measurement

TEST DEFINITION
Measurement of 1,25 dihydroxyvitamin D in serum for the evaluation of calcium and phosphorus homeostasis

REFERENCE RANGE
25-45 pg/mL (60-108 pmol/L)
Pregnant women: Concentrations are 2-fold higher
Please refer to your institution's reference ranges as lab normals may vary.

INDICATIONS
Chronic renal failure
Strength of Recommendation: Class IIb
Strength of Evidence: Category B
Results Interpretation:
Lowered biochemistry findings
Lowered serum levels of vitamin D, 1,25-dihydroxy can be seen in patients with chronic renal failure and can correlate with the severity of the disease.

Suspected vitamin D deficiency
> **Strength of Recommendation:** Class IIb
> **Strength of Evidence:** Category B
> **Results Interpretation:**
> **Lowered biochemistry findings**
>> Decreased serum levels of 1,25-dihydroxyvitamin D can be seen in patients with rickets, osteomalacia, and osteoporosis.
>
> **Raised biochemistry findings**
>> Increased serum levels of 1,25-dihydroxyvitamin D in patients with vitamin D receptor abnormality can be due to hypocalcemia and secondary hyperparathyroidism.
>>
>> An increase in serum levels of 1,25-dihydroxyvitamin D can be seen in patients undergoing vitamin D therapy for treatment of osteomalacia.

COLLECTION/STORAGE INFORMATION
- Specimen Collection and Handling:
  - Collect specimen in red top tube.
  - Store specimen frozen.
  - Specimen is stable at room temperature for 72 hours or indefinitely at $-20°C$.

LOINC CODES
- Code: 1649-3 (*Short Name* - Vit D1,25 Ser-mCnc)
- Code: 14566-4 (*Short Name* - Vit D1,25 Ser-sCnc)

Vitamin D, 25-hydroxy measurement

TEST DEFINITION
Measurement of 25 hydroxyvitamin D in serum or plasma to evaluate suspected vitamin D deficiency or resistance secondary to nutritional or malabsorptive conditions

REFERENCE RANGE
- 25 hydroxyvitamin D (25OHD): 10-68 ng/mL (24.9-169.5 nmol/L)
- Concentrations >32 ng/mL (80 nmol/L) have been recommended for optimizing bone health
  Please refer to your institution's reference ranges as lab normals may vary.

INDICATIONS
Suspected primary nutritional osteomalacia in adults
> **Strength of Recommendation:** Class IIa
> **Strength of Evidence:** Category B
> **Results Interpretation:**
> **Lowered biochemistry findings**
>> Serum 25 hydroxyvitamin D levels less than 10 ng/mL are highly suggestive of osteomalacia.
>> Routine administration of vitamin D supplementation to high risk populations has been suggested.

Suspected rickets in children
> **Strength of Recommendation:** Class IIa
> **Strength of Evidence:** Category B
> **Results Interpretation:**
> **Lowered biochemistry findings**
>> A low 25 hydroxyvitamin D (25OHD) level, in conjunction with clinical and radiographic evidence, is consistent with a diagnosis of rickets.
>>
>> The National Academy of Sciences recommends a daily intake of at least 200 International Units of vitamin D to maintain a serum 25OHD at or above 27.5 nmol/L (11 ng/mL) in infants, children and adolescents.

Suspected vitamin D deficiency
> **Strength of Recommendation:** Class I
> **Strength of Evidence:** Category B

Results Interpretation:
Abnormal laboratory findings

Serum values less than 30 ng/mL indicate vitamin D deficiency, which is common in the elderly. More severe vitamin D deficiency causes osteomalacia. Low serum vitamin D values and weight loss may indicate otherwise asymptomatic celiac disease, a rare secondary cause of osteoporosis. Vitamin D deficiency sometimes leads to secondary hyperparathyroidism with normocalcemia. Hypocalcemia is less common, but can be seen in vitamin D deficiency.

Timing of Monitoring

Measure 25-hydroxyvitamin D when vitamin D deficiency is suspected secondary to low intake or inadequate exposure to sunlight.

CLINICAL NOTES

Significant variations in results have been observed depending upon assay method used and reporting laboratory. International standardization of 25OHD measurement has yet to be established.

Plasma levels decrease with age and pregnancy and vary with sun exposure. The winter season is a significant univariate predictor of hypovitaminosis D. Lower levels have been observed in obese individuals.

COLLECTION/STORAGE INFORMATION
- Specimen Collection and Handling:
  - Obtain venous specimen in heparinized tube.
  - Specimen is stable at room temperature up to 72 hours and indefinitely at -20°C.

LOINC CODES
- Code: 1989-3 (*Short Name* - Vit D25 SerPl-mCnc)
- Code: 35196-5 (*Short Name* - Vit D25 SerPl-msCnc)
- Code: 14635-7 (*Short Name* - Vit D25 SerPl-sCnc)

West Nile virus antibody assay

TEST DEFINITION

Detection of antibodies to West Nile virus in serum to aid in the diagnosis and management of West Nile encephalitis

REFERENCE RANGE
- Hemagglutination inhibition (HI) titer <1:10
  Please refer to your institution's reference ranges as lab normals may vary.

INDICATIONS
Known or suspected West Nile virus (WNV) encephalitis

Strength of Recommendation: Class IIa

Strength of Evidence: Category B

Results Interpretation:

Positive immunology findings

A single positive WNV-specific IgM antibody level with IgM antibody-capture enzyme-linked immunosorbent assay (MAC-ELISA) found in cerebrospinal fluid (CSF) is sufficient to confirm a WNV central nervous system infection as IgM does not cross the blood-brain barrier.

The presence of WNV-specific IgM identified by enzyme-linked immunoassay (EIA)/MAC-ELISA testing plus a WNV-positive IgG antibody in the same or a later specimen by another serologic assay (eg, neutralization or hemagglutination) is diagnostic for WNV disease.

A 4-fold or greater change in a plaque-reduction neutralizing test antibody titer in paired sera specimens is diagnostic for WNV disease.

Due to cross-reactivity and the lingering presence of IgG antibody, a positive IgG finding in serum is not diagnostic of past or present infection. Conversely, the presence of IgM antibody can be considered provisional evidence of infection. Patient age, clinical presentation, season, location of exposure, occurrence of similar cases in the same geographic area and other epidemiological factors must be considered when evaluating serologic results.

Because cross-reactivity of flaviviruses does not permit precise viral identification, a second serum assay is routinely performed to verify the causative virus.

Two-phase testing can also eliminate the possibility of cross-reactivity with St. Louis encephalitis viral antibodies (present in the sera of residents in many areas of the United States). Testing of 2 phases differentiates between a static, possibly cross-reactive titer from a rising titer indicative of current infection.

False Results
False-positive results can occur due to antibody cross-reactivity with other flaviviruses.

Timing of Monitoring
Serum or cerebrospinal fluid (CSF) specimens collected within 7 days of symptom onset (acute phase) in neuroinvasive WNV disease are usually positive. Convalescent serum specimens should be collected 14 to 21 days after illness onset.

Acute phase and convalescent phase testing of sera for WNV antibodies should be performed at least 2 weeks apart to reduce the likelihood of false negative results early in the course of the disease.

WNV IgM may persist for up to a year after infection; therefore, a positive IgM for WNV may not be related to the patient's current illness.

CLINICAL NOTES

For a presumptive diagnosis of recent acute infection by serological testing a 4-fold increase in IgG titer between the acute and the convalescent sera must occur, however definitive diagnosis requires virus isolation. In general, viral-specific IgM appears during the first week of primary infection with levels becoming undetectable within 6 to 8 weeks, although it can remain detectable for extended periods of time. IgM specificity and sensitivity can be improved by removing rheumatoid factor and IgG to reduce competition with IgM for viral antigen. Viral-specific IgG appears 1 to 2 weeks after primary infection and reaches peak levels at 4 to 8 weeks, but remains detectable indefinitely. During reinfection IgM may reappear ephemerally in low levels while IgG will increase rapidly and peak at higher levels than are seen in primary infection. Factors such as infection site and immune status can alter these findings and specific viruses may produce different patterns.

COLLECTION/STORAGE INFORMATION
- Transport immediately to lab
- Freeze specimen if not immediately processed

LOINC CODES
- Code: 29538-6 (*Short Name* - WNV IgM CSF-aCnc)
- Code: 29780-4 (*Short Name* - WNV IgM XXX Ql)
- Code: 33330-2 (*Short Name* - WNV IgM Titr CSF)
- Code: 29537-8 (*Short Name* - WNV IgG CSF-aCnc)
- Code: 29779-6 (*Short Name* - WNV Ab Titr XXX Nt)
- Code: 30178-8 (*Short Name* - WNV IgG XXX Ql EIA)
- Code: 29570-9 (*Short Name* - WNV Ab Titr CSF Nt)
- Code: 29568-3 (*Short Name* - WNV Ab Titr Ser Nt)
- Code: 29569-1 (*Short Name* - WNV IgM CSF Ql EIA)
- Code: 33328-6 (*Short Name* - WNV IgG Titr CSF)
- Code: 31703-2 (*Short Name* - WNV IgM CSF Ql)
- Code: 29778-8 (*Short Name* - WNV IgM XXX Ql EIA)
- Code: 31700-8 (*Short Name* - WNV Ab XXX-aCnc)
- Code: 31702-4 (*Short Name* - WNV IgG XXX Ql)
- Code: 29781-2 (*Short Name* - WNV Ab Titr XXX)
- Code: 29536-0 (*Short Name* - WNV IgM Ser-aCnc)
- Code: 29567-5 (*Short Name* - WNV IgM Ser Ql EIA)
- Code: 33468-0 (*Short Name* - WNV Ab XXX Ql)
- Code: 31704-0 (*Short Name* - WNV IgM Ser Ql)
- Code: 29566-7 (*Short Name* - WNV IgG Ser Ql EIA)
- Code: 33331-0 (*Short Name* - WNV IgM Titr Ser)
- Code: 29535-2 (*Short Name* - WNV IgG Ser-aCnc)
- Code: 31701-6 (*Short Name* - WNV IgG Ser Ql)
- Code: 33329-4 (*Short Name* - WNV IgG Titr Ser)

Western equine encephalitis virus antibody assay

TEST DEFINITION

Detection of antibodies to western equine encephalitis in serum to aid in the diagnosis and management of western equine encephalitis

SYNONYMS

- Serologic test for Western equine encephalitis virus

REFERENCE RANGE

- Complement fixation titer (CF) <1:8
- Hemagglutination inhibition (HI) titer <1:10
  Please refer to your institution's reference ranges as lab normals may vary.

INDICATIONS

Suspected or known Western equine encephalitis
> **Strength of Recommendation:** Class IIb
> **Strength of Evidence:** Category C
> **Results Interpretation:**
> **Positive immunology findings**
>> A single positive WEE-specific IgM antibody level with IgM antibody-capture enzyme-linked immunosorbent assay (MAC-ELISA) found in cerebrospinal fluid (CSF) is sufficient to confirm a WEE central nervous system infection.
>> The presence of WEE-specific IgM identified by enzyme-linked immunoassay (EIA)/MAC-ELISA testing plus a WEE-positive IgG antibody in the same or a later specimen by another serologic assay (eg, neutralization or hemagglutination) is diagnostic for WEE disease.
>> A 4-fold or greater change in a PRNT antibody titer in paired sera specimens is diagnostic for WEE disease.
>> Due to cross-reactivity and the lingering presence of IgG antibody, a positive IgG is not diagnostic of past or present infection. Conversely, the presence of IgM antibody can be considered provisional evidence of infection. Patient age, clinical presentation, season, location of exposure, occurrence of similar cases in the same geographic area and other epidemiologic factors must be considered when evaluating serologic results.
>> A specimen (collected within 45 days of symptom onset) that is positive for IgG but negative for IgM, may indicate a past infection.
> **Timing of Monitoring**
>> Serum specimens should be collected at disease onset and 2 to 4 weeks later for acute and convalescent specimen analysis.
>> IgG antibodies to arboviruses are increased by the 12th day following symptom onset and can persist for years after the acute infection.

CLINICAL NOTES

For a presumptive diagnosis of recent acute infection by serological testing a 4-fold increase in IgG titer between the acute and the convalescent sera must occur, however definitive diagnosis requires virus isolation. In general, viral-specific IgM appears during the first week of primary infection with levels becoming undetectable within 6 to 8 weeks although it can remain detectable for extended periods of time. Enzyme-linked immunoassay (EIA) can detect IgM 2 times longer than immunofluorescent assay. IgM specificity and sensitivity can be improved by removing rheumatoid factor and IgG to reduce competition with IgM for viral antigen. Viral-specific IgG appears 12 days after primary infection, reaches peak levels at 4 to 8 weeks, and remains detectable indefinitely. During reinfection IgM may reappear ephemerally in low levels while IgG will increase rapidly and peak at higher levels than are seen in primary infection. Factors such as infection site and immune status can alter these findings and specific viruses may produce different patterns.

COLLECTION/STORAGE INFORMATION

- Transport immediately to lab
- Freeze specimen if not immediately processed

LOINC CODES
- Code: 9314-6 (*Short Name* - WEEV Ab Titr CSF IF)
- Code: 20983-3 (*Short Name* - WEEV Ab Ser Ql IF)
- Code: 20985-8 (*Short Name* - WEEV Ab Ser Ql CF)
- Code: 31706-5 (*Short Name* - WEEV IgG CSF-aCnc)
- Code: 23583-8 (*Short Name* - WEEV Ab Ser Ql Aggl)
- Code: 9316-1 (*Short Name* - WEEV IgM Titr CSF IF)
- Code: 31705-7 (*Short Name* - WEEV Ab CSF-aCnc)
- Code: 9581-0 (*Short Name* - WEEV Ab Titr Ser IF)
- Code: 8053-1 (*Short Name* - WEEV IgM Ser-aCnc)
- Code: 23586-1 (*Short Name* - WEEV Ab Ser Ql HAI)
- Code: 5406-4 (*Short Name* - WEEV Ab Ser-aCnc)
- Code: 6957-5 (*Short Name* - WEEV IgG Titr Ser IF)
- Code: 22615-9 (*Short Name* - WEEV IgM Titr CSF)
- Code: 23584-6 (*Short Name* - WEEV Ab Titr Ser HAI)
- Code: 17769-1 (*Short Name* - WEEV Ab Titr CSF)
- Code: 6958-3 (*Short Name* - WEEV IgM Titr Ser IF)
- Code: 22610-0 (*Short Name* - WEEV Ab CSF Ql)
- Code: 23585-3 (*Short Name* - WEEV Ab Ser Ql Nt)
- Code: 23588-7 (*Short Name* - WEEV IgM Ser Ql EIA)
- Code: 8052-3 (*Short Name* - WEEV IgG Ser-aCnc)
- Code: 20982-5 (*Short Name* - WEEV Ab Titr Ser Nt)
- Code: 22616-7 (*Short Name* - WEEV IgM Titr Ser)
- Code: 20984-1 (*Short Name* - WEEV Ab CSF Ql IF)
- Code: 23587-9 (*Short Name* - WEEV IgM Ser Ql)
- Code: 20986-6 (*Short Name* - WEEV Ab CSF Ql CF)
- Code: 9315-3 (*Short Name* - WEEV IgG Titr CSF IF)
- Code: 17770-9 (*Short Name* - WEEV Ab Titr Ser)

White blood cell count

TEST DEFINITION
Measurement of circulating leukocytes (white blood cells) in whole blood for the evaluation and management of primary leukocyte disorders and secondary inflammatory or leukocyte suppression responses to physical agents, toxins or disease

SYNONYMS
- WBC count
- WBC - White blood cell count
- WCC - White blood cell count
- White blood cell count - observation

REFERENCE RANGE
- Adults: $4.5\text{-}11 \times 10^3$ cells/mm^3 ($4.5\text{-}11 \times 10^9$ cells/L)
- Blacks: $3.6\text{-}10.2 \times 10^3$ cells/microL ($3.6\text{-}10.2 \times 10^9$ cells/L)
- Infants, 6 months to 2 years: $6\text{-}17.5 \times 10^3$ cells/microL ($6\text{-}17.5 \times 10^9$ cells/L)
- Children, 4-6 years: $5\text{-}15.5 \times 10^3$ cells/microL ($5\text{-}15.5 \times 10^9$ cells/L)
- Children, 8-16 years: $4.5\text{-}13.5 \times 10^3$ cells/microL ($4.5\text{-}13.5 \times 10^9$ cells/L)
  Please refer to your institution's reference ranges as lab normals may vary.

INDICATIONS
Atherosclerotic coronary heart disease
    Strength of Recommendation: Class IIa
    Strength of Evidence: Category B
  Results Interpretation:
  Leukocytosis
    In multiple clinical and epidemiological studies, elevated WBC counts correlate with increased risk of ischemic adverse events and cardiovascular mortality.

Diabetes mellitus
> **Strength of Recommendation:** Class IIb
> **Strength of Evidence:** Category B
> **Results Interpretation:**
> **White blood cell finding**
>> Elevated WBC counts were directly proportional to the risk of developing diabetes mellitus, according to a multivariate adjusted analysis in a longitudinal cohort study. Conversely, the analysis did not show a significant correlation between diabetes incidence and ESR.

Febrile seizure
> **Results Interpretation:**
> **White blood cell number - finding**
>> The peripheral blood leukocyte count was only modestly useful for predicting serious bacterial infections following a febrile seizure in a single prospective study done before the release of the heptavalent pneumococccal vaccine. With rates of pneumococcal disease continuing to fall, the expectation is that this test will continue to have even lower utility.
>> The value of this test does not appear to be affected by the stress imposed by the length of the seizure.

Hantavirus pulmonary syndrome
> **Results Interpretation:**
> **Leukocytosis**
>> The WBC count is typically greater than 12,000/mm^3, with a median peak cell count of 26,000/mm^3 during hospitalization.
>> The combination of a maximally increased WBC count and partial thromboplastin time (PTT) are predictive of death.
> **Leukopenia**
>> Some patients with hantavirus pulmonary syndrome may present with leukopenia (WBC less than 4,000/mm^3).

Hemolytic uremic syndrome (HUS)
> **Results Interpretation:**
> **Raised hematology findings**
>> In hemolytic uremic syndrome (HUS), leukocytosis is usually present, with a mild to moderate left shift and a number of immature cells. The mean WBC count is approximately 17,000/mm^3 and may be as high as 48,500/mm^3.
>> It is uncertain whether the inflammatory response represents a marker of severity of the *Escherichia coli* O157:H7 gastrointestinal infection or whether it is a pathophysiologic marker that leads to hemolytic uremic syndrome (HUS).
>> An elevated polymorphonuclear leukocyte count (particularly greater than 15,000/mm^3) on admission is predictive of severe disease and poor prognosis in patients with HUS.

Hospitalized patients with community-acquired pneumonia or children with suspected pneumonia
> **Results Interpretation:**
> **Leukocytosis**
>> For bacterial pneumonia, a WBC count of 10,000 to 14,000/mm^3 with a marked left shift is typical. A WBC count greater than 15,000/mm^3 strongly suggests a bacterial, particularly a pneumococcal, etiology. A WBC count greater than 20,000/mm^3 is associated with a poor prognosis.
>> In atypical pneumonias, the WBC count usually is only minimally elevated, although in severe cases, counts of 20,000 to 30,000/mm^3 may be present.
>> In Legionnaires disease, a moderately high leukocytosis with a left shift is present in 50% to 80% of patients. This feature may help differentiate Legionella from other causes of atypical pneumonia.
>> In influenza, the WBC count may be moderately high with lymphocytosis, especially early in the course.
>> A WBC count of 20,000/mm^3 or greater in febrile children may indicate an occult pneumonia.
> **White cell count normal**
>> A lack of systemic inflammatory response (ie, absence of fever and leukocytosis) is associated with significantly increased mortality in elderly patients with pneumonia.
> **Leukopenia**
>> Immunosuppressed or elderly patients with overwhelming infection may present with leukopenia and a left shift.
>> Leukopenia, presumably due to overwhelming infection, has been associated with a poor prognosis in patients with pneumococcal pneumonia and Legionnaires disease.

In male patients with bacteremic community-acquired lobar pneumonia, the presence of leukopenia is more suggestive of Klebsiella than of pneumococcal pneumonia.

Leukopenia occasionally can be seen in viral infections. Early in the course of severe acute respiratory syndrome (SARS), the absolute lymphocyte count is often decreased. Overall WBC counts have generally been normal or decreased. At the peak of the respiratory illness, approximately 50% to 70% of patients have a moderate leukopenia.

Initial evaluation of suspected diabetic ketoacidosis
Strength of Recommendation: Class I
Strength of Evidence: Category C
Results Interpretation:
Leukocytosis
An elevated WBC count in diabetic ketoacidosis (DKA) may be due to stress and dehydration, and should not be interpreted as a sign of infection. The majority of patients with DKA present with leukocytosis proportional to the blood ketone body concentration.

The majority of patients in suspected DKA present with WBC counts in the 10,000/mm³ to 15,000/mm³ range without a left shift. A count greater than 25,000/mm³ with a left shift suggests bacterial infection.

Initial evaluation of suspected hyperglycemic hyperosmolar state
Strength of Recommendation: Class I
Strength of Evidence: Category C
Results Interpretation:
Leukocytosis
The majority of patients with hyperglycemic hyperosmolar state (HHS) present with leukocytosis proportional to the blood ketone body concentration.

The majority of patients present with WBC counts in the 10,000 to 15,000/mm³ range without a left shift; counts greater than 25,000/mm³ with a left shift suggest bacterial infection.

Known or suspected hematological malignancies
Strength of Recommendation: Class IIa
Strength of Evidence: Category C
Results Interpretation:
Leukocytosis
Patients with primary bone marrow disorders (eg, leukemia or myeloproliferative disorders) often present with extreme leukocytosis.

In acute myelogenous leukemia (AML), WBC counts are usually above 15,000/microL and may be as high as 1 million cells/mm³ ; rarely, neutropenia is observed. Fewer than 15% of patients have WBC counts less than 100,000 cells/microL. These findings are usually associated with anemia and thrombocytopenia.

In chronic myelogenous leukemia (CML), a WBC count between 30,000 and 400,000/microL is frequently seen, associated with thrombocytosis, mild-to-moderate anemia, and splenomegaly. Hyperleukocytosis at the time of diagnosis is most frequently seen in patients with CML.

In patients with myelogenous or lymphocytic leukemia, signs of pulmonary infiltration (dyspnea, tachypnea, and hypoxia) may be associated with high blast cell counts (WBC counts above 100,000 cells/microL).

Hyperleukocytosis may cause complications arising from leukostasis in cerebral or pulmonary capillary beds. Headache, priapism, blurred vision, and other neurologic symptoms have also been associated with a high blast cell count.

In chronic lymphocytic leukemia (CLL), WBC counts are usually above 20,000 cells/microL.

Metabolic acidosis
Results Interpretation:
Increased white blood cell count
The WBC count is frequently elevated and is probably a nonspecific effect of acidosis. This response may be caused by catecholamine-induced WBC margination.

A marked leukocytosis (WBC count 24,000 to 65,000/mm³) may be seen in cases of significant paraldehyde intoxication.

When leukemia or lymphoma are predisposing factors for lactic acid production, a high WBC count may be seen.

Schizophrenia
Results Interpretation:
Leukopenia
Hematological effects, including inhibition of leukopoiesis, can occur with the use of clozapine or first-generation antipsychotic medications. During clozapine treatment, WBC counts should remain above 3000/mm^3 and absolute neutrophil counts (ANC) should remain above 1500/mm ^{3}.

If the WBC drops below 2,000/mm^3 or the ANC drops to 1000/mm^3, the medication must be stopped immediately and the patient monitored for infection, with daily checks of blood cell counts.

If the WBC drops to 2,000 to 3,000/mm^3 or the ANC drops to 1,000 to 1,500/mm^3, the medication should be stopped immediately and the patient monitored for infection, with daily checks of blood cell counts. Clozapine may be resumed when the patient's WBC is greater than 3,000 or the ANC is greater than 1,500 and there are no signs of infection. Counts should be done biweekly until the WBC is greater than 3,500.

If the WBC is between 3,000 and 3,500/mm^3 or if the WBC has dropped 3,000/mm^3 over 1 to 3 weeks, or if immature cell forms are present, the count should be repeated. If the WBC remains between 3,000 and 3,500/mm^3 and the ANC is greater than 1,500/mm^3, the counts should be monitored, with a differential, bi-weekly until the WBC is greater than 3,500/mm^3. If the counts drop below 3,000/mm^3, or the ANC is below 1,500/mm^3, the guidelines listed above should be followed.

Frequency of Monitoring
In patients treated with clozapine, a WBC count and neutrophil monitoring are required weekly. After a 6-month time period, monitoring may take place every 2 weeks, including during the 4 weeks after medication is stopped.

Timing of Monitoring
For patients treated with clozapine, the risk for hematological effects is highest in the first 6 months for patients treated with clozapine.

Suspected abruptio placentae
Results Interpretation:
White cell count normal
The WBC count is usually normal but may be slightly increased in patients with abruptio placentae.

Leukocytosis
With marked elevation of the WBC count, other causes of abdominal pain (eg, appendicitis) should be considered.

In pregnant trauma patients, an elevated WBC count on admission (greater than 20,000/mm^3) is an indicator of ongoing placental abruption and requires close monitoring.

Suspected acute coronary syndrome
Strength of Recommendation: Class I
Strength of Evidence: Category C
Results Interpretation:
Leukocytosis
Leukocytosis on admission in patients with acute coronary syndrome represents an increased risk of complications and mortality. Leukocytosis (WBC count 12,000 to 15,000/mm^3) is common during the first few hours of acute myocardial infarction; greater increases are often noted when large areas of necrosis are present or when complications occur.

Timing of Monitoring
Leukocyte count is obtained in all patients presenting with acute coronary syndrome, but should not delay implementation of reperfusion therapy in patients with ST-segment elevation myocardial infarction.

Suspected acute mesenteric ischemia
Results Interpretation:
White blood cell number - finding
Leukocytosis (WBC count greater than or equal than 15,000/mm^3) is common in the acute setting of bowel ischemia, but neither its presence nor the degree of WBC elevation is helpful in diagnosis. WBC count is normal in about 15% of cases.

Suspected adrenal insufficiency
Results Interpretation:
Leukocytosis
The total WBC count is usually greater than 10,000/mm^3 in adrenal crisis; however, it also may be normal.

Leukopenia
In chronic adrenal insufficiency, the total WBC count may be less than 5,000/mm^3.

Lymphocytosis
A relative lymphocytosis is common in chronic adrenal insufficiency. Cortisol is necessary for the maintenance of the reticuloendothelial system and normal lymphoid tissue. In the absence of cortisol, lymphocytic infiltration of body tissues has been noted.

This finding may also be seen in adrenal crisis, but a nonspecific leukocytosis is more common.

Suspected and known avian influenza
Results Interpretation:
Leukopenia
Leukopenia is a common finding in avian influenza. In one series, the median total leukocyte count was 2,109 (range 1,200 to 3,400)/mm^3, with a marked inversion of the CD4:CD8 ratio noted in some patients.

A decreased leukocyte count is associated with the development of acute respiratory distress syndrome (ARDS) and an increased risk of death.

Lymphocytopenia
Lymphopenia is a common finding in avian influenza. In one series, the median total lymphocyte count was 700 (range 250 to 1,100)/mm^3.

Lymphopenia is associated with the development of ARDS and an increased risk of death.

Suspected and known blunt abdominal trauma
Results Interpretation:
Leukocytosis
Elevations of the WBC count to 20,000/mm^3 with a moderate left shift occur frequently within several hours of injury and persist for several days. The elevation is the result of stress-caused demargination, tissue injury, acute hemorrhage, and peritoneal irritation.

Suspected and known Kawasaki disease
Results Interpretation:
Leukocytosis
The peripheral WBC count is often greater than 15,000/mm^3 with a left shift in acute Kawasaki disease.

A high toxic neutrophil (peripheral neutrophils with vacuoles and/or toxic granulations) count has been associated with Kawasaki disease.

Increases in WBC and neutrophil counts after intravenous immunoglobulin (IVIG) therapy have been associated with coronary artery aneurysms and may suggest the need for more aggressive treatment.

Timing of Monitoring
Leukocytosis presents in the acute febrile phase, and may persist for 1 to 3 weeks.

Suspected and known mastoiditis
Results Interpretation:
Leukocytosis
The WBC count is greater than 15,000 mm^3 in the majority of patients with mastoiditis.

Suspected and known septic bursitis
Results Interpretation:
Leukocytosis
Leukocytosis is not diagnostic of septic bursitis since it is present in only 30% to 40% of the patients with septic bursitis and may occur in other inflammatory process such as gout.

WBC counts have been found to range from 3,700 to 24,400/mm^3 (mean 11,000 to 12,000/mm^3) in septic bursitis with increases in the band forms more frequent among immunocompromised patients.

Serial peripheral WBC counts, if initially elevated, may be a useful laboratory measurement to substantiate clinical improvement with treatment, although more specific indices of treatment effectiveness are conversion of the bursal fluid cultures from positive to negative and reduction in bursal fluid leukocyte concentration.

Suspected appendicitis
Results Interpretation:
White cell count normal
Although leukocytosis is more common in patients with appendicitis than those without appendicitis, the WBC count may be normal early in the course in nearly 25% of patients with appendicitis.

Acute appendicitis is unlikely in the setting of a normal leukocyte count and C-reactive protein; however, the WBC count should never be used alone to diagnose appendicitis and determine patient disposition, although serial levels may be helpful in equivocal cases.

White blood cell finding

Although the presence of leukocytosis may suggest the diagnosis of appendicitis, racial differences, early normal values, and the inability to differentiate appendicitis from other causes of abdominal pain limits its usefulness as a reliable diagnostic marker.

Blacks tend to have a significantly lower WBC count in acute appendicitis than do whites.

Leukocytosis

The WBC count may be elevated in patients with a normal appendix.

Leukocytosis is noted in 70% to 90% of cases; it is usually mild to moderate (10,000 to 18,000 mm^3), with polymorphonuclear predominance. A marked elevation greater than 18,000 to 20,000/mm^3 suggests rupture, phlegmon, or abscess.

In children, the WBC count with differential is the single most useful laboratory test but is helpful only in supporting the clinical diagnosis; both the total count and percentage of neutrophils are significantly higher in appendicitis.

Appendicitis should be suspected in pregnant patients with abdominal pain and a WBC count greater than 12.5 X 10^9 /L, especially if associated with nausea and abdominal guarding.

In patients older than 60 years, an elevated WBC count or abnormal differential is the most valuable laboratory test. In 1 study, 80% of patients had WBC counts greater than 10,000/mm^3 ; 12% had only a left shift (greater than 10 bands) noted.

The neutrophil to lymphocyte ratio may be a more sensitive indicator of appendicitis than the total WBC count. In 1 study, 88% of patients with appendicitis had a ratio greater than 3.5; however, a normal value for the ratio does not exclude the diagnosis.

Suspected bacterial infection
Results Interpretation:
Leukocytosis

Leukocytosis (WBC count greater than 12,000 cells/mm^3), and in particular neutrophilia, is a characteristic sign of systemic inflammation in response to infection.

In the context of meningitis, the majority of patients have a WBC count greater than 10,000/mm^3 ; however, the peripheral WBC count is not a useful screening test for ruling out meningeal infection, nor should it be used for the purpose of identifying infants in need of diagnostic lumbar puncture.

When combined with 3 other clinical markers (urinary analysis, age, and temperature), elevated WBC count was found to be predictive of serious bacterial infection in infants less than 3 months of age.

Leukopenia

Leukopenia (WBC count less than 4,000/mm^3) is a possible sign of systemic inflammation in response to infection. It may be seen in immunosuppressed or debilitated patients, as well as in patients with overwhelming sepsis.

Suspected bowel obstruction
Results Interpretation:
Leukocytosis

The WBC count is inconsistently elevated with a bowel obstruction. However, it may signify bowel perforation or strangulation.

Normal hematology findings

The absence of leukocytosis does not rule out bowel obstruction or strangulation.

Suspected cholecystitis
Results Interpretation:
Increased level (laboratory finding)

The WBC count is elevated in 85% of patients with acute cholecystitis. Like fever, it is not a reliable indicator in the elderly or immunocompromised patient.

In cholecystitis, the WBC count may be increased to 12,000 to 15,000/mm^3, with a left shift toward neutrophils and band forms. Retrospective chart reviews of pathologically confirmed acute cholecystitis found WBC counts less than 11,000 mm^3 in 25% to 40% of cases.

Suspected choledocholithiasis
Results Interpretation:
Leukocytosis

Combined elevations of the WBC count, alkaline phosphatase, and total bilirubin suggest choledocholithiasis and herald acute toxic cholangitis.

Suspected disseminated gonococcal infection (DGI or gonococcemia)
    Results Interpretation:
    White cell count abnormal
        The WBC may be increased to 12,000/mm^3 with gonococcal arthritis and may reach as high as 17,500/mm^3 during the bacteremic phase of disseminated gonococcal infection.

Suspected diverticulitis
    Results Interpretation:
    Leukocytosis
        Leukocytosis is present in over 80% of patients with acute colonic diverticulitis.
    White cell count normal
        The WBC count may be normal in half to two thirds of patients with acute complications from diverticulitis at surgery. The absence of leukocytosis does not rule out the diagnosis of diverticulitis.

Suspected epididymitis
    Results Interpretation:
    Leukocytosis
        A WBC count greater than 10,000/mm^3 was present in 4 of 8 men over the age of 30 with testicular torsion, 3 of whom were initially diagnosed as having epididymitis. In 25 patients with epididymitis under 18 years of age, only 44% had WBC counts greater than 10,000/mm^3.

Suspected epiglottitis after the airway is secured
    Results Interpretation:
    White cell count abnormal
        Although the white blood cell (WBC) count may be decreased, normal, or increased, most patients will have a WBC count greater than 10,000/mm^3.
        Elevated WBC and tachycardia correlate significantly with airway compromise in adults.
        Leukocytosis with a left shift in the differential may be seen.

Suspected erysipelas
    Results Interpretation:
    Leukocytosis
        Nearly all of these patients have leukocytosis and an elevated erythrocyte sedimentation rate or C-reactive protein, but these findings are nonspecific.
        Leukocytosis, that is, a WBC of 10,000 to 20,000/mm^3, is characteristic, but nonspecific for the diagnosis.

Suspected esophageal perforation
    Results Interpretation:
    Increased level (laboratory finding)
        The WBC count is usually elevated (as reported in 15% to 60% of patients with esophageal perforation); the differential count usually demonstrates a shift to the left
        The WBC count typically doubles within 2 to 6 hours of the injury, making it a reliable early indicator of injury.

Suspected gout
    Results Interpretation:
    Increased
        The serum WBC count is elevated in acute gout, but levels are typically not as high as levels seen in septic arthritis.
        Mild leukocytosis occurs in acute gout attacks, but the WBC count may be as high as 25,000/mm^3.

Suspected hyperventilation
    Results Interpretation:
    Normal laboratory findings
        The WBC is usually normal in patients with hyperventilation syndrome (HVS).
    Increased level (laboratory finding)
        When WBC is elevated, causes other than hyperventilation syndrome (HVS) should be sought, including pneumonia, myocardial infarction, or pulmonary infarction. A patient with HVS may be in a hyperadrenergic state which may elevate the WBC count secondary to demargination.

Suspected hypothermia
Results Interpretation:
Leukopenia
Decreased white blood cells may occur from splenic, hepatic, or splanchnic sequestration.

Leukopenia does not imply an absence of infection. It is a common finding in patients who are at either age extreme, intoxicated, myxedematous, debilitated, or who have secondary hypothermia.

Hypothermia produces an acquired neutrophil dysfunction.
Leukocytosis
An increased white blood cell count is common in neonatal hypothermia and also may occur with associated leukemia, infections, or water depletion.

Suspected infective endocarditis
Results Interpretation:
Leukocytosis
In infective endocarditis, a WBC count of 10,000 to 20,000/mm³ may be present, but it is commonly normal or may even be low. A leukocyte count of greater than 10,000 mm³ is present in about 50% of patients, and occurs more commonly when embolic complications of acute infective endocarditis are present, or when infections are due to organisms other than *S viridans*.
Leukopenia
Leukopenia is uncommon (5% to 15%) and, when present, usually is associated with splenomegaly.

Suspected inhalation anthrax
Results Interpretation:
White blood cell finding
On initial presentation, the total WBC count may be normal or slightly elevated; however, elevation in the percentage of neutrophils with prominent band forms is frequently noted.

Suspected Ludwig's angina
Results Interpretation:
Leukocytosis
Leukocytosis greater than 10,000/mm³ is present in about 85% of patients.

Suspected mumps
Results Interpretation:
Increased level (laboratory finding)
A polymorphonuclear leukocytosis (WBC count of 15,000 to 20,000/mm³) is common with extraparotid manifestations of mumps, particularly meningitis, orchitis, or pancreatitis.

Suspected necrotizing soft tissue infection
Results Interpretation:
Abnormal laboratory findings
In one series of necrotizing soft tissue infections the WBC count was elevated in all patients except those with synergistic gangrene, with an average of 17,303/mm³. An admission WBC count greater than 15,400/mm³ combined with a serum Na less than 135 mmol/L may help distinguish necrotizing fasciitis from non-necrotizing fasciitis, particularly when classic 'hard' signs of necrotizing fasciitis such as hypotension, crepitation, skin necrosis, bullae, or gas on x-ray are absent. A WBC count greater than 30,000/mm³ upon admission is an objective predictor of increased mortality in patients diagnosed with necrotizing fasciitis.

The peripheral WBC count may be depressed in overwhelming wound infections, especially in patients diagnosed with clostridial myonecrosis.

A WBC count less than 4000/mm³ with greater than 10% bands is predictive of an ominous course.

The WBC count should be taken in context with the clinical index of suspicion. An elevated WBC count is consistent with the diagnosis of necrotizing soft tissue infection, whereas a lower WBC count suggests a lower likelihood of the disease.

Suspected neonatal sepsis
Strength of Recommendation: Class IIa
Strength of Evidence: Category B
Results Interpretation:
Abnormal hematology findings
White blood cell counts greater than 21,000 cells/mm³ or less than 5,000 cells/mm³ may be an effective means of detecting sepsis in neonates less than 30 days old. The ability to predict sepsis may be enhanced by combining the WBC count with other CBC-associated measures of inflammation.

Suspected neuroleptic malignant syndrome
Results Interpretation:
Laboratory findings present

A WBC count of 12,000 to 30,000/mm^3 with or without a left shift is characteristic of neuroleptic malignant syndrome (NMS), although it is a nonspecific finding. WBC count does not help to differentiate NMS from NMS-like acute medical illnesses, in particular sepsis.

Suspected or known aspiration pneumonitis
Results Interpretation:
Leukocytosis

Although there is usually an elevation in the WBC count, this is not a helpful finding in the initial diagnosis. Leukocytosis (WBC count greater than 10,000/mm^3) 2 to 3 days after an apparent recovery from aspiration indicates a probable secondary bacterial infection.

Suspected or known myocardial infarction
Results Interpretation:
Leukocytosis

WBCs may be elevated secondary to stress and increased catecholamine production in shock.

Leukocytosis (WBC 12,000 to 15,000/mm^3) during the first few hours of myocardial infarction is common. Greater increases often will be noted when large areas of cardiac necrosis are present or when complications occur.

Leukocytosis may be a response to tissue necrosis, increased secretion of adrenal glucocorticoids, or both.

Suspected or known respiratory failure
Results Interpretation:
Leukocytosis

An increased WBC count may signal infection as the precipitating factor, or it may represent an acute stress reaction from any cause.

Neutropenia

A decreased WBC count, especially neutropenia (WBC count less than 3,000/mm^3), may indicate overwhelming infection, especially in the elderly.

Left shifted white blood cells

A left shift with increased band forms, toxic granulations, or Dohle bodies makes the diagnosis of a coexistent infection more likely.

Suspected or known status epilepticus
Results Interpretation:
Increased level (laboratory finding)

The usual range of the WBC count in status epilepticus is 12,000-28,000/mm^3, even without evidence of infection.

A high WBC count with elevated bands may indicate an underlying infection; however, an elevated WBC level without an increase in band forms is a response to physiologic stress and is often seen in patients with status epilepticus.

Suspected pancreatitis
Results Interpretation:
Leukocytosis

The WBC count is often elevated (10,000 to 30,000/mm^3). Marked leukocytosis or persistent elevation after therapy should alert the clinician to a possible abscess.

Suspected pelvic inflammatory disease
Results Interpretation:
Leukocytosis

Fewer than 50% of patients with pelvic inflammatory disease (PID) have a WBC count greater than 12,000/mm^3 ; however, most will exhibit a left shift (increased ratio of band to segmented forms). In some cases, the WBC count may be increased up to 20,000/mm^3.

Gonococcal PID is associated with a higher WBC count than is chlamydial PID.

Suspected peritonsillar abscess
Results Interpretation:
White blood cell finding
The WBC count will be elevated with a shift to the left in approximately 80% of patients with a peritonsillar abscess, but it may not be helpful in distinguishing peritonsillar abscess from cellulitis.

Suspected post-streptococcal glomerulonephritis
Strength of Recommendation: Class I
Strength of Evidence: Category C
Results Interpretation:
Increased level (laboratory finding)
The WBC count is mildly elevated, with a polymorphonuclear neutrophil shift to the left, in those patients who present during or soon after a streptococcal infection.

Suspected pulmonary embolism
Results Interpretation:
Raised hematology findings
The WBC count may range from normal to 15,000 to 20,000/mm^3 in pulmonary embolism, with higher values possibly suggesting infarction.

Suspected septic arthritis
Strength of Recommendation: Class IIb
Strength of Evidence: Category C
Results Interpretation:
Leukocytosis
Although the WBC count is elevated in up to 90% of patients with septic arthritis, this finding is an unreliable marker of septic arthritis.

A WBC count greater than 11,000 cells/mm^3 has a poor sensitivity in predicting septic arthritis. The WBC count is extremely variable in adults with bacterial arthritis. Laboratory tests do not rule out septic arthritis with any degree of accuracy.

Gonococcal arthritis is more likely to be accompanied by a normal WBC count than is septic arthritis caused by other organisms.

Retrospective and prospective studies have found that an elevated WBC count should not be used to differentiate between septic arthritis of the hip and other more benign causes of hip pain in children.

Suspected Stevens-Johnson syndrome
Results Interpretation:
Leukopenia
A WBC count less than 9,000/mm^3 is a common finding in Stevens-Johnson syndrome, noted within 72 hours of the appearance of skin lesions. The presence of leukopenia significantly increases the risk of sepsis.
Leukocytosis
Leukocytosis is present in about 25% of patients with Stevens-Johnson syndrome.

Suspected subarachnoid hemorrhage
Results Interpretation:
Leukocytosis
An admission WBC count greater than 20,000/mm^3 in spontaneous subarachnoid hemorrhage correlates with a poor clinical grade and poor prognosis (50% morbidity).

A WBC count greater than 15,000/mm^3 is significantly associated with increased risk of cerebral vasospasm following spontaneous subarachnoid hemorrhage.

Suspected testicular torsion
Results Interpretation:
Normal
A normal WBC count is suggestive of testicular torsion, but not diagnostic.
Leukocytosis
Leukocytosis does not exclude the diagnosis of acute testicular torsion because 33% to 67% of patients with testicular torsion have an elevated WBC count.

Suspected torsion of the ovary, ovarian pedicle, or fallopian tube
Strength of Recommendation: Class I
Strength of Evidence: Category C

Results Interpretation:
Leukocytosis
Generally the white blood cell (WBC) count is normal or only mildly elevated to greater than 15,000/mm^3 in about 20% of cases. A shift to the left may also be noted.

Suspected toxic epidermal necrolysis
Results Interpretation:
Leukopenia
A WBC count less than 9,000/mm^3 is a common finding, noted within 72 hours of the appearance of skin lesions, most typically being a lymphopenia. The presence of leukopenia significantly increases the risk of sepsis.
In one study, a lower nadir in the WBC count in patients with toxic epidermal necrolysis was significantly associated with a fatal outcome.
Leukocytosis
Leukocytosis is present in approximately 25% of patients with toxic epidermal necrolysis.

Suspected toxic shock syndrome
Results Interpretation:
Leukocytosis
Varying degrees of leukocytosis are present in toxic shock syndrome.
Leukopenia
Leukopenia may be present in streptococcal toxic shock syndrome.
Left shifted white blood cells
A left shift to immature forms of neutrophils is common in toxic shock syndrome.

Suspected tularemia
Results Interpretation:
Leukocytosis
The WBC count may be elevated to 24,000/mm^3 (mean 11,000/mm^3), regardless of clinical syndrome.
Normal hematology findings
The WBC count is normal in uncomplicated cases and is often normal in toxic-appearing patients despite a high fever.

COMMON PANELS
- Complete blood count

ABNORMAL RESULTS
- Results increased in:
    - Anesthesia
    - Cold exposure
    - Convulsive seizures
    - Electric shock
    - Emotional disturbance
    - Exercise
    - Menstruation
    - Nausea and vomiting
    - Obstetrical labor
    - Paroxysmal tachycardia
    - Ultraviolet irradiation exposure
- Results decreased in:
    - Persons of black African descent

COLLECTION/STORAGE INFORMATION
- Specimen Collection and Handling:
    - Collect specimen in lavender-top (EDTA) or red-top tube
    - May be stored for 24 hours at 23°C and for 48 hours at 4°C
    - Avoid use of heparin

LOINC CODES
- Code: 6690-2 (*Short Name* - WBC # Bld Auto)
- Code: 20584-9 (*Short Name* - WBC # XXX Auto)

White blood cell cytochemistry

Test Definition
Identification of cell markers for diagnosis and classification of hematologic malignancies.

Synonyms
• Leukocyte cytochemistry

Reference Range
Since the test(s) are used to identify cell markers rather than measure quantities, normal ranges do not exist. **Please refer to your institution's reference ranges as lab normals may vary.**

Indications
Acute leukemia
Results Interpretation:
White blood cell finding
• Cytochemical Characteristics of Acute Leukemias

ACUTE LEUKEMIA TYPE	M1	M2	M3	M4
Cytochemical Marker	.	.	.	.
Peroxidase	1-3+	3+	4+	1-3+
Sudan black B	1-3+	3+	4+	1-3+
Chloroacetate esterase	0-2+	1-3+	1-3+	1-3+
Naphthyl butyrate esterase	0	0	0-2+	1-2+ dfs
Acid phosphatase	1-2+ dfs	1-2+ dfs	3+ dfs	1-3+ dfs
Iron stain	0	0	0	0
dfs = diffuse cytoplasmic staining f = focal staining in Golgi area				
Immunochemical Marker	.	.	.	.
Myeloid (CD13, CD33)	+	+	+	+
Monocyte (CD14, CD68)	0	0	0	+
Megakaryocytic (CD41)	0	0	0	0
Red cell antigen (RC 82.4)	0	0	0	0
Lymphoid markers (TdT)	0	0	0	0

ACUTE LEUKEMIA TYPE	M5	M6	M7	T-cell ALL	Non-T cell ALL
Cytochemical Marker	.	.	.	.	.
Peroxidase	0-1+	1-3+	0	0	0
Sudan black B	0-2+	1-3+	0	0	0
Chloroacetate esterase	0	1-3+	0	0	0
Naphthyl butyrate esterase	2-4+ dfs	0-1+ dfs	0-1+ dfs	0-1+ f	0
Acid phosphatase	1-3+ dfs	1-3+ dfs/f	1-2+ dfs	1-3+ f	0-1+ dfs
Iron stain	0	+	0	0	0
dfs = diffuse cytoplasmic staining f = focal staining in Golgi area					
Immunochemical Marker	.	.	.	.	.
Myeloid (CD13, CD33)	+	+	0	0	0
Monocyte (CD14, CD68)	+	0	0	0	0
Megakaryocytic CD41)	0	0	+	0	0
Red cell antigen (RC 82.4)	0	+	0	0	0
Lymphoid markers (TdT)	0	0	0	+	+

Hematologic malignancy
Results Interpretation:
White blood cell finding
- Cytochemical Characteristics of Hematologic Malignancies:

CHRONIC LEUKEMIA TYPE	FANAE	FAcP	TAcP	Sig(Cig)	CD2	CD3	CD4
B-cell lymphocytic	-	-	-	Weak	-	-	-
B-cell prolymphocytic	-	-	+/-	Strong	-	-	-
Hairy cell	-	-	+	Strong	-	-	-
Plasma cell	-	-	-	Strong	-	-	-
T-helper cell	+	+/-	-	-	+	+	+
T-mixed cell	+	+/-	-	-	+	+	+
T-suppressor cell	-	-	-	-	+	+	-
T-lymphoma	+/-	+	-	-	+	+	+/-

FANAE=focal alpha-naphthyl acetate esterase
FAcP=focal acid phosphatase
TAcP=tartrate-resistant acid phosphatase
Sig=Surface immunoglobulin
Cig=Cytoplasmic immunoglobulin

CHRONIC LEUKEMIA TYPE	CD8	CD5	CD20	HLA-DR	CD10	CD25	CD38
B-cell lymphocytic	-	+	Weak	+	-	-	-
B-cell prolymphocytic	-	+/-	Strong	+	-	-	-
Hairy cell	-	-	Strong	+	-	+	+/-
Plasma cell	-	-	-	-	-	-	+
T-helper cell	-	+	-	-	-	-	-
T-mixed cell	+	+	-	-	-	-	-
T-suppressor cell	+	+	-	-	-	-	-
T-lymphoma	+/-	+	-	+	-	+	-

LYMPHOMA TYPE	FANAE	FAcP	TAcP	Sig(Cig)	CD2	CD3	CD4
Follicular center cell	-	-	-	Strong	-	-	-
Mantle zone	-	-	-	Mod	-	-	-
Splenic w/villous lymphocytes	-	-	+/-	Strong	-	-	-
Monocytoid B-cell	-	-	-	Strong	-	-	-

FANAE=focal alpha-naphthyl acetate esterase
FAcP=focal acid phosphatase
TAcP=tartrate-resistant acid phosphatase
Sig=Surface immunoglobulin
Cig=Cytoplasmic immunoglobulin

LYMPHOMA TYPE	CD8	CD5	CD20	HLA-DR	CD10	CD25	CD38
Follicular center cell	-	-	Strong	+	+	-	+/-
Mantle zone	-	+	Mod	+	+/-	-	-
Splenic w/villous lymphocytes	-	-	Strong	+	-	+/-	+/-
Monocytoid B-cell	-	-	Strong	+	-	-	-

- Cytochemical Characteristics of Hematologic Malignancies:

LYMPHOCYTE NEOPLASM	CD5	CD10	CD19	CD20
Clonal B-cell proliferation	+	.	+	Dim
Mantle cell lymphoma	+	.	.	Bright
Nodal marginal zone lymphoma	-	.	.	Bright
Hairy cell leukemia	-	.	+	Bright
Lymphoplasmacytic lymphoma	+/-	.	+	+
Follicular lymphoma (leukemic phase)	-	+/-	+	+

LYMPHOCYTE NEOPLASM	CD11c/CD22	CD23	CD103	Surface immunoglobulin
Clonal B-cell proliferation	.	+	.	Dim
Mantle cell lymphoma	.	Dim or Absent	.	.
Nodal marginal zone lymphoma	.	.	.	.
Hairy cell leukemia	Bright	.	+	.
Lymphoplasmacytic lymphoma	.	.	.	.
Follicular lymphoma (leukemic phase)	.	.	.	.

Zinc protoporphyrin measurement

TEST DEFINITION

Measurement of zinc protoporphyrin (ZPP) to heme (H) ratio in whole blood for evaluation of iron nutrition and metabolism

REFERENCE RANGE

- Adults: <60 micromol ZPP/mol H
- Premature neonates 24 to 26 weeks' gestational age: 53-189 micromol ZPP/mol H
- Premature neonates 27 to 29 weeks' gestational age: 67-139 micromol ZPP/mol H
- Premature neonates 30 to 36 weeks' gestational age: 49-109 micromol ZPP/mol H
- Neonates 37-40 weeks' gestational age: 53 to 189 micromol ZPP/mol H
  Please refer to your institution's reference ranges as lab normals may vary.

INDICATIONS

Screening for suspected chronic lead toxicity in children
> **Strength of Recommendation:** Class III
> **Strength of Evidence:** Category B
> **Results Interpretation:**
> **Normal laboratory findings**
> Although a zinc protoporphyrin (ZPP) assay may be used as an adjunct to blood lead level testing, it is not sensitive enough to detect lead exposure at lower blood lead levels.
> **Increased level (laboratory finding)**
> An elevated ZPP level is poorly correlated with venous lead levels and should not be used as a screening test for suspected chronic lead toxicity.

Suspected ineffective erythropoiesis due to iron deficiency
> **Strength of Recommendation:** Class IIb
> **Strength of Evidence:** Category B
> **Results Interpretation:**
> **Increased level (laboratory finding)**
> - Normal zinc protoporphyrin to heme (ZPP/H) ratio: Effective erythropoiesis
> - Elevated ZPP/H: Ineffective erythropoiesis, most often due to iron deficiency.

> **False Results**
> The zinc protoporphyrin to heme (ZPP/H) ratio may not be an accurate indicator of erythropoiesis in renal failure.

Suspected iron deficiency in infants and young children
    Strength of Recommendation: Class IIb
    Strength of Evidence: Category B
    Results Interpretation:
    Increased level (laboratory finding)
        Zinc protoporphyrin screening may be effective for detecting iron deficiency in young children, particularly when used as an adjunct to hematocrit.
        There is not enough evidence to conclusively correlate elevated zinc protoporphyrin to heme (ZPP/H) ratios with iron deficiency in the neonatal population.

CLINICAL NOTES

The ZPP/H ratio has not found widespread acceptance largely due to criticisms surrounding factors that give rise to false results. Plasma interference from bilirubinemia causes false elevations in the ratio; washing erythrocytes free of plasma eliminates this type of interference issue. Deoxygenated hemoglobin (Hgb) causes a shift in Hgb absorption falsely lowering the ratio. One suggested solution is to use a reagent that converts hemoglobin to cyanomethemoglobin.

COLLECTION/STORAGE INFORMATION

- Collect whole blood in a tube containing either heparin or EDTA.